Critical Care Nursing

made **Incredibly Easy!®**

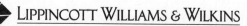

LIPPINCOTT WILLIAMS & WILKINS
A **Wolters Kluwer** Company

Philadelphia • Baltimore • New York • London
Buenos Aires • Hong Kong • Sydney • Tokyo

Staff

Executive Publisher
Judith A. Schilling McCann, RN, MSN

Editorial Director
David Moreau

Clinical Director
Joan M. Robinson, RN, MSN

Senior Art Director
Arlene Putterman

Art Director
Mary Ludwicki

Editorial Project Manager
Jaime L. Stockslager

Clinical Project Manager
Mary Perrong, RN, CRNP, MSN, APRN, BC, CPAN

Editors
Kevin Haworth, Brenna H. Mayer, Julie Munden,
Carol Munson, Liz Schaeffer, Pat Wittig

Clinical Editors
Marcy Caplin, RN, MSN; Tina Dietrich, RN, BSN;
Collette Bishop Hendler, RN, BS, CCRN; Carol A.
Knauff, RN, MSN, CCRN; Pamela Kovach, RN, BSN;
Patricia Berlin Malay, RN, MSN, FNP, MA; Bonnie L.
McGonigle, RN, CRNP, MSN, CRRN; Kate McGovern,
RN, MSN, CCRN

Copy Editors
Kimberly Bilotta (supervisor), Scotti Cohn,
Tom DeZego, Heather Ditch, Amy Furman,
Dorothy P. Terry, Pamela Wingrod

Designers
Lynn Foulk, Jacalyn B. Facciolo

Illustrator
Bot Roda

Digital Composition Services
Diane Paluba (manager), Joyce Rossi Biletz,
Richard Eng

Manufacturing
Patricia K. Dorshaw (senior manager),
Beth Janae Orr

Editorial Assistants
Megan L. Aldinger, Tara L. Carter-Bell, Arlene Claffee,
Linda K. Ruhf

Librarian
Wani Z. Larsen

Indexer
Barbara Hodgson

The clinical treatments described and recommended in this publication are based on research and consultation with nursing, medical, and legal authorities. To the best of our knowledge, these procedures reflect currently accepted practice. Nevertheless, they can't be considered absolute and universal recommendations. For individual applications, all recommendations must be considered in light of the patient's clinical condition and, before administration of new or infrequently used drugs, in light of the latest package-insert information. The authors and the publisher disclaim any responsibility for any adverse effects resulting from the suggested procedures, from any undetected errors, or from the reader's misunderstanding of the text.

CCIE011003 — 070406

06   10 9 8 7

Library of Congress Cataloging-in-Publication Data
Critical care nursing made incredibly easy.
    p. ; cm.
    Includes bibliographical references and index.
    1. Intensive care nursing — Handbooks, manuals, etc.
[DNLM: 1. Critical Care — Handbooks. 2. Nursing Care —
Handbooks. WY 49 C934 2004]
    I. Lippincott Williams & Wilkins.

RT120.I5C766 2004
610.73'61 — dc21
ISBN 1-58255-267-3 (alk. paper)   2003013876

Contents

Contributors and consultants

Deborah Becker, RN, CRNP, MSN, BC, CCRN
Associate Director, Adult Acute Care Nurse Practitioner Program
University of Pennsylvania School of Nursing
Philadelphia

Ellie Z. Franges, RN, MSN, CNRN
Clinical Nurse Specialist—Neurosurgery
St. Luke's Hospital & Health Network
Bethlehem, Pa.

Henry Geiter, Jr., RN, CCRN
Adjunct Instructor
St. Petersburg (Fla.) College
Critical Care Nurse
Bayfront Medical Center
Critical Care Transport Nurse
Sunstar-AMR

Nancy H. Haynes, RN, MN, CCRN
Assistant Professor of Nursing
Saint Luke's College
Kansas City, Mo.

Barbara A. Konopka, RN, MSN, CCRN, CEN
Nursing Instructor
Pennsylvania State University
Worthington-Scranton Campus
Dunmore

Elizabeth Molle, RN, MS
Clinical Educator
Middlesex Hospital
Middletown, Conn.

Ruthie Robinson, RN, MSN, CCRN, CEN
Instructor of Nursing and Staff Nurse
Lamar University
Beaumont, Tex.

Maureen A. Seckel, RN, MSN, CCRN, CES
Medical-Pulmonary Clinical Nurse Specialist
Christiana Care Health System
Newark, Del.

Brenda K. Shelton, RN, MS, AOCN, CCRN
Clinical Nurse Specialist
The Sidney Kimmel Comprehensive Cancer Institute
Johns Hopkins University
Baltimore

Douglas M. Turner, RN, PhD(c), CNS, CRNA
Lead Instructor
Forsyth Technical Community College
Winston-Salem, N.C.

Foreword

Critical care nursing is a demanding and complex specialty. In order to provide safe and proficient care, a nurse entering the field of critical care needs to be able to act fast, processing data from multiple sources in an environment where there's no time to waste. The critical care nurse must also have a thorough understanding of a wide range of interconnected topics, including anatomy and physiology; pathophysiology; diagnostic, electrophysiologic, and laboratory tests; drug therapies; medical devices; and more. A new book from the award-winning *Incredibly Easy* series, *Critical Care Nursing Made Incredibly Easy* presents the essentials of critical care nursing in an easy-to-understand and fun-to-learn format that makes it simple for students coming into the critical care environment. The book can also benefit nurses who are changing specialties or those just looking for a refresher in the field or for some targeted information on difficult topics.

Critical Care Nursing Made Incredibly Easy provides coverage of all major topics related to critical care nursing. This information is presented in a straightforward, concise, easy-to-read, and understandable manner. Each chapter begins with "Just the facts," a list of the major areas to be covered in the text—the first of many features that guide the reader through each chapter and make learning enjoyable. Other features include whimsical cartoons that reinforce important information and mnemonic devices called *Memory joggers* that help the reader remember key points in unique and interesting ways. Numerous quick-scan tables, detailed anatomic drawings (including some beautifully detailed full-color illustrations), and flowcharts throughout the text also contribute to the ease of learning about critical care nursing.

The first chapter focuses on the unique interdisciplinary nature of critical care nursing. It presents the roles and responsibilities of critical care nurses and other team members and introduces the clinical tools necessary to deliver care using best practices and evidence-based techniques. The second chapter provides insight into the breadth of critical care nursing. It helps remind us that patients and their families are the recipients of our care, that managing pain is central to a critical care nurse's role, and that every day we encounter ethical dilemmas and decisions.

The body-system approach used to organize the remaining chapters echoes the way that critical care nurses are trained to think and apply critical thinking skills in the fast-paced critical care environment. Every disorder commonly encountered in the critical care environment, from acute adrenal crisis to septic shock, is covered in complete, but not excessive, detail. For each of the nearly 100 disorders included, you'll find causes, pathophysiology, assessment tips, appropriate diagnostic test results, treatments, and nursing interventions. Incorporated into the nursing interventions are instructions for when collaborative management, a vital aspect of modern clinical practice, is necessary. Quick self-assessment quizzes at the end of each chapter help the reader to determine his or her level of mastery of key concepts.

Logos throughout the book attract attention and point the reader to essential information, including:

Senior moment — guidelines regarding how critically ill geriatric patients differ from the rest of the population and how these differences affect your care

Take charge! — sidebars that point out potentially lethal situations and steps to take when they occur, encouraging vigilance by the nurse

Advice from the experts — tips and tricks for critical care nurses provided by the people who know best — other critical care nurses.

With all of these features, there's no denying that *Critical Care Nursing Made Incredibly Easy* is a wonderful reference for student nurses entering critical care practice who want to become competent in the essentials of critical care nursing as well as a useful review for experienced critical care nurses looking to brush up on the essentials. I hope that you enjoy this book as much as I do!

John M. Clochesy, RN, PhD, CS, FAAN, FCCM
Independence Foundation Professor of Nursing Education
Frances Payne Bolton School of Nursing
Case Western Reserve University
Cleveland

1

Critical care basics

Just the facts

In this chapter, you'll learn:
♦ roles and responsibilities of the critical care nurse
♦ credentials for critical care nurses
♦ ways to work with a multidisciplinary team
♦ ways to incorporate clinical tools and best practices into your care.

What's critical care nursing?

Critical care nursing is the delivery of specialized care to critically ill patients — that is, ones who have life-threatening illnesses or injuries. Such patients may be unstable, have complex needs, and require intensive and vigilant nursing care.

Illnesses and injuries commonly seen in patients on critical care units (CCUs) include:
• gunshot wounds
• traumatic injuries from such events as car collisions and falls
• cardiovascular disorders, such as heart failure and acute coronary syndromes (unstable angina and myocardial infarction [MI])
• surgeries, such as abdominal aortic aneurysm repair and carotid endarterectomy
• respiratory disorders, such as acute respiratory failure and pulmonary embolism
• GI and hepatic disorders, such as acute pancreatitis, acute upper GI bleeding, and acute liver failure
• renal disorders, such as acute and chronic renal failure
• cancers, such as lung, esophageal, and gastric cancer
• shock due to hypovolemia, sepsis, and cardiogenic shock after MI.

Get ready! Patients in your care may be unstable, have complex needs, and require intensive and vigilant care.

Meet the critical care nurse

> Put your best foot forward and strive to deliver the best care possible to patients and their families.

Critical care nurses are responsible for making sure that critically ill patients and members of their families receive close attention and the best care possible.

What do you do?

Critical care nurses fill many roles in the critical care setting, such as staff nurses, nurse-educators, nurse-managers, case managers, clinical nurse specialists, nurse practitioners, and nurse researchers. (See *Role call.*)

Where do you work?

Critical care nurses work wherever critically ill patients are found, including:
- adult, pediatric, and neonatal CCUs
- coronary care and progressive coronary care units
- emergency departments
- postanesthesia care units.

What makes you special?

As a nurse who specializes in critical care, you accept a wide range of responsibilities, including:
- being an advocate
- using sound clinical judgment
- demonstrating caring practices
- collaborating with a multidisciplinary team
- demonstrating an understanding of cultural diversity
- providing patient and family teaching.

> A critical care nurse is perfect for many roles. She can play a nurse-manager, a nurse-educator, a case manager, or another type of specialist.

Advocacy

An advocate is a person who works on another person's behalf. As a patient advocate, you should also address the concerns of family members and the community whenever possible.

As an advocate, the critical care nurse is also responsible for:
- protecting the patient's rights
- assisting the patient and his family members in the decision-making process by providing education and support
- negotiating with other members of the health care team on behalf of the patient and his family members
- keeping the patient and his family members informed about the care plan

Role call

By filling various nursing and management roles, a critical care nurse helps to promote optimum health, prevent illness, and aid coping with illness or death. Here are various capacities in which a critical care nurse may function.

Staff nurse

When a patient is admitted to a critical care unit (CCU), it's because a critical care nurse's technical skills and nursing knowledge are required. The staff nurse functions as a primary caregiver by independently making assessments, planning and implementing patient care, and providing direct nursing care. For example, a staff nurse may make clinical observations and execute interventions, such as administering medications and treatments, as well as promote activities of daily living.

Nurse-educator

As the emphasis on health promotion and illness prevention has increased, the nurse's role as educator has become increasingly important. The nurse-educator's students include patients and family members as well as other health care professionals. The nurse assesses patients' and family members' learning needs, plans and implements teaching strategies to meet those needs, and evaluates the effectiveness of teaching. The critical care nurse also provides education to peers and colleagues, such as other nurses, physical therapists, and occupational therapists.

To be an effective educator, the nurse must have excellent interpersonal skills. She must also be familiar with adult learning principles.

Nurse-manager

All nurses practice leadership and manage time, people, resources, and the environment in which they provide care. They carry out these tasks by directing, delegating, and coordinating activities. The nurse-manager acts as both a staff nurse and an administrative representative of the unit, ensuring that effective and quality nursing care is provided in a timely and fiscally managed environment.

Case manager

To counter the trend toward fragmented, depersonalized nursing care, hospitals have developed the role of case manager.

This expanded capacity enables the nurse to manage comprehensive care of an individual patient.

Case management is a systematic approach to delivering total patient care within specified time frames and economic resources. Case management encompasses the patient's entire illness episode, crosses all care settings, and involves the collaboration of all personnel who provide care. The case manager is involved in discharge planning, making referrals, identifying community and personal resources, and arranging for equipment and supplies needed by the patient on discharge.

Clinical nurse specialist

A clinical nurse specialist is a health care provider who has obtained a Master of Science degree in Nursing and has expertise in a clinical specialty such as critical care. The clinical nurse specialist provides evidence-based nursing care by participating in education and direct patient care, consulting the patient and family members, and collaborating with other nurses and health care team members to deliver high-quality care.

Nurse practitioner

A nurse practitioner also has obtained a Master of Science degree in Nursing and specializes in a clinical area such as critical care. Nurse practitioners provide primary health care to patients and families and can function independently. The nurse practitioner may obtain histories and conduct physical examinations, order laboratory and diagnostic tests and interpret their results, diagnose disorders, treat patients, counsel and educate patients and family members, and provide continuous follow-up care after patients are discharged from the CCU.

Nurse researcher

Nurse researchers promote the science of nursing by investigating problems related to nursing. The goal is to develop and refine nursing knowledge and practice. Staff nurses participate in nursing research by reading current nursing literature, applying the information in practice, and collecting data. Advanced practice nurses (clinical nurse specialists and nurse practitioners) can assist staff nurses by conducting the research study and by serving as a consultant to the nurses during implementation of a research study.

- advocating for flexible visitation on the CCU
- respecting and supporting the patient's and his family members' decisions
- serving as a liaison between the patient and family and other members of the health care team
- respecting the values and cultures of the patient
- acting in the patient's best interest.

> One role of the critical care nurse is liaison between the patient and family members and the health care team.

Stuck in the middle

Being a patient advocate can sometimes cause conflict between you and other members of the health care team. For example, when dialysis is ordered because of a patient's deteriorating renal status, you may need to contact the doctor to relay the patient's request to decline this treatment.

It may also cause conflict between your professional duty and the patient's personal values. For example, the patient may be a Jehovah's Witness and refuse a blood transfusion. In this case, you should consult your facility's ethics committee as well as your facility's policies and procedures.

Clinical judgment

A critical care nurse needs to exercise clinical judgment. To develop sound clinical judgment, you need critical thinking skills. Critical thinking is a complex mixture of knowledge, intuition, logic, common sense, and experience.

> Here's a thought! Critical thinking fosters understanding and enables us to solve difficult problems.

Why be critical?

Critical thinking fosters understanding of issues and enables you to quickly find answers to difficult questions. It isn't a trial-and-error method, yet it isn't strictly a scientific problem-solving method, either.

Critical thinking enhances your ability to identify a patient's needs. It also enables you to use sound clinical decision making and to determine which nursing actions best meet a patient's needs.

Developing critical thinking skills

Critical thinking skills improve with increasing clinical and scientific experience. The best way for you to develop critical thinking skills is by asking questions and learning.

Always asking questions

The first question you should find the answer to is "What's the patient's diagnosis?" If it's a diagnosis with which you aren't familiar, look it up and read about it. Find the answers to questions like these:

* What are the signs and symptoms?
* What's the usual cause?
* What complications can occur?

In addition to finding the answers to diagnosis-related questions, also be sure to find out:

* What are the patient's physical examination findings?
* What laboratory and diagnostic tests are necessary?
* Does the patient have any risk factors? If so, are they significant? What interventions would minimize those risk factors?
* What are the patient's cultural beliefs? How can you best address the patient's cultural concerns?
* What are the possible complications? What type of monitoring is needed to watch for complications?
* What are the usual medications and treatments for the patient's condition? (If you aren't familiar with the medications or treatments, look them up in a reliable source or consult a colleague.)

Critical thinking and the nursing process

Critical thinking skills are necessary when applying the nursing process — assessment, planning, intervention, and evaluation — and making patient-care decisions.

Step 1: Assessment

To obtain assessment data:

* ask relevant questions
* validate evidence or data that has been collected
* identify present and potential concerns.

Then be sure to analyze the assessment data and determine the nursing diagnoses. To do this, you must interpret the collected data and identify any gaps. For example, if laboratory values are missing, call to obtain test results or schedule a test that wasn't performed.

Step 2: Planning

During the planning stage, critical thinking skills come in handy when considering how the patient is expected

It's a workout for the mind. Applying the nursing process requires critical thinking.

OUTCOME EVALUATION

IMPLEMENTATION

PLANNING

ASSESSMENT

to achieve goals. During this stage, consider the consequences of any planned interventions. This is also the time to set priorities of care for the patient.

Step 3: Implementation

During the implementation stage, use critical thinking to involve the patient and other members of the health care team in implementing the care plan.

Step 4: Evaluation

During the evaluation stage, use critical thinking to continually reassess, modify, and individualize care. Evaluation enables you to assess the patient's responses and determine whether expected outcomes have been met.

Caring practice

Caring practice is the use of a therapeutic and compassionate environment to focus on the patient's needs. Although care is based on standards and protocols, it must also be individualized to each patient.

Caring practice also involves:
• maintaining a safe environment
• interacting with the patient and his family members in a compassionate and respectful manner throughout the critical care stay
• supporting the patient and his family in end-of-life issues and decisions.

Collaboration

Collaboration allows a health care team to use all available resources for the patient. A critical care nurse is part of a multidisciplinary team in which each person contributes expertise. The collaborative goal is to optimize patient outcomes. As a nurse, you may often serve as the coordinator of such collaborative teams.

Two ways about it

Models of collaborative care include case management and outcome management:
• *Case management* consists of coordinating and organizing patient care in collaboration with the primary care doctor.
• *Outcome management* uses a quality improvement process and team approach to manage patient outcomes.

Cultural diversity

Culture is defined as the way people live and how they behave in a social group. This behavior is learned and passed on from generation to generation. Acknowledging and respecting patients' diverse cultural beliefs is a necessary part of high-quality care.

Keep an open mind

A critical care nurse is expected to demonstrate awareness and sensitivity toward a patient's religion, lifestyle, family makeup, socioeconomic status, age, gender, and values. Be sure to assess cultural factors and concerns and integrate them into the care plan.

Keep an open mind about cultural factors. It's necessary for delivering high-quality care to all patients.

Education

As an educator, a critical care nurse is the facilitator of patient, family, and staff education. Patient education involves teaching patients and their families about:
- the patient's illness
- the importance of managing comorbid disorders (such as diabetes, arthritis, and hypertension)
- diagnostic and laboratory testing
- planned surgical procedures, including preoperative and postoperative expectations
- instructions on specific patient care, such as wound care and range-of-motion exercises.

Critical care nurses are teachers, too. Their students include patients, family members, and other staff.

Staff as students

Critical care nurses also commonly serve as staff educators. Examples of staff teaching topics you may need to address include:
- how to use new equipment
- how to interpret diagnostic test results
- how to administer a new medication.

Becoming a critical care nurse

Most nursing students are only briefly exposed to critical care nursing. Much of the training required to become a critical care nurse is learned on the job.

Learning by doing

On-the-job training is central to gaining the extensive skills required by a critical care nurse. There are several ways to become trained as a critical care nurse.

One way...

Your facility may provide a critical care course. Such courses vary in duration from 1 month to 3 months. The course consists of both classroom lectures and clinical exposure to the critical care environment.

...or another

Your facility may also provide a competency-based orientation program for new critical care nurses. In a program such as this, you gain knowledge and experience while working on the CCU and a *preceptor* (a staff nurse or clinical nurse specialist with specialized training in critical care nursing) provides guidance.

An orientation period allows the nurse time to acquire knowledge and the technical skills needed to work in the critical care environment. Such technical skills include working with equipment, such as cardiac monitoring systems, mechanical ventilators, hemodynamic monitoring devices, and intracranial pressure (ICP) monitoring devices.

Gaining credentials

The American Association of Critical Care Nurses (AACN) is one of the world's largest specialty nursing organizations, with more than 65,000 members. The primary goal of the AACN is to enhance the education of critical care nurses.

Through AACN, you can become certified as a critical care registered nurse (CCRN) in adult, pediatric, or neonatal critical care. CCRN certification tells everyone you're a professional, with proficiency and skill in a highly specialized area of nursing. Many specialty-nursing organizations offer certification. (See *Organizations offering certifications.*)

CCRN certification requires renewal after 3 years. Nurses can recertify by taking the examination again or by demonstrating continuing education in critical care nursing (by working 432 hours and completing 100 continuing education hours during the certification period).

CCRN certification tells everyone you're highly skilled in a specialized area of nursing. A critical care registered nurse may be certified in adult, pediatric, or neonatal critical care.

Help wanted

Certification isn't mandatory to work as a critical care nurse, but it's certainly encouraged. Many units prefer to hire nurses

Organizations offering certifications

Here's a list of professional organizations that offer certifications of interest to critical care nurses.
- American Association of Critical-Care Nurses, *www.aacn.org*
- American Board of Neuroscience Nurses, *www.aann.org/credential*
- American Board of Perianesthesia Nursing Certification, Inc., *www.cpancapa.org*
- American Nurses Credentialing Center, *www.nursingworld.org/ancc/*
- Board of Certification for Emergency Nursing, *www.ena.org/bcen*
- Certification Board Perioperative Nursing, *www.certboard.org*
- National Certification Corporation for the Obstetric, Gynecologic, Neonatal, and Telephone Nursing Specialties, *www.nccnet.org*
- Nephrology Nursing Certification Commission, *www.nncc-exam.org*

Are you investigating the job market? Many units prefer to hire nurses with certification.

with certification because it means that they have demonstrated expertise and commitment to critical care nursing.

Safety first

The goal of any nursing certification program is to promote safe nursing care. CCRN certification is evidence that a nurse has demonstrated clinical excellence and recognizes the importance of patient safety. Certification validates the nurse's qualifications and specialized clinical knowledge.

What's in it for me?

For most nurses, the main reason for seeking CCRN certification is personal fulfillment, but there are other rewards as well. Many institutions reimburse nurses for taking the examination and others offer monetary incentives to nurses with CCRN certification.

Nursing responsibilities

As a critical care nurse, you're responsible for all parts of the nursing process: assessing, planning, implementing, and evaluating care of critically ill patients. Remember that each of these steps gives you an opportunity to exercise your critical thinking skills.

Assessment

Critical care nursing requires that you constantly assess the patient for subtle changes in condition and monitor all equipment being used. Caring for critically ill patients may involve the use of such highly specialized equipment as cardiac monitors, hemodynamic monitoring devices, intra-aortic balloon pumps, and ICP monitoring devices. As part of the patient assessment, you should also assess the patient's physical and psychological statuses and interpret laboratory data.

Planning

Planning requires you to consider the patient's psychological and physiological needs and set realistic patient goals. The result is an individualized care plan for your patient. To ensure safe passage through the critical care environment, you must also anticipate changes in the patient's condition. For example, for a patient admitted with a diagnosis of MI, you should monitor cardiac rhythm and anticipate rhythm changes. If an arrhythmia such as complete heart block develops, the treatment plan may need to be changed and new goals established.

Critical care assessment involves constantly evaluating the patient's condition and monitoring equipment.

What's the problem?

In planning, be sure to address present and potential problems, such as:
- pain
- cardiac arrhythmias
- altered hemodynamic states
- impaired physical mobility
- impaired skin integrity
- deficient fluid volume.

Gotta run! The wide range of interventions I perform really keeps me on the go!

Implementation

As a nurse, you must implement specific interventions to address existing and potential patient problems.

A call to intervene

Examples of interventions include:
- monitoring and treating cardiac arrhythmias
- assessing hemodynamic parameters, such as pulmonary artery pressure, central venous pressure, and cardiac output
- titrating vasoactive drips
- managing pain
- monitoring responses to therapy.

There's more in store

Some other common interventions are:
- repositioning the patient to maintain joint and body functions
- performing hygiene measures to prevent skin breakdown
- assisting the patient with coughing and deep-breathing exercises to prevent pulmonary complications.

Evaluation

It's necessary for you to continually evaluate a patient's response to interventions. Use such evaluations to change the care plan as needed to make sure that your patient continues to work toward achieving his outcome goals.

Multidisciplinary teamwork

Everyone on the health care team contributes expertise. The goal is to provide effective holistic care.

Nurses working with critically ill patients commonly collaborate with a multidisciplinary team of health care professionals. The team approach enables caregivers to better meet the diverse needs of individual patients.

The goal is holism

The goal of collaboration is to provide effective and comprehensive (holistic) care. Holistic care addresses the biological, psychological, social, and spiritual dimensions of a person.

Team huddle

A multidisciplinary team providing direct patient care may consist of many professionals. Members commonly include:
- registered nurses (RNs)
- doctors
- advanced practice nurses (such as clinical nurse specialists and nurse practitioners)
- licensed practical nurses (LPNs)
- respiratory therapists and others. (See *Meet the team*, page 12.)

Working with registered nurses

Teamwork is essential in the stressful environment of the CCU. The critical care nurse needs to work well with the other professional RNs on the unit.

Meet the team

Various members of the multidisciplinary team have collaborative relationships with critical care nurses. Here are some examples.

Patient-care technician

A patient-care technician, or nursing assistant, is responsible for providing direct patient care to critically ill patients. A registered nurse delegates to and is responsible for supervision of the patient-care technician's daily patient assignment. Types of duties assigned include bathing, obtaining vital signs, and assisting with transportation of patients for testing.

Physical therapist

A physical therapist is involved in assessing muscle groups and mobility and improving motor function of critically ill patients. He develops a specialized care plan and provides care based on the patient's functional abilities and the disease process or physical injury. Such a therapist teaches gait and transfer training to the patient and administers hydrotherapy. A physical therapist may also teach other health care team members about proper transferring and repositioning of patients.

Occupational therapist

An occupational therapist is responsible for assessing a patient's activities of daily living (ADLs) status. Examples of ADLs are bathing, grooming, dressing, and toileting. An occupational therapist teaches the patient and his family members methods for completing these tasks and achieving the discharge plan. For example, an occupational therapist teaches how to use adaptive equipment, such as a long shoehorn and adaptive utensils. An occupational therapist works with you to reinforce patient teaching.

Speech pathologist

The primary responsibility of a speech pathologist is to assess the critically ill patient's ability to swallow and then develop a care plan with appropriate interventions. The speech pathologist also assesses for speech and language disorders. Speech pathologists are involved in teaching about:
• techniques for dealing with swallowing impairment (dysphagia)
• communication methods for those with aphasia, a speech disorder caused by injury to the cerebral cortex that affects the patient's ability to express or comprehend language
• techniques to assist the patient with auditory processing difficulties.

A speech pathologist works with you to reinforce treatment and improve the patient's quality of life.

Wound-ostomy-continence nurse

The primary responsibility of a wound-ostomy-continence nurse is to assess, monitor, and make recommendations to the doctor regarding the patient's skin integrity and bowel and bladder issues. She also helps to develop a treatment plan.

Examples of a wound-ostomy-continence nurse's recommendations include providing a pressure-relieving bed to promote wound healing and applying topical medications to prevent skin breakdown.

Dietitian

A dietitian is responsible for monitoring a critically ill patient's dietary intake. Because many critically ill patients are medically unstable, a dietitian assesses the patient's daily caloric intake and reports deviations to you and the doctor. The doctor orders a specific diet (such as a no-concentrated-sweets diet or a 2-g sodium diet) and the dietitian is responsible for devising a meal plan to meet the patient's needs.

As a critical care nurse, you may collaborate with the dietitian in discussing a patient's intake status. In addition, the dietitian may recommend interventions, such as providing supplemental feedings or decreasing the patient's daily caloric intake.

Pastoral caregiver

A pastoral caregiver — also known as a *chaplain* — is an essential member of the multidisciplinary team in the critical care environment. The goal of pastoral care is to meet the patient's and family members' spiritual and religious needs. Pastoral care consists of providing support and empathy to the patient and his family members. A pastoral caregiver works with you to achieve this goal. As the main caregiver, you spend the most time with the patient, listening to, caring for, and providing empathy to the patient and his family. You should notify the chaplain if a patient or family member requests his services. He should also be notified to deliver the patient's last rites, if appropriate.

Social services

In some facilities, social services and case management are equivalent. Agents of social services provide continuity of care for the patient after discharge.

The buddy system

It's important to have a colleague to look to for moral support, physical assistance with a patient, and problem solving. No one person has all the answers but, together, nurses have a better chance of solving any problem.

Working with doctors

Patients on the CCU rarely have only one doctor. Most have an admitting doctor and several consultants, such as:
- a cardiologist
- a neurologist
- a pulmonologist
- an infectious disease specialist.

In addition, if you work in a teaching institution, you may also interact on a regular basis with medical students, interns, and residents who are under the direction of the attending doctor.

Coordinated efforts

Having a good professional working relationship with doctors involved in patient care is essential. In many cases, a nurse coordinates patient care among the many different specialists.

Short and sweet

Because a doctor is available on the unit for only a short period, it's important that you accurately and succinctly convey important patient information to him during that time. When a doctor is visiting his patient on the unit, you need to relay assessment findings, laboratory data, and patient care issues in a concise report.

You'll often collaborate with doctors on patient care decisions; you may even suggest additional treatments or interventions that may benefit the patient. In addition, you need to know when it's important to call the doctor with a change in the patient's condition. Be sure to have important information at hand before you call. (See *Timesaving tip*, page 14.)

Working with advanced practice nurses

Advanced practice nurses — clinical nurse specialists (CNSs) and acute care nurse practitioners (ACNPs) — are increasingly seen working on CCUs. An advanced practice nurse may be employed by a hospital and assigned to a specific unit or she may be employed by a doctor to assist in caring for and monitoring patients. The advanced practice nurse assists staff nurses in clinical decision making and enhances the quality of patient care, which improves patient care outcomes.

Teamwork requires a lot of coordination!

I rely on nurses to relay assessment findings, laboratory data, and patient care issues to me.

The roles of a lifetime

The traditional roles of a CNS are:
- clinician
- educator
- researcher
- consultant
- manager.

The CNS offers support and guidance to staff nurses as they care for patients. She assists with problem solving when complex care is necessary for patients and their families. In addition, the CNS may develop research projects dealing with problems identified on the unit. In some facilities, a CNS may be a case manager or outcomes manager.

On a role

An ACNP fills the traditional roles of a nurse practitioner. These may include:
- conducting comprehensive health assessments
- diagnosing
- prescribing pharmacologic and nonpharmacologic treatments.

An ACNP may also conduct research, manage care, and perform advanced procedures, such as removing chest tubes and inserting central lines.

Working with licensed practical nurses

On many CCUs, LPNs are members of the health care team. Generally, an LPN collaborates with an RN to deliver patient care. The RN is responsible for and delegates specific tasks to the LPN, which may include caring directly for patients and collecting data. As such, the LPN may administer approved medications, assist with procedures, and record vital signs.

Working with respiratory therapists

A critical care nurse also commonly collaborates with a respiratory therapist in caring for critically ill patients.

Respiration-related roles

The role of a respiratory therapist is to monitor and manage the respiratory status of patients. To do this, the respiratory therapist may:
- administer breathing treatments
- suction patients
- collect specimens

Advice from the experts

Timesaving tip

Make sure that you have everything you need before calling the doctor, including:
- assessment data
- laboratory results
- radiology results.

Be ready to tell the doctor exactly what the patient's status is and the reason for the call. Having all the necessary information at your fingertips before making the phone call saves time for everyone involved.

An RN delegates tasks to an LPN. Together, they deliver the best possible patient care.

- obtain arterial blood gas values
- manage ventilator changes.

   In some cases, you may need to work closely with a respiratory therapist. For example, when weaning a patient from a ventilator, you're both responsible for monitoring the patient's response to ventilator changes and tolerance to weaning.

Clinical tools

The multidisciplinary team uses various tools to promote safe and comprehensive holistic care. These tools include clinical pathways, practice guidelines, and protocols.

Clinical pathways

Clinical pathways (also known as *critical pathways*) are care management plans for patients with a given diagnosis or condition.

Follow the path

Clinical pathways are typically generated and used by facilities that deliver care for similar conditions to many patients. A multidisciplinary committee of clinicians at the facility usually develops clinical pathways. The overall goals are to:
- establish a standard approach to care for all providers in the facility
- establish roles for various members of the health care team
- provide a framework for collecting data on patient outcomes.

Tried and true

Pathways are based on evidence from reliable sources, such as benchmarks, research, and guidelines. The committee gathers and uses information from peer-reviewed literature and experts outside the facility.

Outlines and timelines

Clinical pathways usually outline the duties of all professionals involved with patient care. They follow specific timelines for indicated actions. They also specify expected patient outcomes, which serve as checkpoints for the patient's progress and caregiver's performance.

Clinical pathways lead to similar care for patients with similar conditions.

Practice guidelines

Practice guidelines specify courses of action to be taken in response to a diagnosis or condition. They reflect value judgments about the relative importance of various health and economic outcomes.

Practice guidelines aid decision making by practitioners and patients. They're multidisciplinary in nature and can be used to coordinate care by multiple providers.

> Practice guidelines reflect value judgments about the relative importance of various health and economic outcomes.

Let an expert be your guide

Expert health care providers usually write practice guidelines. They condense large amounts of information into easily usable formats, combining clinical expertise with the best available clinical evidence. Practice guidelines are used to:
- streamline care
- control variations in practice patterns
- distribute health care resources more effectively.

The evidence is in

Practice guidelines are valuable sources of information. They indicate which tests and treatments are appropriate. They also provide a framework for building a standard of care (a statement describing an expected level of care or performance).

Consider the source

Like research-based information, clinical guidelines should be evaluated for the quality of their sources. It's a good idea to read the developers' policy statement about how evidence was selected and what values were applied in making recommendations for care.

Protocols

Protocols are facility-established sets of procedures for a given circumstance. Their purpose is to outline actions that are most likely to produce optimal patient outcomes.

First things first

Protocols describe a sequence of actions a practitioner should take to establish a diagnosis or begin a treatment regimen. For example, a pain management protocol outlines a bedside strategy for managing acute pain.

Protocols facilitate delivery of consistent, cost-effective care. They're also educational resources for clinicians who strive to keep abreast of current best practices. Protocols may be either highly directive or flexible, allowing practitioners to use clinical judgment.

Input from experts

Nursing or medical experts write protocols, commonly with input from other health care providers. They may be approved by legislative bodies, such as boards of nursing or medicine in some states. Hospital committees may approve other types of protocols for various facilities.

Best practices

As new procedures and medicines become available, nurses committed to excellence regularly update and adapt their practices. An approach known as *best practice* is an important tool for providing high-quality care.

Best for all concerned

The term *best practice* refers to clinical practices, treatments, and interventions that result in the best possible outcomes for both the patient and your facility.

The best practice approach is generally a team effort that draws on various types of information. Common sources of information used to identify best practices are research data, personal experience, and expert opinion.

Critical care research

The goal of critical care research is to improve the delivery of care and, thereby, improve patient outcomes. Nursing care is commonly based on evidence that's derived from research. Evidence can be used to support current practices or to change practices. (See *Research and nursing*, page 18.)

The best way to get involved in research is to be a good consumer of nursing research. You can do so by reading nursing journals and being aware of the quality of research and reported results.

Share and share alike

Don't be afraid to share research findings with colleagues. Sharing promotes sound clinical care, and all involved may learn about easier and more efficient ways to care for patients.

Research and nursing

All scientific research is based on the same basic process.

Research steps
The research process consists of the following steps:
1. Identify a problem. Identifying problems in the critical care environment isn't difficult. An example of such a problem is skin breakdown.
2. Conduct a literature review. The goal of this step is to see what has been published about the identified problem.
3. Formulate a research question or hypothesis. In the case of skin breakdown, one question is, "Which type of adhesive is most irritating to the skin of a patient on bed rest?"
4. Design a study. The study may be experimental or nonexperimental. The nurse must decide what data are to be collected and how to collect that data.
5. Obtain consent. The nurse must obtain consent to conduct research from the study participants. Most facilities have an internal review board that must approve such permission for studies.
6. Collect data. After the study is approved, the nurse can begin conducting the study and collecting the data.
7. Analyze the data. The nurse analyzes the data and states the conclusions derived from the analysis.
8. Share the information. Finally, the researcher shares the collected information with other nurses through publications and presentations.

Evidence-based care

Health care professionals have long recognized the importance of laboratory research and have recently developed ways to make research results more useful in clinical practice. One way is by delivering evidence-based care.

Evidence-based care isn't based on tradition, custom, or intuition. It's derived from various concrete sources, such as:
- formal nursing research
- clinical knowledge
- scientific knowledge.

The goal of delivering evidence-based care is to improve nursing care and patient outcomes.

An evidence-based example

Research results may provide insight into the treatment of a patient who, for example, doesn't respond to a medication or treatment that seemed effective for other patients.

In this example, you may believe that a certain drug should be effective for pain relief based on previous experience with that drug. The trouble with such an approach is that other factors can contribute to pain relief, such as the route of administration, the dosage, and concurrent treatments.

First, last, and always

Regardless of the value of evidence-based care, you should always use professional clinical judgment when dealing with critically ill patients and their families. Remember that each patient's condition ultimately dictates treatment.

Quick quiz

1. To work on a CCU, you must:
A. have a baccalaureate degree.
B. have certification in critical care nursing.
C. use the nursing process in delivering nursing care.
D. possess an advanced nursing degree.

Answer: C. The professional nurse uses the nursing process (assessment, planning, implementation, and evaluation) to care for critically ill patients.

2. Professional certification in critical care nursing allows you to:
A. function as an advanced practice nurse.
B. validate knowledge and skills in critical care nursing.
C. obtain an administrative position.
D. obtain a pay raise.

Answer: B. The purpose of professional certifications is to validate knowledge and skill in a particular area. Certification is a demonstration of excellence and commitment to your chosen specialty area.

3. The purpose of the multidisciplinary team is to:
A. assist the nurse in performing patient care.
B. replace the concept of primary care in the acute care setting.
C. minimize lawsuits on the CCU.
D. provide holistic, comprehensive care to the patient.

Answer: D. The purpose of the multidisciplinary team is to provide comprehensive care to the critically ill patient.

4. When alerting a doctor about a change in a patient's status, you need to:
  A. fax all of the vital signs to the office first.
  B. have all assessment data and laboratory and radiology results available.
  C. ask for specific orders.
  D. delegate the phone call to the charge nurse.

Answer: B. Save time by having all assessment data and laboratory and radiology results available when you make the phone call. Let the doctor know why you're calling and what your specific concern is.

5. The easiest way to participate in research is to:
  A. be a good consumer of research.
  B. analyze related studies.
  C. conduct a research study.
  D. participate on your facility's internal review board.

Answer: A. Begin by reading research articles and judging whether they're applicable to your practice. Research findings aren't useful if they aren't incorporated into practice.

6. The purpose of evidence-based practice is to:
  A. validate traditional nursing practices.
  B. improve patient outcomes.
  C. refute traditional nursing practices.
  D. establish a body of knowledge unique to nursing.

Answer: B. Although evidence-based practices may validate or refute traditional practice, the purpose is to improve patient outcomes.

Scoring

☆☆☆ If you answered all six questions correctly, take a bow. You're basically a wiz when it comes to critical care basics.

☆☆ If you answered four or five questions correctly, there's no room for criticism. Your critical thinking skills are basically intact.

☆ If you answered fewer than four questions correctly, the situation is critical. Review the chapter and you'll be on the right pathway.

Holistic care issues

Just the facts

In this chapter, you'll learn:

♦ family dynamics that should be considered as you provide care

♦ issues that affect critically ill patients and their families

♦ ways to assess and manage pain in critically ill patients

♦ eight principles of ethical decision making

♦ concepts related to end-of-life decisions and how they're important to your care.

What's holistic health care?

Holistic health care revolves around a notion of totality. The goal of holistic care is to meet not just the patient's physical needs but also his social and emotional needs.

The whole is the goal

Holistic care addresses all dimensions of a person, including:
- physical
- emotional
- social
- spiritual.

Only by considering all dimensions of a person can the health care team provide high-quality holistic care. You should strive to provide holistic care to all critically ill patients, even though their physical needs may seem to be more pressing than their other needs.

> Here's the whole story about holistic health care.

The issues

The road to the goal of delivering the best holistic care is riddled with various issues (problems or concerns), including:

- patient and family issues
- cognitive issues
- pain control issues
- ethics issues.

Patient and family issues

A family is a group of two or more persons who possibly live together in the same household, perform certain interrelated social tasks, and share an emotional bond. Families can profoundly influence the individuals within them.

Family ties

A family is a dynamic system. During stress-free times, this system tends to maintain homeostasis, meaning that it exists in a stable state of harmony and balance. However, when a crisis sends a family member into a critical care environment, family members may feel a tremendous strain and family homeostasis is thrown off. The major effects of such imbalances are:

- increased stress levels for family members
- fear of death for the patient
- reorganization of family roles.

Unprepared for the worst

The family may be caught off guard by sudden exposure to the hospital environment, causing homeostasis to be disrupted. Family members may worry about the possible death of the ill family member. The suddenness of the illness may overwhelm the family and put it into a crisis state. The ramifications of the patient's illness may cause other family members to feel hopeless and helpless.

Circle out of round

When sudden critical illness or injury disrupts the family circle, the patient can no longer fulfill certain role responsibilities. Such roles are typically:

- financial (if the patient is a major contributor to the family's monetary stability)
- social (if the patient fills such roles as spouse, parent, mediator, or disciplinarian).

Holy mackerel! Holistic care means that you may have to deal with several patient and family issues.

One thing leads to another

A sudden shift in the patient's ability to bear family responsibilities can create havoc and a feeling of overwhelming responsibility for other family members.

Nursing responsibilities

Because a critical illness or injury greatly affects family members as well, be sure to provide care to the family as well as the patient. Members of the patient's family need guidance and support during the patient's hospital stay. The critical care nurse's responsibility to family members is to provide information about:
• nursing care
• the patient's prognosis and expected treatments
• ways to communicate with the patient.

Stand by to answer whatever questions family members have. They may turn to you for guidance and support.

Slipping on emotional turmoil

The critically ill patient's condition may change rapidly (within minutes or hours). The result of such physiological instability is emotional turmoil for the family.

The family may use whatever coping mechanisms they have, such as seeking support from friends or clergy. The longer the patient remains in critical care, however, the more stress increases for both the patient and family members. The result can be slow deterioration of the family system.

Step in and lend a helping hand

Because you're regularly exposed to members of the patient's family, you can help them during their time of crisis. For example, you can observe the anxiety level of family members and, if necessary, refer them to another member of the multidisciplinary team, such as a social service agent.

You can also help family members solve problems by assisting them to:
• verbalize the immediate problem
• identify support systems
• recall how they handled stress in the past.

Such assistance helps family members to focus on the present issue. It also allows them to solve problems and regain a sense of control over their lives.

Lean on me

You can also help the family cope with their feelings during this stressful time. Two ways to do this are by encouraging expression of feelings (such as by crying or discussing the issue) and providing empathy.

Since you asked

During a patient's critical illness, family members come to rely on the opinions of professionals and commonly ask for their input. They need honest information given to them in terms they can understand. In many cases, you're the health care team member who provides this information. (See *Tips for helping the family cope.*)

Tips for helping the family cope

A large role for the nurse is orienting a patient's family to the critical care unit. Here are some useful tips for dealing with family members of critically ill patients.

Please touch
Let family members know that it's okay to touch the patient. Many are afraid to touch a critically ill loved one for fear of interfering with monitoring equipment or invasive lines. Let them know if there are any special considerations when touching the patient.

Watch your language
Tell visitors that patients may not appear to respond, but that they may be able to hear what's going on around them. Therefore, everyone should be careful of what they say in the patient's presence. Let family members know that they should talk to the patient as if he can hear.

How's the weather?
Many family members spend their visitation time looking at equipment in the room and asking the patient questions such as, "Are you in pain?" Let the family know that you ask these questions all day long.

Let family members know how to be visitors. The patient wants to hear about the outside world—not reminders that he's ill and hospitalized. He wants to hear about other family members, the family pet, and who won the latest basketball game.

One at a time, please
Ask the family to appoint one spokesperson for the group. This is especially important when families are large. The spokesperson is the person who should call the unit for updates on the patient's condition. The spokesperson can then spread the word to the rest of the family. It also may be helpful to identify a primary nursing contact for the family.

Should they stay, or should they go?
Allow family members to stay at the patient's bedside when appropriate. For example, a patient may require constant monitoring to keep him from trying to climb out of bed. If a family member is available to stay with such a patient, the use of restraints could be avoided.

On the other hand, some patients appear to be agitated and have adverse changes in their vital signs when certain family members are present. Remember: Your first role is to be a patient advocate and to do what's best for the patient. Ask him whether he wants to have visitors and whom he wants to visit. If having a family member is best for the patient, then allow the visitor to stay. Many units have open visitation policies.

Ensure support
Ensure that support services are available to family members if they need them. If they belong to a particular church, offer to call someone if needed. Most facilities provide spiritual care for families if they request it.

A dose of reality

The best way to respond to concerned family members is to acknowledge their feelings and ambivalences and to lend reality to their statements.

Living with the decision

The nurse can use phrases such as "I know you would like me to decide what's best for your loved one, but I can't make that decision because you're the ones who will have to live with the consequences of your decision." The critical care nurse then needs to reinforce and acknowledge the family's decision and accept their feelings and decisions.

Always honor the cultural beliefs and values of patients and family members.

Cultural considerations

How a family copes with the hospitalization of a loved one can be influenced be cultural characteristics. A patient's cultural background can also affect many aspects of care, such as:
• patient and family roles during illness
• communication between health care providers and the patient and family members
• feelings of the patient and family members about end-of-life issues
• family views regarding health care practices
• pain management
• nutrition
• spiritual support.

Consider culture

Because your knowledge about cultural characteristics impacts care, you should perform a cultural assessment. (See *Assessing cultural considerations*, page 26.)

Conducting a cultural assessment enables you to:
• recognize a patient's cultural responses to illness and hospitalization
• determine how the patient and family members define health and illness
• determine the family's beliefs about the cause of the illness.

To provide effective holistic care, you must honor the patient's cultural beliefs and values.

Although it's good to be aware of cultural considerations, make sure that you don't stereotype patients based on their cultural backgrounds.

CAUTION!

Advice from the experts

Assessing cultural considerations

A cultural assessment yields the information you need to administer high-quality nursing care to members of various cultural populations. The goal of the cultural assessment quest is to gain awareness and understanding of cultural variations and their effects on the care you provide. For each patient, you and other members of the multidisciplinary team use the findings of a cultural assessment to develop an individualized care plan.

When performing a cultural assessment, be sure to ask questions that yield information about the patient's and family members':
- cultural health beliefs
- communication methods
- cultural restrictions
- social networks
- nutritional status
- religion
- values and beliefs.

See examples below of the types of questions you should consider for each patient.

Cultural health beliefs
- What does the patient believe caused his illness? A patient may believe that his illness is the result of an imbalance in yin and yang, punishment for a past transgression, or the result of divine wrath.
- How does the patient express pain?
- What does the patient believe promotes health? Beliefs can range from eating certain foods to wearing amulets for good luck.
- In what types of healing practices (such as herbal remedies and healing rituals) does the patient engage?

Communication differences
- What language does the patient speak?
- Does the patient require an interpreter?
- How does the patient want to be addressed?
- What are the styles of nonverbal communication (eye contact, touching)?

Cultural restrictions
- How does the patient's cultural group express emotion?
- How are feelings about death, dying, and grief expressed?
- How is modesty expressed?
- Does the patient have restrictions related to exposure of any parts of the body?

Social networks
- What are the roles of each family member during health and illness?
- Who makes the decisions?

Nutrition
- What's the meaning of food and eating to the patient?
- What types of food does he eat?
- Does the patient's food need to be prepared a certain way?

Religion
- What's the role of religious beliefs and practices during illness?
- Does the patient believe that special rites or blessings need to be performed?
- Are there healing rituals or practices that must be followed?

Cognitive issues

A patient on a critical care unit (CCU) may feel overwhelmed by the technology around him. Although this equipment is essential for patient care, it can create an environment that's foreign to the patient, which can result in disturbed cognition (thought-related function). In addition, the disease process can affect cognitive function in a critically ill patient. For example, patients with metabolic disturbances or hypoxia can experience confusion and changes in sensorium (mental clarity).

The way things were

When assessing cognitive function, the first question you should ask is, "What was your previous level of functioning?" If the patient can't answer this question, ask a family member. If the patient has been transferred to the CCU from another floor, ask the nurse who provided care before the transfer.

It's a factor

Many factors impact a patient's cognitive function while on the CCU, including:
• medications
• sensory input
• invasion of personal space.

> Uh-oh! It says here that the disease process can affect cognitive function.

Medications

Some medications that can cause adverse central nervous system reactions and affect cognitive function include:
• inotropics—such as digoxin, which can cause agitation, hallucinations, malaise, dizziness, vertigo, and paresthesia
• barbiturates—such as phenobarbital, which can cause drowsiness, lethargy, hangover symptoms, physical and psychological dependence, and paradoxical excitement (in elderly patients)
• corticosteroids—such as prednisone, which can cause euphoria, psychotic behavior, insomnia, vertigo, headache, paresthesia, and seizures
• benzodiazepines—such as lorazepam, which can cause drowsiness, sedation, disorientation, amnesia, unsteadiness, and agitation
• opioid analgesics—such as oxycodone, which can cause sedation, clouded sensorium, euphoria, dizziness, lightheadedness, and somnolence.

> Inotropic medications can cause a patient to become agitated or hallucinate.

Sensory input

Sensory stimulation in any environment may be perceived as pleasant or unpleasant and comfortable or painful. The critical care environment tends to stimulate all five senses:
• auditory
• visual

- gustatory
- olfactory
- tactile.

Too much or too little

Patients on the CCU don't have control over the environmental stimulation around them. They may experience sensory deprivation, sensory overload, or both. Sensory deprivation can result from a reduction in the quantity and quality of normal and familiar sensory input, such as the normal sights and sounds encountered at home. Sensory overload results from an increase in the amount of unfamiliar sounds and sights in the critical care environment, such as beeping cardiac monitors, ringing telephones, overhead paging systems, and voices.

When environmental stimuli exceed the patient's ability to cope with the stimulation, the patient may experience anxiety, confusion, and panic as well as delusions.

Shhh! Keep it down as much as possible because noise can result in delirium.

A sensitive subject

Sensory deprivation or overload can lead to such problems as sleep disturbances, reality disturbances, and delirium.

Sleep disturbances

Because the critical care environment is typically noisy due to staff, other patients, and equipment alarms, patients on CCUs commonly experience sleep disturbances.

Other factors that interfere with sleep on the CCU include nursing interventions, pain, and fear.

Torture chamber

Sleep deprivation can cause anxiety, restlessness, disorientation, depression, irritability, confusion, combativeness, and hallucinations.

In addition, sleep deprivation can cause further medical problems, such as:

- immunosuppression
- decreased pain tolerance
- decreased muscle strength.

In other words, sleep deprivation can impede the recovery process and contribute to new problems.

Sleep deprivation can impede the recovery process and cause other complications.

Quiet time

To promote rest, the critical care nurse can take steps to provide a quieter environment for patients.

For example, the nurse may reduce light and noise by not having loud conversations near the patient and by closing the door to the patient's room if it's safe to do so.

Reality disturbances

Integration of the senses is necessary for a person to process environmental information. Disturbances in reality occur when a patient's ability to interpret the environment is altered. Examples of reality disturbances are:
• disorientation to time
• inability to decipher whether it's night or day
• misinterpretation of environmental stimuli — for example, thoughts that alarms and noises from equipment are phones ringing for the patient.

The surreal world

Hearing or vision loss or loss of consciousness (caused, for example, by a head injury) can make a patient especially vulnerable to reality disturbances. Lack of one or more sensory mechanisms that are necessary to function make it hard for the patient to adapt to the critical care environment.

When any of the senses is lost, reality disturbances result and the abilities to function and adapt are compromised.

Delirium

Delirium (acute confusion) is an altered state of consciousness, consisting of confusion, distractibility, disorientation, delusional thinking, defective perception, and agitation. When it occurs in a critical care environment, it's commonly called *ICU psychosis*. It has a rapid onset and is generally reversible.

Common contributors

In addition to sensory deprivation or overload, contributing factors that affect most patients on the CCU include:
• infection
• immobility.

Anti-ICU psychosis

The nurse can assist the patient suffering from ICU psychosis by:
• promoting rest
• decreasing noise and light in the room
• encouraging mobility when possible
• providing orientation to the patient.

Invasion of personal space

Personal space is the unmarked boundary or territory around a person. Several factors — such as cultural background and social situation — influence a patient's interpretation of personal space. A patient's personal space is limited in many ways by the critical care environment — for example, due to the confines of bed rest, lack of privacy, and use of invasive equipment.

You can try to increase your patient's sense of personal space — even within the critical care environment — by simply remembering to show common courtesy, such as:
• asking permission to perform a procedure or look at a wound or dressing
• pulling the curtain or closing the door
• knocking before you enter the patient's room.

The critical care environment doesn't allow for much personal space — for you or the patient!

Pain control issues

Because fear of pain is a major concern for many critically ill patients, pain management is an important part of your care.

Critical care patients are exposed to many types of procedures — such as I.V. procedures, cardiac monitoring, and intubation — that cause discomfort and pain. Pain is classified as acute or chronic.

Acute pain

Acute pain is caused by tissue damage due to injury or disease. It varies in intensity from mild to severe and lasts briefly (generally up to 6 months).

Acute pain is considered a protective mechanism because it warns of present or potential tissue damage or organ disease. It may result from a traumatic injury, surgical or diagnostic procedure, or medical disorder.

Examples of acute pain are:
• pain experienced during a dressing change
• pain related to surgery
• pain of acute myocardial infarction.

Acute pain can be managed effectively, and it generally subsides when the underlying problem is resolved. That's a relief!

Help is at hand

Acute pain can be managed effectively with analgesics, such as opioids and nonsteroidal anti-inflammatory drugs (NSAIDs). It generally subsides when the underlying problem is resolved.

Chronic pain

Chronic pain is pain that has lasted 6 months or longer and is on-going. It may be as intense as acute pain but it isn't a warning of tissue damage. Some patients on the CCU experience chronic as well as acute pain.

Examples of chronic pain include:
- arthritis pain
- chronic back pain
- chronic pain from cancer.

Don't look for the signs

The nervous system adapts to chronic pain. This means that many typical manifestations of pain—such as abnormal vital signs and facial grimacing—cease to exist. Therefore, chronic pain should be assessed as often as acute pain (generally, at least every 2 hours or more often, depending on the patient's condition). Assess chronic pain by questioning the patient.

Pain assessment

When it comes to pain assessment for critical care patients, it's especially important for the nurse to have good assessment skills. The most valid pain assessment comes from the patient's own reports of pain.

A pain assessment includes questions about:
- *location*—Ask the patient to tell you where the pain is; there may be more than one area of pain.
- *intensity*—Ask the patient to rate the pain using a pain scale.
- *quality*—Ask how the pain feels: sharp, dull, aching, or burning.
- *onset, duration, and frequency*—Ask when the pain started, how long it lasts, and how often it occurs.
- *alleviating and aggravating factors*—Ask what makes the pain feel better and what makes it worse.
- *associated factors*—Ask whether other problems are associated with the pain, such as nausea and vomiting.
- *effects on lifestyle*—Ask whether appetite, sleep, relationships, emotions, and work are affected.

Choose a tool

Many pain assessment tools are available. Whichever you choose, make sure it's used consistently so that everyone on the health care team is speaking the same language when addressing the patient's pain.

Common pain-rating scales

These scales are examples of the rating systems you can use to help a patient quantify pain levels.

Visual analog scale

To use the visual analog scale, ask the patient to place a line across the scale to indicate the current level of pain. The scale is a 10-cm line with "No pain" at one end and "Pain as bad as it can be" at the other end. The pain rating is determined by using a ruler to measure the distance, in millimeters, from "No pain" to the patient's mark.

No pain _____ **Pain as bad as it can be**

Numeric rating scale

To use the numeric rating scale, ask the patient to choose a number from 0 (indicating no pain) to 10 (indicating the worst pain imaginable) to indicate the current pain level. The patient may circle the number on the scale or verbally state the number that best describes the pain.

No pain | 0   1   2   3   4   5   6   7   8   9   10 | **Pain as bad as it can be**

Faces scale

A pediatric or adult patient with language difficulty may not be able to describe the current pain level using the visual analog scale or the numeric rating scale. In that case, use a faces scale like the one below. Ask your patient to choose the face on a scale from 1 to 6 that best represents the severity of current pain.

1   2   3   4   5   6

The three most common pain assessment tools used by clinicians are the visual analog scale, numeric rating scale, and faces scale. (See *Common pain-rating scales.*)

The sounds of silence

Many patients can't verbally express feelings of pain. For example, a patient may be unable to speak due to intubation or have an altered level of consciousness (LOC) ranging from confusion to unresponsiveness. In such cases, it's up to the nurse to ascertain the patient's pain level.

Body and mind

There are many physiologic and psychological responses to pain that the nurse should watch for during a pain assessment.

Some examples of the physiologic responses to pain are:
- tachycardia
- tachypnea
- dilated pupils
- increased or decreased blood pressure
- pallor
- nausea and vomiting
- loss of appetite.

Psychological responses to pain may manifest as:
- fear
- anxiety
- confusion
- depression
- sleep deprivation.

> When a patient can't tell you about feelings of pain, it's up to you to see the unspoken signs.

Pain particulars

When communicating aspects of a patient's pain to his doctor or other health care providers, make sure you:
- describe the pain by location, intensity, and duration
- indicate possible causes of the pain if known
- describe how the patient is responding to the pain or any treatment interventions.

Pain management

Achieving adequate pain control in critical care depends on effective pain assessment and the use of pharmacologic and nonpharmacologic treatments.

To provide the best holistic care possible, work with the doctor and other members of the health care team to develop an individualized pain management program for each patient.

Pharmacologic pain management

Pharmacologic pain management is common on CCUs.

Take three and call in the morning

Three classes of medications commonly used by the critical care nurse are:
- nonopioids
- opioids
- adjuvant medications. (See *The WHO analgesic ladder*, page 34.)

The WHO analgesic ladder

The World Health Organization (WHO) developed a three-step ladder (shown below) to guide pain-relief efforts for patients with cancer. Analgesics are selected based on the intensity of the patient's pain. The ladder includes three categories of drugs: non-opioids, opioids, and adjuvant drugs. Adjuvant drugs can be used on any step of the ladder.

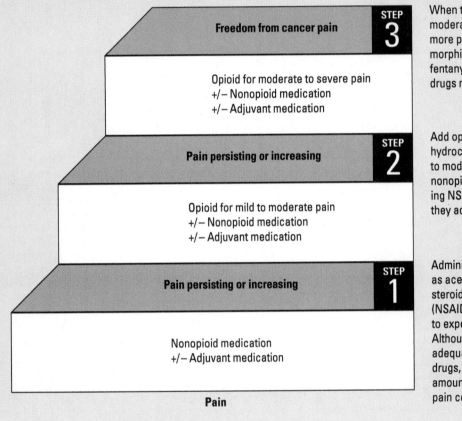

STEP 3

Freedom from cancer pain

Opioid for moderate to severe pain
+/– Nonopioid medication
+/– Adjuvant medication

When the patient's pain reaches the moderate to severe level, administer more potent opioid drugs, including morphine, oxycodone, hydromorphone, fentanyl, and methadone. Nonopioid drugs may be continued.

STEP 2

Pain persisting or increasing

Opioid for mild to moderate pain
+/– Nonopioid medication
+/– Adjuvant medication

Add opioid drugs, such as codeine or hydrocodone, for the patient with mild to moderate pain that isn't relieved by a nonopioid. If the patient is already taking NSAIDs, continue to use them as they add to the analgesic effect.

STEP 1

Pain persisting or increasing

Nonopioid medication
+/– Adjuvant medication

Pain

Administer nonopioid analgesics, such as acetaminophen, aspirin, and non-steroidal anti-inflammatory drugs (NSAIDs), to the patient just beginning to experience discomfort and mild pain. Although the patient's pain might not be adequately controlled with nonopioid drugs, their use may reduce the overall amount of opioids needed to achieve pain control.

Nonopioids

Nonopioids are the first choice for managing mild pain. They decrease pain by inhibiting inflammation at the injury site. Examples of nonopioids are:

- acetaminophen
- NSAIDs, such as ibuprofen and naproxen
- salicylates such as aspirin.

A trio of opioids

Opioids block the release of neurotransmitters that send pain signals to the brain. The three categories of opioids are opioid agonists (narcotic analgesics), opioid antagonists (narcotic reversal agents), and mixed agonist-antagonists.

Opioid agonists

Opioid agonists relieve pain by binding to pain receptors, which, in effect, produces pain relief. Examples of opioid agonists are:
- morphine
- fentanyl
- hydromorphone
- codeine
- oxycodone.

Opioid antagonists

Opioid antagonists attach to opiate receptors without producing agonistic effects. They work by displacing the opioid at the receptor site and reversing the analgesic and respiratory depressant effects of the opioid.

Examples of opioid antagonists are:
- naloxone
- naltrexone.

Mixed opioid agonist-antagonists

Mixed opioid agonist-antagonists relieve pain by binding to opiate receptors to effect varying degrees of agonistic and antagonistic activity. They carry a lower risk of toxic effects and drug dependency than opioid agonists and opioid antagonists.

Examples of mixed opioid agonist-antagonists are:
- buprenorphine
- butorphanol
- pentazocine.

Opioids

Opioids are narcotics that contain a derivative of the opium (poppy) plant and other synthetic drugs that imitate natural narcotics. Opioids work by blocking the release of neurotransmitters involved in transmitting pain signals to the brain. There are three categories of opioids. (See *A trio of opioids*.)

We're ready to fight pain! Opioids work by blocking the release of neurotransmitters that send out pain signals.

Adjuvant analgesics

Adjuvant analgesics are drugs that have other primary indications but are used as analgesics in some circumstances.

Alone or together

Adjuvants may be given in combination with opioids or alone to treat patients with chronic pain. Drugs used as adjuvant analgesics include:
- anticonvulsants, such as carbamazepine, clonazepam, and gabapentin
- tricyclic antidepressants, such as amitriptyline and nortriptyline

- benzodiazepines, such as alprazolam, diazepam, and lorazepam
- corticosteroids, such as dexamethasone and methylprednisolone.

Drug administration

A common route of pain medication administration on the CCU is I.V. bolus on an as-needed basis. It's the preferred route for opioid therapy, especially when short-term pain relief is needed — for example, during procedures such as wound care. The benefit of this method is rapid pain control. On the downside, with I.V. bolus administration, the patient experiences alternating periods of pain control and pain.

'Round-the-clock control

Using around-the-clock dosing ensures that steady levels of drugs prevent exacerbations of pain. This type of dosing has many benefits for critically ill patients who have difficulty communicating their pain because of altered LOC or endotracheal intubation.

Patients overpower pain

Some patients are candidates for patient-controlled analgesia (PCA). PCA provides a constant level of pain medication while allowing the patient to self-administer more pain medication as needed. Controls are set to prevent excessive self-administration. (See *Understanding PCA*.)

> 'Round-the-clock dosing controls pain better than as-needed administration.

Understanding PCA

A patient-controlled analgesia (PCA) system provides an optimal narcotic dose while maintaining a constant serum concentration of the drug.

Pump and port
A PCA system consists of a syringe-type injection pump that's piggybacked into an I.V. or subcutaneous infusion port.

By pressing a button, the patient receives a preset bolus dose of a narcotic. The doctor orders the bolus dose and the lock-out time between boluses, thus preventing overdose. The device automatically records the number of times the patient presses the button, helping the doctor to adjust drug dosage.

Patient at the controls
Using a PCA system may reduce a patient's drug dosage need. This may be because the patient using PCA is more in control of pain and typically feels reassured knowing that an analgesic is quickly available.

Patients usually report that they have more control over pain levels when using PCA. Patients using PCA still require close assessment and evaluation for responses to treatment.

A caveat

Note that PCA may not be appropriate for patients with altered LOC or those with renal or hepatic abnormalities.

Music therapy can be effective in controlling pain for short periods of time.

Nonpharmacologic pain management

Pain control isn't achieved solely with medications. Nonpharmacologic means are useful adjuncts in managing pain.

Some common nonpharmacologic pain control methods are:
- distraction—such as television viewing and reading
- music therapy—a form of sound therapy using rhythmic sound to communicate, relax, and encourage healing (this method works for brief periods of time)
- biofeedback—requires use of a biofeedback machine and allows the patient to recognize and control the relaxation process, thereby exerting conscious control over various autonomic functions

You're getting sleepy

- hypnosis—used to achieve *symptom suppression*, to block awareness of pain, or *symptom substitution*, which allows a positive interpretation of pain
- imagery—in which the patient visualizes a soothing image while the nurse describes pleasant sensations (for example, the patient may picture himself at the beach while you describe the sounds of the waves and birds and the feel of the warm sun and a breeze on the patient's skin)
- relaxation therapy—a form of meditation used to focus attention on a single sound or image or on the rhythm of breathing
- heat application (thermotherapy)—application of dry or moist heat to decrease pain (heat enhances blood flow, increases tissue metabolism, and decreases vasomotor tone; it also may relieve pain due to muscle aches or spasms, itching, or joint pain)
- cold application (cryotherapy)—constricts blood vessels at the injury site, reducing blood flow to the site (cold slows edema development, prevents further tissue damage, and minimizes bruising; it may be more effective than heat in relieving such pain as muscle aches or spasms, itching, incision pain, headaches, and joint pain)
- transcutaneous electrical nerve stimulator (TENS)—in which electrodes transmit mild electrical impulses to the brain to block pain impulses
- massage therapy—used as an aid to relaxation.

Massage therapy helps to control pain by inducing relaxation.

Ethics issues

Nurses who work on CCUs routinely deal with ethical dilemmas. You'll recognize a situation as an ethical dilemma in the following circumstances:
• More than one solution exists. That is, there's no clear "right" or "wrong" way to handle a situation.
• Each solution carries equal weight.
• Each solution is ethically defensible.

The value of values

Ethical dilemmas on CCUs commonly revolve around quality-of-life issues for the patient, especially as they relate to end-of-life decisions—such as do-not-resuscitate orders, life support, and patients' requests for no heroic measures. When considering quality of life, make sure others don't impose their own value system on the patient. Each person has a set of personal values that are influenced by environment and culture. Nurses also have a set of professional values.

Code of ethics

The American Nurses Association (ANA) has established a code of ethics. The ANA Code of Ethics for Nurses provides information that's necessary for the practicing nurse to use her professional skills in providing the most effective holistic care possible, such as serving as a patient advocate and striving to protect the health, safety, and rights of each patient.

End-of-life decisions

The threat of death is common on CCUs. Perhaps at no other time is the holistic care of patients and their families as important as it is during this time.

End-of-life decisions are almost always difficult for patients, families, and health care professionals to make. Nurses are in a unique position as advocates to assist patients and their families through this process.

Unsolvable mysteries

Your primary role as a patient advocate is to promote the patient's wishes. In many instances, however, a patient's wishes aren't known. That's when ethical decision making takes priority. Decisions aren't always easy to make and the answers

End-of-life decisions aren't always easy to make and the answers aren't usually clear-cut.

aren't usually clear-cut. At times, such ethical dilemmas may seem insolvable.

A question of quality

It's sometimes difficult to determine what can be done to achieve good quality of life and what can simply be achieved, technologically speaking. Technological advances sometimes seem to exceed our ability to analyze the ethical dilemmas associated with them.

Years ago, death was considered a natural part of life and most people died at home, surrounded by their families. Today, most people die in hospitals and death is commonly regarded as a medical failure rather than a natural event. Sometimes it's hard for you to know whether you're assisting in extending the patient's life or delaying the patient's death.

Consulting the committee

Most hospitals have ethics committees that review ethical dilemmas. The nurse may consider consulting the ethics committee if:
• the doctor disagrees with the patient or his family regarding treatment of the patient.
• health care providers disagree among themselves about treatment options.
• family members disagree about what should be done.

Futile treatment isn't a good use of health care resources and it doesn't change the patient's outcome.

Determining medical futility

Medical futility refers to treatment that's hopeless or interventions that aren't likely to benefit the patient even though they may appear to be effective. For example, a patient with a terminal illness who's expected to die experiences cardiac arrest. Cardiopulmonary resuscitation may be effective in restoring a heartbeat but may still be deemed futile because it doesn't change the patient's outcome.

Withholding or withdrawing treatment

The issue of withholding or withdrawing treatment on the CCU presents some ethical dilemmas. When withdrawing treatment from a patient—even at the patient's request—controversy over the principle of nonmaleficence (to prevent harm) may arise.

Harm alarm

Such controversy revolves around the definition of harm. Some feel that removing a patient from a ventilator and allowing death is an intentional infliction of harm. Others argue that keeping a person on a ventilator against the patient's will — thus prolonging death — is an intentional infliction of harm. (See *Approaching ethical decisions.*)

Dealing with cardiac arrest

In case of cardiac arrest (sudden stoppage of the heart), a critically ill patient may be described by a code status. This code status describes the orders written by the doctor describing what resuscitation measures should be carried out by the nurse and should be based on the patient's wishes regarding resuscitation measures. When cardiac arrest occurs, you must ensure that resuscitative efforts are initiated or that unwanted resuscitation doesn't occur.

Who decides?

The wishes of a competent, informed patient should always be honored. However, when a patient can't make decisions, the health care team — consisting of the patient's family, nursing staff, and doctors — may have to make end-of-life decisions for the patient.

Advance directives

Most people prefer to make their own decisions regarding end-of-life care. It's important that patients discuss their wishes with their loved ones; however, many don't. Instead, total strangers may be asked to make important health care decisions when a patient can't do so. That's why it's important for people to make choices ahead of time and to make these choices known by developing advance directives.

During cardiac arrest, it's typically up to you to ensure that resuscitation is initiated or that unwanted resuscitation doesn't occur.

The Patient Self-Determination Act of 1990 requires hospitals and other institutions to make information available to patients on advance directives. However, it isn't mandatory for patients to have advance directives.

Where there's a will, there's a law

There are two types of advance directives:
• *a treatment directive*—sometimes known as a living will
• *an appointment directive*—sometimes called a durable power of attorney for health care.

A living will states which treatments a patient will accept and which the patient will refuse in case terminal illness renders the patient unable to make those decisions at the time. For example, a patient may be willing to accept artificial nutrition but not hemodialysis.

Durable power of attorney is the appointment of a person—chosen by the patient—to make decisions on the patient's behalf if the patient can no longer do so. Durable power of attorney for health care doesn't give the chosen individual authority to access business accounts; the power is strictly related to health care decisions.

A living will states which treatments a patient will accept and which the patient will refuse in case of terminal illness.

It takes two

After an advance directive is written, two witnesses must sign it. This document can be altered or canceled at any time. For more information, check the laws regarding advance directives for the state in which you practice.

Organ donation

When asked, most people say that they support organ donation. However, only a small percentage of qualified organs are ever donated. Tens of thousands of names are on waiting lists for organs in the United States alone. Organ transplantation is successful for many patients, giving them additional, high-quality years of life.

The Uniform Anatomical Gift Act governs the donation of organs and tissues. In addition, most states have legislation governing the procurement of organs and tissues. Some require medical staff to ask about organ donation on every death. Other states require staff to notify a regional organ procurement agency that then approaches the family. Become familiar with the laws of your state and the policies of the facility in which you practice.

Who died?

Medical criteria for organ donation vary from state to state. Many organ procurement agencies want to be notified of all deaths and

Assessing brain death

Methods for determining brain death vary, but several of the following criteria are commonly used:
• The patient must be unresponsive to all stimuli.
• Pupillary responses are absent.
• All brain functions cease.
• No eye movements are noted when cold water is instilled into the ears (caloric test). Normally, the eyes move toward the ear irrigated with cold water.

• No corneal reflex is present.
• No gag reflex is present.
• Quick rotation of the patient's head from left to right (doll's eyes test) causes the eyes to remain fixed, suggesting brain death. Normally, the eyes move in the opposite direction of the head movement.
• No response to painful stimuli is present.
• An apnea test reveals no spontaneous breathing.
• EEG shows no brain activity or response.

imminent deaths so that they, not the medical staff, can determine if the patient is a potential candidate for organ donation.

No, thank you

These conditions usually preclude any organ or tissue donation:
• advanced age
• metastatic cancer
• history of hepatitis, human immunodeficiency virus, or acquired immunodeficiency syndrome
• sepsis.

Donations accepted

Any patient who donates organs must first be declared brain dead. Death used to be defined as the cessation of respiratory and cardiac function. However, with developments in technology, this definition has become obsolete. We now rely on brain death criteria in determining death of an individual. (See *Assessing brain death.*)

Complex care

Care of a patient who's to be an organ donor is very complex. It's imperative that hemodynamic variables and electrolyte values be kept within very tight ranges for successful organ transplantation. You have a vital role in caring for the patient and in supporting the patient's family during this difficult time.

When caring for an organ donor, it's essential to:
• maintain hemodynamic stability so that vital organs are perfused adequately
• assess urine output hourly to detect diabetes insipidus
• monitor laboratory results — such as electrolyte levels, complete blood count, liver and renal function tests — to assess organ function.

Quick quiz

1. Which of the following statements regarding a patient's culture and his hospitalization experience is true?
    A. Culture affects a patient's experience during hospitalization because the patient has to adapt to the hospital culture.
    B. Culture doesn't affect the patient's hospitalization.
    C. Cultural factors can affect patient and family roles during illness.
    D. Culture rarely impacts decisions about health.

Answer: C. Cultural factors can have a major impact on patient and family roles during illness. Culture affects the patient's and family members' feelings about illness, pain, and end-of-life issues, among other things.

2. Factors that can impact a critically ill patient's cognitive function include:
    A. medications.
    B. health condition.
    C. sleep disturbances.
    D. all of the above.

Answer: D. All of these factors can impact the patient's cognitive function while on the CCU.

3. When dealing with the family of a patient in critical care, the nurse should:
    A. consider them an integral part of the team.
    B. allow them only to visit during posted visiting times.
    C. refer them to the patient's doctor for all information.
    D. tell them not to touch the patient.

Answer: A. Family members know the patient better than anyone else does and should be considered an important part of the team caring for the patient.

4. Pain assessment in an unconscious patient:
   A. isn't necessary because unconscious patients don't experience pain.
   B. requires astute assessment skills by the nurse.
   C. can be achieved through the use of visual analog scales.
   D. is treated differently from pain in a conscious patient.

Answer: B. Nurses should be especially vigilant in assessing for nonverbal signs of pain in an unconscious patient.

5. The Patient Self-Determination Act of 1990 states that:
   A. all hospitalized patients must have advance directives.
   B. hospitals must make information on advance directives available to all patients.
   C. it's the doctor's responsibility to obtain information about advance directives.
   D. patients may have either a living will or a durable power of attorney for health care, but not both.

Answer: B. This act requires hospitals and other institutions to make information about advance directives available to patients, even though having an advance directive isn't mandatory.

Scoring

☆☆☆ If you answered all five questions correctly, jump for joy. You're wholly well versed in holistic care issues.

☆☆ If you answered four questions correctly, we won't issue a complaint. You're ready to join the team.

☆ If you answered fewer than four questions correctly, don't worry; it isn't an ethical dilemma. Just review the chapter and try again.

Neurologic system

Just the facts

In this chapter, you'll learn:

♦ anatomy and physiology of the neurologic system

♦ assessment of the neurologic system

♦ diagnostic tests and procedures

♦ neurologic disorders and treatments.

Understanding the nervous system

The neurologic (or nervous) system is the organ system that coordinates all body functions. This complex system allows a person to adapt to changes within his body and in the environment.

Two systems in one

The nervous system consists of:

☞ the central nervous system (CNS), which includes the brain and spinal cord

✌ the peripheral nervous system, which includes the cranial nerves, spinal nerves, and autonomic system.

Central nervous system

The organs of the CNS—the brain and spinal cord—collect and interpret motor and sensory stimuli. In the process, voluntary and involuntary sensory impulses travel along neural pathways to the brain. (See *A close look at the CNS*, page 46.)

We're both central features of the central nervous system. I'm the smart one!

I'm the sensitive one!

A close look at the CNS

This illustration depicts a cross section of the brain and spinal cord, which together make up the central nervous system (CNS). The brain joins the spinal cord at the base of the skull and ends near the second lumbar vertebrae. Note the H-shaped mass of gray matter in the spinal cord.

Cross section of the brain

- Cerebellum
- Hypothalamus
- Cerebrum
- Thalamus
- Midbrain
- Pituitary gland
- Pons
- Medulla
- Spinal cord

Cross section of the spinal cord

- Ventral horn (relays motor impulses)
- Dorsal horn (relays sensory impulses)
- White matter (forms ascending and descending tracts)
- Gray matter

Brain

The brain consists of three parts:
- cerebrum
- cerebellum
- brain stem.

Brain work

The brain collects, integrates, and interprets all stimuli and initiates and regulates voluntary and involuntary motor activity. Four major arteries supply the brain with oxygen.

Cerebrum

The cerebrum, or cerebral cortex, is the largest part of the brain.

Nerve Central Station

Tissues of the cerebrum make up a nerve center that controls sensory and motor activities and intelligence. It's encased by the

The cerebrum contains the nerve center that controls sensory and motor activities and intelligence.

bones of the skull and enclosed by three meninges (membrane layers): the dura mater, arachnoid, and pia mater.

Relay and regulate

The diencephalons, another part of the cerebrum, contain the thalamus and hypothalamus. The thalamus is a relay station for sensory impulses.

The hypothalamus has many regulatory functions, such as:
• temperature control
• pituitary hormone production
• sleep and wake cycles
• water balance.

Divided in two

The cerebrum is divided into two hemispheres, left and right. The right hemisphere controls the left side of the body. The left hemisphere controls the right side of the body.

The two hemispheres of the brain are composed of four lobes. Each of the four lobes controls different functions. (See *Basic brain functions*, page 48.)

Golly, am I good? I didn't even know I could walk and chew gum at the same time let alone control the right side of the body with my left hemisphere and vice versa.

Cerebellum

The cerebellum—the brain's second largest region—lies behind and below the cerebrum. Like the cerebrum, it has two hemispheres.

Smooth moves

The cerebellum contains the major motor and sensory pathways. It enables smooth, coordinated muscle movement and helps maintain equilibrium.

The brain stem is a sensory and motor pathway to and from the cerebral cortex. It also regulates automatic functions.

Brain stem

The brain stem lies below the diencephalons and includes the:
• midbrain
• pons
• medulla.

Pathway to the brain

The brain stem contains the nuclei, or cranial nerves III through XII. It's a major sensory and motor pathway for impulses running to and from the cerebral cortex. It also regulates automatic body functions, such as heart rate, breathing, swallowing, and coughing.

Basic brain functions

The basic structures and functions of the brain are depicted here. The cerebrum is divided into four lobes, based on location and function. The lobes—parietal, occipital, temporal, and frontal—are named for the cranial bones over them.

Parietal lobe
Sensations, awareness of body shape

Occipital lobe
Visual stimuli

Temporal lobe
Hearing, language and comprehension, storage and recall of memories

Cerebellum
Controls balance and coordination

Sensory cortex
Sensory impulses

Frontal lobe
Personality, judgment, abstract reasoning, social behavior, language, expression, movement

Motor cortex
Movement

Circulation to the brain
The four major blood vessels of the brain include two vertebral and two carotid arteries.

Two arteries converge

The two vertebral arteries converge to become the basilar artery. The basilar artery supplies oxygenated blood to the posterior parts of the brain.

Two arteries diverge

The common carotid arteries branch into the two internal carotids, which further divide to supply oxygenated blood to the anterior and middle areas of the brain. These vessels interconnect and form the circle of Willis at the base of the brain. The circle of Willis ensures that oxygen is continuously circulated to the brain even if any of the brain's major vessels is interrupted. (See *Arteries of the brain*.)

The circle of Willis ensures a constant supply of oxygen to the brain even if a major vessel is interrupted. Whew!

Arteries of the brain

Here's how the inferior surface of the brain appears. The anterior and posterior arteries join smaller arteries to form the circle of Willis.

Anterior communicating artery

Left internal carotid artery

Middle cerebral artery

Posterior cerebral artery

Superior cerebellar artery

Anterior spinal artery

Anterior cerebral artery

Posterior communicating artery

Basilar artery

Anterior inferior cerebellar artery

Left vertebral artery

Spinal cord

The spinal cord extends from the upper border of the first cervical vertebrae to the lower border of the first lumbar vertebrae. It's encased by the same membrane structure as the brain and is protected by the bony vertebrae of the spine.

Long paths

The spinal cord is the primary pathway for messages traveling between the peripheral parts of the body and the brain.

Short paths

The spinal cord also mediates the sensory-to-motor transmission path known as the *reflex arc*. Because the reflex arc enters and exits the spinal cord at the same level, reflex pathways don't need to travel up and down the way other stimuli do. (See *Understanding the reflex arc*, page 50.)

Understanding the reflex arc

Spinal nerves—which have sensory and motor portions—control deep tendon and superficial reflexes. A simple reflex arc requires a sensory (or afferent) neuron and a motor (or efferent) neuron.

Knee jerk reaction

The knee jerk, or patellar, reflex illustrates the sequence of events in a normal reflex arc:
• First, a sensory receptor detects the mechanical stimulus produced by the reflex hammer striking the patellar tendon.

• Then the sensory neuron carries the impulse along its axon by way of the spinal nerve to the dorsal root, where it enters the spinal column.
• Next, in the anterior horn of the spinal cord, shown below, the sensory neuron joins with a motor neuron, which carries the impulse along its axon by way of the spinal nerve to the muscle. The motor neuron transmits the impulse to muscle fibers through stimulation of the motor end plate. This triggers the muscle to contract and the leg to extend.

Patellar reflex arc

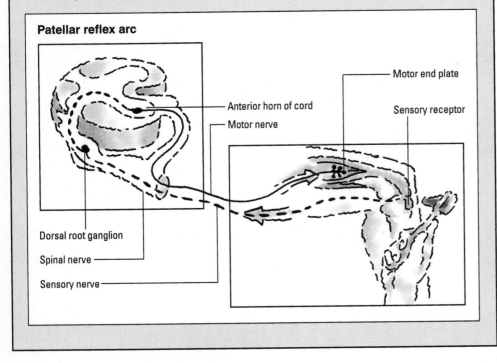

Anterior horn of cord

Motor nerve

Motor end plate

Sensory receptor

Dorsal root ganglion

Spinal nerve

Sensory nerve

Don't stand directly in front of a patient when testing this reflex!

Neural horns

The H-shaped mass of gray matter in the spinal cord is divided into four horns, which consist mainly of neuron cell bodies.

Four horns

The main function of cells in the two dorsal (posterior) horns of the spinal cord is to relay sensations; those in the two ventral (anterior) horns play a part in voluntary and reflex motor activity.

White matter matters

White matter surrounds the four horns. This white matter consists of myelinated nerve fibers grouped in vertical columns, or tracts:
• The *dorsal* white matter contains the ascending tracts, which carry impulses up the spinal cord to higher sensory centers.
• The *ventral* white matter contains the descending tracts, which transmit motor impulses down from higher motor centers to the spinal cord.

Sensory impulse pathways

Sensory impulses travel along the afferent (sensory or ascending) neural pathways to the sensory cortex in the parietal lobe of the brain. There, the impulses are interpreted. The sensory impulses travel along two major pathways:
• dorsal horn
• ganglia.

Dorsal horn

Pain and temperature sensations enter the spinal cord through the dorsal horn. After immediately crossing to the opposite side of the cord, these impulses travel to the thalamus by way of the spinothalamic tract.

Ganglia

Sensations such as touch, pressure, and vibration enter the cord by way of relay stations, called *ganglia*, which are masses of nerve cell bodies on the dorsal roots of spinal nerves. Impulses travel up the dorsal column to the medulla, cross to the opposite side, and enter the thalamus. There, the sensory cortex interprets the impulses.

Sensations of touch, pressure, and vibration enter the spinal cord by way of relay stations called ganglia.

Motor impulse pathways

Motor impulses travel from the brain to muscles by way of the efferent (motor or descending) pathway. Motor impulses begin in the motor cortex of the frontal lobe and travel along the upper motor neurons to reach the lower motor neurons of the peripheral nervous system.

Upper motor neurons originate in the brain and form two major systems:
• the pyramidal system
• the extrapyramidal system.

Pyramidal system

The pyramidal system (corticospinal tract) is responsible for fine and skilled movements of skeletal muscle.

All the right moves

Impulses in this system travel from the motor cortex through the internal capsule to the medulla. At the medulla, they cross to the opposite side and continue down the spinal cord.

Extrapyramidal system

The extrapyramidal system (extracorticospinal tract) controls gross motor movements.

Extra, extra! Read all about it!

Impulses in this system originate in the premotor area of the frontal lobe. They then travel to the pons, where they cross to the opposite side and travel down the spinal cord to the anterior horns. They're then relayed to the lower motor neurons, which carry the impulses to muscles.

The pyramidal system controls fine and skilled movements of skeletal muscle.

Peripheral nervous system

The peripheral nervous system includes the cranial nerves, spinal nerves, and autonomic nervous system.

Cranial nerves

The 12 pairs of cranial nerves are the primary motor and sensory pathways between the brain and the head and neck. All cranial nerves except the olfactory and optic nerves exit from the midbrain, pons, or medulla oblongata of the brain stem. (See *Identifying cranial nerves.*)

Spinal nerves

There are 31 pairs of spinal nerves, each named for the vertebra immediately below its exit point from the spinal cord.

The nerve of nerves

Each spinal nerve consists of afferent (sensory) and efferent (motor) neurons, which carry messages to and from specific body regions, called *dermatomes*.

What's in a name?

Well, each pair of spinal nerves is named for the vertebra below its exit point from the spinal cord.

Identifying cranial nerves

The cranial nerves have either sensory or motor function or both. They're assigned Roman numerals and written this way: CN I, CN II, CN III, and so on. The locations of the cranial nerves as well as their functions are shown below.

Facial (CN VII)
Expressions in forehead, eye, and mouth; taste

Oculomotor (CN III)
Most eye movement, pupillary constriction, upper eyelid elevation

Trochlear (CN IV)
Down and in eye movement

Optic (CN II)
Vision

Acoustic (CN VIII)
Hearing and balance

Abducens (CN VI)
Lateral eye movement

Olfactory (CN I)
Smell

Trigeminal (CN V)
Chewing, corneal reflex, face and scalp sensations

Glossopharyngeal (CN IX)
Swallowing, salivating, and taste

Vagus (CN X)
Swallowing, gag reflex, talking; sensations of the throat, larynx, and abdominal viscera; activities of thoracic and abdominal viscera, such as heart rate and peristalsis

Accessory (CN XI)
Shoulder movement and head rotation

Hypoglossal (CN XII)
Tongue movement

Autonomic nervous system

The large autonomic nervous system supplies nerves to all internal organs. These visceral efferent nerves carry messages to the viscera from the brain stem and neuroendocrine system.

Two sympathetic systems

The autonomic nervous system includes two major parts:

☝ the sympathetic nervous system

✌ the parasympathetic nervous system.

Balancing act

When one part of the autonomic nervous system stimulates smooth muscles to contract or a gland to secrete, the other part of the system inhibits that action. Through such dual innervation, the sympathetic and parasympathetic systems counterbalance each other's activities to keep body systems running smoothly.

> The autonomic nervous system supplies nerves to all internal organs.

Sympathetic nervous system

Sympathetic nerves, called *preganglionic neurons*, exit the spinal cord between the first thoracic and second lumbar vertebrae and enter relay stations (ganglia) near the cord. These ganglia form the links of a chain that sends impulses to postganglionic neurons, which reach the organs and glands.

Enormous responses

The postganglionic neurons of the sympathetic nervous system produce widespread, generalized responses, including:
- vasoconstriction
- elevated blood pressure
- enhanced blood flow to skeletal muscles
- increased heart rate and contractility
- increased respiratory rate
- smooth-muscle relaxation of the bronchioles, GI tract, and urinary tract
- sphincter contraction
- pupillary dilation and ciliary muscle relaxation
- increased sweat gland secretion
- reduced pancreatic secretion.

> The sympathetic and parasympathetic systems counterbalance each other to keep body systems running smoothly.

Parasympathetic nervous system

Fibers of the parasympathetic nervous system leave the CNS by way of the cranial nerves from the midbrain and medulla and the spinal nerves between the second and fourth sacral vertebrae.

After leaving the CNS, the preganglionic fiber of each parasympathetic nerve travels to a ganglion near a specific organ or gland. The postganglionic fiber of the nerve enters that organ or gland.

Subtle responses

The postganglionic fibers of the parasympathetic nervous system produce responses involving one specific organ or gland, such as:
• reductions in heart rate, contractility, and conduction velocity
• bronchial smooth-muscle constriction
• increased GI tract tone and peristalsis, with sphincter relaxation
• increased bladder tone and urinary system sphincter relaxation
• vasodilatation of external genitalia, causing erection
• pupil constriction
• increased pancreatic, salivary, and lacrimal secretions.

> The postganglionic fibers of the parasympathetic nervous system produce responses that involve one specific organ or gland.

Neurologic assessment

Assessment of subtle and elusive changes in the complex nervous system can be difficult. When you assess a patient for possible neurologic impairment, be sure to collect a thorough health history and investigate physical signs of impairment.

Check the records

If you can't interview a critically ill patient due to impairment, you may gather history information from the patient's medical record. In some cases, you may need to ask his family members or the nurse transferring the patient to the critical care unit for information.

Health history

To collect a thorough health history, gather details about the patient's current state of health, previous health status, lifestyle, and family health.

With a little help from his friends (and family)

A patient with neurologic impairment may have trouble remembering. If members of the patient's family or close friends are available, include them in the assessment process. They may be able to corroborate or correct the details of the patient's health history.

Current health

Discover the patient's chief complaint by asking such questions as, "Why did you come to the hospital?" or "What has been bothering you lately?" Use the patient's words when you document such chief complaints.

Common complaints

If your patient is suffering from a neurologic disorder, you may hear reports of headaches, motor disturbances (such as weakness, paresis, and paralysis), seizures, sensory deviations, and altered level of consciousness (LOC).

Details, please

Encourage the patient to describe details of the current condition by asking such questions as:
• Do you have headaches? How often do you have them? What precipitates them?
• Do you feel dizzy from time to time? How often do you feel this way? What seems to precipitate the episodes?
• Do you ever feel a tingling or prickling sensation or numbness? If so, where?
• Have you ever had seizures or tremors? Have you ever had weakness or paralysis in your arms or legs?
• Do you have trouble urinating, walking, speaking, understanding others, reading, or writing?
• How is your memory and ability to concentrate?

Ask members of the patient's family to fill in details of the health history if the patient can't remember.

Previous health

Many chronic diseases affect the neurologic system, so ask questions about the patient's past health and what medications he's taking. Specifically, ask whether the patient has had any:
• major illnesses
• recurrent minor illnesses
• accidents
• injuries
• surgical procedures
• allergies.

Lifestyle

Ask questions about the patient's cultural and social background because these affect care decisions. Note the patient's education level, occupation, and hobbies. As you gather this information, also assess the patient's self-image.

Family health

Information about the patient's family may reveal a hereditary disorder. Ask if anyone in the family has had diabetes, cardiac or renal disease, high blood pressure, cancer, a bleeding disorder, a mental disorder, or a stroke.

Physical examination

A complete neurologic examination can be long and detailed. It's unlikely that you would perform one in its entirety. However, if your initial screening suggests a neurologic problem, you may need to conduct a more detailed assessment.

Top-to-bottom examination

Examine the patient's neurologic system in an orderly way. Beginning with the highest levels of neurologic function and working down to the lowest, assess these five areas:
- mental status
- cranial nerve functions
- sensory function
- motor function
- reflexes.

Mental status

Mental status assessment begins when you talk to the patient during the health history. Responses to your questions reveal clues about the patient's orientation and memory. Use such clues as a guide during the physical assessment.

No easy answers

Make sure that you ask questions that require more than yes-or-no answers. Otherwise, confusion or disorientation might not be apparent. If you have doubts about a patient's mental status, perform a screening examination. (See *Quick check of mental status,* page 58.)

Three-part exam

Use the mental status examination to check these three parameters:
- LOC
- speech
- cognitive function.

Mental status assessment begins with a health history. Your patient's responses reveal clues about his mental status.

Advice from the experts

Quick check of mental status

To quickly screen your patient for disordered thought processes, ask the questions below. An incorrect answer to any question may indicate the need for a complete mental status examination. Make sure that you know the correct answers before asking the questions.

Question	Function screened
What's your name?	Orientation to person
What's your mother's name?	Orientation to other people
What year is it?	Orientation to time
Where are you now?	Orientation to place
How old are you?	Memory
Where were you born?	Remote memory
What did you have for breakfast?	Recent memory
Who is President of the United States?	General knowledge
Can you count backward from 20 to 1?	Attention span and calculation skills

Level of consciousness

Watch for any change in the patient's LOC. It's the earliest and most sensitive indicator that his neurologic status has changed.

Descriptions and definitions

Many terms are used to describe LOC, and definitions differ slightly among practitioners. To avoid confusion, clearly describe the patient's response to various stimuli using these definitions:
• *Alert*—Patient follows commands and responds completely and appropriately to stimuli.
• *Lethargic*—Patient is drowsy, has delayed responses to verbal stimuli, and may drift off to sleep during the examination.
• *Stuporous*—Patient requires vigorous stimulation for a response.
• *Comatose*—Patient doesn't respond appropriately to verbal or painful stimuli and can't follow commands or communicate verbally.

> Watch for a change in the patient's LOC — the earliest and most sensitive indicator of neurologic status change.

Looking at LOC

Start by quietly observing the patient's behavior. If the patient is sleeping, try to rouse him by providing an appropriate stimulus, in this order:

- auditory
- tactile
- painful.

Always start with a minimal stimulus, increasing intensity as necessary. The Glasgow Coma Scale offers an objective way to assess the patient's LOC. (See *Using the Glasgow Coma Scale*, page 60.)

Speech

Listen to how well the patient expresses thoughts. Does he choose the correct words or seem to have problems finding or articulating words?

It's hard to say

To assess for dysarthria (difficulty forming words), ask the patient to repeat the phrase, "No ifs, ands, or buts." Assess speech comprehension by determining the patient's ability to follow instructions and cooperate with your examination.

Language changes

Keep in mind that language performance tends to fluctuate with the time of day and changes in physical condition. A healthy person may have language difficulty when ill or fatigued. However, increasing speech difficulties may indicate deteriorating neurologic status, which warrants further evaluation.

Cognitive function

Assess cognitive function by testing the patient's:
- memory
- orientation
- attention span
- calculation ability
- thought content
- abstract thinking
- judgment
- insight
- emotional status.

Listen up! Increasing speech difficulties may indicate deteriorating neurologic status.

Take charge!

Using the Glasgow Coma Scale

You can use the Glasgow Coma Scale to describe the patient's baseline mental status and detect and interpret changes in the level of consciousness.

To use the scale, test the patient's ability to respond to verbal, motor, and sensory stimulation and base your findings on the scale. A patient who's alert, can follow simple commands, and is oriented to time, place, and person receives a score of 15 points. A lower score in one or more categories may signal an impending neurologic crisis. A total score of 7 or less indicates severe neurologic damage.

Test	Score	Patient's response
Eye-opening response		
Spontaneously	4	Opens eyes spontaneously
To speech	3	Opens eyes when told to
To pain	2	Opens eyes only on painful stimulus
None	1	Doesn't open eyes in response to stimulus
Motor response		
Obeys	6	Shows two fingers when asked
Localizes	5	Reaches toward painful stimulus and tries to remove it
Withdraws	4	Moves away from painful stimulus
Abnormal flexion	3	Assumes a decorticate posture (shown below)
Abnormal extension	2	Assumes a decerebrate posture (shown below)
None	1	No response, just lies flaccid — an ominous sign
Verbal response		
Oriented	5	Tells current date
Confused	4	Tells incorrect year
Inappropriate words	3	Replies randomly with incorrect word
Incomprehensible	2	Moans or screams
None	1	No response
Total score	☐	

Thanks for the memories

Short-term memory is commonly affected first in a patient with neurologic disease. A patient with intact short-term memory can generally remember and repeat five to seven nonconsecutive numbers right away and again 10 minutes later.

When then who

To quickly test your patient's orientation, memory, and attention span, use the mental status screening questions. Orientation to time is usually disrupted first; orientation to person, last.

Always consider the patient's environment and physical condition when assessing orientation. For example, a patient admitted to the critical care unit for several days may not be oriented to time because of the constant activity and noise of the monitoring equipment.

Orientation to time is usually disrupted first; orientation to person, last.

Attention and calculation

When testing attention span and calculation skills, keep in mind that lack of mathematical ability and anxiety can affect the patient's performance. If he has difficulty with numerical computation, ask him to spell the word "world" backwards. While he's performing these functions, note his ability to pay attention.

Thought content

Disordered thought patterns may indicate delirium or psychosis. Assess thought pattern by evaluating the clarity and cohesiveness of the patient's ideas. Is his conversation smooth, with logical transitions between ideas? Does he have hallucinations (sensory perceptions that lack appropriate stimuli) or delusions (beliefs not supported by reality)?

Hypothetically speaking ...

Test the patient's judgment by asking him how he would respond to a hypothetical situation. For example, what would he do if he were in a public building and the fire alarm sounded? Evaluate the appropriateness of his answer.

Test your patient's judgment: Ask how he would respond to a hypothetical situation, and then evaluate his answer.

Insight on insight

Test your patient's insight by finding out:
• whether the patient has a realistic view of himself
• whether he's aware of his illness and circumstances.

Assess insight by asking, for example, "What do you think caused your chest pain?" Expect different patients to have different degrees of insight. For instance, a patient may attribute chest discomfort to indigestion rather than acknowledge that he has had a heart attack.

Lost in emotion

Throughout the interview, assess your patient's emotional status. Note his mood, emotional lability or stability, and the appropriateness of his emotional responses. Also, assess the patient's mood by asking how he feels about himself and his future. Keep in mind that signs and symptoms of depression in an elderly patient may be atypical. (See *Depression and elderly patients.*)

Cranial nerve function

Cranial nerve assessment reveals valuable information about the condition of the CNS, especially the brain stem.

Under pressure

Because of their location, some cranial nerves are more vulnerable to the effects of increasing intracranial pressure (ICP). Therefore, a neurologic screening assessment of the CNS focuses on these key nerves:
• optic (II)
• oculomotor (III)
• trochlear (IV)
• abducens (VI).

Go on

Also evaluate other nerves if the patient's history or symptoms indicate a potential CNS disorder or when performing a complete nervous system assessment. (See *Checking brain stem function.*)

Be nosey

Assess the olfactory nerve (cranial nerve [CN] I) first. Check the patency of each nostril. Then instruct the patient to close his eyes. Occlude one nostril, and hold a familiar, pungent-smelling substance under the patient's nose and ask him to identify it. Repeat this with the other nostril.

See about sight

Next, assess the optic (CN II) and oculomotor (CN III) nerves:
• To assess the optic nerve, check visual acuity, visual fields, and retinal structures. Do this by asking the patient to read a newspaper, starting with large headlines and moving to small print.
• To assess the oculomotor nerve, check pupil size, pupil shape, and pupillary response to light. When assessing pupil size, look for trends such as a gradual increase in the size of one pupil or appearance of unequal pupils. (See *Recognizing pupillary changes*, page 64.)

Senior moment

Depression and elderly patients

Symptoms of depression in elderly patients may be different from those found in other patients. For example, rather than the usual sad affect seen in patients with depression, your elderly patient may exhibit such atypical signs as decreased function and increased agitation.

Assess your patient's olfactory nerve by asking him to identify various substances by smell.

Checking brain stem function

In an unconscious patient, assist the doctor in assessing brain stem function by testing for the oculocephalic (doll's eye) reflex and the oculovestibular reflex. If the patient has a cervical spine injury, expect to use the oculovestibular reflex test as an alternative. The oculovestibular reflex test may also be used to determine the status of the vestibular portion of the acoustic nerve (CN VIII).

Oculocephalic reflex

Before beginning, examine the patient's cervical spine. Don't perform this procedure if you suspect the patient has a cervical spine injury. If the patient has no cervical spine injury, proceed as follows:
• Place both hands on either side of his head and use your thumbs to gently hold his eyelids open.
• While watching the patient's eyes, briskly rotate the head from side to side (as shown at right) or briskly flex and extend the patient's neck.
• Observe how the patient's eyes move in relation to head movement. In a normal response, which indicates an intact brain stem, the eyes appear to move opposite to the movement of the head. For example, if the neck is flexed, the eyes appear to look upward. If the neck is extended, the eyes gaze downward.

Abnormal response

With an abnormal (doll's eye) response, the eyes appear to move passively in the same direction as the head, indicating the absence of oculocephalic reflex. Such a response suggests a deep coma or severe brain stem damage at the level of the pons or midbrain.

Oculovestibular reflex

To assess the oculovestibular reflex, the doctor first determines that the patient has an intact tympanic membrane and a clear external ear canal. Then follow these steps:
• Elevate the head of the bed 30 degrees.
• Using a large syringe with a small catheter on the tip, slowly irrigate the external auditory canal with 20 to 200 ml of cold water or ice water (as shown at right).
• During irrigation, watch the patient's eye movements. In a patient with an intact oculovestibular reflex, the eyes deviate toward the side being irrigated with cold water.

Abnormal responses

If the patient is conscious to some degree, there may be nystagmus (involuntary, rapid movement of the eyeball) with rapid jerking of the eyes away from the side being irrigated. In an abnormal conscious individual, as little as 10 ml of ice water may produce such a response and may also cause nausea. In a comatose patient with an intact brain stem, the eyes tonically deviate toward the stimulated ear. Absence of eye movement suggests a brain stem lesion.

Recognizing pupillary changes

Use this table as a guide to recognize pupillary changes and identify possible causes.

Pupillary change	Possible causes
Unilateral, dilated (4 mm) fixed, and nonreactive 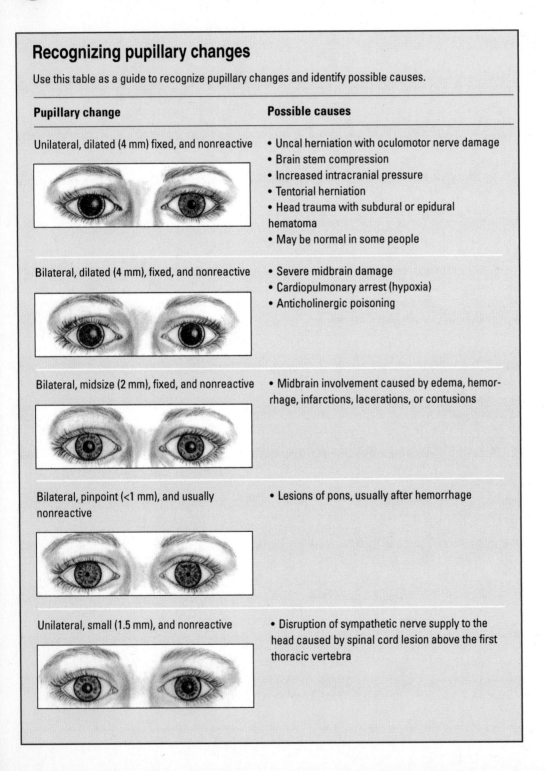	• Uncal herniation with oculomotor nerve damage • Brain stem compression • Increased intracranial pressure • Tentorial herniation • Head trauma with subdural or epidural hematoma • May be normal in some people
Bilateral, dilated (4 mm), fixed, and nonreactive	• Severe midbrain damage • Cardiopulmonary arrest (hypoxia) • Anticholinergic poisoning
Bilateral, midsize (2 mm), fixed, and nonreactive	• Midbrain involvement caused by edema, hemorrhage, infarctions, lacerations, or contusions
Bilateral, pinpoint (<1 mm), and usually nonreactive	• Lesions of pons, usually after hemorrhage
Unilateral, small (1.5 mm), and nonreactive	• Disruption of sympathetic nerve supply to the head caused by spinal cord lesion above the first thoracic vertebra

Check three nerves at once

Assess the coordinated function of the oculomotor (CN III), trochlear (CN IV), and abducens (CN VI) nerves simultaneously. Here's how these nerves normally work:
• The oculomotor nerve controls extraocular movement, pupillary constriction, and raising of the eyelid.
• The trochlear nerve (CN IV) controls downward and inward eye movement.
• The abducens nerve (CN VI) controls lateral eye movement.

Here's how

Make sure that the patient's pupils constrict when exposed to light and that his eyes adapt to seeing objects at various distances. Ask the patient to follow your finger through six cardinal positions of gaze:

left superior

left lateral

left inferior

right superior

right lateral

right inferior.

Pause slightly before moving from one position to the next, to assess the patient for nystagmus, or involuntary eye movement, and the ability to hold gaze in that particular position.

Focus on the face

To assess the sensory portion of the trigeminal nerve (CN V), gently touch the right and left sides of the patient's forehead with a cotton ball while his eyes are closed. Instruct him to tell you the moment the cotton touches each area. Compare the patient's responses on both sides.

Repeat the technique on the right and left cheek and on the right and left jaw. Next, repeat the entire procedure using a sharp object, such as the tip of a safety pin. Ask the patient to describe and compare both sensations.

To assess the motor function of the trigeminal nerve, ask the patient to clench his teeth while you palpate his temporal and masseter muscles.

Look for symmetry when you test the motor portion of the facial nerve.

Make someone smile

To test the motor portion of the facial nerve (CN VII), ask the patient to:
- wrinkle his forehead
- raise and lower his eyebrows
- smile to show his teeth
- puff out his cheeks.

Also, with the patient's eyes tightly closed, attempt to open his eyelids. As you conduct each part of this test, look for symmetry.

Keep it tasteful

The sensory portion of the facial nerve (CN VII) supplies taste sensation to the anterior two-thirds of the tongue. Test the taste sensation by placing items with various flavors on the patient's tongue. Use items such as sugar (sweet), salt, lemon juice (sour), and quinine (bitter). Between items, have the patient wash away each substance with a sip of water.

Use such items as lemon juice and quinine to test your patient's sour and bitter buds.

Now hear this

To assess the acoustic nerve (CN VIII), first test the patient's hearing. Ask the patient to cover one ear. Then stand on the opposite side and whisper a few words. Find out whether the patient can repeat what you said. Test the other ear in the same way.

To test the vestibular portion of the acoustic nerve, observe the patient for nystagmus and disturbed balance. Note reports of the room spinning or dizziness.

Check the pipes

Test the glossopharyngeal nerve (CN IX) and vagus nerve (CN X) together because their innervation overlaps in the pharynx:
- The glossopharyngeal nerve is responsible for swallowing, salivating, and taste perception on the posterior one-third of the tongue.
- The vagus nerve controls swallowing and is responsible for voice quality.

Assess these nerves, first, by listening to the patient's voice. Then check the gag reflex by touching the tip of a tongue blade against the posterior pharynx and asking the patient to open wide and say "ah." Watch for the symmetrical upward movement of the soft palate and uvula and for the midline position of the uvula.

Note shoulder strength and symmetry while inspecting and palpating your patient's trapezius muscles.

Shrug it off

To assess the spinal accessory nerve (CN XI), which controls the sternocleidomastoid muscles and the upper portion of the trapezius muscles, press down on the patient's shoulders while he attempts to shrug against this resistance. Note shoulder strength and symmetry while inspecting and palpating the trapezius muscles.

To further test the trapezius muscles, apply resistance from one side while the patient tries to return his head to midline position. Look for neck strength. Repeat on the other side.

Test tongue toughness

To assess the hypoglossal nerve (CN XII), follow these steps:

Ask the patient to stick out his tongue. Look for any deviation from the midline, atrophy, or fasciculations.

Test tongue strength by asking the patient to push his tongue against his cheek as you apply resistance. Observe the tongue for symmetry.

Test the patient's speech by asking him to repeat the sentence, "Round the rugged rock that ragged rascal ran."

Sensory function

Assess the sensory system to evaluate:
• ability of the sensory receptors to detect stimulus
• ability of the afferent nerves to carry sensory nerve impulses to the spinal cord
• ability of the sensory tracts in the spinal cord to carry sensory messages to the brain.

Five sensations

During your assessment, check five types of sensation, including pain, light touch, vibration, position, and discrimination.

This is gonna hurt

To test for pain sensation, have the patient close his eyes; then touch all the major dermatomes, first with the sharp end of a safety pin and then with the dull end. Proceed in this order:
• fingers
• shoulders
• toes
• thighs
• trunk.

Ouch! To test for pain in a more sensible fashion, touch all the major dermatomes with the sharp end of a safety pin and then with the dull end.

While testing, occasionally alternate sharp and dull ends. Ask the patient to tell you when he feels the sharp stimulus. If the patient has known deficits, start in the area with the least sensation and move toward the area with the most sensation.

Use a light touch

To test for the sense of light touch, follow the instructions for pain sensation, using a wisp of cotton or tissue. Lightly touch the patient's skin; don't swab or sweep the skin. A patient with peripheral neuropathy might retain the sensation for light touch after losing pain sensation.

Find the right vibe

To check for response to vibration, tap a low-pitched tuning fork on the heel of your hand, and then place the base of the fork firmly over the distal interphalangeal joint of the index finger. Then move proximally until the patient feels the vibration; everything above that level is intact.

If the patient's vibratory sense is intact, further testing for position sense isn't necessary because they follow the same pathway.

> If the patient's vibratory sense is intact, you can assume his position sense is intact, too.

Where the toes are

To experience position sense, the patient needs intact vestibular and cerebellar function. To assess for position sense, have the patient close his eyes. Then, grasp the sides of his big toe and move it up and down. Ask the patient what position the toe is in.

To perform the same test on the patient's upper extremities, grasp the sides of his index finger and move it back and forth. Ask the patient what position the finger is in.

Discrimination, integration, and extinction

Discrimination is the cortex's ability to integrate sensory input. Stereognosis is the ability to discriminate the shape, size, weight, texture, and form of an object by touching and manipulating it.

To test stereognosis, ask the patient to close both eyes and open one hand. Then place a common object, such as a key, in the hand and ask the patient to identify it. If the patient can't identify the object, test graphesthesia (ability to identify something by tactile sense). Here's how to do this: While the patient's eyes are closed, draw a large number on the palm of one hand and ask the patient to identify the number.

Extinction is the failure to perceive touch on one side. To test point localization, have the patient close his eyes, touch one of his limbs, and then ask where you touched him. To test two-point dis-

> Discrimination is the ability to integrate sensory input to determine the shape, size, weight, texture, and form of an object.

crimination, touch the patient simultaneously in two contralateral areas and note whether he can identify touch on both sides.

Motor function

Assess motor function to aid evaluation of these structures and functions:
• the cerebral cortex and its initiation of motor activity by way of the pyramidal pathways
• the corticospinal tracts and their capacity to carry motor messages down the spinal cord
• the lower motor neurons and their ability to carry efferent impulses to the muscles
• the muscles and their capacity to carry out motor commands
• the cerebellum and basal ganglia and their capacity to coordinate and fine-tune movement.

> Motor function assessment yields a truckload of information about neurologic structures and functions.

Tone test

Muscle tone represents muscular resistance to passive stretching. To test muscle tone of the arm, move the patient's shoulder through its passive range of motion (ROM); you should feel a slight resistance. When you let the patient's arm drop to his side, it should fall easily.

To test leg muscle tone, guide the patient's hip through its passive ROM, and then let his leg fall to the bed. If it falls in an externally rotated position, note this abnormal finding.

Feats of strength

To assess arm muscle strength, ask the patient to push you away as you apply resistance. Then ask the patient to extend both arms, palms up. Have him close his eyes and maintain this position for 20 to 30 seconds. Observe the arm for downward drifting and pronation.

Strength of feet

Assess leg movement by first asking the patient to move each leg and foot. If he fails to move the leg on command, watch for spontaneous movement.

Grace and gait

Assess the patient's coordination and balance through cerebellar testing. Note whether the patient can sit and stand without support. If appropriate, observe as the patient walks across the room, turns, and walks back.

While observing the patient, note imbalances and abnormalities. When cerebellar dysfunction is present, the patient has a wide-based, unsteady gait. Deviation to one side may indicate a cerebellar lesion on the side.

Synchronized standing

Perform Romberg's test to evaluate cerebellar synchronization of movement with balance. Have the patient stand with his feet together, arms at his sides, and without support. Note his ability to maintain balance with both eyes open and then closed. (Stand nearby in case the patient loses his balance.)

A small amount of swaying normally occurs when the eyes are closed. If the patient has trouble maintaining a steady position with eyes open or closed, cerebellar ataxia may be present.

Extreme coordination

Test the extremities for coordination by having the patient touch his nose and then your outstretched finger as you move it. Have him do this faster and faster. His movements should be accurate and smooth.

Test cerebellar function further by assessing rapid alternating movements. Tell the patient to use the thumb of one hand to touch each finger of the same hand in rapid sequence. Repeat with the other hand.

To assess the legs, have the patient rapidly tap the floor with the ball of one foot. Test each leg separately. Note any slowness or awkwardness. Abnormalities can indicate cerebellar disease or motor weakness associated with extrapyramidal or pyramidal disease.

When assessing coordination and balance, note any imbalance or abnormality.

Present and absent actions

Motor responses in an unconscious patient may be appropriate, inappropriate, or absent. Appropriate responses, such as localization or withdrawal, mean that the sensory and corticospinal pathways are functioning. Inappropriate responses, such as decorticate or decerebrate posturing, indicate a dysfunction.

It can be challenging to assess motor responses in a patient who can't follow commands or is unresponsive. Make sure that you note whether any stimulus produces a response and what that response is.

Reflexes

Assess deep tendon and superficial reflexes to learn about the integrity of the sensory receptor organ. You can also evaluate how well afferent nerves relay sensory messages to the spinal cord or brain stem segment to mediate reflexes.

How deep is your reflex?

Test deep tendon reflexes by checking the responses of the biceps, triceps, brachioradialis, patellar, and Achilles tendons:
• The biceps reflex contracts the biceps muscle and forces flexion of the forearm.
• The triceps reflex contracts the triceps muscle and forces extension of the forearm.
• The brachioradialis reflex causes supination of the hand and flexion of the forearm at the elbow.
• The patellar reflex forces contraction of the quadriceps muscle in the thigh with extension of the leg.
• The Achilles reflex forces plantar flexion of the foot at the ankle.

Superficially speaking

You can elicit superficial reflexes using light, tactile stimulation, such as stroking or scratching the skin.

Because these are cutaneous reflexes, the more you try to elicit them in succession, the less response you'll get. Therefore, observe carefully the first time you stimulate these reflexes.

Superficial reflexes include the pharyngeal, abdominal, and cremasteric reflexes. Here's how to test them:
• Pharyngeal reflex: To test CN IX and CN X, have the patient open his mouth wide. Then, touch the back of the pharynx with a tongue blade. Normally, this causes the patient to gag.
• Abdominal reflex: To test the intactness of thoracic spinal segments T8, T9, and T10, use the tip of the handle on the reflex hammer to stroke one side, and then the opposite side, of the patient's abdomen above the umbilicus. Repeat on the lower abdomen. Normally, the abdominal muscles contract and the umbilicus deviates toward the stimulated side.
• Cremasteric reflex: To test the intactness of lumbar spinal segments L1 and L2: In a male patient, use a tongue blade to scratch the inner aspects of each thigh gently. Normally, this action causes the testicles to lift.

Test deep tendon reflexes of the biceps, triceps, brachioradialis, patellar, and Achilles tendons.

Write it down

After you examine the patient, document your findings using a grading scale to rate each reflex. Document the rating for each reflex at the appropriate site on a stick figure. (See *Documenting reflex findings*, page 72.)

Documenting reflex findings

Use these grading scales to rate the strength of each reflex in a deep tendon and superficial reflex assessment.

Deep tendon reflex grades
0 absent
+ present but diminished
++ normal
+++ increased but not necessarily abnormal
++++ hyperactive or clonic (involuntary contraction and relaxation of skeletal muscle)

Superficial reflex grades
0 absent
+ present

Findings
Record the patient's reflex ratings on a drawing of a stick figure. The figures depict documentation of normal and abnormal reflex responses.

Diagnostic testing can be frightening. Make sure that you prepare the patient and his family members for each test.

Diagnostic tests

Diagnostic testing to evaluate the nervous system typically includes imaging studies, angiography, and electrophysiologic studies. Other tests, such as lumbar puncture and transcranial Doppler studies, may also be used.

Tell it like it is

Diagnostic testing may be routine for you, but it can be frightening for the patient. Make sure that you carefully prepare the patient and his family members for each test and follow-up monitoring procedure. Some tests can be performed at the patient's bedside, but many require transportation to the imaging department.

Thanks to CT scanning, you can see much of what may be wrong in the patient's brain.

Imaging studies

The most common imaging studies used to detect neurologic disorders include computed tomography (CT) scan, magnetic resonance imaging (MRI), positron emission tomography (PET) scan, and skull and spinal X-rays.

Computed tomography scan

CT scanning of intracranial structures combines radiology and computer analysis of tissue density (determined by contrast dye absorption). CT scanning doesn't show blood vessels as well as an angiogram does; however, it carries less risk of complications and causes less trauma than cerebral angiography.

Spine scanning

CT scanning of the spine is used to assess such disorders as herniated disk, spinal cord tumors, and spinal stenosis.

Brain scanning

CT scanning of the brain is used to detect brain contusion, brain calcifications, cerebral atrophy, hydrocephalus, inflammation, space-occupying lesions (tumors, hematomas, edema, and abscesses), and vascular anomalies (arteriovenous malformation [AVM], infarctions, blood clots, and hemorrhage).

Nursing concerns
• Confirm that the patient isn't allergic to iodine or shellfish to avoid an adverse reaction to the contrast medium.
• If the test calls for a contrast medium, tell the patient that it's injected into an existing I.V. line or that a new line may be inserted.
• Preprocedure testing should include evaluation of renal function (serum creatinine and blood urea nitrogen [BUN] levels) because the contrast medium can cause acute renal failure.
• Warn the patient that he may feel flushed or notice a metallic taste in his mouth when the contrast medium is injected.
• Tell him that the CT scanner circles around him for 10 to 30 minutes, depending on the procedure and type of equipment.
• Explain that he must lie still during the test.

Before CT scanning of the brain, make sure that the patient isn't allergic to iodine or shellfish, which may foretell an adverse reaction to the contrast medium.

• Tell him that the contrast medium may discolor his urine for 24 hours. Suggest that he drink more fluids to flush the medium out of his body, unless this is contraindicated or he has oral intake restrictions; otherwise, the doctor may write an order to increase the I.V. flow rate.

Magnetic resonance imaging

MRI generates detailed pictures of body structures. The test may involve the use of a contrast medium such as gadolinium.

Sharper images

Compared with conventional X-rays and CT scans, MRI provides superior contrast of soft tissues, sharply differentiating healthy, benign, and cancerous tissue and clearly revealing blood vessels. In addition, MRI permits imaging in multiple planes, including sagittal and coronal views in regions where bones normally hamper visualization.

MRI is especially useful for studying the CNS because it can reveal structural and biochemical abnormalities associated with such conditions as transient ischemic attack (TIA), tumors, multiple sclerosis (MS), cerebral edema, and hydrocephalus.

Nursing concerns

• Confirm that the patient isn't allergic to the contrast medium (usually gandolinium).
• If the test calls for a contrast medium, tell the patient that it's injected into an existing I.V. line or that a new line may be inserted.
• Explain that the procedure can take up to 1½ hours; tell the patient that he must remain still for intervals of 5 to 20 minutes.
• Instruct the patient to remove all metallic items, such as hair clips, bobby pins, jewelry (including body-piercing jewelry), watches, eyeglasses, hearing aids, and dentures.
• Explain that the test is painless, but that the machinery may seem loud and frightening and the tunnel confining. Tell the patient that he'll receive earplugs to reduce the noise.
• Provide sedation, as ordered, to promote relaxation during the test.
• After the procedure, increase the I.V. flow rate, as ordered, or encourage the patient to increase his fluid intake to flush the contrast medium from his system.

MRI is painless, but the machinery may seem loud, confining, and frightening to your patients.

Positron emission tomography scan

PET scanning provides colorimetric information about the brain's metabolic activity. It works by detecting how quickly tissues consume radioactive isotopes.

PET scanning is used to reveal cerebral dysfunction associated with tumors, seizures, TIA, head trauma, Alzheimer's disease, Parkinson's disease, MS, and some mental illnesses. In addition, a PET scan can be used to evaluate the effect of drug therapy and neurosurgery.

PET scanning is used to gather clues about cerebral blood flow, blood volume, and neuron and neurotransmitter metabolism.

PET project

Here's how PET scanning works:
• A technician administers a radioactive gas or an I.V. injection of glucose or other biochemical substance tagged with isotopes, which act as tracers.
• The isotopes emit positrons that combine with negatively charged electrons in tissue cells to create gamma rays.
• The PET scanner registers the emitted gamma rays and a computer translates the information into patterns that reflect cerebral blood flow, blood volume, and neuron and neurotransmitter metabolism.

Nursing concerns

• Provide reassurance that PET scanning doesn't expose the patient to dangerous levels of radiation.
• Explain that insertion of an I.V. catheter may be required.
• Instruct the patient to lie still during the test.

Skull and spinal X-rays

Skull X-rays are typically taken from two angles: anteroposterior and lateral. The doctor may order other angles, including Waters view, or occipitomental projection, to examine the frontal and maxillary sinuses, facial bones, and eye orbits

Having one's head examined

Skull X-rays are used to detect fractures; bony tumors or unusual calcifications; pineal displacement, which indicates a space-occupying lesion; skull or sella turcica erosion, which indicates a space-occupying lesion; and vascular abnormalities.

Spinal findings

The doctor may order anteroposterior and lateral spinal X-rays when:
• spinal disease is suspected

Skull X-rays are typically taken from the anteroposterior and lateral angles.

• injury to the cervical, thoracic, lumbar, or sacral vertebral segments exists.

Depending on the patient's condition, other X-ray images may be taken from special angles, such as the open-mouth view (to confirm odontoid fracture).

Spinal X-rays are used to detect spinal fracture; displacement and subluxation due to partial dislocation; destructive lesions, such as primary and metastatic bone tumors; arthritic changes or spondylolisthesis; structural abnormalities, such as kyphosis, scoliosis, and lordosis; and congenital abnormalities.

> Critical care nursing seems like backbreaking work, but an X-ray is needed to confirm the diagnosis.

Nursing concerns

• Reassure the patient that X-rays are painless.
• As ordered, administer an analgesic before the procedure if the patient has existing pain, so he'll be more comfortable.
• Remove the patient's cervical collar if cervical X-rays reveal no fracture and the doctor permits it.

Angiography

Angiographic studies include cerebral angiography and digital subtraction angiography (DSA).

Cerebral angiography

During cerebral angiography, the doctor injects a radiopaque contrast medium, usually into the brachial artery (through retrograde brachial injection) or femoral artery (through catheterization).

> Cerebral angiography is used to detect and identify problems affecting the cerebral vessels.

Why it's done

This procedure highlights cerebral vessels, making it easier to:
• detect stenosis or occlusion associated with thrombus or spasm
• identify aneurysms and AVMs
• locate vessel displacement associated with tumors, abscesses, cerebral edema, hematoma, or herniation
• assess collateral circulation.

Nursing concerns

• Explain the procedure to the patient, and answer all questions honestly.

• Confirm that the patient isn't allergic to iodine or shellfish because a person with such allergies may have an adverse reaction to the contrast medium.
• Preprocedure testing should include evaluation of renal function (serum creatinine and BUN levels) and potential risk of bleeding (prothombin time, PTT, and platelet count). Notify the doctor of abnormal results.
• Instruct the patient to lie still during the procedure.
• Explain that he'll probably feel a flushed sensation in his face as the dye is injected.
• Maintain bed rest, as ordered, and monitor the patient's vital signs.
• Monitor the catheter injection site for signs of bleeding.
• As ordered, keep a sandbag over the injection site.
• Monitor the patient's peripheral pulse in the arm or leg used for catheter insertion, and mark the site.
• Unless contraindicated, encourage the patient to drink more fluids to flush the dye from the body; alternatively, increase the I.V. flow rate as ordered.
• Monitor the patient for neurologic changes and such complications as hemiparesis, hemiplegia, aphasia, and impaired LOC.
• Monitor for adverse reactions to the contrast medium, which may include restlessness, tachypnea and respiratory distress, tachycardia, facial flushing, urticaria, and nausea and vomiting.

Encourage fluid consumption to flush out the contrast dye after testing, unless it's contraindicated.

Digital subtraction angiography

Like cerebral angiography, DSA highlights cerebral blood vessels. DSA is done this way:
• Using computerized fluoroscopy, a technician takes an image of the selected area, which is then stored in a computer's memory.
• After administering a contrast medium, the technician takes several more images.
• The computer produces high-resolution images by manipulating the two sets of images.

Sidestep stroke

Arterial DSA requires more contrast medium than cerebral angiography but, because the dye is injected I.V., DSA doesn't increase the patient's risk of stroke and, therefore, the test can be done on an outpatient basis.

Nursing concerns

• Confirm that the patient isn't allergic to iodine or shellfish because a person with these allergies may have an adverse reaction to the contrast medium.

• Preprocedure testing should include evaluation of renal function (serum creatinine and BUN levels) and potential risk of bleeding (prothombin time, PTT, and platelet count). Notify the doctor of abnormal results.
• Restrict the patient's consumption of solid food for 4 hours before the test.
• Explain that the test requires insertion of an I.V. catheter.
• Instruct the patient to remain still during the test.
• Explain that he'll probably feel flushed or have a metallic taste in his mouth as the contrast medium is injected.
• Tell the patient to alert the doctor immediately if he feels discomfort or shortness of breath.
• After the catheter is removed, encourage the patient to resume normal activities.
• Unless contraindicated, encourage the patient to drink more fluids for the rest of the day to flush the contrast medium from the body. Alternatively, increase the I.V. flow rate as ordered.

Electrophysiologic studies

Common electrophysiologic studies include EEG and evoked potential studies.

EEG is used to identify problems that affect the brain's electrical activity.

Electroencephalography

During EEG, the brain's continuous electrical activity is recorded. The results are used to identify seizure disorders; head injury; intracranial lesions, such as abscesses and tumors; TIAs; stroke; and brain death.

Nursing concerns
• Explain that a technician applies paste and attaches electrodes to areas of skin on the patient's head and neck after these areas have been lightly abraded to ensure good contact.
• Instruct the patient to remain still during the test.
• Discuss what the patient may be asked to do during the test, such as hyperventilating for 3 minutes or sleeping, depending on the purpose of the EEG.
• Use acetone to remove any remaining paste from the patient's skin.

Evoked potential studies

Evoked potential studies are used to measure the nervous system's electrical response to a visual, auditory, or sensory stimulus.

The results are used to detect subclinical lesions such as tumors of CN VIII and complicating lesions in a patient with MS.

Showing potential

Evoked potential studies are also useful in diagnosing blindness and deafness in infants.

Nursing concerns
- Explain to the patient that he must remain still during the test.
- Describe how a technician applies paste and electrodes to the head and neck before testing.
- Describe activities—such as gazing at a checkerboard pattern or a strobe light or listening with headphones to a series of clicks—performed during testing. The patient may have electrodes placed on an arm and leg and be asked to respond to a tapping sensation.
- Explain that the test equipment may emit noises.

Other tests

Other neurologic tests include lumbar puncture and transcranial Doppler studies.

Lumbar puncture

During lumbar puncture, a sterile needle is inserted into the sub-arachnoid space of the spinal canal, usually between the third and fourth lumbar vertebrae. A doctor does the lumbar puncture, with a nurse assisting. It requires sterile technique and careful patient positioning.

Why do it?

Lumbar puncture is used to:
- detect blood in cerebrospinal fluid (CSF)
- obtain CSF specimens for laboratory analysis
- inject dyes or gases for contrast in radiologic studies.
  It's also used to administer drugs or anesthetics and to relieve increased ICP by removing CSF.

Contraindications and cautions

Lumbar puncture is contraindicated in patients with lumbar deformity or infection at the puncture site. It's performed cautiously in patients with increased ICP because the rapid decrease of pressure that follows withdrawal of CSF can cause tonsillar herniation and medullary compression.

Be careful! If the patient has increased ICP, the rapid drop in ICP after CSF is withdrawn can lead to serious problems.

CAUTION!

Nursing concerns

• Calmly describe lumbar puncture to the patient, explaining that the procedure may cause some discomfort.
• Reassure the patient that a local anesthetic is administered before the test. Tell him to report any tingling or sharp pain he feels as the anesthetic is injected.
• To prevent headache after the test, instruct the patient to lie flat for 8 to 10 hours after the procedure.
• Monitor the patient for neurologic deficits and complications, such as headache, fever, back spasms, or seizures, according to facility policy.

Transcranial Doppler studies

In transcranial Doppler studies, the velocity of blood flow through cerebral arteries is measured. The results provide information about the presence, quality, and changing nature of blood flow to an area of the brain.

What blood flow tells you

The types of waveforms and velocities obtained by testing indicate whether disease exists. Test results commonly aren't definitive, but this is a noninvasive way to obtain diagnostic information.

High velocities are typically abnormal, suggesting that blood flow is too turbulent or the vessel is too narrow. They may also indicate stenosis or vasospasm. High velocities may also indicate AVM due to the extra blood flow associated with stenosis or vasospasm.

> In transcranial Doppler studies, waveforms and velocities of blood flow are measured. High velocities are typically abnormal.

Nursing concerns

• Tell the patient that the study usually takes less than 1 hour, depending on the number of vessels examined and on any interfering factors.
• Explain that a small amount of gel is applied to the skin and that a probe is then used to transmit a signal to the artery being studied.

Treatments

Treatments for patients with neurologic dysfunction may include medication therapy, surgery, and other forms of treatment.

Medication therapy

For many of your patients with neurologic disorders, medication or drug therapy is essential. For example:

• thrombolytics are used to treat patients with acute ischemic stroke
• anticonvulsants are used to control seizures
• corticosteroids are used to reduce inflammation.
    Types of drugs commonly used to treat patients with neurologic disorders include:
• analgesics
• anticonvulsants
• anticoagulants and antiplatelets
• barbiturates
• benzodiazepines
• calcium channel blockers
• corticosteroids
• diuretics
• thrombolytics.

Watch for severe adverse reactions and interactions with other drugs.

Heads up!

When caring for a patient undergoing medication therapy, stay alert for severe adverse reactions and interactions with other drugs. Some drugs such as barbiturates also carry a high risk of toxicity.

Stay the course

Successful therapy hinges on strict adherence to the medication schedule. Compliance is especially critical for drugs that require steady blood levels for therapeutic effectiveness such as anticonvulsants. (See *Common neurologic drugs*, pages 82 to 85.)

Surgery

Life-threatening neurologic disorders usually call for emergency surgery.

Opening up

Surgery commonly involves craniotomy, a procedure to open the skull and expose the brain.

Be ready before and after

You may be responsible for the patient's care before and after surgery. Here are some general preoperative and postoperative pointers:
• The prospect of surgery usually causes fear and anxiety, so give ongoing emotional support to the patient and his family. Make sure that you're ready to answer their questions.

I feel so exposed. Life-threatening neurologic disorders may call for emergency surgery, beginning with craniotomy.

(Text continues on page 84.)

Common neurologic drugs

Use this table to find out about common neurologic drugs, their indications and adverse effects, and related monitoring measures.

Drug	Indications	Adverse effects
Nonopioid analgesics Acetaminophen	• Mild pain, headache	• Severe liver damage, neutropenia, thrombocytopenia
Opioid analgesics Morphine	• Severe pain	• Respiratory depression, apnea, bradycardia, seizures, sedation
Codeine	• Mild to moderate pain	• Respiratory depression, bradycardia, sedation, constipation
Anticonvulsants Carbamazepine	• Generalized tonic-clonic seizures, complex partial seizures, mixed seizures	• Heart failure, worsening of seizure, atrioventricular block, hepatitis, thrombocytopenia, Stevens-Johnson syndrome
Fosphenytoin	• Status epilepticus, seizures during neurosurgery	• Increased intracranial pressure, cerebral edema, somnolence, bradycardia, QT prolongation, heart block
Phenytoin	• Generalized tonic-clonic seizures, status epilepticus, nonepileptic seizures after head trauma	• Agranulocytosis, thrombocytopenia, toxic hepatitis, slurred speech, Stevens-Johnson syndrome
Primidone	• Generalized tonic-clonic seizures, focal seizures and complex partial seizures	• Thrombocytopenia, drowsiness, ataxia
Valproic acid, valproate	• Complex partial seizures, simple and complex absence seizures	• Thrombocytopenia, pancreatitis, toxic hepatitis, sedation, ataxia
Anticoagulants Heparin	• Embolism prophylaxis after cerebral thrombosis in evolving stroke	• Hemorrhage, thrombocytopenia
Antiplatelets Aspirin	• Transient ischemic attacks, thromboembolic disorders	• GI bleeding, acute renal insufficiency, thrombocytopenia, liver dysfunction
Sulfinpyrazone	• Thrombotic stroke prophylaxis	• Blood dyscrasia, thrombocytopenia, bronchoconstriction
Ticlopidine	• Thrombotic stroke prophylaxis	• Thrombocytopenia, agranulocytosis
Barbiturates Phenobarbital	• All types of seizures except absence seizures and febrile seizures in children; also used for status epilepticus, sedation, and drug withdrawal	• Respiratory depression, apnea, bradycardia, angioedema, Stevens-Johnson syndrome

Practice pointers

• Monitor total daily intake of acetaminophen because of risk of liver toxicity. Use with caution in elderly patients and those with liver disease.

• Monitor for respiratory depression. Use with caution in elderly patients and those with head injury, seizures, or increased intracranial pressure (ICP). Contraindicated in patients with acute bronchial asthma.
• Monitor for respiratory depression. Use with caution in elderly patients and those with head injury, seizures, or increased ICP.

• Use cautiously in patients with mixed seizure disorders because it can increase the risk of seizure. Use cautiously in patients with hepatic dysfunction. Obtain baseline liver function studies, complete blood count, and blood urea nitrogen level. Monitor blood levels of the drug; therapeutic level is 4 to 12 mcg/ml.
• Stop drug with acute hepatotoxicity. May cause hyperglycemia; monitor blood glucose in diabetic patients. Fosphenytoin should be prescribed and dispensed in PE units. Monitor for cardiac arrhythmias and QT prolongation.

• Abrupt withdrawal can trigger status epilepticus. Contraindicated in patients with heart block. Use cautiously in patients with hepatic disease and myocardial insufficiency. Monitor blood levels of the drug; therapeutic range is 10 to 20 mcg/ml. If rash appears, stop the drug.
• Abrupt withdrawal can cause status epilepticus. Reduce dosage in elderly patients.

• Obtain baseline liver function tests. Avoid use in patients at high risk for hepatotoxicity. Abrupt withdrawal may worsen seizures. Monitor blood levels of the drug; therapeutic range is 50 to 100 mcg/ml.

• Monitor for bleeding. Obtain baseline prothrombin time/International Normalized Ratio (PT/INR), and partial thromboplastin time (PTT). Monitor PTT at regular intervals. Protamine sulfate reverses the effects of heparin.

• Monitor for bleeding. Avoid use in patients with active peptic ulcer and GI inflammation.

• Monitor for bleeding. Avoid use in patients with active peptic ulcer and GI inflammation.

• Monitor for bleeding. Avoid use in patients with hepatic impairment and peptic ulcer disease.

• Monitor for respiratory depression and bradycardia. Keep resuscitation equipment on hand when administering I.V. dose; monitor respirations.

(continued)

Common neurologic drugs *(continued)*

Drug	Indications	Adverse effects
Benzodiazepines		
Clonazepam	• Absence and atypical seizures, generalized tonic-clonic seizures, status epilepticus, panic disorders	• Respiratory depression, thrombocytopenia, leukopenia, drowsiness, ataxia
Diazepam	• Status epilepticus, anxiety, acute alcohol withdrawal, muscle spasm	• Respiratory depression, bradycardia, cardiovascular collapse, drowsiness, acute withdrawal syndrome
Lorazepam	• Status epilepticus, anxiety, agitation	• Drowsiness, acute withdrawal syndrome
Calcium channel blockers		
Nimodipine	• Neurologic deficits caused by cerebral vasospasm after congenital aneurysm rupture	• Decreased blood pressure, tachycardia, edema
Corticosteroids		
Dexamethasone, methylprednisolone	• Cerebral edema, severe inflammation	• Heart failure, cardiac arrhythmias, edema, circulatory collapse, thromboembolism, pancreatitis, peptic ulceration
Diuretics		
Furosemide (loop)	• Edema, hypertension	• Renal failure, thrombocytopenia, agranulocytosis, volume depletion, dehydration
Mannitol (osmotic)	• Cerebral edema, increased ICP	• Heart failure, seizures, fluid and electrolyte imbalance
Thrombolytics		
Alteplase (recombinant tissue plasminogen activator)	• Acute ischemic stroke	• Cerebral hemorrhage, spontaneous bleeding, allergic reaction
Streptokinase	• Acute ischemic stroke	• Cerebral hemorrhage, spontaneous bleeding, allergic reaction

• Postoperative care may include teaching about diverse topics, such as ventricular shunt care and tips about cosmetic care after craniotomy. Be ready to give good advice after surgery.

Craniotomy

During craniotomy, a surgical opening into the skull exposes the brain. This procedure allows various treatments, such as ventricular shunting, excision of a tumor or abscess, hematoma aspiration, and aneurysm clipping (placing one or more surgical clips on the neck of an aneurysm to destroy it).

Practice pointers

• Abrupt withdrawal may precipitate status epilepticus. Elderly patients are at a greater risk for central nervous system (CNS) depression and may require a lower dose.
• Monitor for respiratory depression and cardiac arrhythmia. Don't stop suddenly; can cause acute withdrawal in physically dependent persons.

• Don't stop abruptly; can cause withdrawal. Monitor for CNS depressant effects in elderly patients.

• Use cautiously in hepatic failure. Monitor for hypotension and tachycardia.

• Use cautiously in patients with recent myocardial infarction, hypertension, renal disease, and GI ulcer. Monitor blood pressure and blood glucose levels.

• Monitor blood pressure, pulse, and intake and output. Monitor serum electrolyte levels, especially potassium levels. Monitor for cardiac arrhythmias.
• Contraindicated in severe pulmonary congestion and heart failure. Monitor blood pressure, heart rate, and intake and output. Monitor serum electrolyte levels. Use with caution in patients with renal dysfunction.

• Contraindicated in patients with intracranial or subarachnoid hemorrhage. The patient must meet criteria for thrombolytic therapy before initiation of therapy. Monitor baseline laboratory values: hemoglobin level, hematocrit, PTT, PT/INR. Monitor vital signs. Monitor for signs of bleeding. Monitor puncture sites for bleeding.
• Contraindicated in patients with intracranial or subarachnoid hemorrhage. The patient must meet criteria for thrombolytic therapy before initiation of therapy. Monitor baseline laboratory values: hemoglobin level, hematocrit, PTT, PT/INR. Monitor vital signs. Monitor for signs of bleeding. Monitor puncture sites for bleeding.

Condition and complexity count

The degree of risk depends on your patient's condition and the complexity of the surgery. Craniotomy raises the risk of having various complications, such as:

• infection
• hemorrhage
• respiratory compromise
• increased ICP.

Nursing concerns

• Encourage the patient and his family members to ask questions about the procedure. Provide clear, honest answers to reduce their confusion and anxiety and to enhance effective coping.

• Explain that the patient's head will be shaved before surgery.

• Discuss the recovery period so the patient understands what to expect. Explain that he'll awaken with a dressing on his head to protect the incision and may have a surgical drain.

• Tell him to expect a headache and facial swelling for 2 to 3 days after surgery, and reassure him that he'll receive pain medication.

• Monitor the patient's neurologic status and vital signs, and report any acute change immediately. Watch for signs of increased ICP, such as pupil changes, weakness in extremities, headache, and change in LOC.

• Monitor the incision site for signs of infection or drainage.

• Provide emotional support to the patient and his family members as they cope with remaining neurologic deficits.

After craniotomy, provide emotional support to the patient and his family members to help them cope with any remaining deficits.

Cerebral aneurysm repair

Surgical intervention is the only sure way to prevent rupture or re-bleeding of a cerebral aneurysm.

Northern exposure

In cerebral aneurysm repair, a craniotomy is performed to expose the aneurysm. Depending on the shape and location of the aneurysm, the surgeon then uses one of several corrective techniques, such as:

• clamping the affected artery

• wrapping the aneurysm wall with a biological or synthetic material

• clipping or ligating the aneurysm.

Nursing concerns

• Tell the patient and his family members that monitoring is done in the critical care unit before and after surgery. Explain that several I.V. lines, intubation, and mechanical ventilation may be needed.

• Monitor the incision site for signs of infection or drainage.

• Monitor the patient's neurologic status and vital signs, and report acute changes immediately. Watch for signs of increased ICP, such as pupil changes, weakness in extremities, headache, and a change in LOC.

• Give emotional support to the patient and his family members to help them cope with remaining neurologic deficits.

The corrective technique used in cerebral aneurysm repair depends on the shape and location of the aneurysm.

Other treatments

Other treatments include barbiturate coma, CSF drainage, ICP monitoring, and plasmapheresis.

Barbiturate coma

The doctor may order barbiturate coma when conventional treatments, such as fluid restriction, diuretic or corticosteroid therapy, or ventricular shunting, don't correct sustained or acute episodes of increased ICP.

High I.V.

During barbiturate coma, the patient receives high I.V. doses of a short-acting barbiturate (such as pentobarbital) to produce a comatose state. The drug reduces the patient's metabolic rate and cerebral blood flow.

Last resort

The goal of barbiturate coma is to relieve increased ICP and protect cerebral tissue. It's a last resort for patients with:
• acute ICP elevation (over 40 mm Hg)
• persistent ICP elevation (over 20 mm Hg)
• rapidly deteriorating neurologic status that's unresponsive to other treatments.

If barbiturate coma doesn't reduce ICP, the patient's prognosis for recovery is poor.

Nursing concerns

• Focus your attention on the patient's family. The patient's condition and apprehension about the treatment is likely to frighten them. Provide clear explanations of the procedure and its effects, and encourage them to ask questions. Convey a sense of optimism but provide no guarantees of the treatment's success.
• Prepare the family for expected changes in the patient during therapy, such as decreased respirations, hypotension, and loss of muscle tone and reflexes.
• Closely monitor the patient's ICP, electrocardiogram (ECG), and vital signs. Notify the doctor of increased ICP, arrhythmias, or hypotension.
• Check serum barbiturate levels frequently as ordered.
• Because the patient is in a drug-induced coma, devote special care to prevent pressure ulcers.

Devote special care to pressure ulcer prevention when your patient is in a drug-induced coma.

Cerebrospinal fluid drainage

The goal of CSF drainage is to reduce ICP to the desired level and keep it at that level. Fluid is withdrawn from the lateral ventricle through ventriculostomy.

To place the ventricular drain, a doctor inserts a ventricular catheter through a burr hole in the patient's skull. This is usually done in the operating room. (See *CSF closed drainage system.*)

Nursing concerns

• Maintain a continuous hourly output of CSF by raising or lowering the drainage system drip chamber.
• Drain the CSF, as ordered, by putting on gloves and turning the main stopcock on to drainage and allowing the CSF to collect in the drip chamber.
• To stop drainage, turn off the stopcock to drainage. Record the time and the amount of collected CSF.
• Check the patient's dressing frequently for drainage.
• Check the tubing for patency by watching the CSF drops in the drip chamber.
• Observe the CSF for color, clarity, amount, blood, and sediment.
• Maintain the patient on bed rest with the head of the bed at 30 to 45 degrees to promote drainage.
• Observe for complications, such as excessive CSF drainage, characterized by headache, tachycardia, diaphoresis, and nausea. Overly rapid accumulation of drainage is a neurosurgical emergency. Cessation of drainage may indicate clot formation.

Rapid CSF drainage is an emergency! Watch for signs and symptoms, including headache, tachycardia, diaphoresis, and nausea.

EMERGENCY

Intracranial pressure monitoring

In ICP monitoring, pressure exerted by the brain, blood, and CSF against the inside of the skull is measured. ICP monitoring enables prompt intervention, which can avert damage caused by cerebral hypoxia and shifts of brain mass.

Indications for ICP monitoring include:
• head trauma with bleeding or edema
• overproduction or insufficient absorption of CSF
• cerebral hemorrhage
• space-occupying lesions.

Four similar systems

There are four basic types of ICP monitoring systems. (See *Monitoring ICP,* page 90.) Regardless of which system is used, the insertion procedure is always performed by a neurosurgeon in the operating room, emergency department, or critical care

A neurosurgeon always inserts an ICP monitoring device.

unit. Insertion of an ICP monitoring device requires sterile technique to reduce the risk of CNS infection.

Doctors do this

The doctor inserts a ventricular catheter or subarachnoid screw through a twist-drill hole created in the skull. Both devices have

CSF closed drainage system

The goal of cerebrospinal fluid (CSF) drainage is to control intracranial pressure (ICP) during treatment for traumatic injury or other conditions that cause increased ICP. Here's one common procedure.

Ventricular drain
For a ventricular drain, the doctor makes a burr hole in the patient's skull and inserts the catheter into the ventricle. The distal end of the catheter is connected to a closed drainage system.

Closed drainage system

Sample port

To catheter

Drip chamber

Drainage bag

Monitoring ICP

Intracranial pressure (ICP) can be monitored using one of four systems.

 Intraventricular catheter monitoring

In intraventricular catheter monitoring, used to monitor ICP directly, the doctor inserts a small polyethylene or silicone rubber catheter into the lateral ventricles through a burr hole.

Although this method is most accurate for measuring ICP, it carries the greatest risk of infection. This is the only type of ICP monitoring that allows evaluation of brain compliance and significant drainage of cerebrospinal fluid (CSF).

Contraindications usually include stenotic cerebral ventricles, cerebral aneurysms in the path of catheter placement, and suspected vascular lesions.

Ventricular catheter

Subarachnoid bolt monitoring

Subarachnoid bolt monitoring involves insertion of a special bolt into the subarachnoid space through a twist-drill burr hole in the front of the skull, behind the hairline.

Placing the bolt is easier than placing an intraventricular catheter, especially if a computed tomograpy scan reveals that the cerebrum has shifted or the ventricles have collapsed. This type of ICP monitoring also carries less risk of infection and parenchymal damage because the bolt doesn't penetrate the cerebrum.

Subarachnoid bolt

Epidural or subdural sensor monitoring

ICP can also be monitored from the epidural or subdural space. For epidural monitoring, a fiber-optic sensor is inserted into the epidural space through a burr hole. This system's main drawback is its questionable accuracy because ICP isn't being measured directly from a CSF-filled space.

For subdural monitoring, a fiber-optic transducer-tipped catheter is tunneled through a burr hole and is placed on brain tissue under the dura mater. The main drawback to this method is its inability to drain CSF.

Epidural sensor

Intraparenchymal monitoring

In intraparenchymal monitoring, the doctor inserts a catheter through a small subarachnoid bolt and, after punctuating the dura, advances the catheter a few centimeters into the brain's white matter. There's no need to balance or calibrate the equipment after insertion.

This method doesn't provide direct access to CSF, but measurements are accurate because brain tissue pressure correlates well with ventricular pressures. Intraparenchymal monitoring may be used to obtain ICP measurements in patients with compressed or dislocated ventricles.

Dura mater — Arachnoid
White matter

built-in transducers that convert ICP to electrical impulses that allow constant monitoring.

Nursing concerns

• Observe digital ICP readings and waveforms. (See *Interpreting ICP waveforms*, page 92.)
• Assess the patient's clinical status and monitor routine and neurologic vital signs every hour or as ordered.
• Calculate cerebral perfusion pressure (CPP) hourly. To calculate CPP, subtract ICP from mean arterial pressure (MAP).
• Inspect the insertion site at least every 24 hours for redness, swelling, and drainage.

Plasmapheresis

Symptoms of several neurologic disorders are reduced through plasma exchange, or plasmapheresis.

> Looks like I'm movin' out! In plasmapheresis, plasma is filtered to remove toxins and disease mediators from the patient's blood.

Out with the bad

In plasmapheresis, blood from the patient flows into a cell separator, which separates plasma from formed elements. The plasma is then filtered to remove toxins and disease mediators, such as immune complexes and autoantibodies, from the patient's blood.

In with the good

The cellular components are then transfused back into the patient using fresh frozen plasma or albumin in place of the plasma removed.

Who benefits?

Plasmapheresis benefits patients with neurologic disorders such as Guillain-Barré syndrome and, especially, myasthenia gravis. In myasthenia gravis, plasmapheresis is used to remove circulating antiacetylcholine receptor antibodies.

Plasmapheresis is used most commonly for patients with long-standing neuromuscular disease, but it can also be used to treat patients with acute exacerbations. Some acutely ill patients require treatment up to four times per week; others about once every 2 weeks. When it's successful, treatment may relieve symptoms for months, but results vary.

Nursing concerns

• Discuss the treatment and its purpose with the patient and his family members.

Interpreting ICP waveforms

Three waveforms—A, B, and C—are used to monitor intracranial pressure (ICP). A waves are an ominous sign of intracranial decompensation and poor compliance, B waves correlate with changes in respiration, and C waves correlate with changes in arterial pressure.

Normal waveform

A normal ICP waveform typically shows a steep upward systolic slope followed by a downward diastolic slope with a dicrotic notch. In most cases, this waveform is continuous and indicates an ICP between 0 and 15 mm Hg (normal pressure).

A waves

The most clinically significant ICP waveforms are A waves, which may reach elevations of 50 to 100 mm Hg, persist for 5 to 20 minutes, then drop sharply, signaling exhaustion of the brain's compliance mechanisms. A waves may come and go, spiking from temporary increases in thoracic pressure or from any condition that increases ICP beyond the brain's compliance limits. Activities, such as sustained coughing or straining during defecation, can cause temporary elevations in thoracic pressure.

B waves

B waves, which appear sharp and rhythmic with a sawtooth pattern, occur every 1½ to 2 minutes and may reach elevation of 50 mm Hg. The clinical significance of B waves isn't clear; however, the waves correlate with respiratory changes and may occur more frequently with decreasing compensation. Because B waves sometimes precede A waves, notify the doctor if B waves occur frequently.

C waves

Like B waves, C waves are rapid and rhythmic, but they aren't as sharp. They're clinically insignificant and may fluctuate with respirations or systemic blood pressure changes.

Waveform showing equipment problem

A waveform like the one shown at right signals a problem with the transducer or monitor. Check for line obstruction, and determine whether the transducer needs rebalancing.

• Explain that the procedure can take up to 5 hours. During that time, blood samples are taken frequently to monitor calcium and potassium levels. Blood pressure and heart rate are checked regularly. Tell the patient to report any paresthesia (numbness, burning, tingling, prickling, or increased sensitivity) during treatment.

• If possible, give the patient prescribed medications after treatment because they're removed from the blood during treatment.

• Monitor the patient's vital signs according to your facility's policy.

• Check puncture sites for signs of bleeding or extravasation.

> Administer prescribed medications after plasmapheresis; otherwise, they're removed from the blood during treatment.

Disorders

In the critical care unit, you're likely to encounter patients with common neurologic disorders, especially acute spinal cord injury, AVM, cerebral aneurysm, encephalitis, Guillain-Barré syndrome, head injury, meningitis, seizure disorders, and stroke.

Acute spinal cord injury

Spinal injuries include fractures, contusions, and compressions of the vertebral column. They usually result from trauma to the head or neck. Fractures of the 5th, 6th, or 7th cervical; 12th thoracic; and 1st lumbar vertebrae are most common.

Dangerous damage

The real danger with spinal injury is spinal cord damage due to cutting, pulling, twisting, and compression. Spinal cord injury can occur at any level, and the damage it causes may be partial or involve the entire cord.

Complications of spinal cord injury include neurogenic shock and spinal shock. (See *Complications of spinal cord injury*, page 94.)

What causes it

The most serious spinal cord trauma typically results from motor vehicle accidents, falls, sports injuries, diving into shallow water, and gunshot or stab wounds. Less serious injuries commonly occur from lifting heavy objects and minor falls.

> The real danger with spinal injury is spinal cord damage.

Spinal dysfunction may also result from hyperparathyroidism and neoplastic lesions.

Pathophysiology

Spinal cord trauma results from acceleration, deceleration, or other deforming forces. Types of trauma include:
- hyperextension due to acceleration-deceleration forces
- hyperflexion from sudden and excessive force
- vertebral compression from downward force from the top of the cranium, along the vertical axis, and through the vertebra
- rotational twisting, which adds shearing forces.

Careful! The most serious causes of spinal cord trauma are car collisions and other accidents.

Take charge!

Complications of spinal cord injury

When you assess your patient, watch for these two complications related to spinal cord injuries.

Neurogenic shock

Neurogenic shock is an abnormal vasomotor response that occurs secondary to disruption of sympathetic impulses from the brain stem to the thoracolumbar area. It's most common in patients with cervical cord injury. It causes temporary loss of autonomic function below the level of injury and leads to cardiovascular changes.

Signs of neurogenic shock include:
- orthostatic hypotension
- bradycardia
- inability to sweat below the level of the injury.

Spinal shock

Spinal shock is the loss of autonomic, reflex, motor, and sensory activity below the level of the cord lesion. It occurs secondary to damage of the spinal cord.

Signs of spinal shock include:
- flaccid paralysis
- loss of deep tendon and perianal reflexes
- loss of motor and sensory function.

Trauma trail

Here's what happens during spinal cord trauma:
• An injury causes microscopic hemorrhages in the gray matter and pia-arachnoid.
• The hemorrhages gradually increase in size until all of the gray matter is filled with blood, which causes necrosis.
• From the gray matter, the blood enters the white matter, where it impedes circulation within the spinal cord.
• Resulting edema causes compression and decreases the blood supply.
• The spinal cord loses perfusion and becomes ischemic. The edema and hemorrhage are usually greatest in the two segments above and below the injury.
• The edema temporarily adds to the patient's dysfunction by increasing pressure and compressing the nerves. For example, edema near the 3rd to 5th cervical vertebrae may interfere with respiration.

After acute injury

Here's what happens following acute trauma:
• In the white matter, circulation usually returns to normal within 24 hours after injury.
• In the gray matter, an inflammatory reaction prevents restoration of circulation.
• Phagocytes appear at the site within 35 to 48 hours after injury.
• Macrophages engulf degenerating axons and collagen replaces the normal tissue.
• Scarring and meningeal thickening leaves the nerves in the area blocked or tangled.

After acute spinal injury, scarring and meningeal thickening leaves the nerves in the area blocked or tangled.

What to look for

In your assessment, look for:
• history of trauma, a neoplastic lesion, an infection that could produce a spinal abscess, or an endocrine disorder
• muscle spasm and back or neck pain that worsens with movement; in cervical fractures, pain that causes point tenderness; in dorsal and lumbar fractures, pain that may radiate to other areas, such as the legs
• mild paresthesia to quadriplegia and shock, if the injury damages the spinal cord; in milder injury, symptoms that may be delayed several days or weeks.

Types of spinal cord injury

Spinal cord injury may be classified as complete or incomplete. Incomplete injury may be an anterior cord syndrome, central cord syndrome, or Brown-Séquard's syndrome, depending on which area of the cord is affected. Here are the characteristic signs and symptoms of each.

Type	Description	Signs and symptoms
Complete transection	• All tracts of the spinal cord completely disrupted • All functions involving the spinal cord below the level of transection lost • Complete and permanent loss	• Loss of motor function (quadriplegia) with cervical cord transection; paraplegia with thoracic cord transection • Muscle flaccidity • Loss of all reflexes and sensory function below the level of injury • Bladder and bowel atony • Paralytic ileus • Loss of vasomotor tone in lower body parts with low and unstable blood pressure • Loss of perspiration below level of injury • Dry, pale skin • Respiratory impairment
Incomplete transection: Central cord syndrome	• Center position of cord affected • Typically from hyperextension injury	• Motor deficits greater in upper than in lower extremities • Variable degree of bladder dysfunction
Incomplete transection: Anterior cord syndrome	• Occlusion of anterior spinal artery • Occlusion from pressure of bone fragments	• Loss of motor function below the level of injury • Loss of pain and temperature sensations below the level of injury • Intact touch, pressure, position, and vibration senses
Incomplete transection: Brown-Séquard's syndrome	• Hemisection of cord affected • Most common in stabbing and gunshot wounds • Damage to cord on only one side	• Ipsilateral paralysis or paresis below the level of injury • Ipsilateral loss of touch, pressure, vibration, and position sense below the level of injury • Contralateral loss of pain and temperature sensations below the level of injury

Speaking specifically

Specific signs and symptoms depend on the type and degree of injury. (See *Types of spinal cord injury*.)

What tests tell you

Diagnoses of acute spinal cord injuries are based on the results of these diagnostic tests:

• Spinal X-rays (the most important diagnostic measure) reveal fracture.
• Myelography shows the location of fracture and site of compression.
• CT scan and MRI show the location of fracture and the site of compression and reveal spinal cord edema and a possible spinal cord mass.
• Neurologic evaluation is used to locate the level of injury and detect cord damage.
• Lumbar puncture shows increased CSF pressure from a lesion or trauma in spinal compression.

How it's treated

The primary treatment after spinal injury is immediate immobilization to stabilize the spine and prevent cord damage. Other treatment is supportive.

Cervical injuries require immobilization, using sandbags on both sides of the patient's head, a hard cervical collar, or skeletal traction with skull tongs or a halo device.

When a patient shows clinical evidence of a spinal cord injury, high doses of I.V. methylprednisolone (Solu-Medrol) are started to reduce inflammation.

What to do

Here's what you should do for patients with spinal cord injuries:
• Immediately stabilize the patient's spine. As with all spinal injuries, suspect cord damage until proven otherwise.
• Perform a neurologic assessment to establish a baseline and continually reassess neurologic status for changes.
• Assess respiratory status closely at least every hour, initially. Obtain baseline tidal volume, vital capacity, negative inspiratory forces, and minute volume.
• Auscultate breath sounds and check secretions as necessary.
• Monitor oxygen saturation levels as ordered. Administer supplemental oxygen as indicated.
• Assess cardiac status frequently, at least every hour initially. Begin cardiac monitoring. Monitor blood pressure and hemodynamic status frequently. If a pulmonary artery catheter is in place, inform the doctor if there's a decrease in right atrial pressure, pulmonary artery pressure, pulmonary wedge pressure, and systemic vascular resistance that indicates neurogenic shock.
• If your patient becomes hypotensive, prepare to administer vasopressors.
• Prepare the patient for surgical stabilization, if necessary.

After the spine is immobilized, begin a neurologic assessment to establish baselines. Be alert at all times for changes.

• Assess GI status closely for signs of ulceration or bleeding. Anticipate nasogastric (NG) tube insertion and low intermittent suctioning. Assess the abdomen for distention, auscultate bowel sounds, and report any decrease or absence. Be alert for paralytic ileus, which usually occurs 72 hours after injury.
• Monitor intake and output for fluid imbalance.
• Insert an indwelling urinary catheter as ordered.
• Begin measures to prevent skin breakdown due to immobilization, including repositioning, padding, and care of equipment such as halo or traction devices.
• Monitor laboratory and diagnostic test results, including BUN and creatinine levels, complete blood count (CBC), and urine culture (if indicated).
• Monitor the patient for deep vein thrombosis and pulmonary embolism. Apply antiembolism stockings or intermittent sequential compression devices as ordered.
• Provide emotional support to the patient and his family members.
• Begin rehabilitation as soon as possible.

Arteriovenous malformation

AVMs are tangled masses of thin-walled, dilated blood vessels between arteries and veins that aren't connected by capillaries. Abnormal channels between the arterial and venous system mix oxygenated and unoxygenated blood. This prevents adequate perfusion of brain tissue.

Looking for AVMs

AVMs are common in the brain, especially in the posterior parts of the cerebral hemispheres. They range in size from a few millimeters to large malformations extending from the cerebral cortex to the ventricles. More than one AVM is commonly found.

Males and females are affected equally, and some evidence exists that AVMs occur in families. Most AVMs are present at birth, but symptoms typically occur later, when the person is 10 to 20 years old.

Uh-oh

Complications depend on the severity (location and size) of the AVM and include:
• aneurysm development and subsequent rupture
• hemorrhage (intracerebral, subarachnoid, or subdural, depending on the location of the AVM)
• hydrocephalus.

Uh-oh! AVMs are tangled masses of blood vessels that prevent adequate perfusion of brain tissue.

What causes it

Causes of AVMs may be either:
• congenital—due to a hereditary defect
• acquired—due to penetrating injuries such as trauma.

Pathophysiology

AVMs lack the typical structural characteristics of the blood vessels; the vessels of an AVM are very thin.

Blood pressure, aneurysm, and hemorrhage

One or more arteries feed into the AVM; the typically high-pressured arterial blood flow moves into the venous system through connecting channels. This increases venous pressure, engorging and dilating the venous structures, which may result in the development of an aneurysm.

If the AVM is large enough, the shunting can deprive the surrounding tissue of adequate blood flow. Additionally, the thin-walled vessels may ooze small amounts of blood or rupture, causing hemorrhage into the brain or subarachnoid space.

Shunting can deprive tissues of adequate blood flow.

What to look for

Typically, patients exhibit few, if any, signs and symptoms unless the AVM is large or it leaks or ruptures.

Some signs and symptoms

In some patients, signs and symptoms include:
• chronic mild headache and confusion from AVM dilation, vessel engorgement, and increased pressure
• seizures secondary to compression of the surrounding tissues by the engorged vessels
• systolic bruit over the carotid artery, mastoid process, or orbit, indicating turbulent blood flow
• focal neurologic deficits (depending on the location of the AVM) resulting from compression and diminished perfusion
• symptoms of intracranial (intracerebral, subarachnoid, or subdural) hemorrhage, including sudden severe headache, seizures, confusion, lethargy, and meningeal irritation from bleeding into the brain tissue or subarachnoid space
• hydrocephalus from AVM extension into the ventricular lining.

Loss of blood through thin-walled vessels can lead to rupture and hemorrhage.

What tests tell you

The following tests are used to diagnose AVM:

• Cerebral angiography yields the most definitive diagnostic information. It's used to localize the AVM and allow visualization of large feeding arteries and drainage veins.
• CT scan with a contrast medium is used to differentiate AVM from a clot or tumor.
• MRI is used to determine the location and size of AVM.
• EEG is used to locate AVM.
• Doppler ultrasonography of the cerebrovascular system is used to find abnormal and turbulent blood flow.

Check CT scan results to differentiate AVM from a clot or tumor.

How it's treated

The choice of treatment depends on the:
• size and location of the AVM
• feeder vessels supplying it
• age and condition of the patient.

Supportive, corrective, or both

Treatment can be supportive, corrective, or both, including:
• support measures, such as aneurysm precautions to prevent possible rupture
• surgery—block dissection, laser, or ligation—to repair the communicating channels and remove the feeding vessels
• embolization or radiation therapy if surgery isn't possible, to close the communicating channels and feeder vessels and thus reduce blood flow to the AVM.

What to do

If hemorrhage hasn't occurred in your patient with AVM, focus your efforts on bleeding prevention.

Steps to take

To prevent bleeding, follow these steps to control hypertension and seizure activity:
• Maintain a quiet therapeutic environment.
• Monitor and control associated hypertension with drug therapy as ordered.
• Conduct ongoing neurologic assessment.
• Monitor vital signs frequently.
• Assess and monitor characteristics of headache, seizure activity, or bruit as needed.
• Provide emotional support.

Rupture measures

If the AVM ruptures, work to control elevated ICP and intracranial hemorrhage. Follow the steps described above as well as those listed here:

• Provide appropriate preoperative teaching.
• After surgery, monitor neurologic status and vital signs frequently.
• Monitor the wound for signs of infection.
• Monitor fluid balance and electrolyte levels.

Cerebral aneurysm

In intracranial or cerebral aneurysm, a weakness in the wall of a cerebral artery causes that area of the artery to dilate or bulge. The most common form is the berry aneurysm, a saclike outpouching in a cerebral artery.

The usual place

Cerebral aneurysms usually arise at an arterial junction in the circle of Willis, the circular anastomosis forming the major cerebral arteries at the base of the brain. Cerebral aneurysms commonly rupture and cause subarachnoid hemorrhage.

The usual patient

The incidence of cerebral aneurysm is slightly higher in women than in men, especially those in their late 40s or early to mid-50s, but a cerebral aneurysm can occur at any age in either sex.

The usual prognosis

The prognosis for any patient with cerebral aneurysm is guarded. About 50% of all patients who suffer a subarachnoid hemorrhage die immediately.

Of those who survive untreated, 40% die from the effects of hemorrhage and another 20% die later from recurring hemorrhage. New treatments are improving the prognosis.

The major complications of cerebral aneurysm include death from increased ICP and brain herniation, rebleeding, and vasospasm. (See *Signs of increased ICP*, page 102.)

What causes it

Causes of cerebral aneurysm include:
• congenital defect
• degenerative process
• combination of congenital defect and degenerative process
• trauma.

In cerebral aneurysm, blood pressure against a weak arterial wall stretches the vessel like a balloon, making it likely to rupture.

Take charge!

Signs of increased ICP

The earlier you spot signs of increased intracranial pressure (ICP), the quicker you can intervene and the better your patient's chance of recovery. By the time late signs appear, interventions may be useless.

Assessment area	Early signs	Late signs
Level of consciousness	• Requires increased stimulation • Subtle orientation loss • Restlessness and anxiety • Sudden quietness	• Unarousable
Pupils	• Pupil changes on side of lesion • One pupil constricts but then dilates (unilateral hippus) • Sluggish reaction of both pupils • Unequal pupils	• Pupils fixed and dilated or "blown"
Motor response	• Sudden weakness • Motor changes on side opposite the lesion • Positive pronator drift: With palms up, one hand pronates	• Profound weakness
Vital signs	• Intermittent increases in blood pressure	• Increased systolic pressure with widening pulse pressure, bradycardia, and abnormal respirations (Cushing's triad)

Pathophysiology

Blood flow exerts pressure against a weak arterial wall, stretching it like an overblown balloon and making it likely to rupture.

Right after rupture

Rupture is followed by a subarachnoid hemorrhage, in which blood spills into the space normally occupied by CSF. Sometimes, blood also spills into brain tissue, where a clot can cause potentially fatal increased ICP and brain tissue damage.

What to look for

Occasionally, your patient may exhibit signs and symptoms due to blood oozing into the subarachnoid space. The symptoms, which may persist for several days, include:

If your patient reports headache, nausea, and back and leg stiffness lasting for several days, suspect cerebral aneurysm.

- headache
- intermittent nausea
- nuchal rigidity
- stiff back and legs.

Rupture without warning

Aneurysm rupture usually occurs abruptly and without warning, causing:
- sudden severe headache caused by increased pressure from bleeding into a closed space
- nausea and projectile vomiting related to increased ICP
- altered LOC, possibly including deep coma, depending on the severity and location of bleeding, due to increased pressure caused by increased cerebral blood volume
- meningeal irritation due to bleeding into the meninges and resulting in nuchal rigidity, back and leg pain, fever, restlessness, irritability, occasional seizures, photophobia, and blurred vision
- hemiparesis, hemisensory defects, dysphagia, and visual defects due to bleeding into the brain tissues
- diplopia, ptosis, dilated pupil, and inability to rotate the eye caused by compression on the oculomotor nerve if the aneurysm is near the internal carotid artery.

A cerebral aneurysm typically ruptures before symptoms are seen. Signs after rupture are sudden and severe.

Grading severity

Typically, the severity of a ruptured intracranial aneurysm is graded according to the patient's signs and symptoms. (See *Grading cerebral aneurysm rupture*.)

Grading cerebral aneurysm rupture

The severity of symptoms varies from patient to patient, depending on the site and amount of bleeding. Five grades characterize ruptured cerebral aneurysm:
- *Grade I: minimal bleeding*—The patient is alert, with no neurologic deficit; he may have a slight headache and nuchal rigidity.
- *Grade II: mild bleeding*—The patient is alert, with a mild to severe headache and nuchal rigidity; he may have third-nerve palsy.
- *Grade III: moderate bleeding*—The patient is confused or drowsy, with nuchal rigidity and, possibly, a mild focal deficit.
- *Grade IV: severe bleeding*—The patient is stuporous, with nuchal rigidity and, possibly, mild to severe hemiparesis.
- *Grade V: moribund (usually fatal)*—If the rupture is nonfatal, the patient is in a deep coma or decerebrate.

What tests tell you

The following tests aid in the diagnosis of cerebral aneurysm:

• Cerebral angiography confirms a cerebral aneurysm that isn't ruptured and reveals altered cerebral blood flow, vessel lumen dilation, and differences in arterial filling.

• CT scan reveals evidence of aneurysm and possible hemorrhage.

• MRI is used to detect vasospasm and locate the bleeding.

• PET scan shows the chemical activity of the brain and extent of tissue damage.

How it's treated

Emergency treatment begins with oxygenation and ventilation. Then, to reduce the risk of rebleeding, the doctor may attempt to repair the aneurysm. Surgical repair usually includes clipping, ligating, or wrapping the aneurysm neck with muscle.

New and improved

Newer techniques for surgery include *interventional radiology* in conjunction with endovascular balloon therapy. This technique occludes the aneurysm or vessel and uses cerebral angiography to treat arterial vasospasm.

Think fast! Emergency treatment begins with oxygenation and ventilation before the doctor attempts aneurysm repair.

Endovascular aneurysm repair

When surgery isn't appropriate for intracranial aneurysm repair, a recently developed endovascular treatment method called electrothrombosis may be used. Electrothrombosis is most successful in aneurysms with small necks and those without significant intrafundal thrombus.

Electrothrombosis

Here's what happens in electrothrombosis:

• Soft platinum coils soldered to a stainless steel delivery wire are positioned in the aneurysm.

• After the coil is positioned within the fundus of the aneurysm, a 1-mA current is applied to the delivery wire.

• The delivery wire is removed, leaving the platinum coil in place, and another coil is introduced into the fundus.

• The process is continued until the aneurysm is densely packed with platinum and no longer opacifies during diagnostic contrast injections.

How it works

The positively charged platinum left in the aneurysm theoretically attracts negatively charged blood elements, such as white and red blood cells, platelets, and fibrinogen. This induces intra-aneurysmal thrombosis.

The coils provide immediate protection against further hemorrhage by reducing blood pulsations in the fundus and sealing the hole or weak portion of the artery wall. Eventually, clots form and the aneurysm is separated from the parent vessel by the formation of new connective tissue.

In some cases, a type of nonsurgical repair called electro-thrombosis is used. (See *Endovascular aneurysm repair*.)

Conservative whys

The patient may receive conservative treatment when surgical correction poses too much risk, such as when:
• the patient is elderly
• the patient has heart, lung, or other serious disease
• the aneurysm is in a dangerous location
• vasospasm necessitates a delay in surgery.

Conservative ways

Conservative treatment methods include:
• bed rest in a quiet, darkened room with the head of bed flat or raised less than 30 degrees, which may continue for 4 to 6 weeks
• avoidance of coffee, other stimulants, and aspirin to reduce the risk of rupture and elevation of blood pressure
• possible administration of codeine or other analgesic
• administration of hydralazine or another antihypertensive, if the patient is hypertensive
• administration of corticosteroids to reduce edema
• administration of phenobarbital or other sedative
• administration of a vasoconstrictor to maintain an optimum blood pressure level (20 to 40 mm Hg above normal), if necessary
• administration of aminocaproic acid, a fibrinolysis inhibitor, to minimize the risk of rebleeding by delaying blood clot lysis (the effectiveness of this drug is under dispute).

What to do

When caring for a patient with an intact cerebral aneurysm, an accurate neurologic assessment, good patient care, patient and family teaching, and psychological support can speed recovery and reduce complications.

Your next step

During the initial treatment after hemorrhage, follow these steps:
• Establish and maintain a patent airway and anticipate the need for supplementary oxygen or mechanical ventilatory support. Monitor arterial blood gas levels.
• Position the patient to promote pulmonary drainage and prevent upper airway obstruction. If intubated, preoxygenate with 100% oxygen before suctioning.
• Impose aneurysm precautions (such as bed rest, limited visitors, and avoidance of coffee and physical activity) to minimize the risk of rebleeding and avoid increased ICP.

When surgical correction is too risky for your patient, implement these conservative treatment methods.

- Administer a stool softener, as ordered, to prevent straining.
- Monitor LOC and vital signs frequently. Avoid rectal temperatures.
- Determine the CPP. Institute cerebral blood flow monitoring as ordered to determine CPP. If not available, calculate CPP by subtracting the patient's ICP from the MAP (systolic blood pressure plus twice the diastolic pressure divided by three).
- Accurately measure intake and output.
- Be alert for danger signs that may indicate an enlarging aneurysm, rebleeding, intracranial clot, increased ICP, or vasospasm, including decreased LOC, unilateral enlarged pupil, onset or worsening of hemiparesis or motor deficit, increased blood pressure, slowed pulse rate, worsening of headache or sudden onset of a headache, renewed or worsened nuchal rigidity, and renewed or persistent vomiting.
- If the patient develops vasospasm — evidenced by focal motor deficits, increasing confusion, and worsening headache — initiate hypervolemic-hemodilution therapy, as ordered, such as the administration of normal saline, whole blood, packed red cells, albumin plasma protein fraction, and crystalloid solution. The calcium channel blocker, nimodipine, may reduce smooth-muscle spasm and maximize perfusion during spasm. During therapy, assess the patient for fluid overload.
- Turn the patient often, apply antiembolism stockings or intermittent sequential compression devices to the patient's legs, and begin measures to prevent skin breakdown.
- If the patient has facial weakness, assist during meals. If he can't swallow, insert an NG tube, as ordered. Give all tube feedings slowly.
- If mannitol is used, administer as ordered. Be alert for rebound effect and subsequent rebound of increased ICP, which may occur 8 to 12 hours after administration.
- Prepare the patient for surgery, as appropriate, and provide preoperative teaching if the patient's condition permits.
- Teach the patient and his family members about the condition and how to recognize and report signs of rebleeding.

Aneurysm precautions may minimize your patient's risk of rebleeding and prevent increased ICP.

Encephalitis

Encephalitis is severe inflammation of the brain, usually caused by a mosquito-borne or, in some areas, a tick-borne virus. Other means of transmission include ingestion of infected goat's milk and accidental injection or inhalation of the virus.

What causes it

Encephalitis results from infection with arboviruses specific to rural areas. In urban areas, it's most commonly caused by enteroviruses (coxsackievirus, poliovirus, and echovirus).

Other causes include herpesvirus, mumps virus, human immunodeficiency virus, adenoviruses, and demyelinating diseases following measles, varicella, rubella, or vaccination.

Pathophysiology

With encephalitis, intense lymphocytic infiltration of brain tissues and the leptomeninges causes cerebral edema, degeneration of the brain's ganglion cells, and diffuse nerve cell destruction.

What to look for

Watch for the signs and symptoms that signal the beginning of acute illness, including:
- fever (102° to 105° F [38.9° to 40.6° C])
- headache
- vomiting.

When a patient presents with fever, headache, vomiting, and stiff neck and back, suspect encephalitis.

Negative progression

The illness can progress to include signs and symptoms of meningeal irritation, such as stiff neck and back. Be alert for signs of neuron damage, such as:
- drowsiness
- coma
- paralysis
- seizures
- ataxia
- organic psychoses.

Stay alert for changes! Symptoms can escalate to include drowsiness, coma, paralysis, and other signs of neuron damage.

What tests tell you

The following diagnostic tests are used in the diagnosis of encephalitis:
- CSF or blood analysis used to identify the causative virus confirms the diagnosis.
- Technetium-99 scan results may show localized abnormalities.
- CT scan may disclose localized abnormalities.

How it's treated

Most of the treatments for patients with encephalitis are entirely supportive:

• The antiviral agent, acyclovir, is effective in treatment for herpes encephalitis.
• Anticonvulsants and corticosteroids reduce cerebral inflammation and edema.
• Furosemide or mannitol reduces cerebral swelling.
• Sedatives are given to alleviate restlessness.
• Aspirin or acetaminophen relieves headache and reduces fever.
• Fluids and electrolytes prevent dehydration and electrolyte imbalance.
• Antibiotics are used to fight an associated infection such as pneumonia.

What to do

During the acute phase of the illness, follow these guidelines:
• Assess neurologic function frequently. Check for changes in LOC and signs of increased ICP. Watch for signs and symptoms of cranial nerve involvement, such as ptosis, strabismus, diplopia, abnormal sleep patterns, and behavior changes.
• Monitor intake and output carefully to maintain fluid balance. Be aware that fluid overload can increase cerebral edema.
• Position the patient carefully and turn him often to prevent joint stiffness and neck pain.
• Perform ROM exercises to prevent contractures.
• Provide a quiet, darkened room to ease headache and photophobia.
• Maintain adequate nutrition by giving small, frequent meals and NG tube or parenteral feedings, as ordered.
• Reassure the patient and his family members that behavior changes caused by encephalitis usually disappear.
• If the patient is disoriented or confused, attempt to reorient him frequently. Place a calendar or clock in the patient's room to aid in orientation.

If your patient with encephalitis is disoriented, place a calendar or clock in the room.

Guillain-Barré syndrome

Guillain-Barré syndrome, or acute idiopathic polyneuritis, is also known as *infectious polyneuritis*. It's an acute, rapidly progressive, and potentially fatal form of polyneuritis that causes muscle weakness and mild distal sensory loss.

Equal opportunity syndrome

This syndrome can occur at any age but is most common in people between ages 30 and 50. It affects both sexes equally.

Recovery is spontaneous and complete in about 95% of patients; however, mild motor or reflex deficits may persist in the feet and legs. The prognosis is best when symptoms resolve sooner than 15 to 20 days after onset.

Three-phase syndrome

Guillain-Barré syndrome occurs in three phases:

The acute phase begins with the onset of the first definitive symptom and ends 1 to 3 weeks later. Further deterioration doesn't occur after the acute phase.

The plateau phase lasts several days to 2 weeks.

The recovery phase coincides with remyelinization and regrowth of axonal processes. Recovery commonly takes 4 to 6 months, but may take as long as 2 to 3 years in severe cases.

In a severe case, your patient with Guillain-Barré syndrome may take 2 to 3 years to recover.

Commonly complicated syndrome

Common complications include thrombophlebitis, pressure ulcers, muscle wasting, sepsis, joint contractures, respiratory tract infections, respiratory failure, and loss of bladder and bowel control.

What causes it

The precise cause of Guillain-Barré syndrome isn't known, but it may be a cell-mediated immune response to a virus. About 50% of patients with Guillain-Barré syndrome have a recent history of minor febrile illness, usually an upper respiratory tract infection or, less commonly, gastroenteritis. When infection precedes the onset of Guillain-Barré syndrome, signs of infection subside before neurologic features appear.

Possible precipitators

Other possible precipitating factors include:
• surgery
• rabies or swine influenza vaccination
• Hodgkin's or other malignant disease
• systemic lupus erythematosus.

Pathophysiology

The major pathologic feature of Guillain-Barré syndrome is segmental demyelination of the peripheral nerves, which prevents the normal transmission of electrical impulses along the sensorimotor nerve roots.

Double trouble

Guillain-Barré syndrome causes inflammation and degenerative changes in both the posterior (sensory) and the anterior (motor) nerve roots. That's why signs of sensory and motor losses occur simultaneously. Additionally, autonomic nerve transmission may be impaired.

Guillain-Barré syndrome causes sensory and motor losses at the same time...

What to look for

During your assessment, look for symptoms that are progressive and include:
• symmetrical muscle weakness (the major neurologic sign), appearing first in the legs (in the ascending type of the syndrome, which is the most common form) and then extending to the arms and facial nerves within 24 to 72 hours, due to impaired anterior nerve root transmission
• muscle weakness developing in the brainstem, in the cranial nerves, and progressing downward in the arms first (in the descending type of the syndrome) or in the arms and legs simultaneously, due to impaired anterior nerve root transmission
• normal muscle strength (in mild forms of the syndrome) or weakness affecting only the cranial nerves
• paresthesia, sometimes preceding muscle weakness but vanishing quickly, due to impairment of the dorsal nerve root transmission
• diplegia, possibly with ophthalmoplegia (ocular paralysis), from impaired motor nerve root transmission and involvement of cranial nerves III, IV, and VI
• dysphagia or dysarthria and, less commonly, weakness of the muscles supplied by CN XI (the spinal accessory nerve)
• hypotonia and areflexia from interruption of the reflex arc.

...thanks to changes in both the sensory and motor nerve roots. Thanks, but no thanks!

What tests tell you

These diagnostic tests aid in the diagnosis of Guillain-Barré syndrome:
• CSF analysis reveals protein levels that begin to increase several days after the onset of symptoms and peak in 4 to 6 weeks.
• CBC early in illness shows leukocytosis and immature forms of white blood cells (immature neutrophils, called bands).
• Electromyography may show repeated firing of the same motor unit instead of widespread sectional stimulation.
• Nerve conduction velocities slow soon after paralysis develops.
• Serum immunoglobulin levels are elevated due to an inflammatory response.

How it's treated

• Treatments are primarily supportive and include endotracheal (ET) intubation or tracheotomy if respiratory muscle involvement causes difficulty in clearing secretions.
• A trial dose (7 days) of prednisone is given to reduce inflammatory response if the disease is relentlessly progressive; if prednisone produces no noticeable improvement, the drug is discontinued.
• Plasmapheresis is useful during the initial phase, but of no benefit if started 2 weeks after onset.
• Continuous ECG is used to monitor for possible arrhythmias due to autonomic dysfunction. Propranolol is used to reduce tachycardia and hypertension. Atropine is given for bradycardia. Volume replacement is used in treating patients with severe hypotension.

Stand by to provide supportive treatments, such as ET intubation or tracheotomy.

What to do

When caring for a patient with Guillain-Barré syndrome:
• Watch for ascending sensory loss, which precedes motor loss.
• Monitor vital signs and LOC.
• Assess and treat patients with respiratory dysfunction.
• Auscultate breath sounds, turn and position patient, and encourage coughing and deep breathing. Begin respiratory support at the first sign of respiratory failure, which may include ET intubation and mechanical ventilation.
• Provide meticulous skin care to prevent skin breakdown.
• Perform passive ROM exercises within the patient's pain limits.
• To prevent aspiration, test the gag reflex and elevate the head of the bed before the patient eats. If the gag reflex is absent, give NG tube feedings until the gag reflex returns.
• As the patient regains strength and can tolerate a vertical position, be alert for hypotension. Change the patient's position slowly.
• Apply antiembolism stockings and a sequential compression device to the legs.
• If the patient has facial paralysis, provide eye and mouth care every 4 hours.
• Watch for urine retention. Use an indwelling urinary catheter if necessary.
• To prevent constipation, provide a high-fiber diet and offer prune juice. Administer a suppository or bisacodyl (Fleet enema) as ordered.
• Refer the patient to physical therapy.

Head injury

Head injury is any traumatic insult to the brain that causes physical, intellectual, emotional, social, or vocational changes. Children ages 6 months to 2 years, adults ages 15 to 24, and elderly adults are most at risk for head injury.

Ahh! It's no surprise that most patients with head injuries are toddlers, young adults, or elderly people.

To put it bluntly

Head injury is generally categorized as closed trauma or open trauma. Closed (or blunt) trauma is more common. It typically occurs when the head strikes a hard surface or a rapidly moving object strikes the head. The dura is intact, and no brain tissue is exposed to the external environment.

In open trauma, as the name suggests, an opening in the scalp, skull, meninges, or brain tissue (the dura) exposes the cranial contents to the environment. The risk of infection is high.

Complications are possible

Possible complications include:
• increased ICP
• infection (in open trauma)
• respiratory depression and failure
• brain herniation.

On the decline

Mortality from head injury has declined as a result of:
• advances in preventive measures, such as air bags and seat belts
• quicker emergency response and transport times
• improved treatment measures.

What causes it

Head injury commonly results from:
• motor vehicle collisions (the number one cause)
• falls
• sports-related accidents
• assaults and other crimes.

Pathophysiology

The patient's brain is shielded by the cranial vault (comprised of skin, bone, meninges, and CSF), which intercepts the force of a physical blow. Below a certain level of force, the cranial vault prevents energy from affecting the brain.

The degree of traumatic head injury usually is proportional to the amount of force reaching the cranial tissues. In addition, unless it's ruled out, you may presume that neck injuries are present in patients with traumatic head injuries.

Case closed

Closed trauma is typically a sudden acceleration-deceleration or coup-contrecoup injury. In coup-contrecoup injury, the head hits a more stationary object, injuring cranial tissues near the point of impact (coup); the remaining force then pushes the brain against the opposite side of the skull, causing a second impact and injury (contrecoup).

Contusions and lacerations may also occur during contrecoup as the brain's soft tissues slide over the rough bone of the cranial cavity. The cerebrum may endure rotational shear, damaging the upper midbrain and areas of the frontal, temporal, and occipital lobes.

What to look for

Types of head trauma include:
- concussion
- contusion
- epidural hematoma
- subdural hematoma
- intracerebral hematoma
- skull fractures.

Each type is associated with specific signs and symptoms. (See *Types of head injury*, pages 114 to 117.) Signs and symptoms of head trauma in elderly patients may not be readily apparent. (See *Hidden hematoma*.)

What tests tell you

These diagnostic tests are used in diagnosing head injury:
• Skull X-rays show the location of the fracture, unless the cranial vault is fractured. (A CT scan will show a fracture of the cranial vault.)
• Cerebral angiography shows the location of vascular disruption due to internal pressure or injuries that result from cerebral contusion or skull fracture.
• CT scan shows intracranial hemorrhage from ruptured blood vessels, ischemic or necrotic tissue, cerebral edema, a shift in brain tissue, and subdural, epidural, and intracerebral hematomas.
• MRI may show intracranial hemorrhage from ruptured blood vessels in a patient with a skull fracture.

(Text continues on page 118.)

Senior moment

Hidden hematoma

An older person with cerebral atrophy can tolerate a larger subdural hematoma for a longer time than a younger person can before the hematoma causes neurologic changes. That's why a hematoma in an older patient can become rather large before you see any symptoms, even in an acute condition.

Types of head injury

Here's a summary of the signs and symptoms and diagnostic test findings for different types of head injury.

Type	Description
Concussion (closed head injury)	• A blow to the head hard enough to make the brain hit the skull, but not hard enough to cause a cerebral contusion; causes temporary neural dysfunction. • Recovery is usually complete within 24 to 48 hours. • Repeated injuries have a cumulative effect on the brain.
Contusion (bruising of brain tissue; more serious than concussion)	• Most common in 20- to 40-year-olds. • Most result from arterial bleeding. • Blood commonly accumulates between skull and dura. Injury to middle meningeal artery in parietotemporal area is most common and is typically accompanied by linear skull fractures in temporal region over middle meningeal artery. • Less commonly arises from dural venous sinuses.
Epidural hematoma	• Acceleration-deceleration or coup-contrecoup injuries disrupt normal nerve functions in bruised area. • Injury is directly beneath the site of impact when the brain rebounds against the skull from the force of a blow (a beating with a blunt instrument, for example), when the force of the blow drives the brain against the opposite side of the skull, or when the head is hurled forward and stopped abruptly (as in an automobile crash when a driver's head strikes the windshield). • Brain continues moving and slaps against the skull (acceleration), then rebounds (deceleration). Brain may strike bony prominences inside the skull (especially the sphenoidal ridges), causing intracranial hemorrhage or hematoma that may result in tentorial herniation.

Signs and symptoms	Diagnostic test findings
• Short-term loss of consciousness secondary to disruption of reticular activating system, possibly due to abrupt pressure changes in the areas responsible for consciousness, changes in polarity of the neurons, ischemia, or structural distortion of neurons • Vomiting from localized injury and compression • Anterograde and retrograde amnesia (patient can't recall events immediately after the injury or events that led up to the traumatic incident) correlating with severity of injury; all related to disruption of reticular activating system • Irritability or lethargy from localized injury and compression • Behavior out of character due to focal injury • Complaints of dizziness, nausea, or severe headache due to focal injury and compression	• Computed tomography (CT) scan reveals no sign of fracture, bleeding, or other nervous system lesion.
• Severe scalp wounds from direct injury • Labored respiration and loss of consciousness secondary to increased pressure from bruising • Drowsiness, confusion, disorientation, agitation, or violence from increased intracranial pressure (ICP) associated with trauma • Hemiparesis related to interrupted blood flow to the site of injury • Decorticate or decerebrate posturing from cortical damage or hemispheric dysfunction • Unequal pupillary response from brain stem involvement	• CT scan shows changes in tissue density, possible displacement of the surrounding structures, and evidence of ischemic tissue, hematomas, and fractures. • Lumbar puncture with cerebrospinal fluid (CSF) analysis reveals increased pressure and blood (not performed if hemorrhage is suspected). • EEG recordings directly over the area of contusion reveal progressive abnormalities by appearance of high-amplitude theta and delta waves.
• Brief period of unconsciousness after injury reflects the concussive effects of head trauma, followed by a lucid interval varying from 10-15 minutes to hours or, rarely, days • Severe headache • Progressive loss of consciousness and deterioration in neurologic signs results from expanding lesion and extrusion of medial portion of temporal lobe through tentorial opening • Compression of brain stem by temporal lobe causes clinical manifestations of intracranial hypertension • Deterioration in level of consciousness results from compression of brain stem reticular formation as temporal lobe herniates on its upper portion • Respirations, initially deep and labored, become shallow and irregular as brain stem is impacted • Contralateral motor deficits reflect compression of corticospinal tracts that pass through the brain stem	• CT scan or magnetic resonance imaging (MRI) identifies abnormal masses or structural shifts within the cranium.

(continued)

Types of head injury *(continued)*

Type	Description
Epidural hematoma *(continued)*	
Subdural hematoma	• Meningeal hemorrhages, resulting from accumulation of blood in subdural space (between dura mater and arachnoid). • May be acute, subacute, and chronic: unilateral or bilateral. • Usually associated with torn connecting veins in cerebral cortex; rarely from arteries. • Acute hematomas are a surgical emergency.
Intracerebral hematoma	• Subacute hematomas have better prognosis because venous bleeding tends to be slower. • Traumatic or spontaneous disruption of cerebral vessels in brain parenchyma cause neurologic deficits, depending on site and amount of bleeding. • Shear forces from brain movement frequently cause vessel laceration and hemorrhage into the parenchyma. • Frontal and temporal lobes are common sites. Trauma is associated with few intracerebral hematomas; most are caused by hypertension.
Skull fracture	• There are four types: linear, comminuted, depressed, and basilar. • Fractures of anterior and middle fossae are associated with severe head trauma and are more common than those of posterior fossa. • Blow to the head causes one or more of the types. May not be problematic unless the brain is exposed or bone fragments are driven into neural tissue.

Signs and symptoms	Diagnostic test findings
• Ipsilateral (same-side) pupillary dilation due to compression of third cranial nerve • Seizures possible from high ICP • Continued bleeding leads to progressive neurologic degeneration, evidenced by bilateral pupillary dilation, bilateral decerebrate response, increased systemic blood pressure, decreased pulse, and profound coma with irregular respiratory patterns	
• Similar to epidural hematoma but significantly slower in onset because bleeding is typically of venous origin	• CT scan, X-rays, and arteriography reveal mass and altered blood flow in the area, confirming a hematoma. • CT scan or MRI reveals evidence of masses and tissue shifting. • The CSF is yellow and has relatively low protein (chronic subdural hematoma).
• Unresponsive immediately or experiencing a lucid period before lapsing into a coma from increasing ICP and mass effect of hemorrhage • Possible motor deficits and decorticate or decerebrate responses from compression of corticospinal tracts and brain stem	• CT scan or cerebral arteriography identifies the bleeding site. CSF pressure is elevated, and the fluid may appear bloody or xanthochromic (yellow or straw-colored) from hemoglobin breakdown.
• May not produce symptoms, depending on underlying brain trauma • Discontinuity and displacement of bone structure with severe fracture • Motor sensory and cranial nerve dysfunction with associated facial fractures • Persons with anterior fossa basilar skull fractures may have periorbital ecchymosis (raccoon eyes), anosmia (loss of smell due to first cranial nerve involvement) and pupil abnormalities (second and third cranial nerve involvement) • CSF rhinorrhea (leakage through nose), CSF otorrhea (leakage from the ear), hemotympanium (blood accumulation at the tympanic membrane), ecchymosis over the mastoid bone (Battle's sign), and facial paralysis (seventh cranial nerve injury) accompany middle fossa basilar skull fractures • Signs of medullary dysfunction such as cardiovascular and respiratory failure accompany posterior fossa basilar skull fracture	• CT scan and MRI reveal swelling and intracranial hemorrhage from ruptured blood vessels. • Skull X-ray may reveal a fracture. • A lumbar puncture is contraindicated by expanding lesions.

How it's treated

Treatment may be surgical or supportive.

It's surgical

Surgical treatment includes:
- evacuation of a hematoma
- craniotomy.

The goal of surgery is to remove fragments driven into the brain and to extract foreign bodies and necrotic tissue. Such measures reduce the risk of infection and further brain damage due to fractures.

It's supportive

Provide supportive treatment, which includes:
- close observation to detect changes in neurologic status suggesting further damage or expanding hematoma
- cleaning and debridement of any wounds associated with skull fractures
- diuretics such as mannitol and corticosteroids to reduce cerebral edema
- analgesics such as acetaminophen to relieve complaints of headache
- anticonvulsants such as phenytoin to prevent seizures
- respiratory support, including mechanical ventilation and ET intubation for patients with respiratory failure from brain stem involvement
- prophylactic antibiotics to prevent the onset of meningitis from CSF leakage associated with skull fractures.

What to do

- Initially, monitor vital signs continuously and check for additional injuries.
- Continue to check vital signs and neurologic status, including LOC and pupil size, every 15 minutes.
- Maintain a patent airway. Monitor oxygen saturation levels through pulse oximetry and arterial blood gas (ABG) analysis as ordered.
- Assess hemodynamic parameters to aid in evaluating CPP.
- Administer medications as ordered. If necessary, use continuous infusions of such agents as midazolam (Versed), fentanyl (Sublimaze), morphine, or propofol (Diprivan) to reduce metabolic demand and the risk of increased ICP.
- Observe the patient closely for signs of hypoxia or increased ICP, such as headache, dizziness, irritability, anxiety, and changes in behavior such as agitation.

Check skull X-rays for the location of a fracture.

Surgical intervention may be needed to reduce your patient's risk of infection and further brain damage due to fractures.

- Monitor elderly patients especially closely because they may have brain atrophy and, therefore, more space for cerebral edema. This means ICP may increase without showing signs.
- If an ICP monitoring system is inserted, continuously monitor ICP waveforms and pressure.
- Carefully observe the patient for CSF leakage. Check the bed sheets for a blood-tinged spot surrounded by a lighter ring (halo sign). If the patient has CSF leakage or is unconscious, elevate the head of the bed 30 degrees or leave it flat. Such a patient is at risk for jugular compression that leads to increased ICP when not positioned on his back.
- Position the patient so that secretions drain properly. If you detect CSF leakage from the nose, place a gauze pad under the nostrils. Don't suction through the nose, but use the mouth. If CSF leaks from the ear, position the patient so his ear drains naturally.
- Monitor intake and output frequently to maintain fluid balance.
- Institute seizure precautions as necessary. Use safety precautions to minimize the risk of injury.
- Cluster nursing activities to provide rest periods, thus reducing metabolic demands and reducing the risk of sustained increases in ICP.
- Prepare the patient for craniotomy as indicated.
- After the patient is stabilized, clean and dress superficial scalp wounds using strict sterile technique. Monitor wounds for signs and symptoms of infection.
- Explain all procedures and treatments to the patient and his family members.
- Urge the patient with a cerebral contusion not to cough, sneeze, or blow his nose because these activities can increase ICP.

Meningitis

In meningitis, the brain and the spinal cord meninges become inflamed, usually because of bacterial infection. Such inflammation may involve all three meningeal membranes — the dura mater, arachnoid, and pia mater.

Promptness improves the prognosis

If meningitis is recognized early and the infecting organism responds to treatment, the prognosis is good. Complications are rare and may include increased ICP, hydrocephalus, cerebral infarction, cranial nerve deficits causing optic neuritis and deafness, brain abscess, seizures, or coma.

Time matters. Prompt recognition and treatment improves the meningitis patient's prognosis.

What causes it

Meningitis is usually a complication of bacteremia, especially from pneumonia, empyema, osteomyelitis, or endocarditis. Aseptic meningitis may result from a virus or other organism. Sometimes no causative organism can be found.

Uh-oh, other infections

Other infections associated with meningitis include:
- sinusitis
- otitis media
- encephalitis
- myelitis
- brain abscess, usually caused by *Neisseria meningitidis, Haemophilus influenzae, Streptococcus pneumoniae,* and *Escherichia coli.*

Any opening

Meningitis may follow trauma or invasive procedures, including skull fracture, penetrating head wound, lumbar puncture, and ventricular shunting.

> Your patient with meningitis may play host to a whole host of infective organisms.

Pathophysiology

Meningitis commonly begins as inflammation of the pia-arachnoid tissue. It may progress to congestion of adjacent tissues and destroy some nerve cells.

It enters here...

The causative organism typically enters the CNS by one of four routes:

1.   the blood (most common)

2.   a direct opening between the CSF and the environment as a result of trauma

3.   along the cranial and peripheral nerves

4.   through the mouth or nose.

...and triggers a response...

The invading organism triggers an inflammatory response in the meninges. To ward off the invasion, neutrophils gather in the area and produce an exudate in the subarachnoid space, causing the CSF to thicken. The thickened CSF flows less readily around the brain and spinal cord. This can block the arachnoid villi, further obstructing CSF flow and causing hydrocephalus.

> Meningitis that begins as inflammation may progress to congestion of adjacent tissues and destroy some nerve cells.

...and yet more responses

The exudate also:
• exacerbates the inflammatory response, increasing the pressure in the brain
• can extend to the cranial and peripheral nerves, triggering additional inflammation
• irritates the meninges, disrupting their cell membranes and causing edema.

Truth or consequences

The consequences of meningitis are:
• elevated ICP
• engorged blood vessels
• disrupted cerebral blood supply
• possible thrombosis or rupture
• cerebral infarction if ICP isn't reduced
• possible encephalitis (a secondary infection of the brain tissue).

In aseptic meningitis, lymphocytes infiltrate the pia-arachnoid layers, but usually not as severely as in bacterial meningitis; no exudate is formed. Thus, this type of meningitis is self-limiting.

Thickened CSF flows slowly around the brain and spinal cord, sometimes causing hydrocephalus.

What to look for

Look for the signs of meningitis, which typically include:
• fever, chills, and malaise resulting from infection and inflammation
• headache, vomiting and, rarely, papilledema (inflammation and edema of the optic nerve) from increased ICP.

Signs of irritation

Signs of meningeal irritation include:
• nuchal rigidity
• positive Brudzinski's and Kernig's signs
• exaggerated and symmetrical deep tendon reflexes
• opisthotonos (a spasm more common in infants and children in which the back and extremities arch backward so that the body rests on the head and heels).

Further features

Other features of meningitis may include:
• sinus arrhythmias due to irritation of autonomic nerves
• irritability due to increasing ICP
• photophobia, diplopia, and other visual problems due to cranial nerve irritation
• delirium, deep stupor, and coma due to increased ICP and cerebral edema.

What tests tell you

• Lumbar puncture shows elevated CSF pressure (from obstructed CSF outflow at the arachnoid villi), cloudy or milky-white CSF, high protein levels, positive Gram stain and culture (unless a virus is responsible), and decreased glucose concentration.
• Positive Brudzinski's and Kernig's signs indicate meningeal irritation.
• Cultures of blood, urine, and nose and throat secretions reveal the offending organism.
• Chest X-ray may reveal pneumonitis or lung abscess, tubercular lesions, or granulomas secondary to a fungal infection.
• Sinus and skull X-rays may identify paranasal sinusitis as the underlying infectious process or a skull fracture as the mechanism for entrance of microorganisms.
• White blood cell count reveals leukocytosis.

How it's treated

Treatment includes administration of:
• antibiotic therapy, usually for 2 weeks
• digoxin to control arrhythmia
• mannitol to decrease cerebral edema
• anticonvulsant or sedative to reduce restlessness
• acetaminophen to relieve headache and fever.

Supportive measures

Supportive measures include bed rest; fever reduction, which may include tepid baths or cooling the patient with a hyperthermia-hypothermia blanket; and isolation, if necessary.

What to do

Take the following steps when caring for a patient with meningitis:
• Assess neurologic function often.
• Watch for deterioration, especially temperature increase, deteriorating LOC, onset of seizures, and altered respirations.
• Monitor fluid balance. Maintain adequate fluid intake to avoid dehydration, but avoid fluid overload because of the danger of cerebral edema.
• Position the patient to prevent joint stiffness and neck pain. Assist with ROM exercises.
• Maintain adequate nutrition and elimination.
• Maintain a quiet environment.
• Follow strict sterile technique when treating patients with head wounds or skull fractures.
• Provide emotional support.

Remember: Meningitis is usually due to infection, so use sterile technique for patients with a head or skull injury.

Seizure disorder

Seizure disorder, or epilepsy, is a condition of the brain character-ized by recurrent seizures (paroxysmal events associated with ab-normal electrical discharges of neurons in the brain).

Primary and secondary

Primary seizure disorder or epilepsy is idiopathic without appar-ent structural changes in the brain.

Secondary epilepsy, characterized by structural changes or metabolic alterations of the neuronal membranes, causes in-creased automaticity.

Who's affected...

Epilepsy affects 1% to 2% of the population; approximately 2 mil-lion people live with epilepsy. The incidence is highest in child-hood and old age. The prognosis is good if the patient adheres strictly to the prescribed treatment.

...and how

I'm clueless. Primary epilepsy is idiopathic, causing no apparent changes in brain structure.

Complications of epilepsy may include hypoxia or anoxia due to airway occlusion, traumatic injury, brain damage, and depression and anxiety.

What causes it

In about one-half of seizure disorder cases, the cause is unknown. Some possible causes are:
• birth trauma (such as inadequate oxygen supply to the brain, blood incompatibility, or hemorrhage)
• perinatal infection
• anoxia
• infectious diseases (meningitis, encephalitis, or brain abscess)
• head injury or trauma.

Pathophysiology

Some neurons in the brain may depolarize easily or be hyperex-citable, firing more readily than normal when stimulated. On stim-ulation, the electrical current spreads to surrounding cells, which fire in turn. The impulse thus cascades to:
• one side of the brain (a partial seizure)
• both sides of the brain (a generalized seizure)
• cortical, subcortical, and brain stem areas.

Increase O₂, or else

The brain's metabolic demand for oxygen increases dramatically during a seizure. If this demand isn't met, hypoxia and brain damage result.

Firing of inhibitory neurons causes the excited neurons to slow their firing and eventually stop. Without this inhibitory action, the result is status epilepticus (seizures occurring one right after another). Without treatment, resulting anoxia is fatal.

> In epilepsy, some neurons in the brain fire more readily than normal when stimulated.

What to look for

The hallmarks of seizure disorders are recurring seizures, which can be classified as partial or generalized. Some patients are affected by more than one type. (See *Types of seizures.*)

What tests tell you

The results of primary diagnostic tests for seizure disorders may include these:
• CT scan to show density readings of the brain may indicate abnormalities in internal structures.
• MRI may indicate abnormalities in internal brain structures.
• EEG is used to confirm the diagnosis of epilepsy by providing evidence of the continuing tendency to have seizures.

How it's treated

Generally, treatment consists of drug therapy specific to the type of seizures. The goal is to reduce seizures using a combination of the fewest drugs.

> Treatment for a patient with a seizure disorder generally consists of drug therapy specific to the type of seizure.

For tonic-clonic seizures

The most commonly prescribed drugs for generalized tonic-clonic seizures (alternating episodes of muscle spasm and relaxation) include phenytoin, carbamazepine, phenobarbital, and primidone.

For absence seizures

Drugs commonly prescribed for absence seizures (brief changes in LOC) include valproic acid, clonazepam, and ethosuximide.

Surgery and emergencies

If drug therapy fails, treatment may include surgical removal of a focal lesion in an attempt to stop seizures.

Emergency treatment for patients with status epilepticus usually includes:

Types of seizures

Use the guidelines below to understand different seizure types. Keep in mind that some patients may be affected by more than one type.

Partial seizures

Partial seizure activity arising from a localized area in the brain may spread to the entire brain, causing a generalized seizure. There are several types and subtypes of partial seizures:
• simple partial seizures, which include jacksonian and sensory seizures
• complex partial seizures
• secondarily generalized partial seizures (partial onset leading to generalized tonic-clonic seizure).

Jacksonian seizures

A jacksonian seizure begins as a localized motor seizure, characterized by a spread of abnormal activity to adjacent areas of the brain.

The patient experiences stiffening or jerking in one extremity, with a tingling sensation in the same area. The patient seldom loses consciousness, but the seizure may progress to a generalized tonic-clonic seizure.

Sensory seizure

Symptoms of a sensory seizure include hallucinations, flashing lights, tingling sensations, vertigo, déjà vu, and smelling a foul odor.

Complex partial seizure

Signs and symptoms of a complex partial seizure are variable but usually include purposeless behavior, including a glassy stare, picking at clothes, aimless wandering, lip-smacking or chewing motions, and unintelligible speech.

An aura may occur first, and seizures may last a few seconds to 20 minutes. Afterward, mental confusion may last for several minutes and may be mistaken for alcohol or drug intoxication or psychosis. The patient has no memory of his actions during the seizure.

Secondarily generalized partial seizure

A secondarily generalized partial seizure can be simple or complex and can progress to a generalized seizure. An aura may occur first, with loss of concentration immediately or 1 to 2 minutes later.

Generalized seizure

Generalized seizures cause a generalized electrical abnormality in the brain. Types include absence, myoclonic, clonic, tonic, generalized tonic-clonic, and atonic.

Absence seizure

Absence seizure, also known as petit mal seizure, is most common in children. It usually begins with a brief change in the level of consciousness, signaled by blinking or rolling of the eyes, a blank stare, and slight mouth movements. The patient retains his posture and continues preseizure activity without difficulty.

Such seizures last 1 to 10 seconds and impairment is so brief that the patient may be unaware of it. If not properly treated, seizures can recur up to 100 times a day and progress to a generalized tonic-clonic seizure.

Myoclonic seizure

Myoclonic seizure is marked by brief, involuntary muscle jerks of the body or extremities and typically occurs in early morning.

Clonic seizure

Clonic seizure is characterized by bilateral rhythmic movements.

Tonic seizure

Tonic seizure is characterized by a sudden stiffening of muscle tone, usually of the arms but may also include the legs.

Generalized tonic-clonic seizure

Typically, a generalized tonic-clonic seizure begins with a loud cry, caused by air rushing from the lungs and through the vocal cords. The patient falls to the ground, losing consciousness. The body stiffens (tonic phase) and then alternates between episodes of muscle spasm and relaxation (clonic phase). Tongue biting, incontinence, labored breathing, apnea, and cyanosis may also occur.

The seizure stops in 2 to 5 minutes, when abnormal electrical conduction of the neurons is completed. Afterward, the patient regains consciousness but is somewhat confused. He may have difficulty talking and may have drowsiness, fatigue, headache, muscle soreness, and arm or leg weakness. He may fall into a deep sleep afterward.

Atonic seizure

Atonic seizure is characterized by a general loss of postural tone and temporary loss of consciousness. It occurs in children and is sometimes called a "drop attack" because the child falls.

Take charge!

Understanding status epilepticus

Status epilepticus is a continuous seizure state that must be interrupted by emergency measures. It can occur during all types of seizures. For example, generalized tonic-clonic status epilepticus is a continuous generalized tonic-clonic seizure without an intervening return of consciousness.

Always an emergency
Status epilepticus is accompanied by respiratory distress. It can result from withdrawal of antiepileptic medications, hypoxic or metabolic encephalopathy, acute head trauma, or septicemia secondary to encephalitis or meningitis.

Act fast
Emergency treatment usually consists of diazepam, phenytoin, or phenobarbital; I.V. dextrose 50% when seizures are secondary to hypoglycemia; and I.V. thiamine in patients with chronic alcoholism or those who are undergoing withdrawal.

• administration of diazepam, lorazepam, fosphenytoin, or phenobarbital
• 50% dextrose I.V. (when seizures are secondary to hypoglycemia)
• thiamine I.V. (in chronic alcoholism or withdrawal). (See *Understanding status epilepticus.*)

A new approach

There's a new approach for managing seizures: The vagus nerve stimulation device acts on the brain the way a pacemaker acts on the heart. It sends electrical signals to the brain to inhibit seizure activity.

Because the device is implanted in the chest and neck, adverse effects include voice changes, throat discomfort, and shortness of breath, all of which usually occur when the device is turned on.

What to do

• Monitor a patient taking anticonvulsants constantly for signs of toxicity, such as nystagmus, ataxia, lethargy, dizziness, drowsiness, slurred speech, irritability, nausea, and vomiting.
• When administering fosphenytoin I.V., use a large vein, administer according to guidelines (not more than 150 mg/minute), and monitor vital signs often.
• Encourage the patient and his family to express their feelings about the patient's condition.
• Stress the need for compliance with the prescribed drug schedule.

The vagus nerve stimulation device is like a pacemaker for the brain. It sends electrical signals to me to inhibit seizure activity.

• Emphasize the importance of having blood levels of anticonvulsants checked at regular intervals.

Tonic-clonic interventions

Generalized tonic-clonic seizures may necessitate the following interventions:
• Avoid restraining the patient during a seizure.
• Help the patient to a lying position, loosen any tight clothing, and place something flat and soft, such as a pillow, under his head.
• Clear the area of hard objects.
• Don't force anything into the patient's mouth if his teeth are clenched.
• Turn the patient's head or turn him on his side to provide an open airway.
• After the seizure, reassure the patient that he's all right, orient him to time and place, and tell him that he had a seizure.

When caring for seizure patients, stress the need to have blood levels of anticonvulsants checked regularly.

Stroke

Stroke, also known as a *cerebrovascular accident* or *brain attack*, is a sudden impairment of cerebral circulation in one or more blood vessels. A stroke interrupts or diminishes oxygen supply and commonly causes serious damage or necrosis in the brain tissues.

The sooner, the better

The sooner circulation returns to normal after a stroke, the better your patient's chances are for a complete recovery. However, about one-half of the patients who survive a stroke remain permanently disabled and experience a recurrence within weeks, months, or years. It's the leading cause of admission to long-term care.

Numbers three and one

Stroke is the third most common cause of death in the United States and the most common cause of neurologic disability. It affects more than 500,000 people each year and is fatal in about one-half of these cases.

The sooner circulation in the brain returns to normal, the better your patient's chances are for a complete recovery after a stroke.

What causes it

Stroke typically results from one of three causes:

   thrombosis of the cerebral arteries supplying the brain or of the intracranial vessels occluding blood flow

   embolism from thrombus outside the brain, such as in the heart, aorta, or common carotid artery hemorrhage from an intracranial artery or vein, such as from hypertension, ruptured aneurysm, AVM, trauma, hemorrhagic disorder, or septic embolism.

Risk factor facts

Risk factors that predispose patients to stroke include:
• hypertension
• family history of stroke
• history of TIA (see *TIA and elderly patients*)
• cardiac disease, including arrhythmias, coronary artery disease, acute myocardial infarction, dilated cardiomyopathy, and valvular disease
• diabetes
• familial hyperlipidemia
• cigarette smoking
• increased alcohol intake
• obesity, sedentary lifestyle
• use of hormonal contraceptives.

Pathophysiology

Regardless of the cause, the underlying event leading to stroke is oxygen and nutrient deprivation. Here's what happens:
• Normally, if the arteries become blocked, autoregulatory mechanisms maintain cerebral circulation until collateral circulation develops to deliver blood to the affected area.
• If the compensatory mechanisms become overworked or cerebral blood flow remains impaired for more than a few minutes, oxygen deprivation leads to infarction of brain tissue.
• The brain cells cease to function because they can't engage in anaerobic metabolism or store glucose or glycogen for later use.

Ischemic stroke

Here's what happens when a thrombotic or embolic stroke causes ischemia:
• Some of the neurons served by the occluded vessel die from lack of oxygen and nutrients.
• The result is cerebral infarction, in which tissue injury triggers an inflammatory response that in turn increases ICP.
• Injury to the surrounding cells disrupts metabolism and leads to changes in ionic transport, localized acidosis, and free radical formation.
• Calcium, sodium, and water accumulate in the injured cells, and excitatory neurotransmitters are released.
• Consequent continued cellular injury and swelling set up a vicious cycle of further damage.

Senior moment

TIA and elderly patients

During your assessment, ask an elderly patient about recent falls—especially frequent falls. This is important because an older patient is less likely to forget about or minimize frequent falls than he is to report other signs of a transient ischemic attack (TIA).

Regardless of the cause, the underlying event leading to stroke is oxygen and nutrient deprivation.

Hemorrhagic stroke

Here's what happens when a hemorrhage causes a stroke:
• Impaired cerebral perfusion causes infarction, and the blood acts as a space-occupying mass, exerting pressure on the brain tissues.
• The brain's regulatory mechanisms attempt to maintain equilibrium by increasing blood pressure to maintain CPP. The increased ICP forces CSF out, thus restoring equilibrium.
• If the hemorrhage is small, the patient may have minimal neurologic deficits. If the bleeding is heavy, ICP increases rapidly and perfusion stops. Even if the pressure returns to normal, many brain cells die.
• Initially, the ruptured cerebral blood vessels may constrict to limit the blood loss. This vasospasm further compromises blood flow, leading to more ischemia and cellular damage.
• If a clot forms in the vessel, decreased blood flow also promotes ischemia. If the blood enters the subarachnoid space, meningeal irritation occurs.
• Blood cells that pass through the vessel wall into the surrounding tissue may break down and block the arachnoid villi, causing hydrocephalus.

What to look for

Clinical features of stroke vary, depending on the artery affected (and, consequently, the portion of the brain it supplies), the severity of the damage, and the extent of collateral circulation that develops to help the brain compensate for decreased blood supply. (See *Stroke signs and symptoms*, page 130.)

Left is right and right is left

A stroke in the left hemisphere produces symptoms on the right side of the body; in the right hemisphere, symptoms on the left side.
    Common signs and symptoms of stroke include sudden onset of:
• hemiparesis on the affected side (may be more severe in the face and arm than in the leg)
• unilateral sensory defect (such as numbness, or tingling) generally on the same side as the hemiparesis
• slurred or indistinct speech or the inability to understand speech
• blurred or indistinct vision, double vision, or vision loss in one eye (usually described as a curtain coming down or gray-out of vision)

Stroke on the left causes symptoms on the right...

...stroke on the right causes symptoms on the left.

Stroke signs and symptoms

With stroke, functional loss reflects damage to the area of the brain that's normally perfused by the occluded or ruptured artery. Although one patient may experience only mild hand weakness, another may develop unilateral paralysis.

Hypoxia and ischemia may produce edema that affects distal parts of the brain, causing further neurologic deficits. Here are the signs and symptoms that accompany stroke at different sites.

Site	Signs and symptoms	Site	Signs and symptoms
Middle cerebral artery	• Aphasia • Dysphasia • Dyslexia (reading problems) • Dysgraphia (inability to write) • Visual field cuts • Hemiparesis on the affected side, which is more severe in the face and arm than in the leg	Anterior cerebral artery	• Confusion • Weakness • Numbness on the affected side (especially in the arm) • Paralysis of the contralateral foot and leg • Incontinence • Poor coordination • Impaired motor and sensory functions • Personality changes, such as flat affect and distractibility
Internal carotid artery	• Headaches • Weakness • Paralysis • Numbness • Sensory changes • Visual disturbances such as blurring on the affected side • Altered level of consciousness • Bruits over the carotid artery • Aphasia • Dysphagia • Ptosis	Vertebral or basilar artery	• Mouth and lip numbness • Dizziness • Weakness on the affected side • Visual deficits, such as color blindness, lack of depth perception, and diplopia • Poor coordination • Dysphagia • Slurred speech • Amnesia • Ataxia
		Posterior cerebral artery	• Visual field cuts • Sensory impairment • Dyslexia • Coma • Blindness from ischemia in the occipital area

• mental status changes or loss of consciousness (particularly if associated with one of the above symptoms)
• very severe headache (with hemorrhagic stroke).

What tests tell you

Here are some test findings that can help you diagnose a stroke:
• CT scan discloses structural abnormalities, edema, and lesions, such as nonhemorrhagic infarction and aneurysms. Results are

used to differentiate a stroke from other disorders, such as a tumor or hematoma. Patients with TIA generally have a normal CT scan. CT scan shows evidence of hemorrhagic stroke immediately and of ischemic (thrombotic or embolic) stroke within 72 hours after onset of symptoms. CT scan should be obtained within 25 minutes after the patient arrives in the emergency department, and results should be available within 45 minutes of arrival to determine whether hemorrhage is present. If hemorrhagic stroke is present, thrombolytic therapy is contraindicated.

• MRI is used to identify areas of ischemia and infarction and cerebral swelling.

• Cerebral angiography shows details of disruption or displacement of the cerebral circulation by occlusion or hemorrhage.

• DSA is used to evaluate patency of the cerebral vessels and shows evidence of occlusion of the cerebral vessels, a lesion, or vascular abnormalities.

• Carotid duplex scan is a high-frequency ultrasound that shows blood flow through the carotid arteries and reveals stenosis due to atherosclerotic plaque and blood clots.

• Transcranial Doppler studies are used to evaluate the velocity of blood flow through major intracranial vessels, which can indicate vessel diameter.

• Brain scan shows ischemic areas but may not be conclusive for up to 2 weeks after stroke.

• Single photon emission computed tomography scanning and PET scan show areas of altered metabolism surrounding lesions that aren't revealed by other diagnostic tests.

• Lumbar puncture reveals bloody CSF when stroke is hemorrhagic.

• EEG is used to identify damaged areas of the brain and to differentiate seizure activity from stroke.

• No laboratory tests confirm the diagnosis of stroke, but some tests aid diagnosis and some are used to establish a baseline for thrombolytic treatment. A blood glucose test shows whether the patient's symptoms are related to hypoglycemia. Hemoglobin level and hematocrit may be elevated in severe occlusion. Baselines obtained before thrombolytic therapy begins include CBC, platelet count, partial thromboplastin time, prothrombin time, fibrinogen level, and chemistry panel.

How it's treated

The goal is to begin treatment within 60 minutes after your patient arrives in the emergency department.

Drugs of choice

Thrombolytics (also called fibrinolytics) are the drugs of choice in treating a stroke patient. The patient must first meet certain criteria to be considered for this type of treatment. (See *Who's suited for thrombolytic therapy?*)

Drugs of choice for management

Drug therapy for the management of stroke includes:
- thrombolytics for emergency treatment of ischemic stroke (See *Treating suspected stroke.*)
- aspirin or ticlopidine as an antiplatelet agent to prevent recurrent stroke
- benzodiazepines to treat patients with seizure activity
- anticonvulsants to treat patients with seizures or to prevent them after the patient's condition has stabilized
- stool softeners to avoid straining, which increases ICP
- antihypertensives and antiarrhythmics to treat patients with risk factors for recurrent stroke.
- corticosteroids to minimize associated cerebral edema
- analgesics to relieve the headaches that may follow a hemorrhagic stroke.

> Antihypertensives and antiarrhythmics are given to patients with risk factors for recurrent stroke

Medical management

Medical management of stroke commonly includes physical rehabilitation, dietary and drug regimens to reduce risk factors,

---

Who's suited for thrombolytic therapy?

Not every stroke patient is a candidate for thrombolytic therapy. Each is evaluated to see whether established criteria are met.

Criteria that must be present
Criteria that must be present for a patient to be considered for thrombolytic therapy include:
- acute ischemic stroke associated with significant neurologic deficit
- onset of symptoms less than 3 hours before treatment begins.

Criteria that must *not* be present
In addition to meeting the above criteria, the patient must not:
- show evidence of intracranial hemorrhage during pretreatment evaluation
- exhibit evidence of subarachnoid hemorrhage during pretreatment evaluation

- have a history of recent (within 3 months) intracranial or intraspinal surgery, serious head trauma, or previous stroke
- have a history of intracranial hemorrhage
- have uncontrolled hypertension at the time of treatment
- have experienced a seizure at the onset of stroke
- have active internal bleeding
- have an intracranial neoplasm, arteriovenous malformation, or aneurysm
- have known bleeding diathesis involving, but not limited to:
– current use of oral anticoagulants such as warfarin, International Normalized Ratio greater than 1.7, or prothrombin time greater than 15 seconds
– receipt of heparin within 48 hours before the onset of stroke and having an elevated partial thromboplastin time
– platelet count less than 100,000/µl.

Take charge!

Treating suspected stroke

This algorithm is used in cases of suspected stroke, when the patient's survival depends on prompt recognition of symptoms and treatment.

Detection, Dispatch, Delivery to Door

Immediate general assessment: first 10 minutes after arrival
- Assess airway, breathing, circulation, and vital signs.
- Provide oxygen by nasal cannula.
- Obtain I.V. access; obtain blood samples (complete blood count, electrolyte levels, coagulation studies).
- Check blood glucose levels; treat if indicated.
- Obtain 12-lead electrocardiogram, check for arrhythmias.
- Perform general neurologic screening assessment.
- Alert stroke team, neurologist, radiologist, computed tomography (CT) technician.

Immediate neurologic assessment: first 25 minutes after arrival
- Review the patient's history.
- Establish onset (< 3 hours required for fibrinolytics).
- Perform physical examination.
- Perform neurologic examination: Determine level of consciousness (Glasgow Coma Scale) and level of stroke severity (National Institutes of Health Stroke Scale or Hunt and Hess Scale).
- Order an urgent noncontrast CT scan (door-to-CT scan performed: goal < 25 minutes from arrival).
- Read CT scan (door-to-CT scan read: goal < 45 minutes from arrival).
- Perform lateral cervical spine X-ray (if the patient is comatose or has a history of trauma).

Does CT scan show intracerebral or arachnoid hemorrhage?

Check data

No

Yes

Probable acute ischemic stroke
- Review for CT exclusions: Are any observed?
- Repeat neurologic examination: Are deficits variable or rapidly improving?
- Review fibrinolytic exclusions: Are any observed?
- Review patient data: Is symptom onset now > 3 hours?

Consult neurosurgery.

Blood on LP

Initiate actions for acute hemorrhage:
- Reverse any anticoagulants.
- Reverse any bleeding disorder.
- Monitor neurologic condition.
- Treat hypertension in acute patients.

No to all of the above

Check decision

If high suspicion of subarachnoid hemorrhage remains despite normal findings on CT scan, perform lumbar puncture (LP). Fibrinolytic therapy is contraindicated following an LP.

Does the patient remain a candidate for fibrinolytic therapy?

No blood on LP

Yes

Check drug

No

- Review risks and benefits with the patient and his family. If acceptable:
Begin fibrinolytic treatment (door-to-treatment goal < 60 minutes).
- Monitor neurologic status; emergent CT if deterioration.
- Monitor blood pressure; treat as indicated.
- Admit patient to critical care unit.
- Hold anticoagulant or antiplatelet treatment for 24 hours.

- Initiate supportive therapy as indicated.
- Consider admission.
- Consider anticoagulation.
- Consider additional conditions needing treatment.
- Consider alternate diagnosis.

Cincinnati Pre-Hospital Stroke Scale

The Cincinnati Pre-Hospital Stroke Scale is a simplified scale for evaluating stroke patients that was derived from the National Institutes of Health Stroke Scale. It's used to evaluate facial palsy, arm weakness, and speech abnormalities. An abnormality in any one of the categories below is highly suggestive of stroke.

Facial droop (The patient shows teeth or smiles.)
• Normal—Both sides of the face move equally.
• Abnormal—One side of the face doesn't move as well as the other.

Arm drift (The patient closes eyes and extends both arms straight out for 10 seconds.)
• Normal—Both arms move the same or both arms don't move at all.
• Abnormal—One arm either doesn't move or one arm drifts downward as compared with the other.

Speech (The patient repeats, "The sky is blue in Cincinnati.")
• Normal—The patient says the correct words with no slurring of words.
• Abnormal—The patient slurs words, says the wrong words, or can't speak.

Adapted with permission from: Kathari R.U., et al. "Cincinnati Pre-Hospital Stroke Scale: Reproducibility and Validity," *Annals of Emergency Medicine,* 33:373-78, April 1999.

---

surgery, and care measures to help the patient adapt to deficits, such as motor impairment and paralysis.

Under the knife

Depending on the cause and extent of the stroke, the patient may undergo:
• a craniotomy to remove a hematoma
• a carotid endarterectomy to remove atherosclerotic plaques from the inner arterial wall
• an extracranial bypass to circumvent an artery that's blocked by occlusion or stenosis.

Cut it out! Surgical intervention after stroke is called for in some cases.

Call the "S" Team

Your facility may have a stroke protocol and stroke team composed of specially trained nurses who respond to potential stroke patients. When a patient shows signs and symptoms of a stroke, first assess the patient using a stroke assessment tool such as the Cincinnati Stroke Scale. (See *Cincinnati Pre-Hospital Stroke Scale.*)

After your initial assessment, call the stroke team nurse, who will evaluate the patient, complete a neurologic assessment, report findings to the doctor, and facilitate rapid and appropriate care of the patient, including emergency interventions, diagnostic tests, and transfer to the critical care unit.

What to do

- Secure and maintain the patient's airway and anticipate the need for ET intubation and mechanical ventilation.
- Monitor oxygen saturation levels via pulse oximetry and ABG levels as ordered. Administer supplemental oxygen as ordered to maintain oxygen saturation greater than 90%.
- Place the patient on a cardiac monitor, and monitor for cardiac arrhythmias.
- Assess the patient's neurologic status frequently, at least every 15 to 30 minutes, initially, then hourly as indicated. Observe for signs of increased ICP.
- If cerebral edema is suspected, maintain ICP sufficient for adequate cerebral perfusion but low enough to avoid brain herniation. Elevate the head of the bed 20 to 30 degrees.
- Assess hemodynamic status frequently. Give fluids as ordered and monitor I.V. infusions to avoid overhydration, which may increase ICP.
- For a patient receiving thrombolytic therapy, assess the patient for signs and symptoms of bleeding every 15 to 30 minutes and institute bleeding precautions. Monitor results of coagulation studies.
- Monitor the patient for seizures and administer anticonvulsants as ordered. Institute safety precautions to prevent injury.
- If the patient had a TIA, administer antiplatelet agents. Administer anticoagulants such as heparin if he shows signs of stroke progression, unstable signs of stroke (such as TIA), or evidence of embolic stroke. Monitor coagulation studies closely.
- Turn the patient often and position him using careful body alignment. Apply antiembolism stockings or intermittent sequential compression devices.
- Take steps to prevent skin breakdown.
- Begin exercises as soon as possible. Perform passive ROM exercises for both the affected and unaffected sides. Teach and encourage the patient to use his unaffected side to exercise his affected side.
- Manage GI problems. Be alert for signs of straining at stool as it increases ICP. If the patient is receiving steroids, monitor for signs of GI irritation.
- Modify the patient's diet, as appropriate, such as by increasing fiber.
- Provide meticulous eye and mouth care.
- Maintain communication with the patient. If he's aphasic, set up a simple method of communicating.
- Provide psychological support.

Come back soon! For your patient on thrombolytic therapy, check for signs of bleeding every 15 to 30 minutes.

Quick quiz

1. The most sensitive indicator of neurologic status change is:
    A.   LOC.
    B.   speech.
    C.   behavior.
    D.   cognitive function.

Answer: A. Change in LOC is the earliest and most sensitive indicator of neurologic status change.

2. Signs of an adverse reaction to contrast medium include all of the following except:
    A.   restlessness.
    B.   bradycardia.
    C.   urticaria.
    D.   facial flushing.

Answer: B. A sign of adverse reaction to the contrast medium is tachycardia.

3. The major neurologic symptom of Guillain-Barré syndrome is:
    A.   headache.
    B.   nuchal rigidity.
    C.   muscle weakness.
    D.   altered LOC.

Answer: C. Muscle weakness usually appears in the legs first, then extends to the arms and face within 2 weeks or less.

4. Which type of seizure is characterized by brief, involuntary muscle movements?
    A.   Jacksonian
    B.   Myoclonic
    C.   Generalized tonic-clonic
    D.   Akinetic

Answer: B. During myoclonic seizures, the patient has brief, involuntary muscle movements.

Scoring

✰✰✰ If you answered all four questions correctly, you may already know this: You're a brainiac!

✰✰ If you answered three questions correctly, don't feel sad. You have all the brainpower you need to succeed.

✰ If you answered fewer than three questions correctly, don't be nervous. Review the chapter and then take the test again.

Cardiovascular system

Just the facts

In this chapter, you'll learn:

♦ structure and function of the cardiovascular system

♦ assessment of the cardiovascular system

♦ diagnostic tests and procedures for the cardiovascular system

♦ cardiovascular disorders and treatments.

Understanding the cardiovascular system

The cardiovascular system consists of the heart and the blood vessels.

Bring it on...and take it away

This complex system functions to:
• carry life-sustaining oxygen and nutrients in the blood to all cells of the body
• remove metabolic waste products from the cells
• move hormones from one part of the body to another.

> You might say the cardiovascular system is a mover and remover!

Heart

The heart is about the size of a closed fist. It lies beneath the sternum in the mediastinum (the cavity between the lungs), between the second and sixth ribs.

The right border of the heart aligns with the right border of the sternum. The left border aligns with the midclavicular line. The exact position of the heart varies slightly in each patient.

Pericardium

The pericardium is a sac that surrounds the heart. It's composed of an outer (fibrous) layer and inner (serous) layer. The serous layer of the pericardium is composed of a visceral (inner) layer and parietal (outer) layer.

Fluid space

The pericardial space separates the visceral and parietal layers of the serous pericardium. This space contains 10 to 30 ml of thin, clear pericardial fluid, which lubricates the two surfaces of the serous pericardium and cushions the heart.

Heart wall

The heart's wall is composed of three layers:

Epicardium includes the outer layer of the heart wall and the visceral layer of the serous pericardium. It's made up of squamous epithelial cells overlying connective tissue.

Myocardium is the middle and largest portion of the heart wall. This layer of muscle tissue contracts with each heartbeat.

Endocardium is the innermost layer of the heart wall. It contains endothelial tissue made up of small blood vessels and bundles of smooth muscle.

> The myocardium is composed of muscle tissue that contracts with each heartbeat.

Four chambers

The heart has four chambers:
- right atrium
- left atrium
- right ventricle
- left ventricle. (See *A close look at the heart.*)

Blood reservoirs

The right and left atria serve as reservoirs for blood. The right atrium receives deoxygenated blood returning from the body. The left atrium receives oxygenated blood from the lungs. Contraction of the atria forces blood into the ventricles below.

Blood pumps

The right and left ventricles are the pumping chambers of the heart. The ventricles — which have thicker walls and are larger than the atria — are composed of highly developed muscles.

A close look at the heart

This illustration provides a detailed look at the internal structures of the heart.

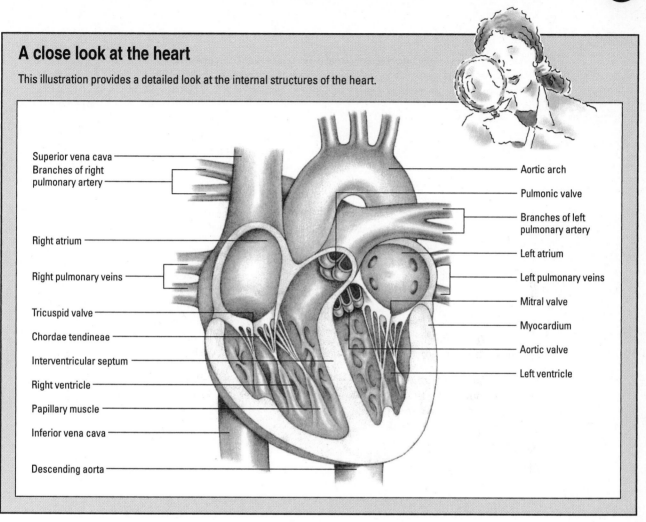

The right ventricle receives blood from the right atrium and pumps it through the pulmonary arteries to the lungs, where it picks up oxygen and drops off carbon dioxide. The left ventricle receives oxygenated blood from the left atrium and pumps it through the aorta and then out to the rest of the body. The interventricular septum separates the ventricles and helps them to pump.

Heart valves

Valves in the heart keep blood flowing in one direction.

One way

Healthy valves open and close passively as a result of pressure changes in the four heart chambers. The valves prevent blood from traveling the wrong way.

Where the valves are

Valves between the atria and ventricles are called *atrioventricular (AV) valves* and include the tricuspid valve on the right side of the heart and the mitral valve on the left side. Valves between the ventricles and the pulmonary artery and the aorta are called *semilunar valves* and include the pulmonic valve on the right (between the right ventricle and the pulmonary artery) and the aortic valve on the left (between the left ventricle and the aorta).

On the cusp

The leaflets, or cusps, of each valve keep the valves tightly closed. The tricuspid valve has three cusps. The mitral valve has two.

The cusps are anchored to the heart wall by cords of fibrous tissue called *chordae tendineae,* which are controlled by papillary muscles.

Great vessels

Leading into and out of the heart are the great vessels:
• The aorta, which carries blood away from the left ventricle, is the main trunk of the systemic artery system.
• The inferior and superior vena cavae carry deoxygenated blood from the body into the right atrium.
• The pulmonary artery is a large artery that carries blood away from the right ventricle. Above the heart, it splits to form the right and left pulmonary arteries, which carry blood to the right and left lungs.
• The four pulmonary veins—two on the left and two on the right—carry oxygenated blood from the left and right lungs to the left atrium.

Coronary arteries

Like all other organs, the heart needs an adequate blood supply to survive. The coronary arteries, which lie on the surface of the heart, supply the heart muscle with blood and oxygen. (See *Heart vessels.*)

Coronary ostium

The coronary ostium is an opening in the aorta near the aortic valve. It feeds blood to the coronary arteries.

The great vessels carry blood into and out of the heart.

Heart vessels

These two views of the heart depict the great vessels and some of the major coronary vessels.

Anterior view

Superior vena cava

Aorta

Pulmonary trunk

Left main coronary artery

Circumflex artery

Great cardiac vein

Right coronary artery

Anterior cardiac veins

Left anterior descending artery

Marginal artery

Posterior view

Aorta

Left pulmonary artery

Pulmonary veins

Circumflex artery

Coronary sinus

Posterior vein of left ventricle

Superior vena cava

Right pulmonary artery

Pulmonary veins

Inferior vena cava

Right coronary artery

Right posterior descending artery

Middle cardiac vein

Ostium action

When the left ventricle is pumping blood through the aorta, the aortic valve is open and the coronary ostium is partly covered. When the left ventricle is filling with blood, the aortic valve is closed and the coronary ostium is open, enabling blood to fill the coronary arteries.

Right coronary artery

The right coronary artery supplies blood to the right atrium, the right ventricle, and part of the left ventricle. It also supplies blood to the bundle of His (muscles that connect the atria with the ventricles) and the AV node (fibers at the base of the interatrial septum that transmit the cardiac impulses from the sinoatrial [SA] node).

What do you SA about that?

In about half the population, the right coronary artery also supplies blood to the SA node of the right atrium. The SA node consists of atypical muscle fibers that establish the rhythm of cardiac contractions.

Left coronary artery

The left coronary artery runs along the surface of the left atrium, where it splits into two major branches: the left anterior descending artery and the left circumflex artery.

The left coronary artery splits into two major branches that supply blood to the rest of the heart.

Left out

The left anterior descending artery supplies blood to the:
- anterior wall of the left ventricle
- interventricular septum
- right bundle branch (a branch of the bundle of His)
- left anterior fasciculus (small cluster) of the left bundle branch.

The branches of the left anterior descending artery — the septal perforators and the diagonal arteries — supply blood to the walls of both ventricles.

Circumflex-ability

The circumflex artery supplies oxygenated blood to the lateral walls of the left ventricle, the left atrium and, in about 50% of the population, the SA node.

Circle left

In addition, the circumflex artery supplies blood to the left posterior fasciculus of the left bundle branch. This artery circles around the left ventricle and provides blood to the ventricle's posterior portion.

Veins

Like other parts of the body, the heart has veins, called *cardiac veins*, that collect deoxygenated blood from the capillaries of the myocardium. These cardiac veins join together to form an enlarged vessel called the *coronary sinus*. The right atrium receives deoxygenated blood from the heart through the coronary sinus.

Pulmonary circulation

During pulmonary circulation, blood travels to the lungs to pick up oxygen in exchange for carbon dioxide.

Heart to lungs to heart

Here's what happens during pulmonary circulation:
• Deoxygenated blood travels from the right ventricle through the pulmonary semilunar valve into the pulmonary arteries.
• Blood passes through smaller arteries and arterioles into the capillaries of the lungs.
• Blood reaches the alveoli and exchanges carbon dioxide for oxygen.
• Oxygenated blood returns through the venules and veins to the pulmonary veins.
• The pulmonary veins carry the oxygenated blood back to the left atrium of the heart.

Cardiac rhythm

Contractions of the heart occur in a rhythm that's regulated by impulses initiated at the SA node.

Nature's pacemaker

The SA node is the heart's pacemaker. Impulses initiated at the SA node are conducted from there throughout the heart. Impulses from the autonomic nervous system affect the SA node and alter its firing rate to meet the body's needs.

The cardiac cycle

The cardiac cycle consists of two phases: systole and diastole.

Out with systole, in with diastole

During systole, the heart contracts and sends blood on its outward journey. During diastole, the heart relaxes and fills with blood; the mitral and tricuspid valves are open, and the aortic and pulmonic valves are closed.

During diastole, the heart relaxes and fills with blood.

Filling and more filling

Diastole consists of ventricular filling and atrial contraction. During ventricular filling, 70% of the blood in the atria drains into the ventricles passively, by gravity. The active period of diastole, atrial contraction (also called *atrial kick*), accounts for the remaining 30% of blood that passes into the ventricles.

The pressure's on

When the pressure in the ventricles is greater than the pressure in the aorta and pulmonary artery, the aortic and pulmonic valves open. Blood then flows from the ventricles into the pulmonary artery, then to the lungs and into the aorta, and then to the rest of the body.

The pressure's off

At the end of ventricular contraction, pressure in the ventricles drops below the pressure in the aorta and pulmonary artery. The difference in pressure forces blood back up toward the ventricles and causes the aortic and pulmonic valves to snap shut.

As the valves shut, the atria fill with blood in preparation for the next period of diastolic filling, and the cycle begins again.

Cardiac output is the amount of blood the heart pumps in 1 minute.

Out in a minute

Cardiac output is the amount of blood the heart pumps in 1 minute. It's equal to the heart rate multiplied by the stroke volume (the amount of blood ejected with each heartbeat).

Stroke volume depends on three major factors:

- preload
- afterload
- contractility. (See *Understanding preload, afterload, and contractility*.)

Understanding preload, afterload, and contractility

If you think of the heart as a balloon, it will help you understand preload, afterload, and contractility.

Blowing up the balloon

Preload is the stretching of muscle fibers in the ventricles. This stretching results from blood volume in the ventricles at end-diastole. According to Starling's law, the more the heart muscles stretch during diastole, the more forcefully they contract during systole. Think of preload as the balloon stretching as air is blown into it. The more air the greater the stretch.

The balloon's stretch

Contractility refers to the inherent ability of the myocardium to contract normally. Contractility is influenced by preload. The greater the stretch the more forceful the contraction—or, the more air in the balloon, the greater the stretch, and the farther the balloon will fly when air is allowed to expel.

The knot that ties the balloon

Afterload refers to the pressure that the ventricular muscles must generate to overcome the higher pressure in the aorta to get the blood out of the heart. *Resistance* is the knot on the end of the balloon, which the balloon has to work against to get the air out.

Blood vessels

The vascular system is the complex network of blood vessels throughout the body that conducts systemic circulation. Blood carries oxygen and other nutrients to body cells and transports waste products for excretion.

Arteries

The major artery—the aorta—branches into vessels that supply blood to specific organs and areas of the body.

Upper blood suppliers

Three arteries arise from the arch of the aorta and supply blood to the brain, arms, and upper chest. These are the:

- left common carotid artery
- left subclavian artery
- innominate artery.

Descending distribution

As the aorta descends through the thorax and abdomen, its branches supply blood to the GI and genitourinary organs, spinal column, and lower chest and abdominal muscles. Then the aorta divides into the iliac arteries, which further divide into the femoral arteries.

Arterioles

As the arteries divide into smaller units, the number of vessels increases, thereby increasing the area of perfusion. These smaller units are known as *arterioles*. Arterioles can dilate to decrease blood pressure or constrict to increase blood pressure.

Capillaries

Where the arterioles end, the capillaries begin. Strong sphincters control blood flow from the capillaries into the tissues. The sphincters open to permit more flow when needed and close to shunt blood to other areas.

Small vessels, large area of distribution

Although the capillary bed contains the smallest vessels, it supplies blood to the largest area. Capillary pressure is extremely low to allow for exchange of nutrients, oxygen, and carbon dioxide with body cells.

Venules and veins

From the capillaries, returning blood flows into venules and, eventually, into veins. Valves in the veins prevent blood backflow, and the pumping action of skeletal muscles assists venous return.

Branching back to the right atrium

The veins merge until they form branches that return blood to the right atrium. The two main branches include the superior venae cavae and the inferior venae cavae.

Dilated arterioles decrease blood pressure. Constricted arterioles increase blood pressure.

Low capillary pressure allows for the exchange of nutrients, oxygen, and carbon dioxide with body cells.

Cardiovascular assessment

Assessment of a patient's cardiovascular system includes a health history and physical examination.

Health history

To obtain a health history of a patient's cardiovascular system, begin by introducing yourself and explaining what happens during the health history and physical examination. Then obtain the following information.

Chief complaint

Ask for details about the patient's chief complaint. Patients with cardiovascular problems typically cite specific complaints, including:
- chest pain
- irregular heartbeat or palpitations
- shortness of breath on exertion, when lying down, or at night
- cough
- weakness or fatigue
- unexplained weight change
- swelling of the extremities
- dizziness
- headache
- peripheral skin changes, such as decreased hair distribution, skin color changes, a thin shiny appearance to the skin, or an ulcer on the lower leg that fails to heal
- pain in the extremities, such as leg pain or cramps.

Personal and family health

Ask the patient for details about his family history and past medical history. Also ask about:
- stressors in the patient's life and coping strategies he uses to deal with them
- current health habits, such as smoking, alcohol intake, caffeine intake, exercise, and dietary intake of fat and sodium
- drugs the patient is taking, including prescription drugs, over-the-counter drugs, and herbal preparations
- previous surgeries
- environmental or occupational considerations
- activities of daily living (ADLs)
- menopause (if applicable).

During your assessment, collect a health history and perform a physical examination.

Advice from the experts

Cardiac questions

To thoroughly assess your patient's cardiac function, be sure to ask these questions:
• Are you in pain?
• Where is the pain located?
• Does the pain feel like a burning, tight, or squeezing sensation?
• Does the pain radiate to your arm, neck, back, or jaw?

• When did the pain begin?
• What relieves or aggravates it?
• Are you experiencing nausea, dizziness, or sweating?
• Do you feel short of breath? Has breathing trouble ever awakened you from sleep?
• Does your heart ever pound or skip a beat? When?

• Do you ever get dizzy or faint? When?
• Do you experience swelling in your ankles or feet. When? Does anything relieve the swelling?
• Do you urinate frequently at night?
• Have you had to limit your activities?

Rating pain

Many patients with cardiovascular problems complain of chest pain. If the patient is experiencing chest pain, ask him to rate the pain on a scale of 0 to 10, in which 0 indicates no pain and 10 indicates the worst chest pain imaginable. It's vital to thoroughly assess pain.

Where, what, and why

If the patient isn't in distress, ask questions that require more than a yes-or-no response. Use familiar expressions rather than medical terms whenever possible. (See *Cardiac questions*.)

In his own words

Let the patient describe his condition in his own words. Ask him to describe the location, radiation, intensity, and duration of pain and any precipitating, exacerbating, or relieving factors to obtain an accurate description of chest pain. (See *Understanding chest pain*.)

Physical examination

Cardiovascular disease affects people of all ages and can take many forms. To best identify abnormalities, use a consistent, methodical approach to the physical examination.

Understanding chest pain

Use this table to help you more accurately assess chest pain.

What it feels like	Where it's located	What makes it worse	What causes it	What makes it better
Aching, squeezing, pressure, heaviness, burning pain; usually subsides within 10 minutes	Substernal; may radiate to jaw, neck, arms, and back	Eating, physical effort, smoking, cold weather, stress, anger, hunger, lying down	Angina pectoris	Rest, nitroglycerin (*Note:* Unstable angina appears even at rest.)
Tightness or pressure; burning, aching pain, possibly accompanied by shortness of breath, diaphoresis, weakness, anxiety, or nausea; sudden onset; lasts ½ hour to 2 hours	Typically across chest but may radiate to jaw, neck, arms, or back	Exertion, anxiety	Acute myocardial infarction	Opioid analgesics such as morphine, nitroglycerin
Sharp and continuous; may be accompanied by friction rub; sudden onset	Substernal; may radiate to neck or left arm	Deep breathing, supine position	Pericarditis	Sitting up, leaning forward, anti-inflammatory drugs
Excruciating, tearing pain; may be accompanied by blood pressure difference between right and left arm; sudden onset	Retrosternal, upper abdominal, or epigastric; may radiate to back, neck, or shoulders	Not applicable	Dissecting aortic aneurysm	Analgesics, surgery
Sudden, stabbing pain; may be accompanied by cyanosis, dyspnea, or cough with hemoptysis	Over lung area	Inspiration	Pulmonary embolus	Analgesics
Sudden and severe pain; sometimes accompanied by dyspnea, increased pulse rate, decreased breath sounds, or deviated trachea	Lateral thorax	Normal respiration	Pneumothorax	Analgesics, chest tube insertion

First things first

Before you begin the physical examination, wash your hands thoroughly. Obtain a stethoscope with a bell and a diaphragm, an appropriate-sized blood pressure cuff, and a penlight. Also, make sure the room is quiet.

Ask the patient to remove all clothing except his underwear and to put on an examination gown. Have the patient lie on his back, with the head of the bed at a 30- to 45-degree angle.

The heart of it

When performing an assessment of a patient's heart health, proceed in this order:

- inspection
- palpation
- percussion
- auscultation.

Inspection

First, take a moment to assess the patient's general appearance.

First impressions

Is the patient too thin or obese? Is he alert? Does he appear anxious? Note the patient's skin color. Are his fingers clubbed? (Clubbing is a sign of chronic hypoxia caused by a lengthy cardiovascular or respiratory disorder.) If the patient is dark-skinned, inspect his mucous membranes for pallor.

Check the chest

Next, inspect the chest. Note landmarks you can use to describe your findings as well as structures underlying the chest wall. (See *Cardiovascular landmarks*.)

Look for pulsations, symmetry of movement, retractions, or heaves (strong outward thrusts of the chest wall that occur during systole).

Inspecting the impulse

Then position a light source, such as a penlight, so that it casts a shadow on the patient's chest. Note the location of the apical impulse. This is also usually the point of maximal impulse (PMI) and should be located in the fifth intercostal space medial to the left midclavicular line.

The apical impulse gives an indication of how well the left ventricle is working because it corresponds to the apex of the heart. To find the apical impulse in a woman with large breasts, displace the breasts during the examination.

Memory jogger

To remember the order in which you should perform assessment of the cardiovascular system, just think, "I'll Properly Perform Assessment."

I — Inspection

P — Palpation

P — Percussion

A — Auscultation

The patient's apical impulse tells you how well the left ventricle is working.

Cardiovascular landmarks

Here's a guide to finding the critical landmarks used in cardiovascular assessment.

Anterior thorax

Lateral thorax

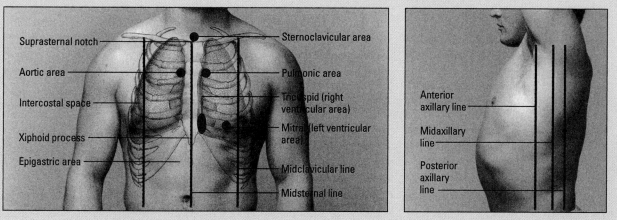

Anterior thorax labels:
- Suprasternal notch
- Aortic area
- Intercostal space
- Xiphoid process
- Epigastric area
- Sternoclavicular area
- Pulmonic area
- Tricuspid (right ventricular area)
- Mitral (left ventricular area)
- Midclavicular line
- Midsternal line

Lateral thorax labels:
- Anterior axillary line
- Midaxillary line
- Posterior axillary line

Abnormal findings on inspection

Here are some of the abnormal findings you may note on inspection and what such findings tell you:
- Inspection may reveal cyanosis, pallor, or cool or cold skin, which may indicate poor cardiac output and tissue perfusion.
- Skin may be flushed if the patient has a fever.
- Absence of body hair on the arms or legs may indicate diminished arterial blood flow to those areas. (See *Assessing arterial and venous insufficiency*, page 152.)
- Swelling, or edema, may indicate heart failure or venous insufficiency. It may also be caused by varicosities or thrombophlebitis.
- Chronic right-sided heart failure may cause ascites and generalized edema.

A chest of clues

- Inspection may reveal barrel chest (rounded thoracic cage caused by chronic obstructive pulmonary disease), scoliosis (lateral curvature of the spine), or kyphosis (convex curvature of the thoracic spine). If severe enough, these conditions can impair cardiac output by preventing chest expansion and inhibiting heart muscle movement.
- Retractions (visible indentations of the soft tissue covering the chest wall) or the use of accessory muscles to breathe typically re-

Edema is a telltale sign of possible heart failure, venous insufficiency, varicosities, or thrombophlebitis.

CAUTION!

Assessing arterial and venous insufficiency

You should be aware of how assessment findings differ between healthy patients and those with arterial insufficiency or chronic venous insufficiency.

Arterial insufficiency

In a patient with arterial insufficiency, pulses may be decreased or absent. The skin is cool, pale, and shiny, and the patient may have pain in his legs and feet. Ulcerations typically occur in the area around the toes, and the foot usually turns deep red when dependent. Nails may be thick and ridged.

Chronic venous insufficiency

In a patient with chronic venous insufficiency, check for ulcerations around his ankle. Pulses are present but may be difficult to find because of pitting edema. The foot may become cyanotic when dependent, and you may see a brown pigmentation and thickening of the skin around the ankle.

sults from a respiratory disorder but may also occur with a congenital heart defect or heart failure.

Palpation

Note skin temperature, turgor, and texture. Using the ball of your hand and then your fingertips, gently palpate over the precordium to find the apical impulse. Note heaves or thrills (fine vibrations that feel like the purring of a cat). (See *Assessing apical impulse.*)

Elusive impulse

The apical impulse may be difficult to palpate in patients who are obese or pregnant and in patients with thick chest walls. If it's difficult to palpate with the patient lying on his back, have him lie of his left side or sit upright.

Plus, palpate

Also palpate the sternoclavicular, aortic, pulmonic, tricuspid, and epigastric areas for abnormal pulsations. Pulsations aren't usually

If the apical impulse is unpalpable with the patient on his back, have him lie on his left side or sit upright.

felt in those areas. However, an aortic arch pulsation in the sternoclavicular area or an abdominal aorta pulsation in the epigastric area may be a normal finding in a thin patient.

Percussion

Percussion is less useful than other assessment methods, but it may help you locate the cardiac borders.

Border patrol

Begin percussing at the anterior axillary line and continue toward the sternum along the fifth intercostal space. The sound changes from resonance to dullness over the left border of the heart, normally at the midclavicular line. The right border of the heart is usually aligned with the sternum and can't be percussed.

Auscultation

You can learn a great deal about the heart by auscultating for heart sounds. Cardiac auscultation requires a methodical approach and lots of practice.

Here's the plan

First, identify the auscultation sites, which include the sites over the four cardiac valves, at Erb's point, and at the third intercostal space at the left sternal border. Use the bell to hear low-pitched sounds and the diaphragm to hear high-pitched sounds. (See *Heart sound sites*, page 154.)

Begin by warming the stethoscope in your hands. Auscultate for heart sounds with the patient in three positions:

lying on his back with the head of the bed raised 30 to 45 degrees

sitting up

lying on his left side.

Upward, downward, zigward, zagward

Use a zigzag pattern over the precordium. Start at the apex and work upward or at the base and work downward. Whichever approach you use, be consistent.

Use the diaphragm to listen as you go in one direction; use the bell as you come back in the other direction. Be sure to listen over the entire precordium, not just over the valves. Note the patient's heart rate and rhythm.

Advice from the experts

Assessing apical impulse

The apical impulse is associated with the first heart sound and carotid pulsation. To ensure that you're feeling the apical impulse and not a muscle spasm or some other pulsation, use one hand to palpate the patient's carotid artery and the other to palpate the apical impulse. Then compare the timing and regularity of the impulses. The apical impulse should roughly coincide with the carotid pulsation.

Note the amplitude, size, intensity, location, and duration of the apical impulse. You should feel a gentle pulsation in an area about ½" to ¾" (1.5 to 2 cm) in diameter.

Heart sound sites

When auscultating for heart sounds, place the stethoscope over the four different sites illustrated below.

Normal heart sounds indicate events in the cardiac cycle, such as the closing of heart valves, and are reflected to specific areas of the chest wall. Auscultation sites are identified by the names of heart valves but aren't located directly over the valves. Rather, these sites are located along the pathway blood takes as it flows through the heart's chambers and valves.

Aortic

Pulmonic

Tricuspid

Mitral

1, 2, 3, 4, and more

Systole is the period of ventricular contraction. As pressure in the ventricles increases, the mitral and tricuspid valves snap closed. The closure produces the first heart sound, S_1.

At the end of ventricular contraction, the aortic and pulmonic valves snap shut. This produces the second heart sound, S_2.

Always identify S_1 and S_2, and then listen for adventitious sounds, such as third and fourth heart sounds (S_3 and S_4). (See *Extra heart sounds in the cardiac cycle.*)

Also listen for murmurs (vibrating, blowing, or rumbling sounds) and rubs (harsh, scratchy, scraping, or squeaking sounds).

Listen for the "dub"

Start auscultating at the aortic area where the S_2 is loudest.

Rubs and dub-lubs, three heart sounds in a tub, and which will sound the loudest?

Extra heart sounds in the cardiac cycle

To understand where extra heart sounds fall in relation to systole, diastole, and normal heart sounds, compare the illustrations of normal and extra heart sounds below.

Normal heart sounds

S_1 S_2 S_1

Systole   Diastole

Extra heart sounds

S_4 S_1 S_2 S_3 S_4 S_1

Systole   Diastole

Those sounds don't belong there!

An S_2 is best heard at the base of the heart at the end of ventricular systole. It occurs when the pulmonic and aortic valves close and is generally described as sounding like "dub." It's a shorter, higher-pitched, and louder sound than S_1.

When the pulmonic valve closes later than the aortic valve during inspiration, you hear a split S_2.

Listen for the "lub"

From the base of the heart, move to the pulmonic area and then down to the tricuspid area. Then move to the mitral area, where S_1 is the loudest.

An S_1 is best heard at the apex of the heart. It occurs with closure of the mitral and tricuspid valves and is generally described as sounding like "lub." It's low-pitched and dull.

An S_1 occurs at the beginning of ventricular systole. It may be split if the mitral valve closes just before the tricuspid valve.

Abnormal findings on heart auscultation

On auscultation, you may detect S_1 and S_2 heart sounds that are accentuated, diminished, or inaudible. Other abnormal heart sounds — such as S_3, S_4, and murmurs — may result from pressure changes, valvular dysfunctions, and conduction defects.

Third heart sound

The third heart sound — known as S_3 or ventricular gallop — is a low-pitched noise best heard by placing the bell of the stethoscope at the apex of the heart.

Kentucky galloper

Its rhythm resembles a horse galloping, and its cadence resembles the word "Ken-tuc-ky" (lub-dub-by). Listen for S_3 with the patient in a supine or left-lateral decubitus position.

An S_3 usually occurs during early diastole to middiastole, at the end of the passive-filling phase of either ventricle. Listen for this sound immediately after S_2. It may signify that the ventricle isn't compliant enough to accept the filling volume without additional force.

Age-related adversity

An S_3 may occur normally in a child or young adult. In a patient older than age 30, however, it usually indicates a disorder, such as:
- right-sided heart failure
- left-sided heart failure
- pulmonary congestion
- intracardiac shunting of blood
- myocardial infarction (MI)
- anemia
- thyrotoxicosis.

Here's a clue: An S_3 heart sound in a person older than age 30 is usually a sign of a disorder.

Fourth heart sound

The fourth heart sound, or S_4, is an abnormal sound that occurs late in diastole, just before the pulse upstroke. It immediately precedes the S_1 of the next cycle. It's known as the atrial or presystolic gallop and it occurs during atrial contraction.

Tennessee walker

An S_4 shares the same cadence as the word "Ten-nes-see" (le-lub-dub). It's heard best with the bell of the stethoscope and with the patient in the supine position.

What S_4 says

An S_4 may indicate cardiovascular disease, such as:
- acute MI
- hypertension
- coronary artery disease (CAD)
- cardiomyopathy
- angina
- anemia
- elevated left ventricular pressure
- aortic stenosis.

If the S_4 sound persists, it may indicate impaired ventricular compliance or volume overload. S_4 commonly appears in elderly patients with age-related systolic hypertension and aortic stenosis.

Ah-hah! Here's another clue: It's an S_4 heart sound — a sign of cardiovascular disease.

Murmurs

A murmur, which is longer than a heart sound, makes a vibrating, blowing, or rumbling noise. Just as turbulent water in a stream babbles as it passes through a narrow point, turbulent blood flow produces a murmur.

If you detect a murmur, identify where it's loudest, pinpoint the time it occurs during the cardiac cycle, and describe its pitch, pattern, quality, and intensity. (See *Identifying heart murmurs*, page 158.)

Location and timing

Murmurs can occur in any cardiac auscultatory site and may radiate from one site to another.

Marking murmurs

To identify the radiation area, auscultate from the site where the murmur seems loudest to the farthest site it's still heard. Note the anatomic landmark of this farthest site.

Pinpoint its presence

Determine if the murmur occurs during systole (between S_1 and S_2) or diastole (between S_2 and the next S_1). Then pinpoint when in the cardiac cycle the murmur occurs — for example, during middiastole or late systole. A murmur heard throughout systole is called a *holosystolic* or *pansystolic* murmur, and a murmur heard throughout diastole is called a *pandiastolic* murmur. Occasionally, murmurs occur during both portions of the cycle (continuous murmur).

Identifying heart murmurs

To identify a heart murmur, first listen closely to determine its timing in the cardiac cycle. Then determine its other characteristics, including quality, pitch, and location as well as possible causes.

Timing	Quality and pitch	Location	Possible causes
Midsystolic (systolic ejection)	Harsh, rough with medium to high pitch	Pulmonic	Pulmonic stenosis
	Harsh, rough with medium to high pitch	Aortic and suprasternal notch	Aortic stenosis
Holosystolic (pansystolic)	Harsh with high pitch	Tricuspid	Ventricular septal defect
	Blowing with high pitch	Mitral, lower left sternal border	Mitral insufficiency
	Blowing with high pitch	Tricuspid	Tricuspid insufficiency
Early diastolic	Blowing with high pitch	Mid-left sternal edge (not aortic area)	Aortic insufficiency
	Blowing with high pitch	Pulmonic	Pulmonic insufficiency
Middiastolic to late diastolic	Rumbling with low pitch	Apex	Mitral stenosis
	Rumbling with low pitch	Tricuspid, lower right sternal border	Tricuspid stenosis

Pitch
Depending on the rate and pressure of blood flow, pitch may be high, medium, or low. You can best hear a low-pitched murmur with the bell of the stethoscope, a high-pitched murmur with the diaphragm, and a medium-pitched murmur with both.

Pattern
Crescendo occurs when the velocity of blood flow increases and the murmur becomes louder. Decrescendo occurs when velocity decreases and the murmur becomes quieter.

Up and down

A crescendo-decrescendo pattern describes a murmur with increasing loudness followed by increasing softness.

Quality
The volume of blood flow, the force of the contraction, and the degree of valve compromise all contribute to murmur quality. Terms used to describe quality include *musical, blowing, harsh, rasping, rumbling,* or *machinelike.*

Describe the quality of your patient's murmur using terms like musical, blowing, harsh, rasping, rumbling, or machinelike.

Intensity

Use a standard, six-level grading scale to describe the intensity of the murmur:

grade I—extremely faint; barely audible even to the trained ear

grade II—soft and low; easily audible to the trained ear

grade III—moderately loud; about equal to the intensity of normal heart sounds

grade IV—loud with a palpable thrill at the murmur site

grade V—very loud with a palpable thrill; audible with the stethoscope in partial contact with the chest

grade VI—extremely loud, with a palpable thrill; audible with the stethoscope over, but not in contact with, the chest.

Rubs

To detect a pericardial friction rub, use the diaphragm of the stethoscope to auscultate in the third left intercostal space along the lower left sternal border.

Rubs the wrong way

Listen for a harsh, scratchy, scraping, or squeaking sound that occurs throughout systole, diastole, or both. To enhance the sound, have the patient sit upright and lean forward or exhale. A rub usually indicates pericarditis.

A rub usually indicates pericarditis. That really rubs me the wrong way!

Assessing the vascular system

Assessment of the vascular system is an important part of a full cardiovascular assessment.

Inspection

Start your assessment of the vascular system the same way you start an assessment of the cardiac system—by making general observations.

To arms!...and legs!

Examination of the patient's arms and legs can reveal arterial or venous disorders. Examine the patient's arms when you take his vital signs. Are the arms equal in size? Evaluate the legs when the patient is standing. Are the legs symmetrical? Check the legs later during the physical examination as well, with the patient lying on his back.

Skimming the skin

Inspect the patient's skin color. Note how body hair is distributed. Note lesions, scars, clubbing, and edema of the extremities. If the patient is confined to bed, be sure to check the sacrum for swelling. Examine the fingernails and toenails for abnormalities.

Checking the neck

Continue your inspection by observing vessels in the neck. Inspection of these vessels can provide information about blood volume and pressure in the right side of the heart.

Picturing pulsations

Check the carotid artery pulsations. The carotid artery should have a brisk, localized pulsation—not weak or bounding. The carotid pulsation doesn't decrease when the patient is upright, when he inhales, or when you palpate the carotid artery.

Inspect the jugular veins. The internal jugular vein has a softer, undulating pulsation. The internal jugular pulsation changes in response to position, breathing, and palpation.

Going for the jugular

To check the jugular venous pulse, have the patient lie on his back. Elevate the head of the bed 30 to 45 degrees and turn the patient's head slightly away from you.

Pulsations a notch above the notch

Normally, the highest pulsation occurs no more than 1½″ (4 cm) above the sternal notch. If pulsations appear higher, it indicates elevation in central venous pressure (CVP) and jugular vein distention.

If you detect pulsations too far above the sternal notch, it's due to elevated CVP and jugular vein distention.

Palpation

The first step in palpation is to assess skin temperature, texture, and turgor.

Note nail beds

Next, check capillary refill by assessing the nail beds on the fingers and toes. Refill time should be no more than 3 seconds, or long enough to say "capillary refill."

Palpate pulses

Palpate for the pulse on each side of the neck, comparing pulse volume and symmetry. Don't palpate both carotid arteries at the same time or press too firmly. If you do, the patient may faint or become bradycardic.

Making the grade

All pulses should be regular in rhythm and equal in strength. Pulses are graded on a scale from 0 to 4+:
- 4+ is bounding.
- 3+ is increased.
- 2+ is normal.
- 1+ is weak.
- 0 is absent.

Abnormal findings

Abnormal findings on palpation may reveal:
- weak pulse, indicating low cardiac output or increased peripheral vascular resistance such as in arterial atherosclerotic disease (note that elderly patients commonly have weak pedal pulses)
- strong bounding pulse, which occurs in hypertension and in high cardiac output states, such as exercise, pregnancy, anemia, and thyrotoxicosis
- apical impulse that exerts unusual force and lasts longer than one-third of the cardiac cycle — a possible indication of increased cardiac output
- displaced or diffuse impulse, which is a possible indication of left ventricular hypertrophy
- pulsation in the aortic, pulmonic, or right ventricular area, which is a sign of chamber enlargement or valvular disease
- pulsation in the sternoclavicular or epigastric area, which is a sign of an aortic aneurysm
- palpable thrill, which is an indication of blood flow turbulence and is usually related to valvular dysfunction; determine how far the thrill radiates and make a mental note to listen for a murmur at this site during auscultation
- heave along the left sternal border, which is an indication of right ventricular hypertrophy
- heave over the left ventricular area, which is a sign of a ventricular aneurysm; a thin patient may experience a heave with exercise, fever, or anxiety because of increased cardiac output and more forceful contraction
- displaced PMI, which is a possible indication of left ventricular hypertrophy caused by volume overload from mitral or aortic stenosis, septal defect, acute MI, or other disorder.

Percussion

Percussion isn't used when assessing the vascular system.

Don't palpate both carotid arteries at once or press too firmly. If you do, the patient may faint or become bradycardic.

CAUTION!

Auscultation

After vascular palpation, use the bell of the stethoscope to begin auscultation. Follow the palpation sequence and listen over each artery.

Abnormal findings

Sounds aren't normally heard over the carotid arteries. A bruit, which sounds like buzzing or blowing, could indicate arteriosclerotic plaque formation.

Brutish bruits

When you auscultate for the femoral and popliteal pulses, check for a bruit or other abnormal sounds. A bruit over the femoral or popliteal artery usually indicates narrowed vessels.

During auscultation of the central and peripheral arteries, you may notice a continuous bruit, caused by turbulent blood flow. A bruit over the abdominal aorta usually indicates an aneurysm (weakness in the arterial wall that allows a sac to form) or a dissection (a tear in the layers of the arterial wall).

Uh-oh! A bruit over the abdominal aorta usually indicates an aneurysm or a dissection.

EMERGENCY

Diagnostic tests

Advances in diagnostic testing allow for earlier and easier diagnosis and treatment of cardiovascular disorders. For example, in some patients, echocardiography—a noninvasive and risk-free test—can provide as much diagnostic information on valvular heart disease as can cardiac catheterization—an invasive and high-risk test.

12-lead electrocardiogram

The 12-lead electrocardiogram (ECG) measures the heart's electrical activity and records it as waveforms. It's one of the most valuable and commonly used diagnostic tools.

A test with 12 views

The standard 12-lead ECG uses a series of electrodes placed on the patient's extremities and chest wall to assess the heart from 12 different views (leads). The 12 leads include three bipolar limb leads (I, II, and III), three unipolar augmented limb leads (aV_R, aV_L, and aV_F), and six unipolar precordial limb leads (V_1 to V_6). The limb leads and augmented leads show the heart from the frontal plane. The precordial leads show the heart from the horizontal plane.

ECG can be used to identify myocardial ischemia and infarction, rhythm and conduction disturbances, chamber enlargement, electrolyte imbalances, and drug toxicity.

Nursing considerations

• Use a systematic approach to interpret the ECG recording. (See *Normal ECG waveforms*, page 164.) Compare the patient's previous ECG with the current one, if available. This will help you identify changes.

Waves of waves

• P waves should be upright; however, they may be inverted in lead aV_R or biphasic or inverted in leads III, aV_L, and V_1.
• PR intervals should always be constant, just like QRS-complex durations.
• QRS-complex deflections vary in different leads. Observe for pathologic Q waves.
• ST segments should be isoelectric or have minimal deviation.
• ST-segment elevation greater than 1 mm above the baseline and ST-segment depression greater than 0.5 mm below the baseline are considered abnormal. Leads facing an injured area have ST-segment elevations, and leads facing away show ST-segment depressions.
• The T wave normally deflects upward in leads I, II, and V_3 through V_6. It's inverted in lead aV_R and variable in the other leads. T-wave changes have many causes and aren't always a reason for alarm. Excessively tall, flat, or inverted T waves occurring with symptoms, such as chest pain, may indicate ischemia.
• A normal Q wave generally has a duration less than 0.04 second. An abnormal Q wave has either a duration of 0.04 second or more, a depth greater than 4 mm, or a height one-fourth of the R wave. Abnormal Q waves indicate myocardial necrosis, developing when depolarization can't follow its normal path because of damaged tissue in the area.
• Remember that aV_R normally has a large Q wave, so disregard this lead when searching for abnormal Q waves.

Abnormal Q waves indicate myocardial necrosis.

Cardiac marker studies

Analysis of cardiac markers (proteins) aids diagnosis of acute MI.

Release the enzymes!

After infarction, damaged cardiac tissue releases significant amounts of enzymes into the blood. Serial measurement of enzyme levels reveals the extent of damage and helps to monitor the progress of healing.

Normal ECG waveforms

Each of the 12 standard leads of an electrocardiogram (ECG) takes a different view of heart activity, and each generates its own characteristic tracing. The tracings shown here represent a normal heart rhythm viewed from each of the 12 leads. Keep in mind:

• An upward (positive) deflection indicates that the wave of depolarization flows toward the positive electrode.

• A downward (negative) deflection indicates that the wave of depolarization flows away from the positive electrode.

• An equally positive and negative (biphasic) deflection indicates that the wave of depolarization flows perpendicularly to the positive electrode.

Each lead represents a picture of a different anatomic area; when you find abnormal tracings, compare information from the different leads to pinpoint areas of cardiac damage.

Heart-zymes

The cardiac enzymes include creatine kinase (CK) and its isoenzyme MB (found specifically in heart muscle) and lactate dehydrogenase (LD) and its isoenzymes LD_1 and LD_2 that occur in heart muscle.

Tests for troponin T and I and myoglobin are more specific to cardiac muscle and can be used to detect damage more quickly, allowing faster and more effective treatment.

Meaning in markers

Here's what the results of cardiac marker studies mean:
• CK-MB levels increase 4 to 8 hours after the onset of acute MI, peak after 20 hours, and may remain elevated for up to 72 hours.
• LD_1 and LD_2 levels increase 8 to 12 hours after acute MI, peak in 24 to 48 hours, and return to normal in 10 to 14 days if tissue necrosis doesn't persist.
• Troponin levels increase within 3 to 6 hours after myocardial damage. Troponin I peaks in 14 to 20 hours, with a return to baseline in 5 to 7 days. Troponin T peaks in 12 to 24 hours, with a return to baseline in 10 to 15 days. Because troponin levels stay elevated for a long time, they can be used to detect an infarction that occurred several days earlier.
• Myoglobin levels may increase within 30 minutes to 4 hours after myocardial damage, peak within 6 to 7 hours, and return to baseline after 24 hours. However, because skeletal muscle damage may cause myoglobin levels to increase, it isn't specific to myocardial injury.

Nursing considerations

• Before CK measurement, withhold alcohol, aminocaproic acid, and lithium as ordered. If the patient must continue taking these substances, note this on the laboratory request. Inform your patient that serial blood tests are necessary.
• Avoid administering I.M. injections because they can cause muscle damage and elevate some cardiac markers.
• After any cardiac enzyme test, handle the collection tube gently to prevent hemolysis and send the sample to the laboratory immediately. A delay can affect test results.

Echocardiography

Echocardiography is used to examine the size, shape, and motion of cardiac structures. It's done using a transducer placed at an acoustic window (an area where bone and lung tissue are absent) on the patient's chest. The transducer directs sound waves toward cardiac structures, which reflect these waves.

Echo, echo

The transducer picks up the echoes, converts them to electrical impulses, and relays them to an echocardiography machine for display on a screen and for recording on a strip chart or video-

Troponin levels stay elevated for a long time and can indicate an infarction that occurred several days earlier.

Echocardiography reflects the size, shape, and motion of cardiac structures.

tape. The most commonly used echocardiographic techniques are M-mode and two-dimensional.

Motion mode

In M-mode (motion mode) echocardiography, a single, pencil-like ultrasound beam strikes the heart, producing an "ice pick," or vertical, view of cardiac structures. This mode is especially useful for precisely viewing cardiac structures.

Echo in 2-D

In two-dimensional echocardiography, the ultrasound beam rapidly sweeps through an arc, producing a cross-sectional, or fan-shaped, view of cardiac structures; this technique is useful for recording lateral motion and providing the correct spatial relationship between cardiac structures. In many cases, both techniques are performed to complement each other.

TEE combination

In transesophageal echocardiography (TEE), ultrasonography is combined with endoscopy to provide a better view of the heart's structures. (See *A closer look at TEE.*)

Echo abnormalities

The echocardiogram may detect mitral stenosis, mitral valve prolapse, aortic insufficiency, wall motion abnormalities, and pericardial effusion (excess pericardial fluid).

Nursing considerations
• Explain the procedure to the patient and advise him to remain still during the test because movement can distort results. Tell him that conductive gel is applied to the chest and a quarter-sized transducer is placed directly over it. Because pressure is exerted to keep the transducer in contact with the skin, warn the patient that he may feel minor discomfort.
• After the procedure, remove the conductive gel from the skin.

Cardiac catheterization

Cardiac catheterization involves passing a catheter into the right, left, or both sides of the heart.

A multipurpose procedure

Cardiac catheterization permits measurement of blood pressure and blood flow in the chambers of the heart. It's used to determine valve competence and cardiac wall contractility and to detect intracardiac shunts.

A closer look at TEE

In transesophageal echocardiography (TEE), ultrasonography is combined with endoscopy to provide a better view of the heart's structures.

How it's done
A small transducer is attached to the end of a gastroscope and inserted into the esophagus so that images of the heart's structure can be taken from the posterior of the heart. This test causes less tissue penetration and interference from chest wall structures and produces high-quality images of the thoracic aorta (except for the superior ascending aorta, which is shadowed by the trachea).

And why
TEE is used to diagnose:
• thoracic and aortic disorders
• endocarditis
• congenital heart disease
• intracardiac thrombi
• tumors.
   It's also used to evaluate valvular disease or repairs.

The procedure also enables collection of blood samples and taking of diagnostic films of the ventricles (contrast ventriculography) and arteries (coronary arteriography or angiography).

Cardiac calculations

Use of thermodilution catheters allows calculation of cardiac output. Such calculations are used to evaluate valvular insufficiency or stenosis, septal defects, congenital anomalies, myocardial function and blood supply, and heart wall motion.

Confirming common problems

Common abnormalities and defects that can be confirmed by cardiac catheterization include CAD, myocardial incompetence, valvular heart disease, and septal defects.

Cardiac catheterization is used to confirm CAD and other common abnormalities.

Nursing considerations

When caring for a patient undergoing a cardiac catheterization, describe the procedure and events after it and take steps to prevent postoperative complications.

Before the procedure

• Explain that this test is used to evaluate the function of the heart and its vessels. Instruct the patient to restrict food and fluids for at least 6 hours before the test. Tell him the procedure takes 1 to 2 hours and that he may receive a mild sedative during the procedure.
• Tell the patient that the catheter is inserted into an artery or vein in the arm or leg. Tell him he'll experience a transient stinging sensation when a local anesthetic is injected to numb the incision site for catheter insertion.
• Inform the patient that injection of the contrast medium through the catheter may produce a hot, flushing sensation or nausea that quickly passes; instruct him to follow directions to cough or breathe deeply. Explain that medication will be given if he experiences chest pain during the procedure, and he may also be given nitroglycerin periodically to dilate coronary vessels and aid visualization. Reassure him that complications, such as MI and thromboembolism, are rare. (See *Cardiac catheterization complications*, page 168.)
• Make sure that the patient or a responsible family member has signed a consent form. Check for and tell the doctor about hypersensitivity to shellfish, iodine, or contrast media used in other diagnostic tests.
• Discontinue anticoagulant therapy, as ordered, to reduce the risk of complications from bleeding.

Reassure your patient that a local anesthetic is used to numb the incision site before catheter insertion.

Cardiac catheterization complications

Cardiac catheterization carries more patient risk than most other diagnostic tests. Although infrequent, complications can become life-threatening. Observe the patient carefully during the procedure. Notify the doctor promptly and carefully document complications such as those listed here.

Left- or right-sided catheterization
• Cardiac tamponade
• Arrhythmias
• Hematoma or blood loss at insertion site
• Hypovolemia
• Infection (systemic or local)

• Myocardial infarction
• Pulmonary edema
• Reaction to contrast medium

Left-sided catheterization
• Arterial embolus or thrombus in limb
• Stroke or transient ischemic attack

Right-sided catheterization
• Pulmonary embolism
• Thrombophlebitis
• Vagal response
• Vagus nerve endings irritated in sinoatrial node, atrial muscle tissue, or atrioventricular junction

• Review activity restrictions that may be required of the patient after the procedure, such as lying flat with the limb extended for 4 to 6 hours and use of sandbags, if a femoral sheath is used.
• Document the presence of peripheral pulses, noting their intensity. Mark the pulses so they may be easily located after the procedure.

After the procedure
• Determine if a hemostatic device, such as a collagen plug or suture closure system, was used to close the vessel puncture site. If either method was used, inspect the site for bleeding or oozing, redness, swelling, or hematoma formation. Maintain the patient on bed rest for 1 to 2 hours.
• Enforce bed rest for 8 hours if no hemostatic device was used. If the femoral route was used for catheter insertion, keep the patient's leg extended for 6 to 8 hours; if the antecubital fossa route was used, keep the arm extended for at least 3 hours.
• Monitor vital signs every 15 minutes for 2 hours, then every 30 minutes for the next 2 hours, and then every hour for 2 hours. If no hematoma or other problems arise, check every 4 hours. If signs are unstable, check every 5 minutes and notify the doctor.
• Continually assess the insertion site for a hematoma or blood loss and reinforce the pressure dressing as needed.
• Check the patient's color, skin temperature, and peripheral pulse below the puncture site.
• Administer I.V. fluids as ordered (usually 100 ml/hour) to promote excretion of the contrast medium. Monitor for signs of fluid overload.

After catheter insertion, continually assess the site for a hematoma or blood loss.

• Watch for signs of chest pain, shortness of breath, abnormal heart rate, dizziness, diaphoresis, nausea or vomiting, or extreme fatigue. Notify the doctor immediately if these complications occur.

Hemodynamic monitoring

Hemodynamic monitoring is used to assess cardiac function and determine the effectiveness of therapy by measuring:
• cardiac output
• mixed venous blood
• oxygen saturation
• intracardiac pressures
• blood pressure. (See *Putting hemodynamic monitoring to use*, page 170.)

The methods behind the monitoring

Follow your facility's procedure for setting up, zero referencing, calibrating, maintaining, and troubleshooting equipment. Common uses of hemodynamic monitoring include arterial blood pressure monitoring and pulmonary artery pressure (PAP) monitoring.

Arterial blood pressure monitoring

In arterial blood pressure monitoring, the doctor inserts a catheter into the radial or femoral artery to measure blood pressure or obtain samples of arterial blood for diagnostic tests such as arterial blood gas (ABG) studies.

A transducer transforms the flow of blood during systole and diastole into a waveform, which appears on an oscilloscope.

Nursing considerations
• Explain the procedure to the patient and his family, including the purpose of arterial pressure monitoring.
• After catheter insertion, observe the pressure waveform to assess arterial pressure.
• Assess the insertion site for signs of infection, such as redness and swelling. Notify the doctor immediately if you note such signs.
• Document the date and time of catheter insertion, catheter insertion site, type of flush solution used, type of dressing applied, and patient's tolerance of the procedure.

Pulmonary artery pressure monitoring

Continuous PAP and intermittent pulmonary artery wedge pressure (PAWP) measurements provide important information about

Putting hemodynamic monitoring to use

Hemodynamic monitoring provides information on intracardiac pressures, arterial pressure, and cardiac output. To understand intracardiac pressures, picture the heart and vascular system as a continuous loop with constantly changing pressure gradients that keep the blood moving. Hemodynamic monitoring records the gradients within the vessels and heart chambers. Cardiac ouput indicates the amount of blood ejected by the heart each minute.

Pressure and description	Normal values	Causes of increased pressure	Causes of decreased pressure
Central venous pressure or right atrial pressure The central venous pressure (CVP) or right atrial pressure (RAP) shows right ventricular function and end-diastolic pressure.	Normal mean pressure ranges from 1 to 6 mm Hg (1.34 to 8 cm H_2O).	• Right-sided heart failure • Volume overload • Tricuspid valve stenosis or insufficiency • Constrictive pericarditis • Pulmonary hypertension • Cardiac tamponade • Right ventricular infarction	• Reduced circulating blood volume
Right ventricular pressure Typically, the doctor measures right ventricular pressure only when initially inserting a pulmonary artery catheter. Right ventricular systolic pressure normally equals pulmonary artery systolic pressure; right ventricular end-diastolic pressure, which reflects right ventricular function, equals RAP.	Normal systolic pressure ranges from 20 to 30 mm Hg; normal diastolic pressure, from 0 to 5 mm Hg.	• Mitral stenosis or insufficiency • Pulmonary disease • Hypoxemia • Constrictive pericarditis • Chronic heart failure • Atrial and ventricular septal defects • Patent ductus arteriosus	• Reduced circulating blood volume
Pulmonary artery pressure Pulmonary artery systolic pressure shows right ventricular function and pulmonary circulation pressures. Pulmonary artery diastolic pressure reflects left ventricular pressures, specifically left ventricular end-diastolic pressure, in a patient without significant pulmonary disease.	Systolic pressure normally ranges from 20 to 30 mm Hg. The mean pressure usually ranges from 10 to 15 mm Hg.	• Left-sided heart failure • Increased pulmonary blood flow (left or right shunting, as in atrial or ventricular septal defects) • Any condition causing increased pulmonary arteriolar resistance (such as pulmonary hypertension, volume overload, mitral stenosis, or hypoxia)	• Reduced circulating blood volume
Pulmonary artery wedge pressure Pulmonary artery wedge pressure (PAWP) reflects left atrial and left ventricular pressures, unless the patient has mitral stenosis. Changes in PAWP reflect changes in left ventricular filling pressure.	The mean pressure normally ranges from 6 to 12 mm Hg.	• Left-sided heart failure • Mitral stenosis or insufficiency • Pericardial tamponade	• Reduced circulating blood volume

left ventricular function and preload. Use this information for monitoring and for aiding diagnosis, refining assessment, guiding interventions, and projecting patient outcomes.

PAP purposes

PAP monitoring is indicated for patients who:
• are hemodynamically unstable
• need fluid management or continuous cardiopulmonary assessment
• are receiving multiple or frequently administered cardioactive drugs.

  PAP monitoring is also crucial for patients experiencing shock, trauma, pulmonary or cardiac disease, or multiple organ dysfunction syndrome.

PAP's parts

A pulmonary artery (PA) catheter has up to six lumens that gather hemodynamic information. In addition to distal and proximal lumens used to measure pressures, a PA catheter has a balloon inflation lumen that inflates the balloon for PAWP measurement and a thermistor connector lumen that allows cardiac output measurement.

  Some catheters also have a pacemaker wire lumen that provides a port for pacemaker electrodes and measures continuous mixed venous oxygen saturation. (See *PA catheter ports*, page 172.)

PAP and PAWP procedures

The doctor inserts the balloon-tipped, multilumen catheter into the patient's internal jugular or subclavian vein. When the catheter reaches the right atrium, the balloon is inflated to float the catheter through the right ventricle into the pulmonary artery. This permits PAWP measurement through an opening at the catheter's tip.

  The deflated catheter rests in the pulmonary artery, allowing diastolic and systolic PAP readings. The balloon should be totally deflated except when taking a PAWP reading because prolonged wedging can cause pulmonary infarction. (See *Normal PA waveforms*, page 173.)

Nursing considerations
• Inform the patient he'll be conscious during catheterization and he may feel temporary local discomfort from the administration of the local anesthetic. Catheter insertion takes about 30 minutes.
• After catheter insertion, you may inflate the balloon with a syringe to take PAWP readings. Be careful not to inflate the balloon

> PA catheters have up to six lumens, so various hemodynamic information can be gathered.

PA catheter ports

A pulmonary artery (PA) catheter contains several lumen ports to allow various catheter functions:

• The balloon inflation lumen inflates the balloon at the distal tip of the catheter for pulmonary artery wedge pressure (PAWP) measurement.

• A distal lumen measures PA pressure when connected to a transducer and measures PAWP during balloon inflation. It also permits drawing of mixed venous blood samples.

• A proximal lumen measures right atrial pressure (central venous pressure).

• The thermistor connector lumen contains temperature-sensitive wires, which feed information into a computer for cardiac output calculation.

• Another lumen may provide a port for pacemaker electrodes or measurement of mixed venous oxygen saturation ($S\tilde{v}o_2$).

Five-lumen PA catheter

Balloon inflation lumen

Distal lumen

Proximal lumen

Thermistor connector lumen

Lumen for pacemaker electrodes or measuring $S\tilde{v}o_2$

with more than 1.5 cc of air. Overinflation could distend the pulmonary artery causing vessel rupture. Don't leave the balloon wedged for a prolonged period because this could lead to a pulmonary infarction.

• After each PAWP reading, flush the line; if you encounter difficulty, notify the doctor.

• Maintain 300 mm Hg pressure in the pressure bag to permit a flush flow of 3 to 6 ml/hour.

• If fever develops when the catheter is in place, inform the doctor; he may remove the catheter and send its tip to the laboratory for culture.

• Make sure stopcocks are properly positioned and connections are secure. Loose connections may introduce air into the system or cause blood backup, leakage of deoxygenated blood, or inaccurate pressure readings. Also make sure the lumen hubs are properly identified to serve the appropriate catheter ports.

Normal PA waveforms

During pulmonary artery (PA) catheter insertion, the waveforms on the monitor change as the catheter advances through the heart.

Right atrium

When the catheter tip enters the right atrium, the first heart chamber on its route, a waveform like the one shown below appears on the monitor. Note the two small upright waves. The *a* waves represent the right ventricular end-diastolic pressure; the *v* waves, right atrial filling.

Right ventricle

As the catheter tip reaches the right ventricle, you'll see a waveform with sharp systolic upstrokes and lower diastolic dips, as shown below.

Pulmonary artery

The catheter then floats into the pulmonary artery, causing a pulmonary artery pressure (PAP) waveform such as the one shown below. Note that the upstroke is smoother than on the right ventricle waveform. The dicrotic notch indicates pulmonic valve closure.

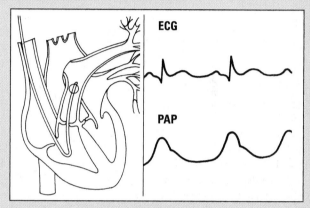

PAWP

Floating into a distal branch of the pulmonary artery, the balloon wedges where the vessel becomes too narrow for it to pass. The monitor now shows a pulmonary artery wedge pressure (PAWP) waveform, with two small upright waves, as shown below. The *a* wave represents left ventricular end-diastolic pressure, the *v* wave, left atrial filling. The balloon is then deflated and the catheter is left in the pulmonary artery.

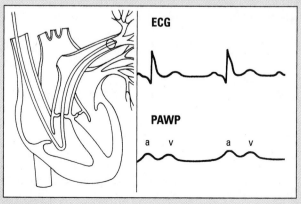

• Because the catheter can slip back into the right ventricle and irritate it, check the monitor for a right ventricular waveform to detect this problem promptly.

• To minimize valvular trauma, make sure the balloon is deflated whenever the catheter is withdrawn from the pulmonary artery to the right ventricle or from the right ventricle to the right atrium.

• Adhere to your facility's policy for dressing, tubing, catheter, and flush changes.

• Document the date and time of catheter insertion, the doctor who performed the procedure, the catheter insertion site, pressure waveforms and values for the various heart chambers, balloon inflation volume required to obtain a wedge tracing, arrhythmias that occured during or after the procedure, type of flush solution used and its heparin concentration (if any), type of dressing applied, and the patient's tolerance of the procedure.

Cardiac output monitoring

Cardiac output—the amount of blood ejected by the heart in one minute—is monitored to evaluate cardiac function. The normal range for cardiac output is 4 to 8 L/minute.

The most widely used method for monitoring cardiac output is the bolus thermodilution technique. Other methods include the Fick method and the dye dilution test. (See *Calculating cardiac output.*)

On the rocks or room temperature

To measure cardiac output, a solution is injected into the right atrium through a port on a PA catheter. Iced or room-temperature injectant may be used depending on your facility's policy and on the patient's status.

> One way to calculate the patient's cardiac output is to use the Fick method.

Calculating cardiac output

One way to calculate cardiac output (CO) is by using the Fick method. In this method, the blood's oxygen content is measured before and after it passes through the lungs. First, blood is removed from the pulmonary and brachial arteries and analyzed for oxygen content. Next, a spirometer is used to measure oxygen consumption (the amount of air entering the lungs each minute).

Use this formula to calculate CO:

$$CO \text{ (L/minute)} = \frac{\text{oxygen consumption (ml/minute)}}{\text{arterial oxygen content} - \text{venous oxygen content (ml/minute)}}$$

This indicator solution mixes with the blood as it travels through the right ventricle into the pulmonary artery, and a thermistor on the catheter registers the change in temperature of the flowing blood. A computer then plots the temperature change over time as a curve and calculates flow based on the area under the curve.

To be continued

Some PA catheters contain a filament that permits continuous cardiac output monitoring. Using such a device, an average cardiac output value is determined over a 3-minute span; the value is updated every 30 to 60 seconds. This type of monitoring allows close scrutiny of the patient's hemodynamic status and prompt intervention in case problems arise.

Better assessor

Cardiac output is better assessed by calculating cardiac index, which takes body size into account. To calculate the patient's cardiac index, divide his cardiac output by his body surface area, a function of height and weight. The normal cardiac index for adults ranges from 2.5 to 4.2 L/minute/m^2; for pregnant women, 3.5 to 6.5 L/minute/m^2.

Continuous cardiac output monitoring allows close scrutiny of the patient's hemodynamic status.

Nursing considerations
• Make sure your patient doesn't move during the procedure because movement can cause an error in measurement.
• Perform cardiac output measurements and monitoring at least every 2 to 4 hours, especially if the patient is receiving vasoactive or inotropic agents or if fluids are being added or restricted.
• Discontinue cardiac output measurements when the patient is hemodynamically stable and weaned from his vasoactive and inotropic medications.
• Monitor the patient for signs and symptoms of inadequate perfusion, including restlessness, fatigue, changes in level of consciousness (LOC), decreased capillary refill time, diminished peripheral pulses, oliguria, and pale, cool skin.
• Add the fluid volume injected for cardiac output determinations to the patient's total intake.
• Record the patient's cardiac output, cardiac index, and other hemodynamic values and vital signs at the time of measurement. Note the patient's position during measurement.

Treatments

Many treatments are available for patients with cardiovascular disease; the dramatic ones, such as heart transplantation and the artificial heart, have received a lot of publicity. Commonly used treatment measures include drug therapy, surgery, balloon catheter treatments, and other treatments, such as defibrillation, synchronized cardioversion, and pacemaker insertion.

Drug therapy

Types of drugs used to improve cardiovascular function include cardiac glycosides and phosphodiesterase (PDE) inhibitors, antiarrhythmic drugs, antianginal drugs, antihypertensive drugs, diuretic drugs, adrenergic drugs, and beta-adrenergic blockers.

Cardiac glycosides and PDE inhibitors

Cardiac glycosides and PDE inhibitors increase the force of the heart's contractions.

More force

Increasing the force of contractions is known as a *positive inotropic effect*, so these drugs are also called *inotropic agents* (effecting the force or energy of muscular contractions). (See *Understanding cardiac glycosides and PDE inhibitors*.)

Slower rate

Cardiac glycosides, such as digoxin, also slow the heart rate (called a *negative chronotropic effect*) and slow electrical impulse conduction through the AV node (called a *negative dromotropic effect*).

The short and long of it

PDE inhibitors, such as inamrinone (Inocor) and milrinone (Primacor), are typically used for short-term management of heart failure or long-term management in patients awaiting heart transplant surgery.

Boosting output

PDE inhibitors improve cardiac output by strengthening contractions. These drugs are thought to help move calcium into the cardiac cell or to increase calcium storage in the sarcoplasmic reticulum.

Cardiac glycosides and PDE inhibitors increase the force of the heart's contractions.

Understanding cardiac glycosides and PDE inhibitors

Cardiac glycosides and phosphodiesterase (PDE) inhibitors have a positive inotropic effect on the heart, meaning they increase the force of contraction. Use this table to learn about the indications, adverse reactions, and practice pointers associated with these drugs.

Drugs	Indications	Adverse reactions	Practice pointers
Cardiac glycoside			
Digoxin	Heart failure, supraventricular arrhythmias	• Digoxin toxicity (nausea, abdominal pain, headache, irritability, depression, insomnia, vision disturbances, arrhythmias)	• If immediate effects are required (as with a supraventricular arrhythmia), a loading dose of digoxin is required. • Check apical pulse for 1 minute before administration; report pulse less than 60 beats/minute. • Therapeutic serum levels are 0.5 to 2 ng/ml.
PDE inhibitors			
Inamrinone, milrinone	Heart failure refractory to digoxin, diuretics, and vasodilators	• Arrhythmias • Nausea • Vomiting • Headache • Fever • Chest pain • Hypokalemia • Thrombocytopenia • Mild increase in heart rate	• These drugs are contraindicated in patients in the acute phase of myocardial infarction (MI) and after an MI. • Serum potassium levels should be within normal limits before and during therapy.

By directly relaxing vascular smooth muscle, they also decrease peripheral vascular resistance (afterload) and the amount of blood returning to the heart (preload).

Antiarrhythmics

Antiarrhythmic drugs are used to treat arrhythmias, which are disturbances of the normal heart rhythm. (See *Understanding antiarrhythmics*, pages 178 and 179.)

Benefits vs. risks

Unfortunately, many antiarrhythmic drugs can worsen or cause arrhythmias, too. In any case, the benefits of antiarrhythmic therapy need to be weighed against its risks.

Understanding antiarrhythmics

Antiarrhythmics are used to restore normal heart rhythm in patients with arrhythmias. Check this table for information about the indications, adverse reactions, and practice pointers associated with these drugs.

Drugs	Indications	Adverse reactions	Practice pointers
Class IA antiarrhythmics			
Disopyramide phosphate, procainamide hydrochloride, quinidine sulfate, quinidine gluconate	• Ventricular tachycardia • Atrial fibrillation • Atrial flutter • Paroxysmal atrial tachycardia	• Diarrhea • Abdominal cramping • Nausea • Vomiting • Anorexia • Bitter taste	• Check apical pulse rate before therapy. If you note extremes in pulse rate, hold the dose and notify the doctor. • Use cautiously in patients with asthma.
Class IB antiarrhythmics			
Lidocaine, mexiletine, tocainide	• Ventricular tachycardia, ventricular fibrillation	• Drowsiness • Light-headedness • Paresthesia • Sensory disturbances • Hypotension • Bradycardia	• IB antiarrhythmics may potentiate the effects of other antiarrhythmics. • Administer I.V. infusions using an infusion pump.
Class IC antiarrhythmics			
Flecainide, moricizine, propafenone	• Ventricular tachycardia, ventricular fibrillation, supraventricular arrhythmias	• New arrhythmias • Bronchospasm (propafenone)	• Correct electrolyte imbalances before administration. • Monitor the patient's electrocardiogram before and after dosage adjustments.
Class II antiarrhythmics			
Acebutolol, esmolol, propranolol	• Atrial flutter, atrial fibrillation, paroxysmal atrial tachycardia	• Arrhythmias • Bradycardia • Heart failure • Hypotension • Nausea and vomiting • Diarrhea • Bronchostriction	• Monitor apical heart rate and blood pressure. • Abruptly stopping these drugs can exacerbate angina and precipitate myocardial infarction.

Understanding antiarrhythmics *(continued)*

Drugs	Indications	Adverse reactions	Practice pointers
Class III antiarrhythmics			
Amiodarone	• Life-threatening arrhythmias resistant to other antiarrhythmics	• Aggravation of arrhythmias • Hypotension • Anorexia • Severe pulmonary toxicity	• Amiodarone increases the risk of digoxin toxicity in patients also taking digoxin. • Monitor blood pressure, heart rate, and rhythm for changes. • Monitor for signs of pulmonary toxicity (dyspnea, nonproductive cough, and pleuritic chest pain).
Class IV antiarrhythmics			
Diltiazem, verapamil	• Supraventricular arrhythmias	• Dizziness • Peripheral edema • Hypotension • Bradycardia • AV block • Flushing (with diltiazem)	• Monitor heart rate and rhythm and blood pressure carefully when initiating therapy or increasing dose. • Calcium supplements may reduce effectiveness.
Miscellaneous			
Adenosine	• Paroxysmal supraventricular tachycardia	• Facial flushing • Shortness of breath • Dyspnea • Chest discomfort	• Adenosine must be administered over 1 to 2 seconds, followed by a 20 ml flush of normal saline solution. • Record rhythm strip during administration.

Four classes plus...

Antiarrhythmics are categorized into four major classes: I (which includes IA, IB, and IC), II, III, and IV. The mechanisms of action of antiarrhythmic drugs vary widely, and a few drugs exhibit properties common to more than one class. One drug, adenosine, doesn't fall into any of these classes.

Class I antiarrhythmics

Class I antiarrhythmics are sodium channel blockers. This is the largest group of antiarrhythmic drugs. Class I agents are commonly subdivided into classes IA, IB, and IC.

Class IA antiarrhythmics

Class IA antiarrhythmics control arrhythmias by altering the myocardial cell membrane and interfering with autonomic nervous system control of pacemaker cells. Class IA antiarrhythmics include:

- disopyramide (Norpace)
- procainamide (Procanbid, Pronestyl)
- quinidine sulfate (Quinidex)
- quinidine gluconate (Quinaglute).

Class IA antiarrhythmics block parasympathetic stimulation and increase the conduction rate of the AV node.

No (para)sympathy

Class IA antiarrhythmics also block parasympathetic stimulation of the SA and AV nodes. Because stimulation of the parasympathetic nervous system causes the heart rate to slow down, drugs that block the parasympathetic nervous system increase the conduction rate of the AV node.

Rhythmic risks

This increase in the conduction rate can produce dangerous increases in the ventricular heart rate if rapid atrial activity is present, as in a patient with atrial fibrillation. In turn, the increased ventricular heart rate can offset the ability of the antiarrhythmics to convert atrial arrhythmias to a regular rhythm.

Class IB antiarrhythmics

Lidocaine (Xylocaine), a class IB antiarrhythmic, is one of the antiarrhythmics commonly used in treating patients with acute ventricular arrhythmias. Other IB antiarrhythmics include mexiletine (Mexitil) and tocainide (Tonocard).

Class IB drugs work by blocking the rapid influx of sodium ions during the depolarization phase of the heart's depolarization-repolarization cycle, resulting in a decreased refractory period, which reduces the risk of arrhythmia.

Class IC antiarrhythmics are used to treat patients with certain severe ventricular arrhythmias.

Make a IB-line for the ventricle

Because class IB antiarrhythmics especially affect the Purkinje fibers (fibers in the conducting system of the heart) and myocardial cells in the ventricles, they're used only in treating patients with ventricular arrhythmias.

Class IC antiarrhythmics

Class IC antiarrhythmics are used to treat patients with certain severe, refractory (resistant) ventricular arrhythmias. Class IC antiarrhythmics include flecainide (Tambocor), moricizine (Ethmozine), and propafenone (Rythmol).

Slowing the seeds of conduction

Class IC antiarrhythmics primarily slow conduction along the heart's conduction system. Moricizine decreases the fast inward current of sodium ions of the action potential. This depresses the depolarization rate and effective refractory period.

Class II antiarrhythmics

Class II antiarrhythmics include the beta-adrenergic antagonists, also known as beta-adrenergic blockers. Beta-adrenergic blockers used as antiarrhythmics include:
- acebutolol (Sectral)
- esmolol (Brevibloc)
- propranolol (Inderal).

Receptor blockers

Class II antiarrhythmics block beta-adrenergic receptor sites in the conduction system of the heart. As a result, the ability of the SA node to fire spontaneously (automaticity) is slowed. The ability of the AV node and other cells to receive and conduct an electrical impulse to nearby cells (conductivity) is also reduced.

Strength reducers

Class II antiarrhythmics also reduce the strength of the heart's contractions. When the heart beats less forcefully, it doesn't require as much oxygen to do its work.

Class III antiarrhythmics

Class III antiarrhythmics are used to treat patients with ventricular arrhythmias. Amiodarone is the most widely used class III antiarrhythmic.

One-way to two-way

Although the exact mechanism of action isn't known, class III antiarrhythmics are thought to suppress arrhythmias by converting a unidirectional block to a bidirectional block. They have little or no effect on depolarization.

Class IV antiarrhythmics

The class IV antiarrhythmics include the calcium channel blockers. These drugs block the movement of calcium during phase 2 of the action potential and slow conduction and the refractory period of calcium-dependent tissues, including the AV node. The calcium channel blockers used to treat patients with arrhythmias are verapamil (Calan) and diltiazem (Cardizem).

Adenosine

Adenosine (Adenocard) is an injectable antiarrhythmic drug indicated for acute treatment for paroxysmal supraventricular tachycardia.

Depressing the pacemaker

Adenosine depresses the pacemaker activity of the SA node, reducing the heart rate and the ability of the AV node to conduct impulses from the atria to the ventricles.

Antianginal drugs

When the oxygen demands of the heart exceed the amount of oxygen being supplied, areas of heart muscle become ischemic (not receiving enough oxygen). When the heart muscle is ischemic, a person experiences chest pain. This condition is known as *angina* or *angina pectoris*.

Reduce demand, increase supply

Although angina's cardinal symptom is chest pain, the drugs used to treat angina aren't typically analgesics. Instead, antianginal drugs correct angina by reducing myocardial oxygen demand (the amount of oxygen the heart needs to do its work), increasing the supply of oxygen to the heart, or both.

The top three

The three classes of commonly used antianginal drugs include:
- nitrates (for acute angina)
- beta-adrenergic blockers (for long-term prevention of angina)
- calcium channel blockers (used when other drugs fail to prevent angina). (See *Understanding antianginal drugs*.)

Nitrates

Nitrates are the drug of choice for relieving acute angina. Nitrates commonly prescribed to correct angina include:
- isosorbide dinitrate (Isordil)
- isosorbide mononitrate (Imdur)
- nitroglycerin (Nitro-Bid).

Anti-angina effect

Nitrates cause the smooth muscle of the veins and, to a lesser extent, the arteries to relax and dilate. This is what happens:
- When the veins dilate, less blood returns to the heart.
- This, in turn, reduces the amount of blood in the ventricles at the end of diastole, when the ventricles are full. (This blood volume in the ventricles just before contraction is called *preload*.)

Angina occurs when I don't receive enough oxygen.

Nitrates cause veins and arteries to relax and dilate, so more blood is delivered to the myocardium.

Understanding antianginal drugs

Antianginal drugs are effective in treating patients with angina because they reduce myocardial oxygen demand, increase the supply of oxygen to the heart, or both. Use this table to learn about the indications, adverse reactions, and practice pointers associated with these drugs.

Drugs	Indications	Adverse reactions	Practice pointers
Nitrates			
Isosorbide dinitrate, isosorbide mononitrate, nitroglycerin	• Relief and prevention of angina	• Headache • Hypotension • Dizziness • Increased heart rate	• Only sublingual and translingual forms should be used to treat an acute angina attack. • Monitor the patient's blood pressure before and after administration.
Beta-adrenergic blockers			
Atenolol, metoprolol tartrate, nadolol, propranolol	• Long-term prevention of angina • First-line therapy for hypertension	• Bradycardia • Fainting • Fluid retention • Shock • Heart failure • Arrhythmias • Angina • Nausea • Vomiting • Diarrhea • Bronchial constriction	• Monitor apical pulse rate before administration. Monitor blood pressure, electrocardiogram, and heart rate and rhythm frequently. • Signs of hypoglycemic shock may be masked; watch diabetic patients for sweating, fatigue, and hunger.
Calcium channel blockers			
Amlodipine, diltiazem, nicardipine, nifedipine, verapamil	• Long-term prevention of angina (especially Prinzmetal's angina)	• Orthostatic hypotension • Heart failure • Hypotension • Arrhythmias • Dizziness • Headache • Flushing • Weakness • Persistent peripheral edema	• Monitor cardiac rate and rhythm and blood pressure carefully when initiating therapy or increasing the dose. • Calcium supplementation may decrease the effects of calcium channel blockers.

- By reducing preload, nitrates reduce ventricular size and ventricular wall tension so the left ventricle doesn't have to stretch as much to pump blood. This, in turn, reduces the oxygen requirements of the heart.
- As the coronary arteries dilate, more blood is delivered to the myocardium, improving oxygenation of the ischemic tissue.

Reducing resistance

The arterioles provide the most resistance to the blood pumped by the left ventricle (called *peripheral vascular resistance*). Nitrates decrease afterload by dilating the arterioles, reducing resistance, easing the heart's workload, and easing oxygen demand.

Beta-adrenergic blockers

Beta-adrenergic blockers are used for long-term prevention of angina, and are one of the main types of drugs used to treat hypertension. Beta-adrenergic blockers include:

- atenolol (Tenormin)
- metoprolol (Lopressor)
- nadolol (Corgard)
- propranolol (Inderal).

Down with everything

Beta-adrenergic blockers decrease blood pressure and block beta-adrenergic receptor sites in the heart muscle and conduction system, decreasing heart rate and reducing the force of the heart's contractions, resulting in lower demand for oxygen.

Calcium channel blockers

Calcium channel blockers are commonly used to prevent angina that doesn't respond to drugs in either of the other antianginal classes. Some calcium channel blockers are also used as antiarrhythmics.

Calcium channel blockers include:

- amlodipine (Norvasc)
- diltiazem (Cardizem)
- nicardipine (Cardene)
- nifedipine (Adalat)
- verapamil (Calan SR).

Preventing passage

Calcium channel blockers prevent the passage of calcium ions across the myocardial cell membrane and vascular smooth muscle cells. This causes dilation of the coronary and peripheral arteries, which decreases the force of the heart's contractions and reduces the workload of the heart.

Rate reduction

By preventing arterioles from constricting, calcium channel blockers also reduce afterload. In addition, decreasing afterload decreases oxygen demands of the heart.

Calcium channel blockers also reduce the heart rate by slowing conduction through the SA and AV nodes. A slower heart rate reduces the heart's need for oxygen.

Calcium channel blockers reduce heart rate, which reduces the heart's need for oxygen.

Antihypertensive drugs

Antihypertensive drugs, which act to reduce blood pressure, are used to treat patients with hypertension, a disorder characterized by high systolic blood pressure, diastolic blood pressure, or both.

Know the program

Treatment for hypertension begins with beta-adrenergic blockers and diuretics. If those drugs aren't effective, treatment continues with sympatholytic drugs (other than beta-adrenergic blockers), vasodilators, angiotensin-converting enzyme (ACE) inhibitors, angiotensin receptor blockers, or a combination of drugs. (See *Understanding antihypertensives*, page 186.)

Sympatholytic drugs

The sympatholytic drugs include several different types of drugs, but work by inhibiting or blocking the sympathetic nervous system, which causes dilation of the peripheral blood vessels or decreases cardiac output, thereby reducing blood pressure.

The sympatholytic drugs are classified by their site or mechanism of action and include:
- central-acting sympathetic nervous system inhibitors, such as clonidine (Catapres), guanabenz (Wytensin), guanfacine (Tenex), and methyldopa (Aldomet)
- alpha blockers, such as doxazosin (Cardura), phentolamine (Regitine), prazosin (Minipress), and terazosin (Hytrin)
- mixed alpha- and beta-adrenergic blockers such as labetalol (Normodyne)
- norepinephrine depletors, such as guanadrel (Hylorel) and guanethidine (Ismelin).

Sympatholytic drugs reduce blood pressure by blocking the sympathetic nervous system.

Vasodilating drugs

The two types of vasodilating drugs include calcium channel blockers and direct vasodilators. These drugs decrease systolic and diastolic blood pressure.

Understanding antihypertensives

Antihypertensives are prescribed to reduce blood pressure in patients with hypertension. Use this table to learn about the indications, adverse reactions, and practice pointers associated with these drugs.

Drugs	Indications	Adverse reactions	Practice pointers
Sympatholytic drugs			
Central-acting sympathetic nervous system inhibitors (such as clonidine, guanabenz, guanfacine, and methyldopa) *Alpha blockers* (such as doxazosin, phentolamine, prazosin, and terazosin) *Mixed alpha- and beta-adrenergic blockers* (such as labetalol) *Norepinephrine depletors* (such as guanadrel and guanethidine)	• Hypertension	• Hypotension (alpha blockers) • Depression • Drowsiness • Edema • Vertigo (central-acting drugs)	• Monitor blood pressure before and after administration.
Vasodilators			
Diazoxide, hydralazine, minoxidil, nitroprusside	• Used in combination with other drugs to treat moderate to severe hypertension	• Vasoconstriction • Tachycardia • Palpitations • Angina • Edema • Breast tenderness • Fatigue • Headache • Rash • Severe pericardial effusion	• Monitor blood pressure before and after administration.
Angiotensin-converting enzyme inhibitors			
Benazepril, captopril, enalapril, fosinopril, lisinopril, quinapril, ramipril	• Hypertension • Heart failure	• Headache • Fatigue • Angioedema • Increased serum potassium concentrations • Persistent cough	• Monitor blood pressure before and after administration.

Calcium stoppers

Calcium channel blockers produce arteriolar relaxation by preventing the entry of calcium into the cells. This prevents the contraction of vascular smooth muscle.

Direct dilators

Direct vasodilators act on arteries, veins, or both. They work by relaxing peripheral vascular smooth muscles, causing the blood vessels to dilate. This decreases blood pressure by increasing the diameter of the blood vessels, reducing total peripheral resistance.

The direct vasodilators include:
- hydralazine (Apresoline)
- minoxidil (Loniten)
- diazoxide (Hyperstat IV)
- nitroprusside (Nitropress).

Hydralazine and minoxidil are usually used to treat patients with resistant or refractory hypertension. Diazoxide and nitroprusside are reserved for use in hypertensive crisis.

ACE inhibitors

ACE inhibitors reduce blood pressure by interrupting the renin-angiotensin-aldosterone system.

Commonly prescribed ACE inhibitors include:
- benazepril (Lotensin)
- captopril (Capoten)
- enalapril (Vasotec)
- fosinopril (Monopril)
- lisinopril (Prinivil)
- quinapril (Accupril)
- ramipril (Altace).

Without ACE interference

Here's how the renin-angiotensin-aldosterone system works:
- Normally, the kidneys maintain blood pressure by releasing the hormone renin.
- Renin acts on the plasma protein angiotensinogen to form angiotensin I.
- Angiotensin I is then converted to angiotensin II.
- Angiotensin II, a potent vasoconstrictor, increases peripheral resistance and promotes the excretion of aldosterone.
- Aldosterone, in turn, promotes the retention of sodium and water, increasing the volume of blood the heart needs to pump.

Vasodilators cause the blood vessels to dilate, which decreases blood pressure.

ACE inhibitors reduce blood pressure by interrupting the renin-angiotensin-aldosterone system.

With ACE interference

ACE inhibitors work by preventing the conversion of angiotensin I to angiotensin II. As angiotensin II is reduced, arterioles dilate, reducing peripheral vascular resistance.

Less water, less work

By reducing aldosterone secretion, ACE inhibitors promote the excretion of sodium and water, reducing the amount of blood the heart needs to pump, resulting in a lowered blood pressure.

Angiotensin II receptor antagonists

Unlike ACE inhibitors, which prevent production of angiotensin, angiotensin II receptor antagonists block the action of angiotensin II by attaching to tissue-binding receptor sites.

Diuretics

Diuretics are used to promote the excretion of water and electrolytes by the kidneys. By doing so, diuretics play a major role in treating hypertension and other cardiovascular conditions. (See *Understanding diuretics*.)

The major diuretics used as cardiovascular drugs include:
- thiazide and thiazide-like diuretics
- loop diuretics
- potassium-sparing diuretics.

Thiazide and thiazide-like diuretics

Thiazide and thiazide-like diuretics are sulfonamide derivatives. Thiazide diuretics include bendroflumethiazide (Naturetin), benzthiazide (Exna), hydrochlorothiazide (HydroDIURIL), hydroflumethiazide (Diucardin), methyclothiazide (Aquatensen), polythiazide (Renese), and trichlormethiazide (Diurese). Thiazide-like diuretics include chlorthalidone (Hygroton) and indapamide (Lozol).

Sodium stoppers

Thiazide and thiazide-like diuretics work by preventing sodium from being reabsorbed in the kidney. As sodium is excreted, it pulls water along with it. Thiazide and thiazide-like diuretics also increase the excretion of chloride, potassium, and bicarbonate, which can result in electrolyte imbalances.

Stability with time

Initially, these drugs decrease circulating blood volume, leading to a reduced cardiac output. However, if the therapy is maintained, cardiac output stabilizes, but plasma fluid volume decreases.

Thiazide and thiazide-like diuretics work by preventing sodium reabsorption in the kidney.

Understanding diuretics

Diuretics are used to treat patients with various cardiovascular conditions. They work by promoting the excretion of water and electrolytes by the kidneys. Use this table to learn about the indications, adverse reactions, and practice pointers associated with these drugs.

Drugs	Indications	Adverse reactions	Practice pointers
Thiazide and thiazide-like diuretics			
Bendroflumethiazide, benzthiazide, chlorthalidone, hydrochlorothiazide, hydroflumethiazide, indapamide, methyclothiazide, polythiazide, trichlormethiazide	• Hypertension • Edema	• Hypokalemia • Orthostatic hypotension • Hyponatremia	• Monitor serum potassium levels. • Monitor intake and output. • Monitor blood glucose values in diabetic patients. Thiazide diuretics can cause hyperglycemia.
Loop diuretics			
Bumetanide, ethacrynate sodium, ethacrynic acid, furosemide	• Hypertension • Heart failure • Edema	• Dehydration • Orthostatic hypotension • Hyperuricemia • Hypokalemia • Hypochloremia • Hyponatremia • Hypocalcemia • Hypomagnesemia	• Monitor for signs of excess diuresis (hypotension, tachycardia, poor skin turgor, and excessive thirst). • Monitor blood pressure, heart rate, and intake and output. • Monitor serum electrolyte levels.
Potassium-sparing diuretics			
Amiloride, spironolactone, triamterene	• Edema • Diuretic-induced hypokalemia in patients with heart failure • Cirrhosis • Nephrotic syndrome • Hypertension	• Hyperkalemia	• Monitor electrocardiogram for arrhythmias. • Monitor serum potassium levels. • Monitor intake and output.

Loop diuretics

Loop (high-ceiling) diuretics are highly potent drugs. They include:
- bumetanide (Bumex)
- ethacrynate sodium and ethacrynic acid (Edecrin)
- furosemide (Lasix).

High potency, big risk

The loop diuretics are the most potent diuretics available, producing the greatest volume of diuresis (urine production). They also have a high potential for causing severe adverse reactions.

Bumetanide is the shortest-acting diuretic. It's even 40 times more potent than another loop diuretic, furosemide.

Locating the loop

Loop diuretics receive their name because they act primarily on the thick ascending loop of Henle (the part of the nephron responsible for concentrating urine) to increase the secretion of sodium, chloride, and water. These drugs may also inhibit sodium, chloride, and water reabsorption.

Potassium-sparing diuretics

Potassium-sparing diuretics have weaker diuretic and antihypertensive effects than other diuretics, but they have the advantage of conserving potassium.

The potassium-sparing diuretics include:
- amiloride (Midamor)
- spironolactone (Aldactone)
- triamterene (Dyrenium).

Potassium-sparing diuretics have weaker diuretic and antihypertensive effects than other diuretics.

Potassium-sparing effects

The direct action of the potassium-sparing diuretics on the distal tubule of the kidneys produces:
- increased urinary excretion of sodium and water
- increased excretion of chloride and calcium ions
- decreased excretion of potassium and hydrogen ions.

These effects lead to reduced blood pressure and increased serum potassium levels.

Aping aldosterone

Spironolactone, one of the main potassium-sparing diuretics, is structurally similar to aldosterone and acts as an aldosterone antagonist.

Aldosterone promotes the retention of sodium and water and loss of potassium; spironolactone counteracts these effects by competing with aldosterone for receptor sites. As a result, sodium, chloride, and water are excreted and potassium is retained.

Anticoagulants

Anticoagulants are used to reduce the ability of the blood to clot. (See *Understanding anticoagulants*.) Major categories of antico-

Understanding anticoagulants

Anticoagulants reduce the blood's ability to clot and are included in the treatment plans for many patients with cardiovascular disorders. Use this table to learn about the indications, adverse reactions, and practice pointers associated with these drugs.

Drugs	Indications	Adverse reactions	Practice pointers
Heparins			
Heparin and low-molecular-weight heparins, such as dalteparin and enoxaparin	• Deep vein thrombosis • Embolism prophylaxis • Disseminated intravascular coagulation • Prevention of complications after myocardial infarction (MI)	• Bleeding	• Monitor thromboplastin time; the therapeutic range is $1\frac{1}{2}$ to $2\frac{1}{2}$ times the control. • Monitor the patient for signs of bleeding. • Concomitant administration with nonsteroidal anti-inflammatory drugs, iron dextran, or an antiplatelet drug increases the risk of bleeding. • Protamine sulfate reverses the effects of heparin.
Oral anticoagulants			
Warfarin	• Deep vein thrombosis prophylaxis • Prevention of complications of prosthetic heart valves or diseased mitral valves • Atrial arrhythmias	• Bleeding (may be severe)	• Monitor prothrombin time and International Normalized Ratio in patients receiving warfarin. • Monitor the patient for signs of bleeding. • The effects of oral anticoagulants can be reversed with phytonadione (vitamin K_1).
Antiplatelet drugs			
Aspirin, dipyridamole, sulfinpyrazone, ticlopidine	• Decreases the risk of death post-MI • Prevention of complications of prosthetic heart valves	• GI distress • Bleeding	• Monitor the patient for signs of bleeding. • Aspirin, sulfinpyrazone, and ticlopidine should be taken with meals to prevent GI irritation. • Dipyridamole should be taken with a full glass of fluid at least 1 hour before meals.

agulants include heparin, oral anticoagulants, and antiplatelet drugs.

Heparin

Heparin, prepared commercially from animal tissue, is used to prevent clot formation. Low-molecular-weight heparin, such as dalteparin (Fragmin) and enoxaparin (Lovenox), prevents deep vein thrombosis (a blood clot in the deep veins, usually of the legs) in surgical patients.

No new clots

Because it doesn't affect the synthesis of clotting factors, heparin can't dissolve already formed clots. It does prevent the formation of new thrombi, though. Here's how it works:
• Heparin inhibits the formation of thrombin and fibrin by activating antithrombin III.
• Antithrombin III then inactivates factors IXa, Xa, XIa, and XIIa in the intrinsic and common pathways. The end result is prevention of a stable fibrin clot.
• In low doses, heparin increases the activity of antithrombin III against factor Xa and thrombin and inhibits clot formation. Much larger doses are necessary to inhibit fibrin formation after a clot has formed. This relationship between dose and effect is the rationale for using low-dose heparin to prevent clotting.
• Whole blood clotting time, thrombin time, and partial thromboplastin time are prolonged during heparin therapy. However, these times may be only slightly prolonged with low or ultra-low preventive doses.

Circulate freely

Heparin can be used to prevent clotting when a patient's blood must circulate outside the body through a machine, such as a cardiopulmonary bypass machine or hemodialysis machine.

Oral anticoagulants

Oral anticoagulants alter the ability of the liver to synthesize vitamin K–dependent clotting factors, including prothrombin and factors VII, IX, and X. Clotting factors already in the bloodstream continue to coagulate blood until they become depleted, so anticoagulation doesn't begin immediately.

Warfarin vs. coagulation

The major oral anticoagulant used in the United States is warfarin (Coumadin).

Antiplatelet drugs

Examples of antiplatelet drugs are:
• aspirin
• dipyridamole (Persantine)
• sulfinpyrazone (Anturane)
• ticlopidine (Ticlid).

> Oral anticoagulants alter my ability to synthesize vitamin K–dependent clotting factors.

Thromboembolism prevention

Antiplatelet drugs are used to prevent arterial thromboembolism, especially in patients at risk for MI, stroke, and arteriosclerosis (hardening of the arteries). They interfere with platelet activity in different drug-specific and dose-related ways.

Low dose

Low dosages of aspirin (81 mg/day) appear to inhibit clot formation by blocking the synthesis of prostaglandin, which in turn prevents formation of the platelet-aggregating substance thromboxane A_2. Dipyridamole may inhibit platelet aggregation.

Single dose

Sulfinpyrazone appears to inhibit several platelet functions. At dosages of 400 to 800 mg/day, it lengthens platelet survival; dosages of more than 600 mg/day prolong the patency of arteriovenous shunts used for hemodialysis. A single dose rapidly inhibits platelet aggregation.

Broken bindings

Ticlopidine inhibits the binding of fibrinogen to platelets during the first stage of the clotting cascade.

All right you platelets, break it up!

Thrombolytic drugs

Thrombolytic drugs are used to dissolve a preexisting clot or thrombus, and are commonly used in an acute or emergency situation. They work by converting plasminogen to plasmin, which lyse (dissolves) thrombi, fibrinogen, and other plasma proteins. (See *Understanding thrombolytics*, page 194.)

Some commonly used thrombolytic drugs include:
- alteplase (Activase)
- anistreplase (Eminase)
- reteplase (Retavase)
- streptokinase (Streptase).

Adrenergic drugs

Adrenergic drugs are also called *sympathomimetic drugs* because they produce effects similar to those produced by the sympathetic nervous system.

Classified by chemical

Adrenergic drugs are classified into two groups based on their chemical structure — catecholamines (both naturally occurring

Understanding thrombolytics

Sometimes called *clot busters,* thrombolytic drugs are prescribed to dissolve a preexisting clot or thrombus. These drugs are typically used in acute or emergency situations. Use this table to learn about the indications, adverse reactions, and practice pointers associated with these drugs.

Drugs	Indications	Adverse reactions	Practice pointers
Thrombolytics			
Alteplase, anistreplase, reteplase, streptokinase	• Acute myocardial infarction • Acute ischemic stroke • Pulmonary embolus • Catheter occlusion • Arterial thrombosis	• Bleeding • Allergic reaction	• Monitor partial thromboplastin time, prothrombin time, International Normalized Ratio, hemoglobin, and hematocrit before, during, and after administration. • Monitor vital signs frequently during and immediately after administration. Don't use an automatic blood pressure cuff to monitor blood pressure. • Monitor puncture sites for bleeding. Don't use a tourniquet when obtaining blood specimens. • Monitor for signs of bleeding.

and synthetic) and noncatecholamines. (See *Understanding adrenergics.*)

Which receptor?

Therapeutic use of adrenergic drugs depends on which receptors they stimulate and to what degree. Adrenergic drugs can affect:
- alpha-adrenergic receptors
- beta-adrenergic receptors
- dopamine receptors.

Mimicking norepinephrine and epinephrine

Most of the adrenergic drugs produce their effects by stimulating alpha- and beta-adrenergic receptors. These drugs mimic the action of norepinephrine or epinephrine.

Doing it like dopamine

Dopaminergic drugs act primarily on receptors in the sympathetic nervous system that are stimulated by dopamine.

Catecholamines

Because of their common basic chemical structure, catecholamines share certain properties. They stimulate the nervous sys-

Most adrenergic drugs mimic the action of norepinephrine or epinephrine.

Understanding adrenergics

Adrenergic drugs produce effects similar to those produced by the sympathetic nervous system. Adrenergic drugs can affect alpha-adrenergic receptors, beta-adrenergic receptors, or dopamine receptors. However, most of the drugs stimulate the alpha- and beta-receptors, mimicking the effects of norepinephrine and epinephrine. Dopaminergic drugs act on receptors typically stimulated by dopamine.

Use this table to learn about the indications, adverse reactions, and practice pointers associated with these drugs.

Drugs	Indications	Adverse reactions	Practice pointers
Catecholamines			
Dobutamine	• Increase cardiac output in short-term treatment of cardiac decompensation from depressed contractility	Headache, paresthesia, tingling sensation, bronchospasm, palpitations, tachycardia, cardiac arrhythmias (PVCs), hypotension, hypertension and hypertensive crisis, angina, skin rash, fever, nausea, vomiting, tissue necrosis and sloughing (if catecholamine given I.V. leaks into surrounding tissue)	• Correct hypovolemia before administering drug. • Incompatible with alkaline solution (sodium bicarbonate); don't mix or give through same line; don't mix with other drugs. • Administer continuous drip on infusion pump. • Give drug into a large vein to prevent irritation or extravasation at site. • Monitor cardiac rate and rhythm and blood pressure carefully when initiating therapy or increasing the dose.
Dopamine	• Adjunct in shock to increase cardiac output, blood pressure, and urine flow	Anxiety, headache, paresthesia, tingling sensation, dyspnea, bradycardia, palpitations, tachycardia, conduction disturbance, cardiac arrhythmias (ventricular), hypotension, hypertension and hypertensive crisis, azotemia, angina, skin rash, fever, nausea, vomiting, may elevate serum glucose, gangrene of extremities in high dose, tissue necrosis and sloughing (if catecholamine given I.V. leaks into surrounding tissue)	• Correct hypovolemia before administering drug. • Incompatible with alkaline solution (sodium bicarbonate); don't mix or give through same line; don't mix with other drugs. • Administer continuous drip on infusion pump. • Give drug into a large vein to prevent extravasation, if extravasation occurs, stop infusion and treat site with phentolamine infiltrate to prevent tissue necrosis. • Monitor cardiac rate and rhythm and blood pressure carefully when initiating therapy or increasing the dose.
Epinephrine	• Bronchospasm • Hypersensitivity reactions • Anaphylaxis	Restlessness, anxiety, dizziness, headache, tachycardia, palpitations, cardiac arrhythmias (ventricular fibrillation), hypotension, hypertension and hypertensive crisis, stroke, cerebral hemorrhage, angina,	• Correct hypovolemia before administering drug. • Incompatible with alkaline solution (sodium bicarbonate); don't mix or give through same line; don't mix with other drugs. • Administer continuous drip on infusion pump. • Give drug into a large vein to prevent irritation or extravasation at site.

(continued)

Understanding adrenergics (continued)

Drugs	Indications	Adverse reactions	Practice pointers
Catecholamines (continued)			
Epinephrine (continued)	• Restoration of cardiac rhythm in cardiac arrest	increased blood glucose levels, tissue necrosis and sloughing (if catecholamine given I.V. leaks into surrounding tissue)	• Monitor cardiac rate and rhythm and blood pressure carefully when initiating therapy or increasing the dose.
Norepinephrine	• Maintain blood pressure in acute hypotensive states • GI bleeding	Restlessness, anxiety, dizziness, headache, bradycardia, tachycardia, palpitations, cardiac arrhythmias (ventricular tachycardia and fibrillation), hypotension, hypertension and hypertensive crisis, stroke, cerebral hemorrhage, angina, gangrene of extremities in high doses, tissue necrosis and sloughing (if catecholamine given I.V. leaks into surrounding tissue)	• Correct hypovolemia before administering drug. • Incompatible with alkaline solution (sodium bicarbonate); don't mix or give through same line; don't mix with other drugs. • Administer continuous drip on infusion pump. • Give drug into a large vein to prevent extravasation; if extravasation occurs, stop infusion and treat site with phentolamine infiltrate to prevent tissue necrosis. • Monitor cardiac rate and rhythm and blood pressure carefully when initiating therapy or increasing the dose.
Noncatecholamines			
Ephedrine	• Maintain blood pressure in acute hypotensive states, especially with spinal anesthesia • Treatment of orthostatic hypotension and bronchospasm	Restlessness, anxiety, dizziness, headache, palpitations, cardiac arrhythmias (ventricular fibrillation), hypotension, hypertension, nausea, vomiting	• Correct hypovolemia before administering drug. • Give drug into a large vein to prevent irritation or extravasation at site. • Monitor cardiac rate and rhythm and blood pressure carefully when initiating therapy or increasing the dose.
Phenylephrine	• Maintain blood pressure in hypotensive states, especially hypotensive emergencies with spinal anesthesia	Restlessness, anxiety, dizziness, headache, palpitations, cardiac arrhythmias, hypertension, tissue necrosis and sloughing (if catecholamine given I.V. leaks into surrounding tissue)	• Correct hypovolemia before administering drug. • Don't mix with other drugs. • Administer continuous drip on infusion pump. • Give drug into a large vein to prevent extravasation; if extravasation occurs, stop infusion and treat site with phentolamine infiltrate to prevent tissue necrosis. • Monitor cardiac rate and rhythm and blood pressure carefully when initiating therapy or increasing the dose.

tem, constrict peripheral blood vessels, increase heart rate, and dilate the bronchi. They can be manufactured in the body or in a laboratory. Common catecholamines include:
- dobutamine (Dobutrex)
- dopamine (Intropin)
- epinephrine
- norepinephrine.

Direct-acting and excitatory or inhibitory

Catecholamines are primarily direct-acting. When catecholamines combine with alpha- or beta-receptors, they cause either an excitatory or inhibitory effect. Typically, activation of alpha-receptors generates an excitatory response except for intestinal relaxation. Activation of the beta-receptors mostly produces an inhibitory response except in the cells of the heart, where norepinephrine produces excitatory effects.

How heartening

The clinical effects of catecholamines depend on the dosage and the route of administration. Catecholamines are potent inotropes, meaning they make the heart contract more forcefully. As a result, the ventricles empty more completely with each heartbeat, increasing the workload of the heart and the amount of oxygen it needs to do this harder work.

Rapid rates

Catecholamines also produce a positive chronotropic effect, which means they cause the heart to beat faster. That's because the pacemaker cells in the SA node of the heart depolarize at a faster rate. As catecholamines cause blood vessels to constrict and blood pressure to increase, the heart rate decreases as the body tries to prevent an excessive increase in blood pressure.

Fascinating rhythm

Catecholamines can cause the Purkinje fibers (an intricate web of fibers that carry electrical impulses into the ventricles of the heart) to fire spontaneously, possibly producing abnormal heart rhythms, such as premature ventricular contractions and fibrillation. Epinephrine is likelier than norepinephrine to produce this spontaneous firing.

Noncatecholamines

Noncatecholamine adrenergic drugs have a variety of therapeutic uses because of the many effects these drugs can have on the body, such as the local or systemic constriction of blood vessels by phenylephrine.

Catecholamines make the heart contract more forcefully so the ventricles empty more completely with each heartbeat.

Alpha active

Direct-acting noncatecholamines that stimulate alpha activity include methoxamine and phenylephrine.

Those that selectively exert beta$_2$ activity include:
- albuterol (Proventil)
- isoetharine (Bronkosol)
- metaproterenol (Alupent).

Dual-acting noncatecholamines combine both actions and include ephedrine and mephentermine (Wyamine).

Adrenergic blocking drugs

Adrenergic blocking drugs, also called *sympatholytic drugs*, are used to disrupt sympathetic nervous system function. (See *Understanding adrenergic blockers*.)

Impeding impulses

These drugs work by blocking impulse transmission (and thus sympathetic nervous system stimulation) at adrenergic neurons or adrenergic receptor sites. The action of the drugs at these sites can be exerted by:
- interrupting the action of sympathomimetic (adrenergic) drugs
- reducing available norepinephrine
- preventing the action of cholinergic drugs.

Classified information

Adrenergic blocking drugs are classified according to their site of action as alpha-adrenergic blockers or beta-adrenergic blockers.

Alpha-adrenergic blocking drugs

Alpha-adrenergic blocking drugs work by interrupting the actions of sympathomimetic drugs at alpha-adrenergic receptors. This results in:
- relaxation of the smooth muscle in the blood vessels
- increased dilation of blood vessels
- decreased blood pressure.

Drugs in this class include phentolamine (Regitine) and prazosin (Minipress).

A mixed bag

Ergotamine is a mixed alpha agonist and antagonist. At high doses, it acts as an alpha-adrenergic blocker.

Alpha-adrenergic blockers work in one of two ways:

Adrenergic blocking drugs block impulse transmission, thus disrupting sympathetic nervous system function.

Understanding adrenergic blockers

Adrenergic blockers block impulse transmission at adrenergic receptor sites by interrupting the action of adrenergic drugs, reducing the amount of norepinephrine available, and blocking the action of cholinergics.

Use this table to learn the indications, adverse reactions, and practice pointers needed to safely administer these drugs.

Drugs	Indications	Adverse reactions	Practice pointers
Alpha-adrenergic blockers			
Phentolamine, prazosin	• Hypertension • Peripheral vascular disorders • Pheochromocytoma	Orthostatic hypotension, severe hypertension, bradycardia, tachycardia, edema, difficulty breathing, light-headedness, flushing, arrhythmias, angina, heart attack, shock	• Monitor vital signs and heart rhythm before, during, and after administration. • Instruct the patient to rise slowly to a standing position to avoid orthostatic hypotension.
Beta-adrenergic blockers			
Nonselective Carvedilol, labetalol, nadolol, penbutolol, pindalol, propranolol, sotalol, timolol *Selective* Acebututolol, atenolol, betaxolol, bisoprolol, esmolol, metoprolol	• Prevention of complications after myocardial infarction, angina, hypertension, supraventricular arrhythmias, anxiety, essential tremor, cardiovascular symptoms associated with thyrotoxicosis, migraine headaches, pheochromocytoma	Hypotension, bradycardia, peripheral vascular insufficiency, heart failure, bronchospasm, sore throat, atrioventricular block	• Monitor vital signs and heart rhythm frequently. • Beta-adrenergic blockers can alter the requirements for insulin and oral antidiabetic agents.

They interfere with or block the synthesis, storage, release, and reuptake of norepinephrine by neurons.

They antagonize epinephrine, norepinephrine, or adrenergic (sympathomimetic) drugs at alpha-receptor sites.

Not very discriminating

Alpha-receptor sites are either alpha$_1$ or alpha$_2$ receptors. Alpha-adrenergic blockers include drugs that block stimulation of alpha$_1$ receptors and that may block alpha$_2$ stimulation.

Reducing resistance

Alpha-adrenergic blockers occupy alpha-receptor sites on the smooth muscle of blood vessels.

This prevents catecholamines from occupying and stimulating the receptor sites. As a result, blood vessels dilate, increasing local blood flow to the skin and other organs. The decreased peripheral vascular resistance (resistance to blood flow) helps to decrease blood pressure.

Beta-adrenergic blockers

Beta-adrenergic blockers, the most widely used adrenergic blockers, prevent stimulation of the sympathetic nervous system by inhibiting the action of catecholamines and other sympathomimetic drugs at beta-adrenergic receptors.

Selective (or not)

Beta-adrenergic drugs are selective or nonselective. Nonselective beta-adrenergic drugs affect:
- beta$_1$-receptor sites (located mainly in the heart)
- beta$_2$-receptor sites (located in the bronchi, blood vessels, and the uterus).

Nonselective beta-adrenergic drugs include carvedilol (Coreg), labetalol (Normodyne), nadolol (Corgard), penbutolol (Levatol), pindolol (Visken), propranolol, sotalol (Betapace), and timolol (Blocadren).

Highly discriminating

Selective beta-adrenergic drugs primarily affect the beta$_1$-adrenergic sites. They include acebutolol (Sectral), atenolol (Tenormin), esmolol (Brevibloc), and metoprolol tartrate (Lopressor).

Intrinsically sympathetic

Some beta-adrenergic blockers, such as pindolol and acebutolol, have intrinsic sympathetic activity. This means that instead of attaching to beta-receptors and blocking them, these beta-adrenergic blockers attach to beta-receptors and stimulate them. These drugs are sometimes classified as partial agonists.

Widely effective

Beta-adrenergic blockers have widespread effects in the body because they produce their blocking action not only at the adrenergic nerve endings but also in the adrenal medulla. Effects on the heart include:

- increased peripheral vascular resistance
- decreased blood pressure
- decreased force of contractions of the heart
- decreased oxygen consumption by the heart
- slowed conduction of impulses between the atria and ventricles
- decreased cardiac output.

Selective or nonselective

Some of the effects of beta-adrenergic blocking drugs depend on whether the drug is classified as selective or nonselective. Selective beta-adrenergic blockers, which preferentially block beta$_1$ receptor sites, reduce stimulation of the heart. They're commonly called *cardioselective beta-adrenergic blockers.*

Nonselective beta-adrenergic blockers, which block both beta$_1$ and beta$_2$ receptor sites, reduce stimulation of the heart and cause the bronchioles of the lungs to constrict. This can cause bronchospasm in patients with chronic obstructive lung disorders.

Nonselective beta-adrenergic blockers can cause bronchospasm in a patient with a chronic obstructive lung disorder.

Surgery

Surgeries for treatment of cardiovascular system disorders include coronary artery bypass graft (CABG), heart transplantation, valve surgery, vascular repair, and insertion of a ventricular assist device (VAD).

Coronary artery bypass graft

CABG circumvents an occluded coronary artery with an autogenous graft (usually a segment of the saphenous vein from the leg or internal mammary artery), thereby restoring blood flow to the myocardium.

CABG is one of the most commonly performed surgeries because it's done to prevent MI in a patient with acute or chronic myocardial ischemia. The need for CABG is determined from the results of cardiac catheterization and patient symptoms. (See *Bypassing coronary occlusions*, page 202.)

Why bypass?

If successful, CABG can relieve anginal pain, improve cardiac function, and possibly enhance the patient's quality of life.

CABG varieties

CABG techniques vary according to the patient's condition and the number of arteries being bypassed.

Newer surgical techniques, such as the mini-CABG and direct coronary artery bypass, can reduce the risk for cerebral complica-

Bypassing coronary occlusions

After the patient receives general anesthesia, surgery begins with graft harvesting. The surgeon makes a series of incisions in the patient's thigh or calf and removes a saphenous vein segment for grafting. Most surgeons prefer to use a segment of the internal mammarian artery.

Exposing the heart

Once the autografts are obtained, the surgeon performs a medial sternotomy to expose the heart, and then initiates cardiopulmonary bypass.

To reduce myocardial oxygen demands during surgery and to protect the heart, the surgeon induces cardiac hypothermia and standstill by injecting a cold cardioplegic solution (potassium-enriched saline solution) into the aortic root.

One fine sewing lesson

After the patient is prepared, the surgeon sutures one end of the venous graft to the ascending aorta and the other end to a patent coronary artery that's distal to the occlusion. The graft is sutured in a reversed position to promote proper blood flow. The surgeon repeats this procedure for each occlusion to be bypassed.

In the example depicted below, saphenous vein segments bypass occlusions in three sections of the coronary artery.

Finishing up

Once the grafts are in place, the surgeon flushes the cardioplegic solution from the heart and discontinues cardiopulmonary bypass. He then implants epicardial pacing electrodes, inserts a chest tube, closes the incision, and applies a sterile dressing.

Aorta

Vein segment

Right coronary artery
Occlusion

Anterior descending branch

Vein segments

Occlusion

Left coronary artery

tions and accelerate recovery for patients requiring grafts of only one or two arteries.

In some patients it's possible to perform the CABG procedure without using a heart-lung bypass machine. This increases recovery time but decreases complications.

Nursing considerations

When caring for a CABG patient, your major roles include patient instruction and caring for the patient's changing cardiovascular needs.

Before surgery

- Reinforce the doctor's explanation of the surgery.
- Explain the complex equipment and procedures used in the critical care unit (CCU) or postanesthesia care unit (PACU).
- Explain that the patient awakens from surgery with an endotracheal (ET) tube in place and connected to a mechanical ventilator. He'll also be connected to a cardiac monitor and have in place a nasogastric (NG) tube, a chest tube, an indwelling urinary catheter, arterial lines, epicardial pacing wires and, possibly, a PA catheter. Tell him that discomfort is minimal and that the equipment is removed as soon as possible.
- Review incentive spirometry techniques and range of motion (ROM) exercises with the patient.
- Make sure that the patient or a responsible family member has signed a consent form.
- Before surgery, prepare the patient's skin as ordered.
- Immediately before surgery, begin cardiac monitoring and then assist with PA catheterization and insertion of arterial lines. Some facilities insert PA catheters and arterial lines in the operating room, before surgery.

After surgery

- After CABG, look for signs of hemodynamic compromise, such as severe hypotension, decreased cardiac output, and shock.
- Begin warming procedures according to your facility's policy.
- Check and record vital signs and hemodynamic parameters every 5 to 15 minutes until the patient's condition stabilizes. Administer medications and titrate according to the patient's response, as ordered
- Monitor ECGs continuously for disturbances in heart rate and rhythm. If you detect serious abnormalities, notify the doctor and be prepared to assist with epicardial pacing or, if necessary, cardioversion or defibrillation.
- To ensure adequate myocardial perfusion, keep arterial pressure within the limits set by the doctor. Usually, mean arterial pressure (MAP) less than 70 mm Hg results in inadequate tissue perfusion; pressure greater than 110 mm Hg can cause hemorrhage and graft

After CABG, be ready to assist with epicardial pacing, cardioversion, or defibrillation.

rupture. Monitor PAP, CVP, left atrial pressure, and cardiac output as ordered.

• Frequently evaluate the patient's peripheral pulses, capillary refill time, and skin temperature and color and auscultate for heart sounds; report abnormalities.

• Evaluate tissue oxygenation by assessing breath sounds, chest excursion, and symmetry of chest expansion. Check ABG results every 2 to 4 hours, and adjust ventilator settings to keep ABG values within ordered limits.

• Maintain chest tube drainage at the ordered negative pressure (usually –10 to –40 cm H_2O), and assess regularly for hemorrhage, excessive drainage (greater than 200 ml/hour), and sudden decrease or cessation of drainage.

• Monitor the patient's intake and output, and assess for electrolyte imbalance, especially hypokalemia and hypomagnesemia. Assess urine output at least hourly during the immediate postoperative period and then less frequently as the patient's condition stabilizes.

• As the patient's incisional pain increases, give an analgesic as ordered. Give other drugs as ordered.

• Throughout the recovery period, assess for symptoms of stroke, pulmonary embolism, and impaired renal perfusion.

• After weaning the patient from the ventilator and removing the ET tube, provide chest physiotherapy. Start with incentive spirometry, and encourage the patient to cough, turn frequently, and deep-breathe. Assist with ROM exercises, as ordered, to enhance peripheral circulation and prevent thrombus formation.

• Explain that postpericardiotomy syndrome commonly develops after open-heart surgery. Instruct the patient about signs and symptoms, such as fever, muscle and joint pain, weakness, and chest discomfort.

• Prepare the patient for the possibility of postoperative depression, which may not develop until weeks after discharge. Reassure him that this depression is normal and should pass quickly.

• Maintain nothing-by-mouth status until bowel sounds return. Then begin clear liquids and advance diet as tolerated and as ordered. Expect sodium and cholesterol restrictions. Explain that this diet can help reduce the risk of recurrent arterial occlusion.

Heart transplantation

Heart transplantation involves the replacement of a person's heart with a donor heart. It's the treatment of choice for patients with end-stage cardiac disease who have a poor prognosis, estimated survival of 6 to 12 months, and poor quality of life. A heart transplant can-

After heart transplantation, most patients experience infection, tissue rejection, or both.

didate typically has uncontrolled symptoms and no other surgical options.

No guarantee

Transplantation doesn't guarantee a cure. Serious postoperative complications include infection and tissue rejection. Most patients experience one or both of these complications postoperatively.

Rejection and infection

Rejection typically occurs in the first 6 weeks after surgery. The patient is treated with monoclonal antibodies and potent immuno-suppressants. The resulting immunosuppression places the patient at risk for life-threatening infection.

Nursing considerations

• Provide emotional support to the patient and his family. Begin to address their fears by discussing the procedure, possible complications, and the impact of transplantation and a prolonged recovery period on the patient's life.
• After surgery maintain reverse isolation.
• Administer immunosuppressants and monitor the patient closely for signs of infection. Transplant recipients may exhibit subtle signs because immunosuppressants mask obvious signs.
• Monitor vital signs every 15 minutes until stabilized and assess the patient for signs of hemodynamic compromise, such as hypotension, decreased cardiac output, and shock.
• If necessary, administer nitroprusside during the first 24 to 48 hours to control blood pressure. An infusion of dopamine can improve contractility and renal perfusion.
• Volume replacement with normal saline, plasma expanders, or blood products may be necessary to maintain CVP.
• Your patients with elevated PAP may receive prostaglandin E to produce pulmonary vasodilation and reduced right ventricular afterload.
• Monitor ECG for rhythm disturbances.
• Maintain the chest tube drainage system at the prescribed negative pressure. Regularly assess for hemorrhage or sudden cessation of drainage.
• Continually assess the patient for signs of tissue rejection (decreased electrical activity on the ECG, right axis shift, atrial arrhythmias, conduction defects, weight gain, lethargy, ventricular failure, jugular vein distention, and increased T-cell count).
• Keep in mind that the effects of denervated heart muscle or denervation (in which the vagus nerve is cut during heart transplant surgery) makes such drugs as edrophonium and anticholinergics (such as atropine) ineffective.

Administer volume replacement to maintain central venous pressure.

Types of valve surgery

When a patient with valve disease develops severe symptoms, surgery may be necessary. Several surgical procedures are available.

Commissurotomy

During commissurotomy, the surgeon incises fused mitral valve leaflets and removes calcium deposits to improve valve mobility.

Valve repair

Valve repair includes resection or patching of valve leaflets, stretching or shortening of chordae tendineae, or placing a ring in a dilated annulus (annuloplasty). Valve repair is done to avoid the complications associated with the use of prosthetic valves.

Valve replacement

Valvular replacement involves replacement of the patient's diseased valve with a mechanical or biological valve.

In the Ross procedure, the patient's own pulmonic valve is excised and used to replace the diseased aortic valve. An allograft from a human cadaver is then used to replace the pulmonic valve. Advantages of this procedure include the potential for the pulmonary autograft to grow when used in children, anticoagulation isn't necessary, and increased durability.

Minimally invasive valve surgery

Minimally invasive valve surgery can be performed without a large median sternotomy incision to repair of replace aortic and mitral valves. Port access techniques may also be used for mitral valve surgery using endovascular cardiopulmonary bypass. Advantages of these types of surgery include a less invasive procedure, shorter hospital stays, fewer postoperative complications, reduced costs, and smaller incisions.

> To prevent heart failure, a patient may need a valve replacement or another type of surgical repair.

Valve surgery

To prevent heart failure, a patient with valvular stenosis or insufficiency accompanied by severe, unmanageable symptoms may require valve replacement (with a mechanical or prosthetic valve), valvular repair, or commissurotomy. (See *Types of valve surgery*.)

Why valve surgery?

Because of the high pressure generated by the left ventricle during contraction, stenosis and insufficiency most commonly affect the mitral and aortic valves. Other indications for valve surgery depend on the patient's symptoms and affected valve:

• In aortic insufficiency, the patient undergoes valve replacement after symptoms — palpitations, dizziness, dyspnea on exertion, angina, and murmurs — have developed or if the chest X-ray and ECG reveal left ventricular hypertrophy.

• In aortic stenosis, which may be asymptomatic, the doctor may recommend valve replacement if cardiac catheterization reveals significant stenosis.

• In mitral stenosis, surgery is indicated if the patient develops fatigue, dyspnea, hemoptysis, arrhythmias, pulmonary hypertension, or right ventricular hypertrophy.
• In mitral insufficiency, surgery is usually done when the patient's symptoms — dyspnea, fatigue, and palpitations — interfere with ADLs or if insufficiency is acute, as in papillary muscle rupture.

Nursing considerations
Provide these care measures after valve replacement surgery or balloon valvuloplasty.

After valve replacement surgery
• Closely monitor the patient's hemodynamic status for signs of compromise. Watch especially for severe hypotension, decreased cardiac output, and shock. Check and record vital signs every 15 minutes until his condition stabilizes. Frequently assess heart sounds; report distant heart sounds or new murmurs, which may indicate prosthetic valve failure.
• Monitor the ECG continuously for disturbances in heart rate and rhythm, such as bradycardia, ventricular tachycardia, and heart block. Such disturbances may signal injury of the conduction system, which may occur during valve replacement from proximity of the atrial and mitral valves to the atrioventricular node. Arrhythmias may also result from myocardial irritability or ischemia, fluid and electrolyte imbalance, hypoxemia, or hypothermia. If you detect serious abnormalities, notify the doctor and be prepared to assist with temporary epicardial pacing.
• Take steps to maintain the patient's MAP between 70 and 100 mm Hg. Also, monitor PAP and left atrial pressure as ordered.
• Frequently assess the patient's peripheral pulses, capillary refill time, and skin temperature and color and auscultate for heart sounds. Evaluate tissue oxygenation by assessing breath sounds, chest excursion, and symmetry of chest expansion. Report any abnormalities.
• Check ABG values every 2 to 4 hours, and adjust ventilator settings as needed.
• Maintain chest tube drainage at the prescribed negative pressure (usually –10 to –40 cm H_2O for adults). Assess chest tubes frequently for signs of hemorrhage, excessive drainage (greater than 200 ml/hour), and a sudden decrease or cessation of drainage.
• As ordered, administer analgesic, anticoagulant, antibiotic, antiarrhythmic, inotropic, and pressor medications as well as I.V. fluids and blood products. Monitor intake and output and assess for electrolyte imbalances, especially hypokalemia. When anticoagu-

If you detect serious abnormalities in the patient's heart rate and rhythm, be ready to assist with temporary epicardial pacing.

lant therapy begins, evaluate its effectiveness by monitoring prothrombin time and International Normalized Ratio daily.
• Throughout the patient's recovery period, observe carefully for complications.
• After weaning from the ventilator and removing the ET tube, promote chest physiotherapy. Start the patient on incentive spirometry and encourage him to cough, turn frequently, and deep-breathe.

Vascular repair

Vascular repair may be needed to treat patients with:
• vessels damaged by arteriosclerotic or thromboembolic disorders trauma, infections, or congenital defects
• vascular obstructions that severely compromise circulation
• vascular disease that doesn't respond to drug therapy or nonsurgical treatments such as balloon catheterization
• life-threatening dissecting or ruptured aortic aneurysms
• limb-threatening acute arterial occlusion.

Repair review

Vascular repair methods include aneurysm resection, grafting, embolectomy, vena caval filtering, and endarterectomy. The surgery used depends on the type, location, and extent of vascular occlusion or damage. (See *Types of vascular repair.*)

Nursing considerations

Provide care measures before and after vascular repair surgery.

Before surgery

• Make sure the patient and his family understand the doctor's explanation of the surgery and possible complications.
• Tell the patient that he'll receive a general anesthetic and will awaken from the anesthetic in the CCU or PACU. Explain that he'll have an I.V. line in place, ECG electrodes for continuous cardiac monitoring, and possibly an arterial line or a PA catheter to provide continuous pressure monitoring. He may also have a urinary catheter in place to allow accurate output measurement. If appropriate, explain that he'll be intubated and placed on mechanical ventilation.

You'll receive a general anesthetic before surgery,

Flow check

• Before surgery, perform a complete vascular assessment. Take vital signs to provide a baseline. Evaluate the strength and sound of the blood flow and the symmetry of the pulses, and note bruits. Record the temperature of the extremities, their sensitivity to mo-

Types of vascular repair

There are several surgical options to repair damaged or diseased vessels. Some of these options are aortic aneurysm repair, vena caval filter insertion, embolectomy, and bypass grafting.

Aortic aneurysm repair

Aortic aneurysm repair is done to remove an aneurysmal segment of the aorta. The surgeon first makes an incision to expose the aneurysm site. The patient is placed on a cardio-pulmonary bypass ma-chine, if necessary. The surgeon then clamps the aorta. The aneurysm is resected and the dam-aged portion of the aorta is repaired.

Vena caval filter insertion

A vena caval filter is in-serted to trap emboli in the vena cava, prevent-ing them from reaching the pulmonary vessels. A vena caval filter or umbrella is inserted transvenously by catheter. Once in place in the vena cava, the umbrella or filter traps emboli but allows ve-nous blood flow.

Umbrella

Direction of blood flow

Embolectomy

An embolectomy is done to re-move an embolism from an artery. During this procedure, the surgeon inserts a balloon-tipped indwelling catheter into the artery and passes it through the thrombus (top). He then inflates the balloon and withdraws the catheter to re-move the thrombus (bottom).

Indwelling catheter
Thrombus
Balloon

Direction of blood flow
Balloon
Thrombus
Indwelling catheter

Bypass grafting

Bypass grafting is used to by-pass an arterial obstruction re-sulting from arteriosclerosis. After exposing the affected artery, the surgeon anasto-moses a synthetic or autoge-nous graft to divert blood flow around the occluded arterial segment. The autogenous graft may be a vein or artery har-vested from elsewhere in the patient's body. A femoro-popliteal bypass is depicted.

tor and sensory stimuli, and pallor, cyanosis, or redness. Rate pe-ripheral pulse volume and strength on a scale of 0 (pulse absent) to 4 (bounding and strong pulse), and check capillary refill time by blanching the fingernail or toenail; normal refill time is less than 3 seconds.

• As ordered, instruct the patient to restrict food and fluids for at least 12 hours before surgery.

Be on guard!

• If the patient is awaiting surgery for aortic aneurysm repair, be on guard for signs and symptoms of acute dissection or rupture. Note especially sudden severe pain in the chest, abdomen, or lower back; severe weakness; diaphoresis; tachycardia; or a precipitous drop in blood pressure. If any of these occur, notify the doctor immediately.

After surgery
• Check and record the patient's vital signs every 15 minutes until his condition stabilizes; then every 30 minutes for 1 hour, and hourly thereafter for 2 to 4 hours. Report hypotension and hypertension immediately.
• Auscultate heart, breath, and bowel sounds and report abnormal findings. Monitor the ECG for abnormalities in heart rate or rhythm. Also monitor other pressure readings and carefully record intake and output.
• Check the patient's dressing regularly for excessive bleeding.
• Assess the patient's neurologic and renal function and report abnormalities.
• Provide analgesics, as ordered, for incisional pain.
• Frequently assess peripheral pulses, using Doppler ultrasonography if palpation is difficult. Check all extremities bilaterally for muscle strength and movement, color, temperature, and capillary refill time.
• Change dressings and provide incision care, as ordered. Position the patient to avoid pressure on grafts and to reduce edema. Administer antithrombotics, as ordered, and monitor appropriate laboratory values to evaluate effectiveness.
• Assess for complications, and immediately report relevent signs and symptoms. (See *Vascular repair complications.*)
• As the patient's condition improves, take steps to wean him from the ventilator, if appropriate. To promote good pulmonary hygiene, encourage the patient to cough, turn, and deep-breathe frequently.
• Assist the patient with ROM exercises, as ordered, to prevent thrombus formation. Assist with early ambulation to prevent complications of immobility.

Ventricular assist device insertion

A VAD is a device that's implanted to provide support to a failing heart. A VAD consists of:
• blood pump

If your patient's awaiting surgery for aortic aneurysm repair, be on guard for signs and symptoms of acute dissection or rupture.

Help your patient with ROM exercises and early ambulation to prevent complications.

Vascular repair complications

After a patient has undergone vascular repair surgery, monitor for these potential complications.

Complication	Signs and symptoms
Pulmonary infection	• Fever • Cough • Congestion • Dyspnea
Infection	• Redness • Warmth • Drainage • Pain • Fever
Renal dysfunction	• Low urine output • Elevated blood urea nitrogen and serum creatinine levels
Occlusion	• Reduced or absent peripheral pulses • Paresthesia • Severe pain • Cyanosis
Hemorrhage	• Hypotension • Tachycardia • Restlessness and confusion • Shallow respirations • Abdominal pain • Increased abdominal girth

• cannulas
• pneumatic or electrical drive console.

More output, less work

VADs are designed to decrease the heart's workload and increase cardiac output in patients with ventricular failure.

A temporary diversion

A VAD is commonly used while a patient waits for a heart transplant. In a surgical procedure, blood is diverted from a ventricle to an artificial pump. This pump, which is synchronized to the pa-

VAD: Help for a failing heart

A ventricular assist device (VAD), which is commonly called a "bridge to transplant," is a mechanical pump that relieves the workload of the ventricle as the heart heals or until a donor heart is located.

Implantable

The typical VAD is implanted in the upper abdominal wall. An inflow cannula drains blood from the left ventricle into a pump, which then pushes the blood into the aorta through the outflow cannula.

Pump options

VADs are available as continuous-flow or pulsatile pumps. A continuous flow pump fills continuously and returns blood to the aorta at a constant rate. A pulsatile pump may work in one of two ways: It may fill during systole and pump blood into the aorta during diastole, or it may pump irrespective of the patient's cardiac cycle.

Many types of VAD systems are available. This illustration shows a VAD (from Baxter Novacor) implanted in the left abdominal wall and connected to an external controller by a percutaneous lead. The patient also has a reserve power pack. The monitor is a backup power source that can run on electricity.

Potential complications

Despite the use of anticoagulants, the VAD may cause thrombi formation, leading to pulmonary embolism or stroke. Other complications may include heart failure, bleeding, cardiac tamponade, or infection.

Implanted left VAD

- Ascending aorta
- Pulmonary artery
- Left ventricle
- Outflow cannula
- Inflow cannula
- Pump unit
- Percutaneous lead
- Primary power pack

tient's ECG, then functions as the ventricle. (See *VAD: Help for a failing heart.*)

Right or left?

A VAD is used to provide systemic or pulmonary support, or both:
• A right VAD (RVAD) provides pulmonary support by diverting blood from the failing right ventricle to the VAD, which then pumps the blood to the pulmonary circulation by way of the VAD connection to the pulmonary artery.
• With a left VAD (LVAD), blood flows from the left ventricle to the VAD, which then pumps blood back to the body by way of the VAD connection to the aorta.
• When RVAD and LVAD are used, biventricular support is provided.

Nursing considerations

Follow these care measures before and after insertion of a VAD.

Before insertion
• Prepare the patient and his family for insertion, reinforcing explanations about the device, its purpose, and what to expect after insertion.
• Make sure that informed consent is obtained.
• Continue close patient monitoring, including continuous ECG, pulmonary artery and hemodynamic status, and intake and output.

After insertion
• Assess the patient's cardiovascular status at least every 15 minutes until stable and then hourly. Monitor blood pressure and hemodynamic parameters, including cardiac output and cardiac index, ECG, and peripheral pulses.
• Inspect the incision and dressing at least every hour initially and then every 2 to 4 hours as indicated by the patient's condition.
• Monitor urine output hourly and maintain I.V. fluid therapy as ordered. Watch for signs of fluid overload or decreasing urine output.
• Assess chest tube drainage and function frequently. Notify the doctor if drainage is greater than 150 ml over 2 hours. Auscultate lungs for evidence of abnormal breath sounds. Evaluate oxygen saturation or mixed venous oxygen saturation levels and administer oxygen as needed and ordered.
• Obtain hemoglobin levels, hematocrit, and coagulation studies as ordered. Administer blood component therapy as indicated and ordered.
• Assess for signs and symptoms of bleeding.

Evaluate oxygen saturation or mixed venous oxygen saturation levels and administer oxygen as needed and ordered.

• Turn the patient every 2 hours and begin ROM exercises when stable
• Administer antibiotics prophylactically, if ordered.

Balloon catheter treatments

Balloon catheter treatments of cardiovascular system disorders include intra-aortic balloon pump counterpulsation (IABP) and percutaneous transluminal coronary angioplasty (PTCA).

IABP counterpulsation

IABP counterpulsation temporarily reduces left ventricular workload and improves coronary perfusion.

What for?

IABP counterpulsation may benefit patients with:
• cardiogenic shock due to acute MI
• septic shock
• intractable angina before surgery
• intractable ventricular arrhythmias
• ventricular septal or papillary muscle ruptures.
    It's also used for patients who suffer pump failure before or after cardiac surgery.

How so?

The doctor may perform balloon catheter insertion at the patient's bedside as an emergency procedure or in the operating room. (See *Understanding a balloon pump.*)

Nursing considerations

• Explain to the patient that the doctor is going to place a catheter in the aorta to help his heart pump more easily. Tell him that, while the catheter is in place, he can't sit up, bend his knee, or flex his hip more than 30 degrees.
• Attach the patient to a continuous ECG monitor and make sure he has an arterial line, a PA catheter, and a peripheral I.V. line in place.
• Gather a surgical tray for percutaneous catheter insertion, heparin, normal saline solution, the IABP catheter, and the pump console. Connect the ECG monitor to the pump console. Then prepare the femoral site.
• After the IABP catheter is inserted, select either the ECG or arterial waveform to regulate inflation and deflation of the balloon. With the ECG waveform, the pump inflates the balloon in the middle of the T wave (diastole) and deflates with the R wave (before

IABP counterpulsation temporarily reduces left ventricular workload and improves coronary perfusion.

Understanding a balloon pump

An intra-aortic balloon pump consists of a polyurethane balloon attached to an external pump console by means of a large-lumen catheter. It's inserted percutaneously through the femoral artery and positioned in the descending aorta just distal to the left subclavian artery and above the renal arteries.

This external pump works in precise counterpoint to the left ventricle, inflating the balloon with helium early in diastole and deflating it just before systole. As the balloon inflates, it forces blood toward the aortic valve, thereby raising pressure in the aortic root and augmenting diastolic pressure to improve coronary perfusion. It also improves peripheral circulation by forcing blood through the brachiocephalic, common carotid, and subclavian arteries arising from the aortic trunk.

The balloon deflates rapidly at the end of diastole, creating a vacuum in the aorta. This reduces aortic volume and pressure, thereby decreasing the resistance to left ventricular ejection (afterload). This decreased workload, in turn, reduces the heart's oxygen requirements and, combined with the improved myocardial perfusion, helps prevent or diminish myocardial ischemia.

Diastole   **Systole**

The balloon inflates during early diastole.

The balloon deflates just before systole.

systole). With the arterial waveform, the upstroke of the arterial wave triggers balloon inflation. (See *Timing IABP counterpulsation*, page 216.)

• Frequently assess the insertion site. Don't elevate the head of the bed more than 30 degrees, to prevent upward migration of the catheter and occlusion of the left subclavian artery. If the balloon

Timing IABP counterpulsation

Intra-aortic balloon pump (IABP) counterpulsation is synchronized with either the electrocardiogram or arterial waveform. Ideally, balloon inflation should begin when the aortic valve closes — at the dicrotic notch on the arterial waveform. Deflation should occur just before systole.

Proper timing is crucial

Early inflation can damage the aortic valve by forcing it closed, whereas late inflation permits most of the blood emerging from the ventricle to flow past the balloon, reducing pump effectiveness.

Late deflation increases the resistance against which the left ventricle must pump, possibly causing cardiac arrest.

Arterial waveforms

The illustration below depicts how IABP counterpulsation boosts peak diastolic pressure and lowers peak systolic and end-diastolic pressures.

How timing affects waveforms

The arterial waveforms below show correctly and incorrectly timed balloon inflation and deflation.

Inflation

Early	Normal	Late

Deflation

Early	Normal	Late

occludes the artery, you may see a diminished left radial pulse, and the patient may report dizziness. Incorrect balloon placement may also cause flank pain or a sudden decrease in urine output.

• Assess distal pulses, color, temperature, and capillary refill of the patient's extremities every 15 minutes for the first 4 hours after insertion. After 4 hours, assess hourly for the duration of IABP therapy.

• Watch for signs of thrombus formation, such as a sudden weakening of pedal pulses, pain, and motor or sensory loss.

• If indicated, apply antiembolism stockings.

- Encourage active ROM exercises every 2 hours for the arms, the unaffected leg, and the affected ankle.
- Maintain adequate hydration to help prevent thrombus formation.
- If bleeding occurs at the catheter insertion site, apply direct pressure and notify the doctor.
- An alarm on the console may indicate a gas leak from a damaged catheter or ruptured balloon. If the alarm sounds or you see blood in the catheter, shut down the pump console and immediately place the patient in Trendelenburg's position to prevent an embolus from reaching the brain. Then notify the doctor.
- After the signs and symptoms of left-sided heart failure diminish and the patient requires only minimal drug support, the doctor begins weaning him from IABP counterpulsation. This may be accomplished by reducing the frequency of pumping or decreasing the balloon volume; a minimum volume or pumping ratio must be maintained to prevent thrombus formation. Most consoles have a flutter function that moves the balloon to prevent clot formation. Use the flutter function when the patient has been weaned from counterpulsation but the catheter hasn't yet been removed.
- To discontinue the IABP, the doctor deflates the balloon, clips the sutures, removes the catheter, and allows the site to bleed for 5 seconds to expel clots.
- After the doctor discontinues the IABP, apply direct pressure for 30 minutes and then apply a pressure dressing. Evaluate the site for bleeding and hematoma formation hourly for the next 4 hours.

PTCA

PTCA is a nonsurgical way to open coronary vessels narrowed by arteriosclerosis. It's usually used with cardiac catheterization to assess the stenosis and efficacy of angioplasty. It can also be used as a visual tool to direct the balloon-tipped catheter through a vessel's area of stenosis.

PTCA for pain

In PTCA, a balloon-tipped catheter is inserted into a narrowed coronary artery. This procedure, performed in the cardiac catheterization laboratory under local anesthesia, relieves pain due to angina and myocardial ischemia. (See *Understanding angioplasty,* page 218.)

Through one artery and into another

After coronary angiography confirms the presence and location of the occlusion, the doctor threads a guide catheter through the patient's femoral artery and into the coronary artery under fluoroscopic guidance.

Understanding angioplasty

Percutaneous transluminal coronary angioplasty is used to open an occluded coronary artery without opening the chest. This illustration shows what happens during the procedure.

First, the doctor threads the catheter. When angiography shows the guide catheter positioned at the occlusion site, the doctor carefully inserts a smaller double-lumen balloon catheter through the guide catheter and directs the balloon through the occlusion.

After the balloon is directed through the occlusion, the balloon is inflated, resulting in arterial stretching and plaque fracture. The balloon may need to be inflated and deflated several times until successful dilation occurs.

The guide catheter enters the coronary artery.

The balloon catheter is advanced to the occlusion in the coronary artery.

The balloon is inflated, flattening the plaque.

When the balloon is inflated, the plaque is compressed against the vessel wall, allowing coronary blood to flow more freely.

Plaque, meet Balloon

When the guide catheter's position at the occlusion site is confirmed by angiography, the doctor carefully introduces a double-lumen balloon into the catheter and through the lesion, where a marked pressure gradient is obvious. The doctor alternately inflates and deflates the balloon until arteriography verifies successful arterial dilation and decrease in the pressure gradient. With balloon inflation, the plaque is compressed against the vessel wall, allowing coronary blood to flow more freely.

Nursing considerations

Provide these care measures before and after cardiac catheterization.

Before the procedure

• Describe the procedure to the patient and his family and tell them the procedure takes 1 to 4 hours to complete.

• Explain that a catheter will be inserted into an artery or a vein in the patient's groin and that he may feel pressure as the catheter moves along the vessel.

• Reassure the patient that although he'll be awake during the procedure, he'll be given a sedative. Instruct him to report any angina during the procedure.

• Explain that the doctor injects a contrast medium to outline the lesion's location. Warn the patient that he may feel a hot, flushing sensation or transient nausea during the injection.

• Check the patient's history for allergies; if he has had allergic reactions to shellfish, iodine, or contrast media, notify the doctor.

• Give 650 mg of aspirin the evening before the procedure, as ordered, to prevent platelet aggregation.

• Make sure the patient signs an informed consent form.

• Restrict food and fluids for at least 6 hours before the procedure.

• Make sure that the results of coagulation studies, complete blood count (CBC), serum electrolyte studies, blood typing and crossmatching, blood urea nitrogen (BUN), and serum creatinine are available.

• Obtain baseline vital signs and assess peripheral pulses.

• Apply ECG electrodes and insert an I.V. line if not already in place.

• Administer oxygen through a nasal cannula.

• Perform skin preparation according to your facility's policy.

• Give the patient a sedative as ordered.

Instruct the patient to report any angina felt during cardiac catheterization.

After the procedure

• Assess the patient's vital signs and oxygen saturation every 15 minutes for the first hour and then every 30 minutes for 4 hours, unless his condition warrants more frequent checking. Monitor I.V. infusions, such as heparin or nitroglycerin, as indicated.

• Assess peripheral pulses distal to the catheter insertion site as well as the color, sensation, temperature, and capillary refill time of the affected extremity.

• Monitor ECG rhythm continuously and assess hemodynamic parameters closely for changes.

• Instruct the patient to remain in bed for 8 hours and to keep the affected extremity straight. Maintain sandbags in position if used to apply pressure to the catheter site. Elevate the head of the bed 15 to 30 degrees. If a hemostatic device was used to close the catheter insertion site, anticipate that the patient may be allowed out of bed in only a few hours.

• Assess the catheter site for hematoma, ecchymosis, and hemorrhage. If bleeding occurs, locate the artery and apply manual pressure; then notify the doctor.

• Administer I.V. fluids as ordered (usually 100 ml/hour) to promote excretion of the contrast medium. Be sure to assess for signs of fluid overload.

• After the doctor removes the catheter, apply direct pressure for at least 10 minutes and monitor the site often.

• Document the patient's tolerance of the procedure and status after it, including vital signs, hemodynamic parameters, appearance of catheter site, ECG findings, condition of the extremity distal to the insertion site, complications and necessary interventions.

> After the doctor removes the catheter, apply direct pressure for at least 10 minutes.

Other therapy

Other treatments for cardiovascular disorders include synchronized cardioversion, defibrillation, and pacemaker insertion.

Synchronized cardioversion

Cardioversion (synchronized countershock) is an elective or emergency procedure used to correct tachyarrhythmias (such as atrial tachycardia, atrial flutter, atrial fibrillation, and symptomatic ventricular tachycardia). It's also the treatment of choice for patients with arrhythmias that don't respond to drug therapy.

Electrifying experience

In synchronized cardioversion, an electric current is delivered to the heart to correct an arrhythmia. Compared with defibrillation, it uses much lower energy levels and is synchronized to deliver an electric charge to the myocardium at the peak R wave.

The procedure causes immediate depolarization, interrupting reentry circuits (abnormal impulse conduction that occurs when cardiac tissue is activated two or more times, causing reentry arrhythmias) and allowing the SA node to resume control.

Synchronizing the electrical charge with the R wave ensures that the current won't be delivered on the vulnerable T wave and disrupt repolarization. Thus, it reduces the risk that the current will strike during the relative refractory period of a cardiac cycle and induce ventricular fibrillation.

> Cardioversion is used to correct tachyarrhythmias as well as arrhythmias that don't respond to drug therapy. What a jolt!

Nursing considerations

• Describe this elective procedure to the patient and make sure an informed consent is obtained.

- Withhold all food and fluids for 6 to 12 hours before the procedure. If cardioversion is urgent, withhold food beginning as soon as possible.
- Obtain a baseline 12-lead ECG.
- Connect the patient to a pulse oximeter and blood pressure cuff.
- If the patient is awake, administer a sedative as ordered.
- Place the leads on the patient's chest and assess his cardiac rhythm.
- Apply conductive gel to the paddles or attach defibrillation pads to the chest wall; position the pads so that one pad is to the right of the sternum, just below the clavicle, and the other is at the fifth or sixth intercostal space in the left anterior axillary line.
- Turn on the defibrillator and select the ordered energy level, usually between 50 and 100 joules. (See *Choosing the correct cardioversion energy level.*)
- Activate the synchronized mode by depressing the synchronizer switch.
- Check that the machine is sensing the R wave correctly.
- Place the paddles on the chest and apply firm pressure.
- Charge the paddles.
- Instruct other personnel to stand clear of the patient and the bed to avoid the risk of an electric shock.
- Discharge the current by pushing both paddles' DISCHARGE buttons simultaneously.
- If cardioversion is unsuccessful, repeat the procedure two or three times, as ordered, gradually increasing the energy with each additional counter-shock.
- If normal rhythm is restored, continue to monitor the patient and provide supplemental ventilation as long as needed.
- If the patient's cardiac rhythm changes to ventricular fibrillation, switch the mode from synchronized to defibrillate and defibrillate the patient immediately after charging the machine.
- When using handheld paddles, continue to hold the paddles on the patient's chest until the energy is delivered.
- Remember to reset the SYNC MODE on the defibrillator after each synchronized cardioversion. Resetting this switch is necessary because most defibrillators automatically reset to an unsynchronized mode.
- Document the use of synchronized cardioversion, the rhythm before and after cardioversion, amperage used, and how the patient tolerated the procedure.

Defibrillation

In defibrillation, electrode paddles are used to direct an electric current through the patient's heart. The current causes the myo-

---

Choosing the correct cardioversion energy level

When choosing an energy level for cardioversion, try the lowest energy level first. If the arrhythmia isn't corrected, repeat the procedure using the next energy level. Repeat this procedure until the arrhythmia is corrected or until the highest energy level is reached. The monophasic energy dose (or clinically equivalent biphasic energy dose) used for cardioversion are:
- 100, 200, 300, 360 joules for unstable ventricular tachycardia with a pulse
- 50, 100, 200, 300, 360 joules for unstable paroxysmal supraventricular tachycardia
- 100, 200, 300, 360 joules for unstable atrial fibrillation with a rapid ventricular response
- 50, 100, 200, 300, 360 joules for unstable atrial flutter with a rapid ventricular response.

Biphasic defibrillators

Most hospital defibrillators are monophasic, delivering a single current of electricity that travels in one direction between the two pads or paddles on the patient's chest. A large amount of electrical current is required for effective monophasic defibrillation.

Current flows to and fro

Biphasic defibrillators have recently been introduced into hospitals. Pad or paddle placement is the same as with the monophasic defibrillator. The difference is that during biphasic defibrillation, the electrical current discharged from the pads or paddles travels in a positive direction for a specified duration and then reverses and flows in a negative direction for the remaining time of the electrical discharge.

Energy efficient

The biphasic defibrillator delivers two currents of electricity and lowers the defibrillation threshold of the heart muscle, making it possible to successfully defibrillate ventricular fibrillation with smaller amounts of energy. Instead of using 200 joules, an initial shock of 150 joules is often effective.

Adjustable

The biphasic defibrillator is able to adjust for differences in impedance or the resistance of the current through the chest. This reduces the number of shocks needed to terminate ventricular fibrillation.

Less myocardial damage

Because the biphasic defibrillator requires lower energy levels and fewer shocks, damage to the myocardial muscle is reduced. Biphasic defibrillators used at the clinically appropriate energy level may be used for defibrillation and, in the synchronized mode, for synchronized cardioversion.

cardium to depolarize, which in turn encourages the SA node to resume control of the heart's electrical activity.

The electrode paddles delivering the current may be placed on the patient's chest or, during cardiac surgery, directly on the myocardium. (See *Biphasic defibrillators.*)

Act early and quickly

Because some arrhythmias, such as ventricular fibrillation, can cause death if not corrected, the success of defibrillation depends on early recognition and quick treatment.

In addition to treating ventricular fibrillation, defibrillation may also be used to treat ventricular tachycardia that doesn't produce a pulse.

Nursing considerations

• Assess the patient to determine if he lacks a pulse. Call for help and perform cardiopulmonary resuscitation (CPR) until the defibrillator and other emergency equipment arrive. (See *Automated external defibrillator.*)
• Connect the monitoring leads of the defibrillator to the patient and assess his cardiac rhythm in two leads.
• Expose the patient's chest and apply conductive pads at the paddle placement positions. (See *Defibrillator paddle placement, page 224.*)

Automated external defibrillator

An automated external defibrillator (AED) has a cardiac rhythm analysis system. The AED interprets the patient's cardiac rhythm and gives the operator step-by-step directions on how to proceed if defibrillation is indicated. Most AEDs have a "quick-look" feature that allows visualization of the rhythm with the paddles before electrodes are connected.

Computer-assisted system
The AED is equipped with a microcomputer that senses and analyzes a patient's heart rhythm at the push of a button. It then audibly or visually prompts you to deliver a shock.

All models have the same basic functions but offer different operating options. For example, all AEDs communicate directions by displaying messages on a screen, giving voice commands, or both. Some AEDs simultaneously display a patient's heart rhythm.

All devices record your interactions with the patient during defibrillation, either on a cassette tape or in a solid-state memory module. Some AEDs have an integral printer for immediate event documentation.

Before discharging the defibrillator, tell everyone to stand clear of the patient and the bed.

CAUTION!

• Turn on the defibrillator and, if performing external defibrillation, set the energy level at 200 joules for an adult patient.
• Charge the paddles by pressing the CHARGE buttons, which are located either on the machine or paddles.
• Place the paddles over the conductive pads and press firmly against the patient's chest, using 25 lb (11.3 kg) of pressure.
• Reassess the patient's cardiac rhythm in two leads.
• If the patient remains in ventricular fibrillation or pulseless ventricular tachycardia, instruct all personnel to stand clear of the patient and the bed. Also make a visual check to make sure everyone is clear of the patient and the bed.
• Discharge the current by pressing both paddle DISCHARGE buttons simultaneously.
• Leave the paddles in position on the patient's chest while you reassess his cardiac rhythm; have someone else assess his pulse.
• If necessary, prepare to defibrillate a second time. Instruct someone to reset the energy level on the defibrillator to 300 joules. Announce that you're preparing to defibrillate and follow the procedure described above.
• Reassess the patient. If defibrillation is again necessary, instruct someone to reset the energy level to 360 joules. Then follow the same procedure as before.
• Perform the three countershocks in rapid succession, reassessing the patient's rhythm before each attempt.
• If the patient still has no pulse after three initial defibrillations, resume CPR, give supplemental oxygen, and begin administering

---

Defibrillator paddle placement

Here's a guide to correct paddle placement for defibrillation.

Anterolateral placement

For anterolateral placement, place one paddle to the right of the upper sternum, just below the right clavicle, and the other over the fifth or sixth intercostal space at the left anterior axillary line.

Anteroposterior placement

For anteroposterior placement, place the anterior paddle directly over the heart at the precordium, to the left of the lower sternal border. Place the flat posterior paddle under the patient's body beneath the heart and immediately below the scapulae (but not under the vertebral column).

---

appropriate medications such as epinephrine. Also, consider possible causes for failure of the patient's rhythm to convert, such as acidosis and hypoxia.

• If defibrillation restores a normal rhythm, assess the patient. Obtain baseline ABG levels and a 12-lead ECG. Provide supplemental oxygen, ventilation, and medications as needed. Prepare the defibrillator for immediate reuse.

• Document the procedure, including the patient's ECG rhythms before and after defibrillation; the number of times defibrillation was performed; the voltage used during each attempt; whether a pulse returned; the dosage, route, and time of any drugs administered; whether CPR was used; how the airway was maintained; and the patient's outcome. (See *Implantable cardioverter-defibrillator.*)

Permanent pacemaker insertion

A permanent pacemaker is a self-contained device surgically implanted in a pocket under the patient's skin. This is usually done in an operating room or cardiac catheterization laboratory.

Permanent pacemakers function in the demand mode, allowing the patient's heart to beat on its own but preventing it from falling below a preset rate.

A permanent pacemaker prevents my rate from falling below a preset level.

Implantable cardioverter-defibrillator

An implantable cardioverter-defibrillator (ICD) is implanted to continually monitor a patient's heart for bradycardia, ventricular tachycardia, and ventricular fibrillation. The device also administers either shocks or paced beats.

ICDs are generally indicated when drug therapy, surgery, or catheter ablation fails to prevent the patient's dangerous arrhythmia.

What it is

An ICD system consists of a programmable pulse generator and one or more leadwires. The pulse generator is a small battery-powered computer that monitors the heart's electrical signals and delivers electrical therapy when an abnormal rhythm is identified.

It also stores information on the heart's activity before, during, and after an arrhythmia, along with tracking which treatment was delivered and the outcome of that treatment. Many devices also store electrograms (electrical tracings similar to electrocardiograms). With an interrogation device, a doctor can retrieve this information to evaluate ICD function and battery status and to adjust ICD system settings.

How it's programmed

When caring for a patient with an ICD, it's important to know how the device is programmed. This information is available through a status report that can be obtained and printed when the doctor or specially trained technician interrogates the device. This involves placing a specialized piece of equipment over the implanted pulse generator to retrieve pacing function.

If the patient experiences an arrhythmia or if the device delivers a therapy, the program information is used to evaluate the functioning of the device. Program information includes:
• type and model of ICD
• status of the device (on or off)
• detection rates
• therapies that will be delivered (pacing, antitachycardia pacing, cardioversion, and defibrillation).

What you should know

• If the patient experiences cardiac arrest, initiate cardiopulmonary resuscitation and advanced cardiac life support.
• If the ICD delivers a shock while you're performing chest compressions, you may feel a slight shock. Wear gloves to eliminate this.
• It's safe to also externally defibrillate a patient with an ICD as long as the paddles aren't placed directly over the pulse generator. The anteroposterior paddle position is preferred.

And the nominees for insertion are...

Permanent pacemakers are indicated for patients with:
• persistent bradycardia
• complete heart block
• congenital or degenerative heart disease
• Stokes-Adams syndrome
• Wolff-Parkinson-White syndrome
• sick sinus syndrome.

Setting the pace

Pacing electrodes can be placed in the atria, ventricles, or both chambers (atrioventricular sequential or dual chamber). Biventricular pacemakers are also available for cardiac resynchronization therapy in some patients with heart failure. (See *Understanding pacemaker codes*, page 226.)

Understanding pacemaker codes

The capabilities of pacemakers are described by a five-letter coding system, although typically only the first three letters are used.

First letter
The first letter identifies which heart chambers are paced. Here are the letters used to signify these options:
• V = Ventricle
• A = Atrium
• D = Dual (ventricle and atrium)
• 0 = None.

Second letter
The second letter signifies the heart chamber where the pacemaker senses the intrinsic activity:
• V = Ventricle
• A = Atrium
• D = Dual
• 0 = None.

Third letter
The third letter shows the pacemaker's response to the intrinsic electrical activity it senses in the atrium or ventricle:
• T = Triggers pacing
• I = Inhibits pacing
• D = Dual; can be triggered or inhibited depending on the mode and where intrinsic activity occurs
• 0 = None; the pacemaker doesn't change its mode in response to sensed activity.

Fourth letter
The fourth letter denotes the pacemaker's programmability; it tells whether the pacemaker can be modified by an external programming device:
• P = Basic functions programmable
• M = Multiprogrammable parameters
• C = Communicating functions such as telemetry
• R = Rate responsiveness (rate adjusts to fit the patient's metabolic needs and achieve normal hemodynamic status)
• 0 = None.

Fifth letter
The fifth letter denotes the pacemaker's response to a tachyarrhythmia:
• P = Pacing ability— pacemaker's rapid burst paces the heart at a rate above its intrinsic rate to override the tachycardia source
• S = Shock—an implantable cardioverter-defibrillator identifies ventricular tachycardia and delivers a shock to stop the arrhythmia
• D = Dual ability to shock and pace
• 0 = None.

The most common pacing codes are VVI for single-chamber pacing and DDD for dual-chamber pacing. To keep the patient healthy and active, newer pacemakers are designed to increase the heart rate with exercise.

Good news for active patients! Newer pacemakers are designed to increase the heart rate with exercise.

Nursing considerations
Provide care measures before and after pacemaker placement. Nursing responsibilities during surgical placement involve monitoring ECG and maintaining sterile technique.

Preoperative care
• Explain the procedure to the patient.
• Before pacemaker insertion, shave the patient's chest from the axilla to the midline and from the clavicle to the nipple line on the side selected by the doctor.
• Establish an I.V. line.
• Obtain baseline vital signs and a baseline ECG.
• Provide sedation, as ordered.

Postoperative care

• Monitor the patient's ECG to check for arrhythmias and to ensure correct pacemaker functioning.
• Check the dressing for signs of bleeding and infection.
• Change the dressing according to facility policy.
• Check vital signs and LOC every 15 minutes for the first hour, every hour for the next 4 hours then every 4 hours.
• Provide the patient with an identification card that lists the pacemaker type and manufacturer, serial number, pacemaker rate setting, date implanted, and the doctor's name.

Temporary pacemaker insertion

A temporary pacemaker is usually inserted in an emergency. The device consists of an external, battery-powered pulse generator and a lead or electrode system.

Temporary pacemakers typically come in three types, including:

- transcutaneous

- transvenous

- epicardial.

Transcutaneous pacing is used only until transvenous pacing is established.

Dire straits

In a life-threatening situation, a transcutaneous pacemaker is the best choice. This device works by sending an electrical impulse from the pulse generator to the patient's heart by way of two electrodes, which are placed on the front and back of the patient's chest.

Transcutaneous pacing is quick and effective, but it's used only until the doctor can institute transvenous pacing.

More comfortable and more reliable

Besides being more comfortable for the patient, a transvenous pacemaker is more reliable than a transcutaneous pacemaker.

Transvenous pacing involves threading an electrode catheter through a vein into the patient's right atrium or right ventricle. The electrode is attached to an external pulse generator that can provide an electrical stimulus directly to the endocardium.

Transvenous pacemaker basics

Indications for a temporary transvenous pacemaker include:
• management of bradycardia
• presence of tachyarrhythmias
• other conduction system disturbances.

The purpose of temporary transvenous pacemaker insertion is:
• to maintain circulatory integrity by providing for standby pacing in case of sudden complete heart block
• to increase heart rate during periods of symptomatic bradycardia
• occasionally, to control sustained supraventricular or ventricular tachycardia.

Pacing options

During cardiac surgery, the surgeon may insert electrodes through the epicardium of the right ventricle and, if he wants to institute AV sequential pacing, the right atrium. From there, the electrodes pass through the chest wall, where they remain available if temporary pacing becomes necessary. This is called *epicardial pacing.*

Transvenous pacemaker no-no's

Among the contraindications to pacemaker therapy are electro-mechanical dissociation and ventricular fibrillation.

Nursing considerations

• Teach measures to prevent microshock; warn the patient not to use any electrical equipment that isn't grounded.
• Use other safety measures such as placing a plastic cover (supplied by the manufacturer) over the pacemaker controls to avoid an accidental setting change. If the patient needs emergency defibrillation, make sure the pacemaker can withstand the procedure. If you're unsure, disconnect the pulse generator to avoid damage.
• When using a transcutaneous pacemaker, don't place the electrodes over a bony area because bone conducts current poorly. With a female patient, place the anterior electrode under the patient's breast but not over her diaphragm.
• If the doctor inserts the transvenous pacer wire through the brachial or femoral vein, immobilize the patient's arm or leg to avoid putting stress on the pacing wires.
• After insertion of any temporary pacemaker, assess the patient's vital signs, skin color, LOC, and peripheral pulses to determine the effectiveness of the paced rhythm. Perform a 12-lead ECG to serve as a baseline, and then perform additional ECGs daily or with clinical changes. Also, if possible, obtain a rhythm strip before, during, and after pacemaker placement; anytime the pacemaker settings are changed; and whenever the patient receives treatment because of a complication due to the pacemaker.
• Continuously monitor the ECG reading, noting capture, sensing, rate, intrinsic beats, and competition of paced and intrinsic

Teach measures to prevent microshock such as using only electrical equipment that's grounded.

rhythms. If the pacemaker is sensing correctly, the sense indicator on the pulse generator should flash with each beat.

• Record the date and time of pacemaker insertion, the type of pacemaker, the reason for insertion, and the patient's response. Note the pacemaker settings. Document any complications and the interventions taken.

• If the patient has epicardial pacing wires in place, clean the insertion site and change the dressing daily. At the same time, monitor the site for signs of infection. Always keep the pulse generator nearby in case pacing becomes necessary.

Disorders

Common cardiovascular disorders include acute coronary syndromes, aneurysms, cardiac arrhythmias, cardiac tamponade, cardiogenic shock, cardiomyopathy, heart failure, hypertensive crisis, pericarditis, and valvular heart disease.

Acute coronary syndromes

Patients with acute coronary syndromes have some degree of coronary artery occlusion. The degree of occlusion defines whether the acute coronary syndrome is:
• unstable angina
• non–Q-wave MI
• Q-wave MI.

Plaque's place

The development of any acute coronary syndrome begins with a rupture or erosion of plaque—an unstable and lipid-rich substance. The rupture results in platelet adhesions, fibrin clot formation, and activation of thrombin.

What causes it

Patients with certain risk factors appear to face a greater likelihood of developing an acute coronary syndrome. These factors include:
• family history of heart disease
• obesity
• smoking
• high-fat, high-carbohydrate diet
• sedentary lifestyle
• menopause

We stick together! That's why an acute coronary syndrome results in platelet adhesions, fibrin clot formation, and thrombin activation.

- stress
- diabetes
- hypertension
- hyperlipoproteinemia.

Pathophysiology

An acute coronary syndrome most commonly results when a thrombus progresses and occludes blood flow. (An early thrombus doesn't necessarily block blood flow.) The effect is an imbalance in myocardial oxygen supply and demand.

Degree and duration

The degree and duration of blockage dictate the type of infarct that occurs:
- If the patient has unstable angina, a thrombus partially occludes a coronary vessel. This thrombus is full of platelets. The partially occluded vessel may have distal microthrombi that cause necrosis in some myocytes.
- If smaller vessels infarct, the patient is at higher risk for MI, which may progress to a non–Q-wave MI. Usually, only the innermost layer of the heart is damaged.
- Q-wave MI results when reduced blood flow through one of the coronary arteries causes myocardial ischemia, injury, and necrosis. The damage extends through all myocardial layers.

What to look for

A patient with angina typically experiences:
- burning
- squeezing
- crushing tightness in the substernal or precordial chest that may radiate to the left arm, neck, jaw, or shoulder blade.

Any patient may experience atypical chest pain, but it's more common in women. (See *Atypical chest pain in women*.)

It hurts when I do this

Angina most frequently follows physical exertion but may also follow emotional excitement, exposure to cold, or a large meal. Angina is commonly relieved by nitroglycerin. It's less severe and shorter-lived than the pain of acute MI.

Four forms

Angina has four major forms:

stable—predictable pain, in frequency and duration, which can be relieved with nitrates and rest

---

Atypical chest pain in women

Women with coronary artery disease may experience typical chest pain, but commonly experience atypical chest pain, vague chest pain, or a lack of chest pain. They're more likely than men to experience a toothache or pain in the arm, shoulder, jaw, neck, throat, back, breast, or stomach.

A patient with MI experiences severe, persistent chest pain that isn't relieved by rest or nitroglycerin.

✌ unstable — increased pain, which is easily induced

✊ Prinzmetal's or a variant — pain from unpredictable coronary artery spasm

🖐 microvascular — angina-like chest pain due to impairment of vasodilator reserve in a patient with normal coronary arteries.

My, my, MI pain

A patient with MI experiences severe, persistent chest pain that isn't relieved by rest or nitroglycerin. He may describe pain as crushing or squeezing. The pain is usually substernal, but may radiate to the left arm, jaw, neck, or shoulder blades.

And many more

Other signs and symptoms of MI include:
- a feeling of impending doom
- fatigue
- nausea and vomiting
- shortness of breath
- cool extremities
- perspiration
- anxiety
- hypotension or hypertension
- palpable precordial pulse
- muffled heart sounds.

What tests tell you

These tests are used to diagnose CAD:
- ECG during an anginal episode shows ischemia. Serial 12-lead ECGs may be normal or inconclusive during the first few hours after an MI. Abnormalities include serial ST-segment depression in non–Q-wave MI and ST-segment elevation and Q waves, representing scarring and necrosis, in a Q-wave MI. (See *Pinpointing infarction.*)
- Coronary angiography reveals coronary artery stenosis or obstruction and collateral circulation and shows the condition of the arteries beyond the narrowing.
- Myocardial perfusion imaging with thallium-201 during treadmill exercise discloses ischemic areas of the myocardium, visualized as "cold spots."
- With MI, serial serum cardiac marker measurements show elevated CK, especially the CK-MB isoenzyme (the cardiac muscle fraction of CK), troponin T and I, and myoglobin.

Pinpointing infarction

The site of myocardial infarction (MI) depends on the vessels involved:
- Occlusion of the circumflex branch of the left coronary artery causes a lateral wall infarction.
- An occlusion of the anterior descending branch of the left coronary artery leads to an anterior wall infarction.
- True posterior or inferior wall infarctions generally result from occlusion of the right coronary artery or one of its branches.
- Right ventricular infarctions can also result from right coronary artery occlusion, can accompany inferior infarctions, and may cause right-sided heart failure.
- In a Q-wave MI, tissue damage extends through all myocardial layers; in a non–Q-wave MI, damage occurs only in the innermost layer.

• With a Q-wave MI, echocardiography shows ventricular wall dyskinesia.

How it's treated

For patients with angina, the goal of treatment is to reduce myocardial oxygen demand or increase oxygen supply.

These treatments are used to manage angina:
• Nitrates reduce myocardial oxygen consumption.
• Beta-adrenergic blockers may be administered to reduce the workload and oxygen demands of the heart.
• If angina is caused by coronary artery spasm, calcium channel blockers may be given.
• Antiplatelet drugs minimize platelet aggregation and the danger of coronary occlusion.
• Antilipemic drugs can reduce elevated serum cholesterol or triglyceride levels.
• Obstructive lesions may necessitate CABG or PTCA. Other alternatives include laser angioplasty, minimally invasive surgery, rotational atherectomy, or stent placement.

For patients with angina, the goal is to reduce oxygen demand or increase oxygen supply.

MI relief

The goals of treatment for MI are to relieve pain, stabilize heart rhythm, revascularize the coronary artery, preserve myocardial tissue, and reduce cardiac workload.

Here are some guidelines for treatment:
• Thrombolytic therapy should be started within 3 hours of the onset of symptoms (unless contraindications exist). Thrombolytic therapy involves administration of streptokinase, alteplase, anistreplase, or reteplase.
• PTCA is an option for opening blocked or narrowed arteries.
• Oxygen is administered to increase oxygenation of the blood.
• Nitroglycerin is administered sublingually to relieve chest pain, unless systolic blood pressure is less than 90 mm Hg or heart rate is less than 50 or greater than 100 beats/minute.
• Morphine is administered as analgesia because pain stimulates the sympathetic nervous system, leading to an increase in heart rate and vasoconstriction.
• Aspirin is administered to inhibit platelet aggregation.
• I.V. heparin is given to patients who have received tissue plasminogen activator to increase the chances of patency in the affected coronary artery.
• Lidocaine, transcutaneous pacing patches (or a transvenous pacemaker), defibrillation, or epinephrine may be used if arrhythmias are present.

- Physical activity is limited for the first 12 hours to reduce cardiac workload, thereby limiting the area of necrosis.
- I.V. nitroglycerin is administered for 24 to 48 hours in patients without hypotension, bradycardia, or excessive tachycardia, to reduce afterload and preload and relieve chest pain.
- Glycoprotein IIb/IIIa inhibitors (such as abciximab [ReoPro]) are administered to patients with continued unstable angina or acute chest pain, or following invasive cardiac procedures, to reduce platelet aggregation.
- I.V. beta-adrenergic blocker is administered early to patients with evolving acute MI; it's followed by oral therapy to reduce heart rate and contractibility and reduce myocardial oxygen requirements.
- ACE inhibitors are administered to those with evolving MI with ST-segment elevation or left bundle-branch block, to reduce afterload and preload and prevent remodeling.
- Laser angioplasty, atherectomy, stent placement, or transmyocardial revascularization may be initiated.
- Lipid-lowering drugs are administered to patients with elevated low-density lipoprotein and cholesterol levels.

Physical activity is limited for the first 12 hours after MI to reduce the cardiac workload and limit necrosis.

What to do

- During anginal episodes, monitor blood pressure and heart rate. Take an ECG before administering nitroglycerin or other nitrates. Record duration of pain, amount of medication required to relieve it, and accompanying symptoms.
- On admission to the coronary care unit, monitor and record the patient's ECG, blood pressure, temperature, and heart and breath sounds. Also, assess and record the severity, location, type, and duration of pain.
- Obtain a 12-lead ECG and assess heart rate and blood pressure when the patient experiences acute chest pain.
- Monitor the patient's hemodynamic status closely. Be alert for indicators suggesting decreased cardiac output, such as decreased blood pressure, increased heart rate, increased PAP, increased PAWP, decreased cardiac output measurements, and decreased right atrial pressure.
- Assess urine output hourly.
- Monitor the patient's oxygen saturation levels and notify the doctor if oxygen saturation falls below 90%.
- Check the patient's blood pressure after giving nitroglycerin, especially the first dose.
- During episodes of chest pain, monitor ECG, blood pressure, and PA catheter readings (if applicable) to determine changes.

During episodes of chest pain, monitor ECG, blood pressure, and PA catheter readings for changes.

- Frequently monitor ECG rhythm strips to detect heart rate changes and arrhythmias.
- Obtain serial measurements of cardiac enzyme levels as ordered.
- Watch for crackles, cough, tachypnea, and edema, which may indicate impending left-sided heart failure. Carefully monitor daily weight, intake and output, respiratory rate, serum enzyme levels, ECG waveforms, and blood pressure. Auscultate for S_3 or S_4 gallops.
- Prepare the patient for reperfusion therapy as indicated.
- Administer and titrate medications as ordered. Avoid giving I.M. injections; I.V. administration provides more rapid symptom relief.
- Organize patient care and activities to allow rest periods. If the patient is immobilized, turn him often and use intermittent compression devices. Gradually increase the patient's activity level as tolerated.
- Provide a clear-liquid diet until nausea subsides. Anticipate a possible order for a low-cholesterol, low-sodium diet without caffeine.
- Provide a stool softener to prevent straining during defecation.

I.V. administration of medications provides more rapid relief.

Aortic aneurysm

An aortic aneurysm is a localized outpouching or an abnormal dilation in a weakened arterial wall. Aortic aneurysm typically occurs in the aorta between the renal arteries and the iliac branches, but the abdominal, thoracic, or ascending arch of the aorta may be affected.

What causes it

The exact cause of an aortic aneurysm is unclear, but several factors place a person at risk, including:
- advanced age
- history of hypertension
- smoking
- atherosclerosis
- connective tissue disorders
- diabetes mellitus
- trauma.

Pathophysiology

Aneurysms arise from a defect in the middle layer of the arterial wall (tunica media, or medial layer). Once the elastic fibers and collagen in the middle layer are damaged, stretching and segmental dilation occur. As a result, the medial layer loses some of its elasticity, and it fragments. Smooth muscle cells are lost and the wall thins.

Thin and thinner

The thinned wall may contain calcium deposits and atherosclerotic plaque, making the wall brittle. As a person ages, the elastin in the wall decreases, further weakening the vessel. If hypertension is present, blood flow slows, resulting in ischemia and additional weakening.

Wide vessel, slow flow

Once an aneurysm begins to develop, lateral pressure increases, causing the vessel lumen to widen and blood flow to slow. Over time, mechanical stressors contribute to elongation of the aneurysm.

Blood forces

Hemodynamic forces may also play a role, causing pulsatile stresses on the weakened wall and pressing on the small vessels that supply nutrients to the arterial wall. In aortic aneurysms, this causes the aorta to become bowed and tortuous.

Most patients with aortic aneurysms are asymptomatic until an enlarging aneurysm compresses surrounding tissue.

What to look for

Most patients with aortic aneurysms are asymptomatic until the aneurysms enlarge and compress surrounding tissue.

A large aneurysm may produce signs and symptoms that mimic those of MI, renal calculi, lumbar disk disease, and duodenal compression.

When symptoms arise

Usually, if the patient exhibits symptoms, it's because of rupture, expansion, embolization, thrombosis, or pressure from the mass on surrounding structures. Rupture is more common if the patient also has hypertension or if the aneurysm is larger than 6 cm.

Thoracic aortic aneurysm

If the patient has a suspected thoracic aortic aneurysm, assess for:
• complaints of substernal pain possibly radiating to the neck, back, abdomen, or shoulders
• hoarseness or coughing
• difficulty swallowing
• difficulty breathing
• hemoptysis
• hematemesis

• unequal blood pressure and pulse when measured in both arms
• aortic insufficiency murmur.

Acute expansion

When there's an acute expansion of a thoracic aortic aneurysm, assess for:
• severe hypertension
• neurologic changes
• a new murmur of aortic sufficiency
• right sternoclavicular lift
• jugular vein distention
• tracheal deviation.

In a patient suspected of having a thoracic aortic aneurysm, the blood pressure in each arm may not be equal.

Abdominal aortic aneurysm

The patient with an abdominal aortic aneurysm may experience:
• gnawing, generalized, steady abdominal pain
• lower back pain that's unaffected by movement
• gastric or abdominal fullness
• pulsating mass in the periumbilical area (if the patient isn't obese)
• systolic bruit over the aorta on auscultation of the abdomen
• bruit over the femoral arteries
• hypotension (with aneurysm rupture).

What tests tell you

No specific laboratory test to diagnose an aortic aneurysm exists. However, the following tests may be helpful:
• If blood is leaking from the aneurysm, leukocytosis and a decrease in hemoglobin and hematocrit may be noted.

Telltale TEE

• TEE allows visualization of the thoracic aorta. It's commonly combined with Doppler flow studies to provide information about blood flow.
• Abdominal ultrasonography or echocardiography can be used to determine the size, shape, length, and location of the aneurysm.
• Anteroposterior and lateral X-rays of the chest or abdomen can be used to detect aortic calcification and widened areas of the aorta.
• Computed tomography (CT) scan and magnetic resonance imaging (MRI) can disclose the aneurysm's size and effect on nearby organs.
• Serial ultrasonography at 6-month intervals reveals any growth of small aneurysms.

Unless blood is leaking from the aneurysm, there's no specific laboratory test to aid the diagnosis.

• Aortography is used in determining the aneurysm's approximate size and patency of the visceral vessels.

How it's treated

Aneurysm treatment usually involves surgery and appropriate drug therapy. Aortic aneurysms usually require resection and replacement of the aortic section using a vascular or Dacron graft. However, keep these points in mind:
• If the aneurysm is small and produces no symptoms, surgery may be delayed, with regular physical examination and ultrasonography performed to monitor its progression.
• Large or symptomatic aneurysms are at risk for rupture and need immediate repair.
• Endovascular grafting may be an option for a patient with an abdominal aortic aneurysm. This procedure, which can be done using local or regional anesthesia, is a minimally invasive procedure whereby the walls of the aorta are reinforced to prevent expansion and rupture of the aneurysm.
• Medications to control blood pressure, relieve anxiety, and control pain are also prescribed.

Rush to respond to rupture

Rupture of an aortic aneurysm is a medical emergency requiring prompt treatment, including:
• resuscitation with fluid and blood replacement
• I.V. propranolol to reduce myocardial contractility
• I.V. nitroprusside to reduce blood pressure and maintain it at 90 to 100 mm Hg systolic
• analgesics to relieve pain
• an arterial line and indwelling urinary catheter to monitor the patient's condition preoperatively.

Rupture of an aortic aneurysm is a medical emergency requiring prompt treatment.

What to do

• Assess the patient's vital signs, especially blood pressure, every 2 to 4 hours or more frequently, depending on the severity of his condition. Monitor blood pressure and pulse in extremities and compare findings bilaterally. If the difference in systolic blood pressure exceeds 10 mm Hg, notify the doctor immediately.
• Assess cardiovascular status frequently, including heart rate, rhythm, ECG, and cardiac enzyme levels. MI can occur if an aneurysm ruptures along the coronary arteries.
• Obtain blood samples to evaluate kidney function by assessing BUN, creatinine, and electrolyte levels. Measure intake and output, hourly if necessary, depending on the patient's condition.

• Monitor CBC for evidence of blood loss, including decreased hemoglobin, hematocrit, and red blood cell (RBC) count.
• If the patient's condition is acute, obtain an arterial sample for ABG analysis, as ordered, and monitor cardiac rhythm. Assist with arterial line insertion to allow for continuous blood pressure monitoring. Assist with insertion of a PA catheter to assess hemodynamic balance.
• Administer ordered medications to control aneurysm progression. Provide analgesics to relieve pain, if present.
• Observe the patient for signs of rupture, which may be immediately fatal. Watch closely for any signs of acute blood loss: decreasing blood pressure; increasing pulse and respiratory rates; cool, clammy skin; restlessness; and decreased LOC.

Rupture response

• If rupture occurs, insert a large-bore I.V. catheter, begin fluid resuscitation, and administer nitroprusside I.V. as ordered, usually to maintain a MAP of 70 to 80 mm Hg. Also administer propranolol I.V. (to reduce left ventricular ejection velocity) as ordered until the heart rate ranges from 60 to 80 beats per minute. Expect to administer additional doses every 4 to 6 hours until oral medications can be used.
• If the patient is experiencing acute pain, administer morphine I.V. as ordered.
• Prepare the patient for emergency surgery.

After surgery

• Administer nitroprusside or nitroglycerin and titrate to maintain a normotensive state.
• Perform meticulous pulmonary hygiene measures, including suctioning, chest physiotherapy, and deep breathing.
• Provide continuous cardiac monitoring.
• Assess urine output hourly.
• Maintain NG tube patency to ensure gastric decompression.
• Assist with serial Doppler examination of all extremities to evaluate the adequacy of vascular repair and presence of embolization.
• Assess for signs of poor arterial perfusion, such as pain, paresthesia, pallor, pulselessness, paralysis and poikilothermy (coldness).

Remember the six signs of poor arterial perfusion: pain, paresthesia, pallor, pulselessness, paralysis, and poikilothermy.

Cardiac arrhythmias

In cardiac arrhythmia, abnormal electrical conduction or automaticity changes heart rate and rhythm.

Asymptomatic to catastrophic

Cardiac arrhythmias vary in severity, from those that are mild, asymptomatic, and require no treatment (such as sinus arrhythmia, in which heart rate increases and decreases with respiration) to catastrophic ventricular fibrillation, which requires immediate resuscitation.

Organized by origin and effects

Cardiac arrhythmias are generally classified according to their origin (ventricular or supraventricular). Their effect on cardiac output and blood pressure, partially influenced by the site of origin, determines their clinical significance. Lethal arrhythmias, such as ventricular tachycardia and ventricular fibrillation, are a major cause of sudden cardiac death.

Arrhythmias are generally classified according to whether their origin is ventricular or supraventricular.

What causes it

Common causes of cardiac arrhythmias include:
- congenital defects
- myocardial ischemia or infarction
- organic heart disease
- drug toxicity
- degeneration of the conductive tissue
- connective tissue disorders
- electrolyte imbalances
- cellular hypoxia
- hypertrophy of the heart muscle
- acid-base imbalances
- emotional stress.

Pathophysiology

Cardiac arrhythmias may result from:
- enhanced automaticity
- reentry
- escape beats (additional abnormal heart beats that occur when the heart rate is very slow)
- abnormal electrical conduction.

What to look for

When a patient presents with a history of symptoms suggestive of cardiac arrhythmias, or has been treated for a cardiac arrhythmia, be alert for:
- reports of precipitating factors, such as exercise, smoking, sleep, emotional stress, exposure to heat or cold, caffeine intake, position changes, or recent illnesses

• attempts to alleviate the symptoms, such as coughing, rest, medications, or deep breathing
• reports of sensing the heart's rhythm, such as palpitations, irregular beating, skipped beats, or rapid or slow heart rate.

A matter of degree

Physical examination findings vary depending on the arrhythmia and the degree of hemodynamic compromise.

Circulatory failure along with an absence of pulse and respirations is found with asystole, ventricular fibrillation, and sometimes with ventricular tachycardia.

That's not all

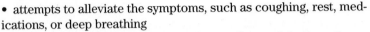

Dizziness may indicate a cardiac arrhythmia.

Additional findings may include:
• pallor
• cold and clammy extremities
• reduced urine output
• dyspnea
• hypotension
• weakness
• chest pains
• dizziness
• syncope (with severely impaired cerebral circulation).

What tests tell you

• A 12-lead ECG is the standard test for identifying cardiac arrhythmias. A 15-lead ECG (in which additional leads are applied to the right side of the chest) or an 18-lead ECG (in which additional leads are also added to the posterior scapular area) may be done to provide more definitive information about the patient's right ventricle and posterior wall of the left ventricle. (See *Understanding cardiac arrhythmias*, pages 242 to 249.)
• Laboratory testing may reveal electrolyte abnormalities, hypoxemia or acid-base abnormalities (with ABG analysis), or drug toxicities as the cause of arrhythmias.
• Exercise testing may reveal exercise-induced arrhythmias.
• Electrophysiologic testing may be used to identify the mechanism of an arrhythmia and location of accessory pathways and to assess the effectiveness of antiarrhythmic drugs.

How it's treated

The goals of treatment are to return pacer function to the sinus node, increase or decrease ventricular rate to normal, regain AV synchrony, and maintain normal sinus rhythm.

Treatments to correct abnormal rhythms include therapy with:

- antiarrhythmic drugs
- electrical conversion with defibrillation and cardioversion
- Valsalva's maneuver
- temporary or permanent placement of a pacemaker to maintain heart rate
- implantable cardioverter-defibrillator (ICD), if indicated
- surgical removal or cryotherapy of an irritable ectopic focus to prevent recurring arrhythmias
- management of the underlying disorder such as correction of hypoxia.

What to do

Care for the patient experiencing a cardiac arrhythmia as follows:
- Evaluate the patient's ECG regularly for arrhythmia and assess hemodynamic parameters as indicated. Document arrhythmias and notify the doctor immediately.
- When life-threatening arrhythmias develop, rapidly assess the patient's LOC, pulse and respiratory rates, and hemodynamic parameters. Monitor his ECG continuously. Be prepared to initiate CPR, if indicated.
- Assess the patient for predisposing factors, such as fluid and electrolyte imbalance, and signs of drug toxicity, especially with digoxin.
- Administer medications as ordered, monitor for adverse effects, and monitor vital signs, hemodynamic parameters (as appropriate), and appropriate laboratory studies. Prepare to assist with or perform cardioversion or defibrillation, if indicated.
- If you suspect drug toxicity, report it to the doctor immediately and withhold the next dose.
- If a temporary pacemaker needs to be inserted, make sure that a fresh battery is installed to avoid temporary pacemaker malfunction and carefully secure the external catheter wires and the pacemaker box.
- After pacemaker insertion, monitor the patient's pulse rate regularly and watch for signs of pacemaker failure and decreased cardiac output.

Cardiac tamponade

Cardiac tamponade is a rapid, unchecked increase in pressure in the pericardial sac. This compresses the heart, impairs diastolic filling, and reduces cardiac output.

If I'm compressed, cardiac output decreases.

(Text continues on page 248.)

Understanding cardiac arrhythmias

Here's an outline of many common cardiac arrhythmias and their features, causes, and treatments. Use a normal electrocardiogram strip, if available, to compare normal cardiac rhythm configurations with the rhythm strips shown here. Characteristics of normal sinus rhythm include:

- ventricular and atrial rates of 60 to 100 beats/minute
- regular and uniform QRS complexes and P waves
- PR interval of 0.12 to 0.20 second
- QRS duration < 0.12 second
- identical atrial and ventricular rates, with constant PR intervals.

Arrhythmia and features

Sinus tachycardia

- Atrial and ventricular rhythms regular
- Rate >100 beats/minute; rarely, >160 beats/minute
- Normal P waves preceding each QRS complex

Sinus bradycardia

- Atrial and ventricular rhythms regular
- Rate < 60 beats/minute
- Normal P waves preceding each QRS complex

Paroxysmal supraventricular tachycardia

- Atrial and ventricular rhythms regular
- Heart rate >160 beats/minute; rarely exceeds 250 beats/minute
- P waves regular but aberrant; difficult to differentiate from preceding T waves
- P waves preceding each QRS complex
- Sudden onset and termination of arrhythmia

Atrial flutter

- Atrial rhythm regular; rate 250 to 400 beats/minute
- Ventricular rate variable, depending on degree of AV block (usually 60 to 100 beats/minute)
- No P waves, atrial activity appears as flutter waves (F waves); saw-tooth configuration common in lead II
- QRS complexes are uniform in shape but often irregular in rhythm

Causes	Treatment
• Normal physiologic response to fever, exercise, anxiety, pain, dehydration; may also accompany shock, left-sided heart failure, cardiac tamponade, hyperthyroidism, anemia, hypovolemia, pulmonary embolism, and anterior wall myocardial infarction (MI) • May also occur with atropine, epinephrine, isoproterenol, quinidine, caffeine, alcohol, cocaine, amphetamine, and nicotine use	• Correction of underlying cause • Beta-adrenergic blockers or calcium channel blocker
• Normal, in well-conditioned heart, as in an athlete • Increased intracranial pressure; increased vagal tone due to straining during defecation, vomiting, intubation, or mechanical ventilation; sick sinus syndrome; hypothyroidism; and inferior wall MI • May also occur with anticholinesterase, beta-adrenergic blocker, digoxin, and morphine use	• Correction of underlying cause • For low cardiac output, dizziness, weakness, altered level of consciousness, or low blood pressure; advanced cardiac life support (ACLS) protocol for administration of atropine • Temporary or permanent pacemaker • Dopamine or epinephrine infusion
• Intrinsic abnormality of atrioventricular (AV) conduction system • Physical or psychological stress, hypoxia, hypokalemia, cardiomyopathy, congenital heart disease, MI, valvular disease, Wolff-Parkinson-White syndrome, cor pulmonale, hyperthyroidism, and systemic hypertension • Digoxin toxicity; use of caffeine, marijuana, or central nervous system stimulants	• If patient is unstable, immediate cardioversion • If patient is stable, vagal stimulation, Valsalva's maneuver, and carotid sinus massage or adenosine • If cardiac function is preserved, treatment priority: calcium channel blocker, beta-adrenergic blocker, digoxin, and cardioversion; then consider procainamide, or amiodarone if each preceding treatment is ineffective in rhythm conversion • If the ejection fracture is less than 40% or if the patient is in heart failure, treatment order: digoxin, amiodarone, then diltiazem
• Heart failure, tricuspid or mitral valve disease, pulmonary embolism, cor pulmonale, inferior wall MI, and pericarditis • Digoxin toxicity	• If patient is unstable with a ventricular rate >150 beats/minute, immediate cardioversion • If patient is stable, follow ACLS protocol for cardioversion and drug therapy, which may include calcium channel blockers, beta-adrenergic blockers, amiodarone, or digoxin • Anticoagulation therapy may also be necessary • Radio frequency ablation to control rhythm

(continued)

Understanding cardiac rhythms (continued)

Arrhythmia and features

Atrial fibrillation

- Atrial rhythm grossly irregular; rate > 400 beats/minute
- Ventricular rhythm grossly irregular
- QRS complexes of uniform configuration and duration
- PR interval indiscernible
- No P waves, atrial activity appears as erratic, irregular, baseline fibrillatory waves (f waves)

Junctional rhythm

- Atrial and ventricular rhythms regular; atrial rate 40 to 60 beats/minute; ventricular rate usually 40 to 60 beats/minute (60 to 100 beats/minute is accelerated junctional rhythm)
- P waves preceding, hidden within (absent), or after QRS complex; usually inverted if visible
- PR interval (when present) < 0.12 second
- QRS complex configuration and duration normal, except in aberrant conduction

First-degree AV block

- Atrial and ventricular rhythms regular
- PR interval > 0.20 second
- P wave precedes QRS complex
- QRS complex normal

Second-degree AV block
Mobitz I (Wenckebach)

- Atrial rhythm regular
- Ventricular rhythm irregular
- Atrial rate exceeds ventricular rate
- PR interval progressively longer with each cycle until QRS complex disappears (dropped beat); PR interval shorter after dropped beat

Second-degree AV block
Mobitz II

- Atrial rhythm regular
- Ventricular rhythm regular or irregular, with varying degree of block
- PR interval constant for conducted beats
- P waves normal size and shape, but some aren't followed by a QRS complex

Causes	Treatment
• Heart failure, chronic obstructive pulmonary disease, thyro-toxicosis, constrictive pericarditis, ischemic heart disease, sepsis, pulmonary embolus, rheumatic heart disease, hypertension, mitral stenosis, atrial irritation, or complication of coronary bypass or valve replacement surgery • Nifedipine and digoxin use	• If patient is unstable with a ventricular rate > 150 beats/minute, immediate cardioversion • If patient is stable, follow ACLS protocol and drug therapy, which may include calcium channel blockers, beta-adrenergic blockers, amiodarone, or digoxin • Anticoagulation therapy may also be necessary • In some patients with refractory atrial fibrillation uncontrolled by drugs, radio frequency catheter ablation
• Inferior wall MI or ischemia, hypoxia, vagal stimulation, and sick sinus syndrome • Acute rheumatic fever • Valve surgery • Digoxin toxicity	• Correction of underlying cause • Atropine for symptomatic slow rate • Pacemaker insertion if patient doesn't respond to drugs • Discontinuation of digoxin if appropriate
• May be seen in healthy persons • Inferior wall MI or ischemia, hypothyroidism, hypokalemia, and hyperkalemia • Digoxin toxicity; use of quinidine, procainamide, beta-adren-ergic blockers, calcium channel blockers, or amiodarone	• Correction of underlying cause • Possibly atropine if severe symptomatic bradycardia develops • Cautious use of digoxin, calcium channel blockers, and beta-adrenergic blockers
• Inferior wall MI, cardiac surgery, acute rheumatic fever, and vagal stimulation • Digoxin toxicity; use of propranolol, quinidine, or pro-cainamide	• Treatment of underlying cause • Atropine or temporary pacemaker for symptomatic brady-cardia • Discontinuation of digoxin if appropriate
• Severe coronary artery disease, anterior wall MI, and acute myocarditis • Digoxin toxicity	• Temporary or permanent pacemaker • Atropine, dopamine, or epinephrine for a symptomatic brady-cardia • Discontinuation of digoxin if appropriate

(continued)

Understanding cardiac rhythms *(continued)*

Arrhythmia and features

Third-degree AV block
(complete heart block)

- Atrial rhythm regular
- Ventricular rhythm regular and rate slower than atrial rate
- No relation between P waves and QRS complexes
- No constant PR interval
- QRS duration normal (junctional pacemaker) or wide and bizarre (ventricular pacemaker)

Premature ventricular contraction (PVC)

- Atrial rhythm regular
- Ventricular rhythm irregular
- QRS complex premature, usually followed by a complete compensatory pause
- QRS complex wide and distorted, usually > 0.12 second
- Premature QRS complexes occurring alone, in pairs, or in threes, alternating with normal beats; focus from one or more sites
- Ominous when clustered, multifocal, with R wave on T pattern

Ventricular tachycardia

- Ventricular rate 100 to 220 beats/minute, rhythm usually regular
- QRS complexes wide, bizarre, and independent of P waves
- P waves not discernible
- May start and stop suddenly

Causes	Treatment
• Inferior or anterior wall MI, congenital abnormality, rheumatic fever, hypoxia, postoperative complication of mitral valve replacement, postprocedure complication of radiofrequency ablation in or near AV nodal tissue, Lev's disease (fibrosis and calcification that spreads from cardiac structures to the conductive tissue), and Lenégre's disease (conductive tissue fibrosis) • Digoxin toxicity	• Atropine, dopamine, or epinephrine for symptomatic bradycardia • Temporary or permanent pacemaker
• Heart failure; old or acute MI, ischemia, or contusion; myocardial irritation by ventricular catheter or a pacemaker; hypercapnia; hypokalemia; hypocalcemia; and hypomagnesemia • Drug toxicity (digoxin, aminophylline, tricyclic antidepressants, beta-adrenergic blockers, isoproterenol, or dopamine) • Caffeine, tobacco, or alcohol use • Psychological stress, anxiety, pain, or exercise	• If warranted, procainamide, amiodarone, or lidocaine I.V. • Treatment of underlying cause • Discontinuation of drug causing toxicity • Potassium chloride I.V. if PVC induced by hypokalemia • Magnesium sulfate I.V. if PVC induced by hypomagnesemia
• Myocardial ischemia, MI, or aneurysm; coronary artery disease; rheumatic heart disease; mitral valve prolapse; heart failure; cardiomyopathy; ventricular catheters; hypokalemia; hypercalcemia; hypomagnesemia; and pulmonary embolism • Digoxin, procainamde, epinephrine, or quinidine toxicity • Anxiety	• With pulse: If hemodynamically stable with monomorphic QRS complexes administration of procainamide, sotolol, amiodarone, or lidocaine (follow ACLS protocol); if drugs are ineffective, cardioversion • If polymorphic QRS complexes and normal QT interval, administer beta-adrenergic blockers, lidocaine, amiodarone, procainamide, or sotalol (follow ACLS protocol); if drug is unsuccessful, cardioversion • If polymorphic QRS and QT interval is prolonged, magnesium I.V., then overdrive pacing if rhythm persists; may also administer isoproterenol, phenytoin, or lidocaine • Pulseless: Initiate CPR; follow ACLS protocol for defibrillation, endotracheal (ET) intubation, and administration of epinephrine or vasopressin, followed by amiodarone or lidocaine and, if ineffective, magnesium sulfate or procainamide • Implantable cardioverter-defibrillator (ICD) if recurrent ventricular tachycardia

(continued)

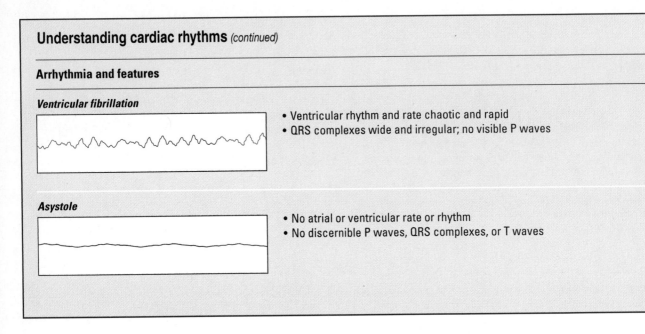

Understanding cardiac rhythms (continued)

Arrhythmia and features

Ventricular fibrillation

- Ventricular rhythm and rate chaotic and rapid
- QRS complexes wide and irregular; no visible P waves

Asystole

- No atrial or ventricular rate or rhythm
- No discernible P waves, QRS complexes, or T waves

Pericardial pressure

The increase in pressure usually results from blood or fluid accumulation in the pericardial sac. Even a small amount of fluid (50 to 100 ml) can cause a serious tamponade if it accumulates rapidly.

If fluid accumulates rapidly, cardiac tamponade requires emergency lifesaving measures to prevent death. A slow accumulation and increase in pressure may not produce immediate symptoms because the fibrous wall of the pericardial sac can gradually stretch to accommodate as much as 1 to 2 L of fluid.

What causes it

Cardiac tamponade may result from:
- idiopathic causes (such as Dressler's syndrome)
- effusion (from cancer, bacterial infections, tuberculosis and, rarely, acute rheumatic fever)
- hemorrhage due to trauma (such as gunshot or stab wounds of the chest)
- hemorrhage due to nontraumatic causes (such as anticoagulant therapy in patients with pericarditis or rupture of the heart or great vessels)
- viral or postirradiation pericarditis
- chronic renal failure requiring dialysis

> Cardiac tamponade may result from a slew of causative conditions and disorders.

Causes	Treatment
• Myocardial ischemia, MI, untreated ventricular tachycardia, R-on-T phenomenon, hypokalemia, hyperkalemia, hypercalcemia, hypoxemia, alkalosis, electric shock, and hypothermia • Digoxin, epinephrine, or quinidine toxicity	• CPR; follow ACLS protocol for defibrillation, ET intubation, and administration of epinephrine or vasopressin, amiodarone, or lidocaine and, if ineffective, magnesium sulfate or procainamide • ICD if risk for recurrent ventricular fibrillation
• Myocardial ischemia, MI, aortic valve disease, heart failure, hypoxia, hypokalemia, severe acidosis, electric shock, ventricular arrhythmia, AV block, pulmonary embolism, heart rupture, cardiac tamponade, hyperkalemia, and electromechanical dissociation • Cocaine overdose	• Continue CPR, follow ACLS protocol for ET intubation, temporary pacing, and administration of epinephrine and atropine.

• drug reaction from procainamide, hydralazine, minoxidil, isoniazid, penicillin, or daunorubicin
• connective tissue disorders (such as rheumatoid arthritis, systemic lupus erythematosus, rheumatic fever, vasculitis, and scleroderma)
• acute MI.

Pathophysiology

In cardiac tamponade, accumulation of fluid in the pericardial sac causes compression of the heart chambers. This compression obstructs blood flow into the ventricles and reduces the amount of blood that can be pumped out of the heart with each contraction. (See *Understanding cardiac tamponade*, page 250.)

What to look for

Cardiac tamponade has three classic features known as Beck's triad:

elevated CVP with jugular vein distention

muffled heart sounds

pulsus paradoxus (inspiratory drop in systemic blood pressure greater that 15 mm Hg).

Understanding cardiac tamponade

The pericardial sac, which surrounds and protects the heart, is composed of several layers:
- The fibrous pericardium is the tough outermost membrane.
- The inner membrane, called the *serous membrane,* consists of the visceral and parietal layers.
- The visceral layer clings to the heart and is also known as the *epicardial layer* of the heart.
- The parietal layer lies between the visceral layer and the fibrous pericardium.

- The pericardial space—between the visceral and parietal layers—contains 10 to 30 ml of pericardial fluid. This fluid lubricates the layers and minimizes friction when the heart contracts.

In cardiac tamponade, shown below right, blood or fluid fills the pericardial space, compressing the heart chambers, increasing intracardiac pressure, and obstructing venous return. As blood flow into the ventricles decreases, so does cardiac output. Without prompt treatment, low cardiac output can be fatal.

Normal heart and pericardium

Aorta
Superior vena cava
Fibrous pericardium
Parietal pericardium
Visceral pericardium
Attachment of fibrous pericardium to diaphragm
Diaphragm

Cardiac tamponade

Aorta
Superior vena cava
Fibrous pericardium
Parietal pericardium
Visceral pericardium
Pericardial space filled with excess fluid
Compressed heart
Diaphragm

That's not all

Other signs include:
- narrowed pulse pressure
- orthopnea
- diaphoresis
- anxiety
- restlessness
- cyanosis
- weak, rapid peripheral pulse.

What tests tell you

- Chest X-ray shows a slightly widened mediastinum and an enlarged cardiac silhouette.

In cardiac tamponade, a chest X-ray reveals a widened mediastinum and enlarged cardiac silhouette.

• ECG may show low-amplitude QRS complex and electrical alternans, an alternating beat-to-beat change in amplitude of the P wave, QRS complex, and T wave. Generalized ST-segment elevation is noted in all leads. An ECG is used to rule out other cardiac disorders; it may reveal changes produced by acute pericarditis.
• PA catheterization discloses increased right atrial pressure, right ventricular diastolic pressure, and CVP.
• Echocardiography may reveal pericardial effusion with signs of right ventricular and atrial compression.
• CT scan or MRI may be used to identify pericardial effusions or pericardial thickening caused by constrictive pericarditis.

How it's treated

The goal of treatment is to relieve intrapericardial pressure and cardiac compression by removing accumulated blood or fluid. This can be done three different ways:

pericardiocentesis (needle aspiration of the pericardial cavity)

surgical creation of an opening, called a *pericardial window*

insertion of a drain into the pericardial sac to drain the effusion.

When pressure's low

If the patient is hypotensive, trial volume loading with crystalloids such as I.V. normal saline solution may be used to maintain systolic blood pressure. An inotropic drug, such as dopamine, may be necessary to improve myocardial contractility until fluid in the pericardial sac can be removed.

Additional treatments

Additional treatment may necessary, depending on the cause. Examples of such causes and treatments are:
• traumatic injury — blood transfusion or a thoracotomy to drain reaccumulating fluid or to repair bleeding sites
• heparin-induced tamponade — administration of the heparin antagonist protamine sulfate
• warfarin-induced tamponade — vitamin K administration.

What to do

• Monitor the patient's cardiovascular status frequently, at least every hour, noting extent of jugular vein distention, quality of heart sounds, and blood pressure.

To correct heparin-induced tamponade, administer the heparin antagonist protamine sulfate.

- Assess hemodynamic status, including CVP, right atrial pressure, and PAP, and determine cardiac output.
- Monitor for pulsus paradoxus.
- Be alert for ST-segment and T-wave changes on ECG. Note rate and rhythm and report evidence of any arrhythmias.
- Watch closely for signs of increasing tamponade, increasing dyspnea, and arrhythmias and report immediately.
- Infuse I.V. solutions and inotropic drugs, such as dopamine, as ordered to maintain the patient's blood pressure.
- Administer oxygen therapy as needed and assess oxygen saturation levels. Monitor the patient's respiratory status for signs of respiratory distress, such as severe tachypnea and changes in the patient's LOC. Anticipate the need for ET intubation and mechanical ventilation if the patient's respiratory status deteriorates.
- Prepare the patient for pericardiocentesis or thoracotomy.
- If the patient has trauma-induced tamponade, assess for other signs of trauma and institute appropriate care, including the use of colloids, crystalloids, and blood component therapy under pressure or by rapid volume infuser if massive fluid replacement is needed; administration of protamine sulfate for heparin-induced tamponade; and vitamin K administration for warfarin-induced tamponade.
- Assess renal function status closely, monitoring urine output every hour and notifying the doctor if output is less than 0.5 mg/kg/hour.
- Monitor capillary refill time, LOC, peripheral pulses, and skin temperature for evidence of diminished tissue perfusion.

> Anticipate the need for ET and mechanical ventilation if the patient's respiratory status deteriorates.

Cardiogenic shock

Cardiogenic shock is a condition of diminished cardiac output that severely impairs tissue perfusion. It's sometimes called *pump failure.*

Shocking stats

Cardiogenic shock is a serious complication in nearly 15% of all patients hospitalized with acute MI. It typically affects patients whose area of infarction involves 40% or more of left ventricular muscle mass; in such patients, mortality may exceed 85%.

What causes it

Cardiogenic shock can result from any condition that causes significant left ventricular dysfunction with reduced cardiac output, such as:
- MI (most common)

- myocardial ischemia
- papillary muscle dysfunction
- end-stage cardiomyopathy.

Other offenders

Other causes include myocarditis and depression of myocardial contractility after cardiac arrest and prolonged cardiac surgery.

Mechanical abnormalities of the ventricle, such as acute mitral or aortic insufficiency or an acutely acquired ventricular septal defect or ventricular aneurysm, may also result in cardiogenic shock.

Pathophysiology

Regardless of the cause, here's what happens:
- Left ventricular dysfunction initiates a series of compensatory mechanisms that attempt to increase cardiac output and, in turn, maintain vital organ function.
- As cardiac output falls, baroreceptors in the aorta and carotid arteries initiate responses in the sympathetic nervous system. These responses, in turn, increase heart rate, left ventricular filling pressure, and peripheral resistance to flow to enhance venous return to the heart.
- These compensatory responses initially stabilize the patient but later cause the patient to deteriorate as the oxygen demands of the already compromised heart increase.

Lower and lower output

- The events involved in cardiogenic shock comprise a vicious cycle of low cardiac output, sympathetic compensation, myocardial ischemia, and even lower cardiac output.

What to look for

Cardiogenic shock produces signs of poor tissue perfusion, such as:
- cold, pale, clammy skin
- drop in systolic blood pressure to 30 mm Hg below baseline or a sustained reading below 80 mm Hg that isn't attributable to medication
- tachycardia
- rapid, shallow respirations
- oliguria (urine output less than 20 ml/hour)
- restlessness
- confusion
- narrowing pulse pressure
- cyanosis

Compensatory mechanisms that increase cardiac output eventually cause the patient to deteriorate because of increased oxygen demands.

• gallop rhythm, faint heart sounds, and possibly a holosystolic murmur.

What tests tell you

• Pulmonary artery pressure monitoring reveals increased PAP and PAWP, reflecting an increase in left ventricular end-diastolic pressure (preload) and heightened resistance to left ventricular emptying (afterload) caused by ineffective pumping and increased peripheral vascular resistance. Thermodilution catheterization reveals a reduced cardiac index.
• Invasive arterial pressure monitoring shows systolic arterial pressure less than 80 mm Hg caused by impaired ventricular ejection.
• ABG analysis may show metabolic and respiratory acidosis and hypoxia.
• ECG demonstrates possible evidence of acute MI, ischemia, or ventricular aneurysm.
• Echocardiography is used to determine left ventricular function and reveals valvular abnormalities.
• Serum enzyme measurements display elevated levels of CK, LD, aspartate aminotransferase, and alanine aminotransferase, which indicate MI or ischemia and suggest heart failure or shock. CK-MB (an isoenzyme of CK that occurs in cardiac tissue) and LD isoenzyme levels may confirm acute MI.
• Cardiac catheterization and echocardiography may reveal other conditions that can lead to pump dysfunction and failure, such as cardiac tamponade, papillary muscle infarct or rupture, ventricular septal rupture, pulmonary emboli, venous pooling (associated with venodilators and continuous or intermittent positive-pressure breathing), and hypovolemia.

How it's treated

The goal of treatment is to enhance cardiovascular status by increasing cardiac output, improving myocardial perfusion, and decreasing cardiac workload. Treatment consists of administering a combination of cardiovascular drugs and mechanical-assist techniques.

Treatment ABCs

Treatment begins with these measures:
• maintaining a patent airway; preparing for intubation and mechanical ventilation if the patient develops respiratory distress
• supplemental oxygen to increase oxygenation
• continuous cardiac monitoring to detect changes in heart rate and rhythm; administration of antiarrhythmics, as necessary

Cardiovascular drugs and mechanical-assist techniques are used to treat cardiogenic shock.

• initiating and maintaining at least two I.V. lines with large-gauge needles for fluid and drug administration
• I.V. fluids, crystalloids, colloids, or blood products, as necessary, to maintain intravascular volume.

Cardiovascular drugs

Drug therapy may include I.V. dopamine, phenylephrine, or norepinephrine to increase blood pressure and blood flow to kidneys. Inamrinone or dobutamine—inotropic agents that increase myocardial contractility and cardiac output—are commonly used.

Decrease resistance and pressure

A vasodilator, nitroglycerin or nitroprusside, may be used with a vasopressor to further improve cardiac output by decreasing peripheral vascular resistance (afterload) and reducing left ventricular end-diastolic pressure (preload). However, the patient's blood pressure must be adequate to support nitroprusside therapy and must be monitored closely.

Diuretics also may be used to reduce preload in patients with fluid volume overload.

Mechanical assistance

Treatment may also include mechanical assistance by IABP to improve coronary artery perfusion and decrease cardiac workload. The IABP is inserted through the femoral artery into the descending thoracic aorta. The balloon inflates during diastole to increase coronary artery perfusion pressure and deflates before systole (before the aortic valve opens) to reduce resistance to ejection (afterload) and therefore reduce cardiac workload.

Improved ventricular ejection significantly improves cardiac output. Subsequent vasodilation in the peripheral vessels leads to lower preload volume and reduced workload of the left ventricle. This is because of decreasing systemic vascular resistance.

End-stage effort

When drug therapy and IABP insertion fail, a VAD may be inserted to assist the pumping action of the heart. When all other medical and surgical therapies fail, heart transplantation may be considered.

More measures

Additional treatment measures for cardiogenic shock may include:
• thrombolytic therapy or coronary artery revascularization to restore coronary artery blood flow, if cardiogenic shock is due to acute MI

Improved ventricular ejection significantly improves cardiac output.

• emergency surgery to repair papillary muscle rupture or ventricular septal defect, if either is the cause of cardiogenic shock.

What to do

• Begin I.V. infusions of normal saline solution or lactated Ringer's solution, using a large-bore (14G to 18G) catheter, which allows easier administration of later blood transfusions.
• Administer oxygen by face mask or artificial airway to ensure adequate oxygenation of tissues. Adjust the oxygen flow rate to a higher or lower level, as ABG measurements indicate. Many patients need 100% oxygen, and some require 5 to 15 cm H_2O of positive end-expiratory or continuous positive airway pressure ventilation.

Monitor, record, and then monitor more

• Monitor and record blood pressure, pulse, respiratory rate, and peripheral pulses every 1 to 5 minutes until the patient stabilizes. Monitor cardiac rhythm continuously. Systolic blood pressure less than 80 mm Hg usually results in inadequate coronary artery blood flow, cardiac ischemia, arrhythmias, and further complications of low cardiac output.
• Using a PA catheter, closely monitor PAP, PAWP and cardiac output. A high PAWP indicates heart failure, increased systemic vascular resistance, decreased cardiac output, and decreased cardiac index and should be reported immediately.
• Determine how much fluid to give by checking blood pressure, urine output, CVP, or PAWP. (To increase accuracy, measure CVP at the level of the right atrium, using the same reference point on the chest each time.) Whenever the fluid infusion rate is increased, watch for signs of fluid overload, such as an increase in PAWP. If the patient is hypovolemic, preload may need to be increased, typically accomplished with I.V. fluids. However, I.V. fluids must be given cautiously, being increased gradually while hemodynamic parameters are closely monitored. In this situation, diuretics aren't given.
• Insert an indwelling urinary catheter to measure hourly urine output. If output is less than 30 ml/hour in adults, increase the fluid infusion rate but watch for signs of fluid overload, such as an increase in PAWP. Notify the doctor if urine output doesn't improve.
• Administer a diuretic, such as furosemide or bumetanide, as ordered, to decrease preload and improve stroke volume and cardiac output.
• Monitor ABG values, CBC, and electrolyte levels. Expect to administer sodium bicarbonate by I.V. push if the patient is acidotic. Administer electrolyte replacement therapy as ordered.

Report a high PAWP immediately. It indicates heart failure, increased systemic vascular resistance, decreased cardiac output, and decreased cardiac index.

• During therapy, assess skin color and temperature and note any changes. Cold, clammy skin may be a sign of continuing peripheral vascular constriction, indicating progressive shock.

Don't move

• When your patient is on the IABP, move him as little as possible. Never flex the patient's "ballooned" leg at the hip because this may displace or fracture the catheter. Never place the patient in a sitting position for any reason (including chest X-rays) while the balloon is inflated; the balloon will tear through the aorta and result in immediate death.

• During use of the IABP, assess pedal pulses and skin temperature and color to ensure adequate peripheral circulation. Check the dressing over the insertion site frequently for bleeding, and change it according to facility protocol. Also check the site for hematoma or signs of infection, and culture any drainage.

• If the patient becomes hemodynamically stable, gradually reduce the frequency of balloon inflation to wean him from the IABP.

• When weaning the patient from the IABP, watch for ECG changes, chest pain, and other signs of recurring cardiac ischemia as well as for shock.

• Prepare the patient for possible emergency cardiac catheterization to determine eligibility for PTCA or CABG to reperfuse (restore blood flow to) areas with reversible injury patterns.

• To ease emotional stress, plan care measures to allow frequent rest periods and provide as much privacy as possible. Allow family members to visit and comfort the patient as much as possible.

To ease emotional stress, allow frequent rest periods and allow family members to comfort the patient as much as possible.

Cardiomyopathy

Cardiomyopathy generally refers to disease of the heart muscle fibers. It takes three main forms:

- dilated

- hypertrophic

- restrictive (extremely rare).

Cardiomyopathy is the second most common direct cause of sudden death; CAD is first. Because dilated cardiomyopathy usually isn't diagnosed until its advanced stages, the prognosis is generally poor.

Dilated cardiomyopathy usually isn't diagnosed until it's advanced, so the prognosis is generally poor.

What causes it

Males and blacks are at greatest risk for cardiomyopathy; other
risk factors include hypertension, pregnancy, viral infections, and
alcohol use.

Pathophysiology

Most patients with cardiomyopathy have idiopathic, or primary,
disease, but some cases are secondary to identifiable causes. Hypertrophic cardiomyopathy is almost always inherited as a non-
sex-linked autosomal dominant trait.

Dilated cardiomyopathy

Dilated cardiomyopathy primarily affects systolic function. It results from extensively damaged myocardial muscle fibers. Consequently, contractility in the left ventricle decreases.

Poor compensation

As systolic function declines, stroke volume, ejection fraction, and
cardiac output decrease. As end-diastolic volumes increase, pulmonary congestion may occur. The elevated end-diastolic volume
is a compensatory response to preserve stroke volume despite a
reduced ejection fraction.

The sympathetic nervous system is also stimulated to increase
heart rate and contractility.

Kidneys kick in

The kidneys are stimulated to retain sodium and water to maintain cardiac output, and vasoconstriction also occurs as the renin-
angiotensin system is stimulated. When these compensatory
mechanisms can no longer maintain cardiac output, the heart begins to fail.

Detrimental dilation

Left ventricular dilation occurs as venous return and systemic
vascular resistance increases. Eventually, the atria also dilate,
as more work is required to pump blood into the full ventricles.
Cardiomegaly is a consequence of dilation of the atria and ventricles. Blood pooling in the ventricles increases the risk of emboli.

Hypertrophic cardiomyopathy

Hypertrophic cardiomyopathy primarily affects diastolic function.
The features of hypertrophic cardiomyopathy include:
- asymmetrical left ventricular hypertrophy
- hypertrophy of the intraventricular septum

In dilated
cardiomyopathy, I
try to help
maintain cardiac
output by
retaining water
and sodium.

- rapid, forceful contractions of the left ventricle
- impaired relaxation
- obstruction of left ventricular outflow.

Fouled-up filling

The hypertrophied ventricle becomes stiff, noncompliant, and unable to relax during ventricular filling. Consequently, ventricular filling is reduced and left ventricular filling pressure rises, causing increases in left atrial and pulmonary venous pressures and leading to venous congestion and dyspnea.

Ventricular filling time is further reduced as a compensatory response to tachycardia. Reduced ventricular filling during diastole and obstruction to ventricular outflow lead to low cardiac output.

Hypertrophy hazards

If papillary muscles become hypertrophied and don't close completely during contraction, mitral insufficiency occurs. Moreover, intramural coronary arteries are abnormally small and may not be sufficient to supply the hypertrophied muscle with enough blood and oxygen to meet the increased needs of the hyperdynamic muscle.

Restrictive cardiomyopathy

Restrictive cardiomyopathy is characterized by stiffness of the ventricle caused by left ventricular hypertrophy and endocardial fibrosis and thickening. The ability of the ventricle to relax and fill during diastole is reduced. Furthermore, the rigid myocardium fails to contract completely during systole. As a result, cardiac output decreases.

What to look for

Generally, for patients with dilated or restrictive cardiomyopathy, the onset is insidious. As the disease progresses, exacerbations and hospitalizations are frequent regardless of the type of cardiomyopathy.

Dilated cardiomyopathy

For a patient with dilated cardiomyopathy, signs and symptoms may be overlooked until left ventricular failure occurs. Be sure to evaluate the patient's current condition and then compare it with that over the past 6 to 12 months. Signs and symptoms of dilated cardiomyopathy may include:

• shortness of breath, orthopnea, dyspnea on exertion, paroxysmal nocturnal dyspnea, fatigue, and a dry cough at night due to left-sided heart failure
• peripheral edema, hepatomegaly, jugular vein distention, and weight gain caused by right-sided heart failure
• peripheral cyanosis
• tachycardia
• pansystolic murmur associated with mitral and tricuspid insufficiency
• S_3 and S_4 gallop rhythms
• irregular pulse if atrial fibrillation exists.

Hypertrophic cardiomyopathy

Signs and symptoms vary widely among patients with hypertrophic cardiomyopathy. The presenting symptom is commonly syncope or sudden cardiac death. Other possible signs and symptoms include:
• angina
• dyspnea
• fatigue
• systolic ejection murmur along the left sternal border and apex
• peripheral pulse with a characteristic double impulse (pulsus biferiens)
• abrupt arterial pulse
• irregular pulse with atrial fibrillation.

Restrictive cardiomyopathy

A patient with restrictive cardiomyopathy presents with signs of heart failure and other signs and symptoms, including:
• fatigue
• dyspnea
• orthopnea
• chest pain
• edema
• liver engorgement
• peripheral cyanosis
• pallor
• S_3 or S_4 gallop rhythms
• systolic murmurs.

What tests tell you

These tests are used to diagnose cardiomyopathy:
• Echocardiography confirms dilated cardiomyopathy.
• Chest X-ray may reveal cardiomegaly associated with any of the cardiomyopathies.

Oh, dear! The first clue to hypertrophic cardiomyopathy may be syncope or sudden cardiac death.

Look for heart failure and other signs and symptoms to find a patient with restrictive cardiomyopathy.

• Cardiac catheterization with possible heart biopsy can be definitive in hypertrophic cardiomyopathy.

How it's treated

There's no known cure for cardiomyopathy. Treatment is individualized based on the type of cardiomyopathy and the patient's condition.

Dilated cardiomyopathy

For a patient with dilated cardiomyopathy, treatment may involve:
• management of the underlying cause, if it's known.
• ACE inhibitors, as first-line therapy, to reduce afterload through vasodilation
• diuretics, taken with ACE inhibitors, to reduce fluid retention
• digoxin, for patients not responding to ACE inhibitor and diuretic therapy, to improve myocardial contractility
• hydralazine and isosorbide dinitrate, in combination, to produce vasodilation
• beta-adrenergic blockers for patients with mild or moderate heart failure
• antiarrhythmics, such as amiodarone, used cautiously to control arrhythmias
• cardioversion to convert atrial fibrillation to sinus rhythm
• pacemaker insertion to correct arrhythmias
• anticoagulants to reduce the risk of emboli (controversial)
• revascularization, such as CABG surgery, if dilated cardiomyopathy is due to ischemia
• valvular repair or replacement, if dilated cardiomyopathy is due to valve dysfunction
• lifestyle modifications, such as smoking cessation; low-fat, low-sodium diet; physical activity; and abstinence from alcohol
• heart transplantation in patients resistant to medical therapy.

Hypertrophic cardiomyopathy

For a patient with hypertrophic cardiomyopathy, treatment may involve:
• beta-adrenergic blockers to slow the heart rate, reduce myocardial oxygen demands, and increase ventricular filling by relaxing the obstructing muscle, thereby increasing cardiac output
• antiarrhythmic drugs, such as amiodarone, to reduce arrhythmias
• cardioversion to treat atrial fibrillation
• anticoagulation to reduce risk of systemic embolism with atrial fibrillation

If your patient's condition doesn't improve with medical measures, a heart transplant may be needed.

• verapamil and diltiazem to reduce ventricular stiffness and elevated diastolic pressures
• ablation of the AV node and implantation of a dual-chamber pacemaker (controversial), in patients with obstructive hypertrophic cardiomyopathy and ventricular tachycardias, to reduce the outflow gradient by altering the pattern of ventricular contraction
• ICD to correct ventricular arrhythmias
• ventricular myotomy or myectomy (resection of the hypertrophied septum) to ease outflow tract obstruction and relieve symptoms
• mitral valve replacement to correct mitral insufficiency
• heart transplantation for intractable symptoms.

Restrictive cardiomyopathy

For the patient with restrictive cardiomyopathy, treatment may involve:
• management of the underlying cause such as administering deferoxamine to bind iron in restrictive cardiomyopathy due to hemochromatosis
• digoxin, diuretics, and a restricted sodium diet may ease the symptoms of heart failure, although no therapy exists for patients with restricted ventricular filling
• oral vasodilators to control intractable heart failure.

Treatment of your patient with restrictive cardiomyopathy may begin with management of the underlying cause.

What to do

• Administer drugs, as ordered, to promote adequate heart function.
• Assess hemodynamic status every 2 hours or more frequently, if necessary.
• Monitor intake and output closely and obtain daily weights; institute fluid restrictions as ordered.
• Institute continuous cardiac monitoring to evaluate for arrhythmias.
• Assess the patient for possible adverse drug reactions, such as orthostatic hypotension with vasodilators, diuretics, or ACE inhibitors.
• Urge the patient to change positions slowly.
• Auscultate heart and lung sounds, being alert for S_3 heart sounds or murmurs, or crackles, rhonchi, and wheezes indicative of heart failure. Monitor vital signs for changes, especially a heart rate greater than 100 beats/minute, respiratory rate greater than 20 breaths/minute, and a systolic blood pressure less than 90 mm Hg, all of which suggest heart failure.
• Assist patient with ADLs to decrease oxygen demand.

Oxygen orders

- Administer supplemental oxygen as ordered. Assess for changes in LOC, such as restlessness or decreased responsiveness, indicating diminished cerebral perfusion. If the patient has a PA catheter in place, evaluate mixed venous oxygen saturation levels; if not, monitor oxygen saturation levels using pulse oximetry.
- Organize care to promote periods of rest for the patient.
- Prepare the patient, as indicated for insertion of pacemaker, ICD, IABP, or cardiac transplantation.

Heart failure

Heart failure occurs when the heart can't pump enough blood to meet the metabolic needs of the body.

Heart failure results in intravascular and interstitial volume overload and poor tissue perfusion. An individual with heart failure experiences reduced exercise tolerance, a reduced quality of life, and a shortened life span.

What causes it

The most common cause of heart failure is CAD, but it also occurs in infants, children, and adults with congenital and acquired heart defects.

Pathophysiology

Heart failure may be classified into four general categories:

- left-sided heart failure
- right-sided heart failure
- systolic dysfunction
- diastolic dysfunction.

When the left loses its faculties

Left-sided heart failure is a result of ineffective left ventricular contractile function.

As the pumping ability of the left ventricle fails, cardiac output drops. Blood is no longer effectively pumped out into the body; it backs up into the left atrium and then into the lungs, causing pulmonary congestion, dyspnea, and activity intolerance.

If the condition persists, pulmonary edema and right-sided heart failure may result. Common causes include:

- left ventricular infarction

Uh-oh! Blood backs up into the left atrium and then into the lungs when the left ventricle can't pump well.

- hypertension
- aortic and mitral valve stenosis.

When right goes wrong

Right-sided heart failure results from ineffective right ventricular contractile function.

When blood isn't pumped effectively through the right ventricle to the lungs, blood backs up into the right atrium and into the peripheral circulation. The patient gains weight and develops peripheral edema and engorgement of the kidney and other organs.

Blame it on the left

Right-sided heart failure may be due to an acute right ventricular infarction or a pulmonary embolus. However, the most common cause is profound backward flow due to left-sided heart failure.

Just can't pump enough

Systolic dysfunction occurs when the left ventricle can't pump enough blood out to the systemic circulation during systole and the ejection fraction falls. Consequently, blood backs up into the pulmonary circulation and pressure increases in the pulmonary venous system. Cardiac output decreases; weakness, fatigue, and shortness of breath may occur.

Causes of systolic dysfunction include MI and dilated cardiomyopathy.

Watch out for systolic dysfunction in your patients with MI and dilated cardiomyopathy.

Can't relax. Can't fill. It all goes to swell from here.

Diastolic dysfunction occurs when the ability of the left ventricle to relax and fill during diastole is reduced and the stroke volume falls. Therefore, higher volumes are needed in the ventricles to maintain cardiac output. Consequently, pulmonary congestion and peripheral edema develop.

Diastolic dysfunction may occur as a result of left ventricular hypertrophy, hypertension, or restrictive cardiomyopathy.

This type of heart failure is less common than that due to systolic dysfunction, and treatment isn't as clear.

Compensatory mechanisms

All types of heart failure eventually lead to reduced cardiac output, which triggers compensatory mechanisms that improve cardiac output at the expense of increased ventricular work. The compensatory mechanisms include:

- increased sympathetic activity
- activation of the renin-angiotensin-aldosterone system
- ventricular dilation
- ventricular hypertrophy.

Increased sympathetic activity

Increased sympathetic activity — a response to decreased cardiac output and blood pressure — enhances peripheral vascular resistance, contractility, heart rate, and venous return. Signs of increased sympathetic activity, such as cool extremities and clamminess, may indicate impending heart failure.

Renin-angiotensin-aldosterone system

Increased sympathetic activity also restricts blood flow to the kidneys, causing them to secrete renin which, in turn, converts angiotensinogen to angiotensin I, which then becomes angiotensin II — a potent vasoconstrictor. Angiotensin causes the adrenal cortex to release aldosterone, leading to sodium and water retention and an increase in circulating blood volume.

This renal mechanism is helpful; however, if it persists unchecked, it can aggravate heart failure as the heart struggles to pump against the increased volume.

Ventricular dilation

In ventricular dilation, an increase in end-diastolic ventricular volume (preload) causes increased stroke work and stroke volume during contraction. This stretches cardiac muscle fibers so that the ventricle can accept the increased volume. Eventually, the muscle becomes stretched beyond optimum limits and contractility declines.

Ventricular hypertrophy

In ventricular hypertrophy, an increase in ventricular muscle mass allows the heart to pump against increased resistance to the outflow of blood, improving cardiac output. However, this increased muscle mass also increases the myocardial oxygen requirements.

Compromising situation

An increase in the ventricular diastolic pressure necessary to fill the enlarged ventricle may compromise diastolic coronary blood flow, limiting the oxygen supply to the ventricle, and causing ischemia and impaired muscle contractility.

Counterregulatory substances

In heart failure, counterregulatory substances — prostaglandins and atrial natriuretic factor — are produced in an attempt to reduce the negative effects of volume overload and vasoconstriction caused by the compensatory mechanisms.

Kidneys' contributions

The kidneys release the prostaglandins, prostacyclin and prostaglandin E2, which are potent vasodilators. These vasodilators also

Such signs as cool extremities and clamminess may indicate impending heart failure.

I do my best, but ventricular hypertrophy eventually leads to ischemia and impaired contractility.

act to reduce volume overload produced by the renin-angiotensin-aldosterone system by inhibiting sodium and water reabsorption by the kidneys.

Counteracting hormone

Atrial natriuretic factor is a hormone that's secreted mainly by the atria in response to stimulation of the stretch receptors in the atria caused by excess fluid volume.

Atrial natriuretic factor works to counteract the negative effects of sympathetic nervous system stimulation and the renin-angiotensin-aldosterone system by producing vasodilation and diuresis.

What to look for

Early signs and symptoms of left-sided heart failure include:
- dyspnea
- orthopnea
- paroxysmal nocturnal dyspnea
- fatigue
- nonproductive cough.

Later, on the left

Later clinical manifestations of left-sided heart failure may include:
- crackles on auscultation
- hemoptysis
- displacement of the PMI toward the left anterior axillary line
- tachycardia
- S_3 heart sound
- S_4 heart sound
- cool, pale skin
- restlessness and confusion.

On the right side

Clinical manifestations of right-sided heart failure include:
- jugular vein distention
- hepatojugular reflux and hepatomegaly
- right upper quadrant pain
- anorexia, fullness, and nausea
- nocturia
- weight gain
- edema
- ascites or anasarca.

Learn to recognize both early and later signs of left-sided heart failure.

What tests tell you

These tests are used to diagnose heart failure:
• Chest X-ray shows increased pulmonary vascular markings, interstitial edema, or pleural effusion and cardiomegaly.
• ECG may indicate hypertrophy, ischemic changes, or infarction, and may also reveal tachycardia and extrasystoles.
• Laboratory testing may reveal abnormal liver function and elevated BUN and creatinine levels.
• ABG analysis may reveal hypoxemia from impaired gas exchange and respiratory alkalosis because the patient blows off more carbon dioxide as respiratory rate increases in compensation.
• Echocardiography may reveal left ventricular hypertrophy, dilation, and abnormal contractility.
• Pulmonary artery monitoring typically demonstrates elevated PAP and PAWP, left ventricular end-diastolic pressure in left-sided heart failure, and elevated right atrial pressure or CVP in right-sided heart failure.
• Radionuclide ventriculography may reveal an ejection fraction less than 40%; in diastolic dysfunction, the ejection fraction may be normal.

Check echocardiography results for signs of left ventricular hypertrophy, dilation, and abnormal contractility.

How it's treated

The goal of therapy is to improve pump function. Correction of heart failure may involve:
• treatment of the underlying cause, if it's known
• ACE inhibitors for patients with left ventricle dysfunction to reduce production of angiotensin II, resulting in preload and afterload reduction
• digoxin for patients with heart failure due to left ventricular systolic dysfunction to increase myocardial contractility, improve cardiac output, reduce the volume of the ventricle, and decrease ventricular stretch
• diuretics to reduce fluid volume overload, venous return, and preload
• beta-adrenergic blockers in patients with mild to moderate heart failure caused by left ventricular systolic dysfunction, to prevent remodeling
• diuretics, nitrates, morphine, and oxygen to treat pulmonary edema
• lifestyle modifications to reduce symptoms of heart failure, such as weight loss if obese; limited sodium (to 2 g/day) and alcohol intake; reduced fat intake; smoking cessation; stress reduction; and development of an exercise program

Teach your patient about lifestyle changes that can reduce symptoms of heart failure.

• CABG surgery or angioplasty for patients with heart failure due to CAD
• heart transplantation in patients receiving aggressive medical treatment but still experiencing limitations or repeated hospitalizations
• other surgery or invasive procedures, such as cardiomyoplasty, insertion of an IABP, partial left ventriculectomy, use of a mechanical ventricular assist device, and implantation of an ICD or a biventricular pacemaker.

What to do

• Place the patient in Fowler's position to maximize chest expansion and give supplemental oxygen, as ordered, to ease his breathing. Monitor oxygen saturation levels and ABGs as indicated. If respiratory status deteriorates, anticipate the need for ET intubation and mechanical ventilation.
• Institute continuous cardiac monitoring and notify the doctor of changes in rhythm and rate. If the patient develops tachycardia, administer beta-adrenergic blockers as ordered; if atrial fibrillation is present, administer anticoagulants or antiplatelet agents as ordered to prevent thrombus formation.
• If the patient develops a new arrhythmia, obtain a 12-lead ECG immediately.
• Monitor hemodynamic status, including cardiac output, cardiac index, pulmonary and systemic vascular pressures closely, at least hourly, noting trends. If available, institute continuous cardiac output monitoring.
• Administer medications as ordered. Check apical heart rate before administering digoxin.
• Assess respiratory status frequently, at least every 1 to 2 hours. Auscultate lungs for abnormal breath sounds, such as crackles, wheezes, and rhonchi. Encourage coughing and deep breathing.
• Obtain daily weights and observe for peripheral edema.
• Assess hourly urine output. Also, monitor fluid intake, including I.V. fluids.
• Frequently monitor BUN and serum creatinine, liver function studies, and serum potassium, sodium, chloride, and magnesium levels daily.
• Organize all activities to provide maximum rest periods. Assess for signs of activity intolerance, such as increased shortness of breath, chest pain, increased arrhythmias, heart rate greater than 120 beats/minute, and ST-segment changes, and have the patient stop activity.
• To prevent deep vein thrombosis caused by vascular congestion, assist the patient with ROM exercises. Enforce bed rest and apply antiembolism stockings or intermittent compression devices.

If your patient's respiratory status deteriorates, be ready to institute intubation and mechanical ventilation.

Check your patient's apical heart rate before you administer digoxin.

- Prepare the patient for surgical intervention or insertion of IABP or ICD, if indicated.

Hypertensive crisis typically strikes patients with long histories of chronic, poorly controlled, or untreated hypertension.

Hypertensive crisis

A hypertensive emergency, commonly called *hypertensive crisis*, refers to the abrupt, acute, and marked increase in blood pressure from the patient's baseline that ultimately leads to acute and rapidly progressing end-organ damage.

Rapid rise

Typically, the patient's diastolic blood pressure is greater than 120 mm Hg. The increased blood pressure value, although important, is probably less important than how rapidly the blood pressure increases.

What causes it

Most patients who develop hypertensive crisis have long histories of chronic, poorly controlled, or untreated primary hypertension. Conditions that cause secondary hypertension, such as pheochromocytoma or Cushing's syndrome, may also be responsible.

Pathophysiology

Arterial blood pressure is a product of total peripheral resistance and cardiac output:
- Cardiac output is increased by conditions that increase heart rate or stroke volume, or both.
- Peripheral resistance is increased by factors that increase blood viscosity or reduce the lumen size of vessels, especially the arterioles.

Faulty mechanisms

Hypertension may result from a disturbance in one of the body's intrinsic mechanisms, including:
- renin-angiotensin system
- autoregulation
- sympathetic nervous system
- antidiuretic hormone.

Up with pressure

The renin-angiotensin system increases blood pressure in these ways:

- Sodium depletion, reduced blood pressure, and dehydration stimulate renin release.
- Renin reacts with angiotensinogen, a liver enzyme, and converts it to angiotensin I, which increases preload and afterload.
- Angiotensin I converts to angiotensin II in the lungs; angiotensin II is a potent vasoconstrictor that targets the arterioles.
- Circulating angiotensin II increases preload and afterload by stimulating the adrenal cortex to secrete aldosterone. This increases blood volume by conserving sodium and water.

Maintaining flow

In autoregulation, several intrinsic mechanisms together change an artery's diameter to maintain tissue and organ perfusion despite fluctuations in systemic blood pressure.

These mechanisms include stress relaxation and capillary fluid shifts:
- In stress relaxation, blood vessels gradually dilate when blood pressure increases, reducing peripheral resistance.
- In capillary fluid shift, plasma moves between vessels and extravascular spaces to maintain intravascular volume.

Autoregulation mechanisms maintain tissue and organ perfusion despite blood pressure changes.

Taking control

Sympathetic nervous system mechanisms control blood pressure. When blood pressure decreases, baroreceptors in the aortic arch and carotid sinuses decrease their inhibition of the medulla's vasomotor center.

Consequent increases in sympathetic stimulation of the heart by norepinephrine increases cardiac output by:
- strengthening the contractile force
- raising the heart rate
- augmenting peripheral resistance by vasoconstriction.

Stress can also stimulate the sympathetic nervous system to increase cardiac output and peripheral vascular resistance. The release of antidiuretic hormone can regulate hypotension by increasing reabsorption of water by the kidney. In reabsorption, blood plasma volume increases, thus raising blood pressure. In hypertensive crisis, one or more of these regulating mechanisms is disrupted.

Strain for the brain

Hypertensive crisis can result in hypertensive encephalopathy because of cerebral vasodilation from an inability to maintain autoregulation. Blood flow increases, causing an increase in pressure and subsequent cerebral edema. This increase in pressure damages the intimal and medial lining of the arterioles.

This is serious trouble! Hypertensive crisis can result in hypertensive encephalopathy because of cerebral vasodilation.

What to look for

Your assessment of a patient in hypertensive crisis almost always reveals a history of hypertension that's poorly controlled or hasn't been treated. Signs and symptoms may include:
• severe, throbbing headache in the back of the head
• nausea
• vomiting
• anorexia
• irritability
• confusion, somnolence, or stupor
• vision loss, blurred vision, or diplopia
• dizziness
• dyspnea on exertion, orthopnea, or paroxysmal nocturnal dyspnea
• edema
• angina
• possible left ventricular heave palpated at the mitral valve area
• S_4 heart sound
• acute retinopathy and hemorrhage, retinal exudates, and papilledema.

Check the head

If the patient has hypertensive encephalopathy, you may note:
• decreased LOC
• disorientation
• seizures
• focal neurologic deficits, such as hemiparesis, and unilateral sensory deficits.

Kidney-related consequences

If the hypertensive emergency has affected the kidneys, you may note reduced urine output as well as elevated BUN and creatinine levels.

What tests tell you

• Blood pressure measurement confirms the diagnosis of hypertensive emergency. Blood pressure measurement, obtained several times at an interval of at least 2 minutes, reveals an elevated diastolic pressure greater than 120 mm Hg.
• RBC count may be decreased secondary to hematuria if there's kidney involvement.
• If there's renal involvement, BUN may be greater than 20 mg/dl and serum creatinine level may be greater than 1.3 mg/dl.
• ECG may reveal ischemic changes or left ventricular hypertrophy; ST segment depression and T wave inversion suggest repolar-

Hypertensive crisis may affect the kidneys, causing reduced urine output and elevated BUN and creatinine levels.

ization problems from endocardial fibrosis associated with left ventricular hypertrophy.
- Echocardiography may reveal increased wall thickness with or without an increase in left ventricular size.
- Chest X-ray may reveal enlargement of the cardiac silhouette with left ventricular dilation, or pulmonary congestion and pleural effusions with heart failure.
- Urinalysis results may be normal unless there's renal impairment; then specific gravity is low (less than 1.010); hematuria, casts, and proteinuria may also be found. If the patient's condition is due to a disease condition, such as pheochromocytoma, a 24-hour urine test reveals increases in vanillylmandelic acid and urinary catecholamines.

How it's treated

Treatment is focused immediately on reducing the patient's blood pressure with I.V. antihypertensive therapy. However, care must be taken not to reduce the patient's blood pressure too rapidly because the patient's autoregulatory control is impaired.

Slow pressure cuts

The current recommendation is to reduce the blood pressure by no more than 25% of the MAP over the first 2 hours. Further reductions should occur over the next several days.

> Take steps to reduce your patient's blood pressure gradually, over several days.

More measures

- Sodium nitroprusside given as an I.V. infusion and titrated according to the patient's response is the drug of choice. It has a rapid onset of action and its effects cease within 1 to 5 minutes of stopping the drug. Thus, if the patient's blood pressure drops too low, stopping the drug almost immediately allows the blood pressure to increase.
- Other agents that may be used include labetalol, nitroglycerin (the drug of choice for treating hypertensive emergency when myocardial ischemia, acute MI, or pulmonary edema is present), and hydralazine (specifically indicated for treating hypertension in pregnant women with preeclampsia).
- Lifestyle changes may include weight reduction, smoking cessation, exercise, and dietary changes.
- After the acute episode is controlled, maintenance pharmacotherapy to control blood pressure plays a key role.

What to do

- Immediately obtain the patient's blood pressure.

- If not already in place, institute continuous cardiac and arterial pressure monitoring to assess blood pressure directly; determine the patient's MAP.
- Assess ABGs. Monitor the patient's oxygen saturation level using pulse oximetry; if you're monitoring the patient hemodynamically, assess mixed venous oxygen saturation. Administer supplemental oxygen, as ordered, based on the findings.
- Administer I.V. antihypertensive therapy, as ordered; if using nitroprusside, wrap the container in foil to protect it from the light and titrate the dose based on specified target ranges for systolic and diastolic pressures. Immediately stop the drug if the patient's blood pressure drops below the target range.
- Monitor blood pressure every 1 to 5 minutes while titrating drug therapy, then every 15 minutes to 1 hour as the patient's condition stabilizes.
- Continuously monitor ECG and institute treatment as indicated if arrhythmias occur. Auscultate the patient's heart, noting signs of heart failure, such as S_3 or S_4 heart sounds.
- Assess the patient's neurologic status every hour initially and then every 4 hours as the patient's condition stabilizes.
- Monitor urine output every hour and notify the doctor if output is less than 0.5 ml/kg/hour. Evaluate BUN and serum creatinine levels for changes and monitor daily weights.
- Obtain serum thiocyanate levels after 48 hours of therapy and then regularly thereafter while the patient is receiving nitroprusside.
- Administer other antihypertensives as ordered. As patient's condition stabilizes, expect to begin oral antihypertensive therapy while gradually weaning I.V. drugs to prevent hypotension. If the patient is experiencing fluid overload, administer diuretics as ordered.
- Assess the patient's vision and report changes, such as increased blurred vision, diplopia, or loss of vision.
- Administer analgesics as ordered for headache; keep your patient's environment quiet, with low lighting.

If your patient's blood pressure drops below the target range, stop I.V. hypertensive therapy.

Pericarditis

Pericarditis is an inflammation of the pericardium, the fibroserous sac that envelops, supports, and protects the heart. It occurs in acute and chronic forms. Acute pericarditis can be fibrinous or effusive, with purulent, serous, or hemorrhagic exudate. Chronic constrictive pericarditis is characterized by dense fibrous pericardial thickening.

What causes it

Pericarditis may result from:
• bacterial, fungal, or viral infection (infectious pericarditis)
• neoplasms (primary disease or metastases from lungs, breasts, or other organs)
• high-dose radiation to the chest
• uremia
• hypersensitivity or autoimmune disease, such as acute rheumatic fever (the most common cause of pericarditis in children), systemic lupus erythematosus, and rheumatoid arthritis
• previous cardiac injury, such as MI (Dressler's syndrome), trauma, or surgery (postcardiotomy syndrome) that leaves the pericardium intact but causes blood to leak into the pericardial cavity
• drugs, such as hydralazine or procainamide
• idiopathic factors (most common in acute pericarditis)
• aortic aneurysm with pericardial leakage (less common)
• myxedema with cholesterol deposits in the pericardium (less common).

Pathophysiology

Here's what happens in pericarditis:
• Pericardial tissue damaged by bacteria or other substances results in the release of chemical mediators of inflammation (prostaglandins, histamines, bradykinins, and serotonin) into the surrounding tissue, thereby initiating the inflammatory process.
• Friction occurs as the inflamed pericardial layers rub against each other.
• Histamines and other chemical mediators dilate vessels and increase vessel permeability. Vessel walls then leak fluids and protein (including fibrinogen) into tissues, causing extracellular edema.
• Macrophages already present in the tissue begin to phagocytize the invading bacteria and are joined by neutrophils and monocytes.
• After several days, the area fills with an exudate composed of necrotic tissue and dead and dying bacteria, neutrophils, and macrophages.
• Eventually, the contents of the cavity autolyze and are gradually reabsorbed into healthy tissue.
• A pericardial effusion develops if fluid accumulates in the pericardial cavity.
• Cardiac tamponade results when there's a rapid accumulation of fluid in the pericardial space, compressing the heart and preventing it from filling during diastole, and resulting in a drop in cardiac output.

> Pericardial effusion develops if fluid accumulates in the pericardial cavity.

• Chronic constrictive pericarditis develops if the pericardium becomes thick and stiff from chronic or recurrent pericarditis, encasing the heart in a stiff shell and preventing the heart from properly filling during diastole. This causes an increase in both left- and right-sided filling pressures, leading to a drop in stroke volume and cardiac output.

What to look for

The patient with acute pericarditis typically complains of sharp, sudden pain, usually starting over the sternum and radiating to the neck, shoulders, back, and arms.

The pain is usually pleuritic, increasing with deep inspiration and decreasing when the patient sits up and leans forward. This decrease occurs because leaning forward pulls the heart away from the diaphragmatic pleurae of the lungs.

Cardiac complications

Pericardial effusion, the major complication of acute pericarditis, may produce effects of heart failure, such as dyspnea, orthopnea, and tachycardia. It may also produce ill-defined substernal chest pain and a feeling of chest fullness.

If fluid accumulates rapidly, cardiac tamponade may occur, causing pallor, clammy skin, hypotension, pulsus paradoxus, jugular vein distention and, eventually, cardiovascular collapse and death.

Chronic constrictive pericarditis causes a gradual increase in systemic venous pressure and produces symptoms similar to those of chronic right-sided heart failure, including fluid retention, ascites, and hepatomegaly.

What tests tell you

These tests are used to diagnose pericarditis:
• ECG may reveal diffuse ST-segment elevation in the limb leads and most precordial leads that reflects the inflammatory process. Upright T waves are present in most leads. QRS segments may be diminished when pericardial effusion exists. Arrhythmias, such as atrial fibrillation and sinus arrhythmias may occur. In chronic constrictive pericarditis, there may be low-voltage QRS complexes, T-wave inversion or flattening, and P mitral waves (wide P waves) in leads I, II, and V_6.
• Laboratory testing may reveal an elevated erythrocyte sedimentation rate as a result of the inflammatory process or a normal or elevated WBC count, especially in infectious pericarditis; BUN may point to uremia as a cause of pericarditis.
• Blood cultures may be used to identify an infectious cause.

That hurts! A patient with acute pericarditis typically reports sharp, sudden pain, usually starting over the sternum and radiating to the neck, shoulders, back, and arms.

• Antistreptolysin-O titers may be positive if pericarditis is due to rheumatic fever.
• Purified protein derivative skin test may be positive if pericarditis is due to tuberculosis.
• Echocardiography may show an echo-free space between the ventricular wall and the pericardium, and reduced pumping action of the heart.
• Chest X-rays may be normal with acute pericarditis. The cardiac silhouette may be enlarged, with a water bottle shape caused by fluid accumulation, if pleural effusion is present.

How it's treated

Treatment for a patient with pericarditis is done to:
• relieve symptoms
• prevent or correct pericardial effusion and cardiac tamponade
• manage the underlying disease.

Bed rest and drug therapy

In idiopathic pericarditis, post-MI pericarditis, and postthoracotomy pericarditis, treatment is twofold, including:
• bed rest as long as fever and pain persist
• nonsteroidal anti-infammatory drugs, such as aspirin and indomethacin, to relieve pain and reduce inflammation.

If symptoms continue, the doctor may prescribe corticosteroids to provide rapid and effective relief. Corticosteroids must be used cautiously because pericarditis may recur when drug therapy stops.

Further treatments

When infectious pericarditis results from disease of the left pleural space, mediastinal abscesses, or septicemia, the patient requires antibiotics, surgical drainage, or both.

If cardiac tamponade develops, the doctor may perform emergency pericardiocentesis and may inject antibiotics directly into the pericardial sac.

Heavy-duty treatments

Recurrent pericarditis may necessitate partial pericardiectomy, which creates a window that allows fluid to drain into the pleural space. In constrictive pericarditis, total pericardiectomy may be necessary to permit the heart to fill and contract adequately.

Patients should be placed in an upright position to relieve dyspnea and chest pain.

What to do

• Maintain the patient on bed rest until fever and pain diminish. Assist the patient with bathing if necessary. Provide a bedside commode to reduce myocardial oxygen demand.

• Place the patient in an upright position to relieve dyspnea and chest pain. Auscultate lung sounds at least every 2 hours. Administer supplemental oxygen as needed based on oxygen saturation or mixed venous oxygen saturation levels.

• Administer analgesics to relieve pain and nonsteroidal anti-inflammatory drugs (NSAIDs), as ordered, to reduce inflammation. Administer steroids if the patient fails to respond to NSAIDs.

• If your patient has a PA catheter, monitor hemodynamic status. Assess the patient's cardiovascular status frequently, watching for signs of cardiac tamponade.

• Administer antibiotics on time to maintain consistent drug levels in the blood.

• Institute continuous cardiac monitoring to evaluate for changes in ECG. Look for the return of ST segments to baseline with T-wave flattening by the end of the first 7 days.

• Keep a pericardiocentesis set available if pericardial effusion is suspected, and prepare the patient for pericardiocentesis, as indicated.

• Provide appropriate postoperative care, similar to that given after cardiothoracic surgery.

Valvular heart disease

In valvular heart disease, three types of mechanical disruption can occur:

stenosis, or narrowing, of the valve opening

incomplete closure of the valve

prolapse of the valve.

What causes it

Valvular heart disease in children and adolescents most commonly results from congenital heart defects. In adults, rheumatic heart disease is a common cause.

Pathophysiology

Valvular heart disease may result from numerous conditions, which vary and are different for each type of valve disorder.

In adults, rheumatic heart disease is a common cause of valvular heart disease.

Pathophysiology of valvular heart disease varies according to the valve and the disorder.

Mitral insufficiency

In mitral insufficiency, blood from the left ventricle flows back in to the left atrium during systole, causing the atrium to enlarge to accommodate the backflow. As a result, the left ventricle also dilates to accommodate the increased volume of blood from the atrium and to compensate for diminishing cardiac output.

Ventricular hypertrophy and increased end-diastolic pressure result in increased PAP, eventually leading to left-sided and right-sided heart failure.

With mitral insufficiency, pressure problems eventually lead to left- and right-sided heart failure.

Mitral stenosis

In mitral stenosis, the valve narrows as a result of valvular abnormalities, fibrosis, or calcification. This obstructs blood flow from the left atrium to the left ventricle. Consequently, left atrial volume and pressure increase and the chamber dilates.

Greater resistance to blood flow causes pulmonary hypertension, right ventricular hypertrophy, and right-sided heart failure. Also, inadequate filling of the left ventricle produces low cardiac output.

Aortic insufficiency

In aortic insufficiency, blood flows back into the left ventricle during diastole, causing fluid overload in the ventricle which, in turn, dilates and hypertrophies. The excess volume causes fluid overload in the left atrium and, finally, the pulmonary system. Left-sided heart failure and pulmonary edema eventually result.

Aortic stenosis

In aortic stenosis, elevated left ventricular pressure tries to overcome the resistance of the narrowed valvular opening. The added workload increases the demand for oxygen, and diminished cardiac output causes poor coronary artery perfusion, ischemia of the left ventricle, and left-sided heart failure.

In pulmonic stenosis, the ultimate result is right-sided heart failure.

Pulmonic stenosis

In pulmonic stenosis, obstructed right ventricular outflow causes right ventricular hypertrophy in an attempt to overcome resistance to the narrow valvular opening. The ultimate result is right-sided heart failure.

What to look for

The history and physical examination findings vary according to the type of valvular defects.

Mitral insufficiency

Signs and symptoms of mitral insufficiency include:
- orthopnea
- dyspnea
- fatigue
- angina
- palpitations
- right-sided heart failure (jugular vein distention, peripheral edema, hepatomegaly
- systolic murmur.

Mitral stenosis

Signs and symptoms of mitral stenosis include:
- dyspnea on exertion, paroxysmal nocturnal dyspnea, orthopnea
- fatigue, weakness
- right-sided heart failure
- crackles on auscultation
- cardiac arrhythmias.

Aortic insufficiency

Signs and symptoms of aortic insufficiency include:
- dypsnea
- cough
- left-sided heart failure
- pulsus biferiens (rapidly rising and collapsing pulses)
- blowing diastolic murmur or S_3.

Aortic stenosis

Signs and symptoms of aortic stenosis include:
- dyspnea on exertion and paroxysmal nocturnal dyspnea
- fatigue
- syncope
- angina
- palpitations and cardiac arrhythmias
- left-sided heart failure
- systolic murmur at the base of the carotids
- decreased cardiac output.

Pulmonic stenosis

Although a patient with pulmonic stenosis may be asymptomatic, possible signs and symptoms include:

Your patient with pulmonic stenosis may be asymptomatic.

- dyspnea on exertion
- right-sided heart failure
- systolic murmur.

What tests tell you

The diagnosis of valvular heart disease can be based on the results of:
- cardiac catheterization
- chest X-rays
- echocardiography
- ECG.

How it's treated

Treatments for patients with valvular heart disease commonly include:
- digoxin, a low-sodium diet, diuretics, vasodilators, and especially ACE inhibitors to correct left-sided heart failure
- oxygen administration in acute situations, to increase oxygenation
- anticoagulants to prevent thrombus formation around diseased or replaced valves
- prophylactic antibiotics before and after surgery or dental care to prevent endocarditis
- nitroglycerin to relieve angina in conditions such as aortic stenosis
- beta-adrenergic blockers or digoxin to slow the ventricular rate in atrial fibrillation or atrial flutter
- cardioversion to convert atrial fibrillation to sinus rhythm
- open or closed commissurotomy to separate thick or adherent mitral valve leaflets
- balloon valvuloplasty to enlarge the orifice of a stenotic mitral, aortic, or pulmonic valve
- annuloplasty or valvuloplasty to reconstruct or repair the valve in mitral insufficiency
- valve replacement with a prosthetic valve for mitral and aortic valve disease.

What to do

- Assess the patient's vital signs, ABG values, pulse oximetry, intake and output, daily weights, blood chemistry studies, chest X-rays, and ECG.
- Place the patient in an upright position to relieve dyspnea, if needed. Administer oxygen to prevent tissue hypoxia, as needed and indicated by ABGs and pulse oximetry.

• Institute continuous cardiac monitoring to evaluate for arrhythmias; if any occur, administer appropriate therapy according to facility policy and the doctor's order.
• For a patient with aortic insufficiency, observe ECG for arrhythmias, which can increase the risk of pulmonary edema, and for fever and infection.
• If the patient has mitral stenosis, watch closely for signs of pulmonary dysfunction caused by pulmonary hypertension, tissue ischemia caused by emboli, and adverse reactions to drug therapy.
• For a patient with mitral insufficiency, observe for signs and symptoms of left-sided heart failure, pulmonary edema, and adverse reactions to drug therapy.

Quick quiz

Watch those valves. If your patient has mitral stenosis, observe closely for signs of pulmonary dysfunction, emboli, and adverse reactions to drug therapy.

1. Which sign is characteristic of cardiac tamponade?
    A.   Shortness of breath
    B.   Pulsus paradoxus
    C.   Holosystolic murmur
    D.   Bounding peripheral pulse

Answer: B. Pulsus paradoxus (inspiratory drop in systemic blood pressure greater that 15 mm Hg) is one of the three classic signs of cardiac tamponade. The other classic signs are elevated CVP with jugular vein distention and muffled heart sounds.

2. Identify the arrhythmia in the rhythm strip below.

    A.   Atrial flutter
    B.   Sinus tachycardia
    C.   AV junctional rhythm
    D.   Atrial fibrillation

Answer: D. The rhythm strip reveals atrial fibrillation. No P waves are identifiable; ventricular rate is varied; QRS complexes are uniform in shape but occur at irregular intervals.

3. Which drug is effective in managing mild to moderate hypotension?

A.   Phenylephrine
B.   Amiodarone
C.   Ibutilide
D.   Milrinone

Answer: A. Phenylephrine is indicated for mild to moderate hypotension.

4. Which parameter is elevated in right-sided heart failure?
    A.   CVP
    B.   Left-ventricular end-diastolic pressure
    C.   PAWP
    D.   Cardiac output

Answer: A. CVP is elevated in right-sided heart failure.

5. ACE inhibitors correct heart failure by:
    A.   increasing preload.
    B.   causing vasoconstriction.
    C.   increasing afterload.
    D.   reducing afterload.

Answer: D. ACE inhibitors reduce afterload through vasodilation, thereby reducing heart failure.

Scoring

☆☆☆ If you answered all five questions correctly, you're all heart! (You'd have to be to make it through this cardiovascular workout!)

☆☆ If you answered four questions correctly, take heart. You have all the blood and gumption you need to succeed.

☆ If you answered fewer than four questions correctly, bless your heart. Review the chapter and try again.

Good job! Take a breather and then move on to the respiratory system.

Respiratory system

Just the facts

In this chapter, you'll learn:

♦ structure and function of the respiratory system

♦ assessment of the respiratory system

♦ diagnostic tests and procedures for the respiratory system

♦ respiratory disorders and treatments.

Understanding the respiratory system

The respiratory system delivers oxygen to the bloodstream and removes excess carbon dioxide from the body.

> What a system the body has going! The upper airways warm, filter, and humidify air before sending it to the lower airways.

Respiratory system structures

The structures of the respiratory system include the airways and lungs, bony thorax, and respiratory muscles. (See *A close look at the respiratory system*, page 284.)

Airways and lungs

The airways of the respiratory system consist of two parts: the upper and lower airways. The two lungs are parts of the lower airway and share space in the thoracic cavity with the heart and great vessels, trachea, esophagus, and bronchi.

Upper airway

The upper airway warms, filters, and humidifies inhaled air and then sends it to the lower airway. It also contains the structures that enable a person to make sounds. Upper airway structures include the nasopharynx (nose), oropharynx (mouth), laryngopharynx, and larynx.

Advice from the experts

A close look at the respiratory system

Get to know the basic structures and functions of the respiratory system so you can perform a comprehensive respiratory assessment and identify abnormalities. The major structures of the upper and lower airways are illustrated below. An alveolus, or acinus, is shown in the inset.

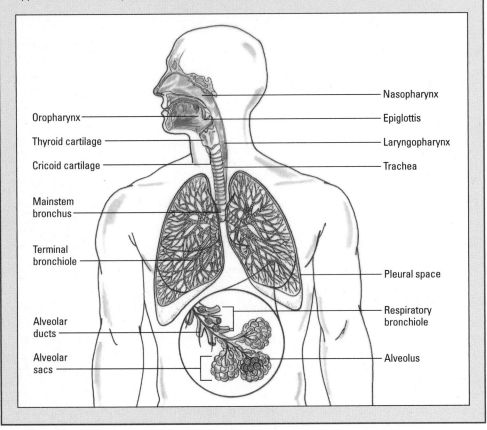

In the zone

The larynx, which is located at the top of the trachea, houses the vocal cords. It's the transition point between the upper and lower airways.

The larynx is composed of nine cartilage segments. The largest is the shield-shaped thyroid cartilage. The cricoid cartilage, which is the only complete ring at the lower end of the larynx, attaches to the first cartilaginous ring of the trachea.

To flap and protect

The epiglottis is a flap of tissue that closes over the top of the larynx when the patient swallows. This protects the patient from aspirating food or fluid into the lower airways.

Lower airway

The lower airway includes the:
- trachea
- bronchi
- lungs.

Lowdown on lower airway

The lower airway begins with the trachea, which divides at the carina to form the right and left mainstem bronchi of the lungs. The right mainstem bronchus is shorter, wider, and more vertical than the left.

The mainstem bronchi branch out in the lungs, forming the:
- lobar bronchi
- tertiary bronchi
- terminal bronchioles
- respiratory bronchioles
- alveolar ducts
- alveoli.

> The mainstem bronchi branch out in the lungs to form smaller airways.

Lungs and lobes

The right lung is larger and has three lobes: upper, middle, and lower. The left lung is smaller and has only two lobes: upper and lower.

Plenty of pleura

Each lung is wrapped in a lining called the *visceral pleura* and all areas of the thoracic cavity that come in contact with the lungs are lined with parietal pleura.

A small amount of pleural fluid fills the area between the two layers of the pleura. This allows the layers to slide smoothly over each other as the chest expands and contracts. The parietal pleura also contain nerve endings that transmit pain signals when inflammation occurs.

All about alveoli

The alveoli are the gas-exchange units of the lungs. The lungs in a typical adult contain about 300 million alveoli.

Alveoli consist of type I and type II epithelial cells:
- Type I cells form the alveolar walls, through which gas exchange occurs.

• Type II cells produce surfactant, a lipid-type substance that coats the alveoli. During inspiration, the alveolar surfactant allows the alveoli to expand uniformly. During expiration, the surfactant prevents alveolar collapse.

Hundreds of millions of tiny alveoli conduct gas exchange in the lungs.

In circulation

Oxygen-depleted blood enters the lungs from the pulmonary artery of the right ventricle, then flows through the main pulmonary arteries into the smaller vessels of the pleural cavities and the main bronchi, through the arterioles and, eventually, to the capillary networks in the alveoli.

Trading gases

Gas exchange (oxygen and carbon dioxide diffusion) takes place in the alveoli. After passing through the pulmonary capillaries, oxygenated blood flows through progressively larger vessels, enters the main pulmonary veins and, finally, flows into the left atrium. (See *Tracking pulmonary circulation.*)

Bony thorax

The bony thorax is composed of:
• clavicles
• sternum

Tracking pulmonary circulation

The right and left pulmonary arteries carry deoxygenated blood from the right side of the heart to the lungs. These arteries divide to form distal branches called *arterioles,* which terminate as a concentrated capillary network in the alveoli and alveolar sac, where gas exchange occurs.

Venules—the end branches of the pulmonary veins—collect oxygenated blood from the capillaries and transport it to larger vessels, which carry it to the pulmonary veins. The pulmonary veins enter the left side of the heart and distribute oxygenated blood throughout the body.

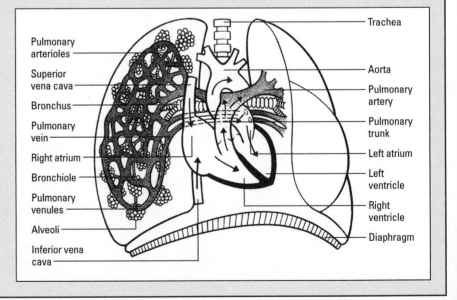

- scapula
- 12 sets of ribs
- 12 thoracic vertebrae.

Parts of the thorax and some imaginary vertical lines on the chest are used to describe the locations of pulmonary assessment findings. (See *Respiratory assessment landmarks*, page 288.)

Can you take a ribbing?

Ribs are made of bone and cartilage and allow the chest to expand and contract during each breath. All ribs are attached to vertebrae. The first seven ribs also are attached directly to the sternum. The eighth and ninth ribs are attached to the seventh rib. The eleventh and twelfth ribs are called *floating ribs* because they aren't attached to any other bones in the front.

Respiratory muscles

The primary muscles used in breathing are the diaphragm and the external intercostal muscles. These muscles contract when the patient inhales and relax when the patient exhales.

Brain-breath connection

The respiratory center in the medulla initiates each breath by sending messages over the phrenic nerve to the primary respiratory muscles. Impulses from the phrenic nerve regulate the rate and depth of breathing, depending on the carbon dioxide and pH levels in the cerebrospinal fluid.

Accessory inspiratory muscles

Here's how other muscles assist in breathing:

In on inspiration

Accessory inspiratory muscles (the trapezius, sternocleidomastoid, and scalenes) elevate the scapula, clavicle, sternum, and upper ribs. This expands the front-to-back diameter of the chest when use of the diaphragm and intercostal muscles isn't effective.

Out on expiration

Expiration occurs when the diaphragm and external intercostal muscles relax. If the patient has an airway obstruction, he may also use the abdominal muscles and internal intercostal muscles to exhale. (See *Understanding the mechanics of breathing*, page 289.)

Ho-hum. The diaphragm and the external intercostal muscles contract on inhalation and relax on exhalation.

Respiratory assessment landmarks

Look at these figures to find the common landmarks used in respiratory assessment.

Anterior view

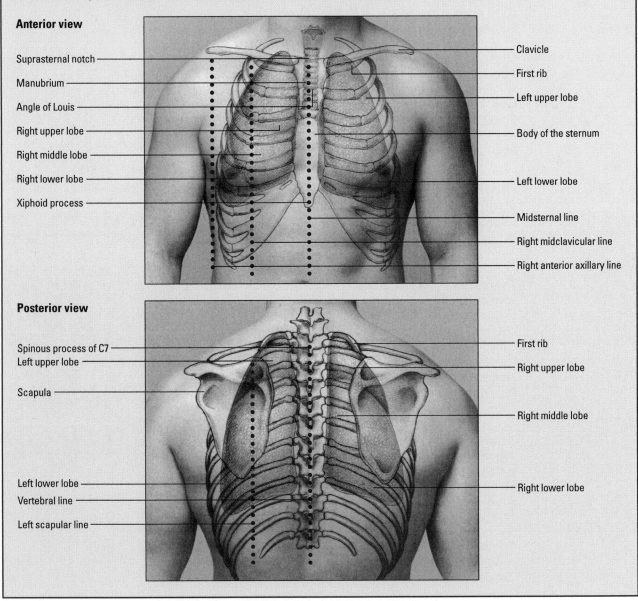

Suprasternal notch

Manubrium

Angle of Louis

Right upper lobe

Right middle lobe

Right lower lobe

Xiphoid process

Clavicle

First rib

Left upper lobe

Body of the sternum

Left lower lobe

Midsternal line

Right midclavicular line

Right anterior axillary line

Posterior view

Spinous process of C7

Left upper lobe

Scapula

Left lower lobe

Vertebral line

Left scapular line

First rib

Right upper lobe

Right middle lobe

Right lower lobe

Understanding the mechanics of breathing

Mechanical forces, such as movement of the diaphragm and intercostal muscles, drive the breathing process. In these depictions, a plus sign (+) indicates positive pressure and a minus sign (−) indicates negative pressure.

At rest

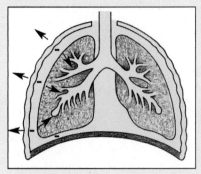

- Inspiratory muscles relax.
- Atmospheric pressure is maintained in the tracheobronchial tree.
- No air movement occurs.

Inhalation

- Inspiratory muscles contract.
- The diaphragm descends.
- Negative alveolar pressure is maintained.
- Air moves into the lungs.

Exhalation

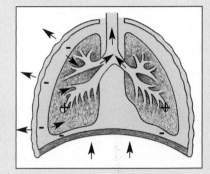

- Inspiratory muscles relax, causing lungs to recoil to their resting size and position.
- The diaphragm ascends.
- Positive alveolar pressure is maintained.
- Air moves out of the lungs.

Respiration

Effective respiration requires gas exchange in the lungs (external respiration) and in the tissues (internal respiration).

O_2 to lungs

Three external respiration processes are needed to maintain adequate oxygenation and acid-base balance:

☝ ventilation (gas distribution into and out of the pulmonary airways)

✌ pulmonary perfusion (blood flow from the right side of the heart, through the pulmonary circulation, and into the left side of the heart)

🖐 diffusion (gas movement from an area of greater to lesser concentration through a semipermeable membrane).

O₂ to tissues

Internal respiration occurs only through diffusion, when the red blood cells (RBCs) release oxygen and absorb carbon dioxide.

Ventilation and perfusion

Gravity affects oxygen and carbon dioxide transport in a positive way by causing more unoxygenated blood to travel to the lower and middle lung lobes than to the upper lobes. That's why ventilation and perfusion differ in various parts of the lungs.

> Gas exchange is most efficient where perfusion and ventilation match.

Match game

Areas where perfusion and ventilation are similar have a ventilation-perfusion ($\dot{V}/\dot{Q}$) match; gas exchange is most efficient in such areas.

For example, in normal lung function, the alveoli receive air at a rate of about 4 L/minute while the capillaries supply blood to the alveoli at a rate of about 5 L/minute, creating a $\dot{V}/\dot{Q}$ ratio of 4:5 or 0.8. (See *Understanding ventilation and perfusion*.)

Mismatch mayhem

A $\dot{V}/\dot{Q}$ mismatch, resulting from ventilation-perfusion dysfunction or altered lung mechanics, causes most of the impaired gas exchange in respiratory disorders.

Ineffective gas exchange between the alveoli and pulmonary capillaries can affect all body systems by changing the amount of oxygen delivered to living cells. Ineffective gas exchange causes three outcomes:

• *Shunting* (reduced ventilation to a lung unit) causes unoxygenated blood to move from the right side of the heart to the left side of the heart and into systemic circulation. Shunting may result from a physical defect that allows unoxygenated blood to bypass fully functioning alveoli. It may also result when airway obstruction (caused by acute conditions, such as atelectasis and pneumonia) prevents oxygen from reaching an adequately perfused area of the lung.

• *Dead-space ventilation* (reduced perfusion to a lung unit) occurs when alveoli don't have adequate blood supply for gas exchange to occur, such as with pulmonary emboli and pulmonary infarction.

Understanding ventilation and perfusion

Effective gas exchange depends on the relationship between ventilation and perfusion or the $\dot{V}/\dot{Q}$ ratio. The diagrams below show what happens when the $\dot{V}/\dot{Q}$ ratio is normal and abnormal.

Normal ventilation and perfusion

When ventilation and perfusion are matched, unoxygenated blood from the venous system returns to the right side of the heart through the pulmonary artery to the lungs, carrying carbon dioxide (CO_2). The arteries branch into the alveolar capillaries. Gas exchange takes place in the alveolar capillaries.

Inadequate perfusion (dead-space ventilation)

When the $\dot{V}/\dot{Q}$ ratio is high, as shown here, ventilation is normal, but alveolar perfusion is reduced or absent. Note the narrowed capillary, indicating poor perfusion. This commonly results from a perfusion defect, such as pulmonary embolism or a disorder that decreases cardiac output.

Inadequate ventilation (shunt)

When the $\dot{V}/\dot{Q}$ ratio is low, pulmonary circulation is adequate but not enough oxygen (O_2) is available to the alveoli for normal diffusion. A portion of the blood flowing through the pulmonary vessels doesn't become oxygenated.

Inadequate ventilation and perfusion (silent unit)

The silent unit indicates an absence of ventilation and perfusion to the lung area. The silent unit may help compensate for a $\dot{V}/\dot{Q}$ balance by delivering blood flow to better ventilated lung areas.

KEY

▨ Blood with CO_2 ▨ Blood with O_2 ▨ Blood with CO_2 and O_2

• A *silent unit* (a combination of shunting and dead-space ventilation) occurs when little or no ventilation and perfusion are present, such as in cases of pneumothorax and acute respiratory distress syndrome (ARDS).

Oxygen transport

Most oxygen collected in the lungs binds with hemoglobin to form oxyhemoglobin; however, a small portion of it dissolves in the plasma. The portion of oxygen that dissolves in the plasma can be measured as the partial pressure of arterial oxygen in blood (Pao_2).

Riding the RBC express

After oxygen binds to hemoglobin, RBCs carry it by way of the circulatory system to tissues throughout the body. Internal respiration occurs by cellular diffusion when RBCs release oxygen and absorb the carbon dioxide produced by cellular metabolism. The RBCs then transport the carbon dioxide back to the lungs for removal during expiration.

Acid-base balance

Because carbon dioxide is 20 times more soluble than oxygen, it dissolves in the blood, where most of it forms bicarbonate (a base) and smaller amounts form carbonic acid.

Acid-base controller

The lungs control bicarbonate levels by converting bicarbonate to carbon dioxide and water for excretion. In response to signals from the medulla, the lungs can change the rate and depth of ventilation. This controls acid-base balance by adjusting the amount of carbon dioxide that's lost.

In metabolic alkalosis, which results from excess bicarbonate retention, the rate and depth of ventilation decrease so that carbon dioxide is retained. This increases carbonic acid levels.

In metabolic acidosis (resulting from excess acid retention or excess bicarbonate loss), the lungs increase the rate and depth of ventilation to exhale excess carbon dioxide, thereby reducing carbonic acid levels.

Off balance

Inadequately functioning lungs can produce acid-base imbalances. For example, *hypoventilation* (reduced rate and depth of ventilation) results in carbon dioxide retention, causing respiratory acidosis. Conversely, *hyperventilation* (increased rate and depth of ventilation) leads to increased exhalation of carbon dioxide and causes respiratory alkalosis.

> Poorly functioning lungs can produce acid-base imbalances.

Respiratory assessment

Respiratory assessment is a critical nursing responsibility. Conduct a thorough assessment to detect subtle and obvious respiratory changes.

History

Build your patient's health history by asking short, open-ended questions. Conduct the interview in several short sessions if you have to, depending on the severity of your patient's condition. Ask his family to provide information if your patient can't.

Respiratory disorders may be caused or exacerbated by obesity, smoking, and workplace conditions so be sure to ask about these conditions.

Respiratory disorders may be caused or worsened by obesity, smoking, and workplace conditions.

Current health status

Begin by asking why your patient is seeking care. Because many respiratory disorders are chronic, ask how the patient's latest acute episode compares with the previous episode and what relief measures are helpful and unhelpful.

Patients with respiratory disorders commonly report such complaints as:
- shortness of breath
- cough
- sputum production
- wheezing
- chest pain
- sleep disturbance.

Shortness of breath

Assess your patient's shortness of breath by asking him to rate his usual level of dyspnea on a scale of 1 to 10, in which 1 means no dyspnea and 10 means the worst he has experienced. Then ask him to rate the level that day. Other scales grade dyspnea as it relates to activity, such as climbing a set of stairs or walking a city block. (See *Grading dyspnea*, page 294.)

In addition to using a severity scale, ask these questions: What do you do to relieve the shortness of breath? How well does it usually work?

Grading dyspnea

To assess dyspnea as objectively as possible, ask your patient to briefly describe how various activities affect his breathing. Then document his response using this grading system:

• *Grade 0:* not troubled by breathlessness except with strenuous exercise

• *Grade 1:* troubled by shortness of breath when hurrying on a level path or walking up a slight hill

• *Grade 2:* walks more slowly on a level path because of breathlessness than people of the same age or has to stop to breathe when walking on a level path at his own pace

• *Grade 3:* stops to breathe after walking about 100 yards (91 m) on a level path

• *Grade 4:* too breathless to leave the house or breathless when dressing or undressing

The number of pillows you need to sleep indicates the severity of your orthopnea.

Orthopnea

A patient with orthopnea (shortness of breath when lying down) tends to sleep with his upper body elevated. Ask this patient how many pillows he uses. The answer reflects the severity of the orthopnea. For instance, a patient who uses three pillows can be said to have "three-pillow orthopnea."

Cough

Ask the patient with a cough these questions: At what time of day do you cough most often? Is the cough productive? If the cough is a chronic problem, has it changed recently? If so, how? What makes the cough better? What makes it worse?

Sputum

If a patient produces sputum, ask him to estimate the amount produced in teaspoons or some other common measurement. Also ask these questions: What's the color and consistency of the sputum? If sputum is a chronic problem, has it changed recently? If so, how? Do you cough up blood? If so, how much and how often?

Wheezing

If a patient wheezes, ask these questions: When does wheezing occur? What makes you wheeze? Do you wheeze loudly enough for others to hear it? What helps stop your wheezing?

Ask detailed questions to assess your patient's complaints.

Chest pain

If the patient has chest pain, ask these questions: Where's the pain? What does it feel like? Is it sharp, stabbing, burning, or aching? Does it move to another area? How long does it last? What causes it? What makes it better?

Pain provocations

Chest pain due to a respiratory problem is usually the result of pleural inflammation, inflammation of the costochondral junctions, soreness of chest muscles because of coughing, or indigestion. Less common causes of pain include rib or vertebral fractures caused by coughing or osteoporosis.

Sleep disturbance

Sleep disturbances may be related to obstructive sleep apnea or other sleep disorder requiring additional evaluation.

Daytime drowsiness

If the patient complains of being drowsy or irritable in the daytime, ask these questions: How many hours of continuous sleep do you get at night? Do you wake up often during the night? Does your family complain about your snoring or restlessness?

Previous health status

Look at the patient's health history, being especially watchful for:
• a smoking habit
• exposure to secondhand smoke
• allergies
• previous operations
• respiratory diseases, such as pneumonia and tuberculosis (TB).

Ask about current immunizations, such as a flu shot or pneumococcal vaccine. Also determine if the patient uses any respiratory equipment, such as oxygen or nebulizers, at home.

Family history

Ask the patient if he has a family history of cancer, sickle cell anemia, heart disease, or chronic illness, such as asthma or emphysema. Determine whether the patient lives with anyone who has an infectious disease, such as TB or influenza.

Lifestyle patterns

Ask about the patient's workplace because some jobs, such as coal mining and construction work, expose workers to substances that can cause lung disease.

Also ask about the patient's home, community, and other environmental factors that may influence how he deals with his respiratory problems. For example, you may ask questions about interpersonal relationships, stress management, and coping methods. Ask about the patient's sex habits or drug use, which may be connected with acquired immunodeficiency syndrome–related pulmonary disorders.

Physical examination

In most cases, you should begin the physical examination after you take the patient's history. However, you may not be able to take a complete history if the patient develops an ominous sign such as acute respiratory distress. If your patient is in respiratory distress, establish the priorities of your nursing assessment, progressing from the most critical factors (airway, breathing, and circulation [the ABCs]) to less critical factors. (See *Emergency respiratory assessment.*)

Four steps

Use a systematic approach to detect subtle and obvious respiratory changes. The four steps for conducting a physical examination of the respiratory system are:
- inspection
- palpation
- percussion
- auscultation.

Back, then front

Examine the back of the chest first, using inspection, palpation, percussion, and auscultation. Always compare one side with the other. Then examine the front of the chest using the same sequence. The patient can lie back when you examine the front of the chest if that's more comfortable for him.

Making introductions

Before you begin the physical examination, make sure the room is well lit and warm. Introduce yourself to the patient and explain why you're there.

Advice from the experts

Emergency respiratory assessment

If your patient is in acute respiratory distress, immediately assess the ABCs—airway, breathing, and circulation. If these are absent, call for help and start cardiopulmonary resuscitation.

Next, quickly check for these signs of impending crisis:

- Is the patient having trouble breathing?
- Is the patient using accessory muscles to breathe? If chest excursion is less than the normal 1⅛″ to 2⅜″ (3 to 6 cm), look for evidence that the patient is using accessory muscles when he breathes, including shoulder elevation, intercostal muscle retraction, and use of scalene and sternocleidomastoid muscles.
- Has the patient's level of consciousness diminished?
- Is he confused, anxious, or agitated?

- Does he change his body position to ease breathing?
- Does his skin look pale, diaphoretic, or cyanotic?

Setting priorities

If your patient is in respiratory distress, establish priorities for your nursing assessment. Don't assume the obvious. Note positive and negative factors, starting with the most critical factors (the ABCs) and progressing to less critical factors.

If you don't have time to go through each step of the nursing process, make sure you gather enough data to answer vital questions. A single sign or symptom has many possible meanings, so gather a group of findings to assess the patient and develop interventions.

Inspection

Make a few observations about the patient as soon as you enter the room and include these observations in your assessment. Note the patient's position in the bed. Does he appear comfortable? Is he sitting up or lying quietly or shifting about? Does he appear anxious? Is he having trouble breathing? Does he require oxygen? Is he on a ventilator?

Chest inspection

Help the patient into an upright position if possible. Ideally, the patient should be undressed from the waist up or clothed in a hospital gown. Inspect the patient's chest configuration, tracheal position, chest symmetry, skin condition, nostrils (for flaring), and accessory muscle use.

Beauty in symmetry

Look for chest wall symmetry. Both sides of the chest should be equal at rest and expand equally as the patient inhales. The diame-

Your first observations of the patient are important parts of the assessment.

ter of the chest, from front to back, should be about one-half of the width of the chest.

A new angle

Also, look at the angle between the ribs and the sternum at the point immediately above the xiphoid process. This angle, the costal angle, should be less than 90 degrees in an adult. The angle is larger if the chest wall is chronically expanded because of an enlargement of the intercostal muscles, as can happen with chronic obstructive pulmonary disease (COPD).

Muscles in motion

When the patient inhales, his diaphragm should descend and the intercostal muscles should contract. This dual motion causes the abdomen to push out and the lower ribs to expand laterally. (See *Types of breathing*.)

When the patient exhales, his abdomen and ribs return to their resting positions. The upper chest shouldn't move much. Accessory muscles may hypertrophy, indicating frequent use. This may be normal in some athletes, but for most patients it indicates a respiratory problem, especially when the patient purses his lips and flares his nostrils when breathing.

Chest wall abnormalities

Inspect for chest wall abnormalities, keeping in mind that a patient with a deformity of the chest wall might have completely normal lungs that might be cramped in the chest. The patient might have a smaller-than-normal lung capacity and limited exercise tolerance.

Barrels, pigeons, and curves

Common abnormalities include:
• *Barrel chest*—A barrel chest looks like the name implies; it's abnormally round and bulging. Barrel chest may be normal in infants and elderly patients. In other patients, barrel chest occurs as a result of COPD due to lungs that have lost their elasticity. The patient typically uses accessory muscles to breathe and easily becomes breathless. Also note kyphosis of the thoracic spine.
• *Pigeon chest*—A patient with pigeon chest, or pectus carinatum, has a chest with a sternum that protrudes beyond the front of the abdomen. The displaced sternum increases the front-to-back diameter of the chest but is a minor deformity that doesn't require treatment.

> ## Types of breathing
>
> Men, children, and infants usually use abdominal, or diaphragmatic, breathing. Athletes and singers do as well. Most women, however, usually use chest, or intercostal, breathing.

A deformity of the patient's chest wall can limit lung capacity and exercise tolerance.

• *Funnel chest* — A patient with funnel chest, or pectus excavatum, has a funnel-shaped depression on all of or part of the sternum. This may cause disruptions in respiratory or cardiac function. Compression of the heart and great vessels may cause murmurs.

• *Thoracic kyphoscoliosis* — The patient's spine curves to one side and the vertebrae are rotated. Because the rotation distorts lung tissues, it may be more difficult to assess respiratory status.

Raising a red flag

Watch for paradoxical, or uneven, movement of the patient's chest wall. Paradoxical movement may appear as an abnormal collapse of part of the chest wall when the patient inhales or an abnormal expansion when the patient exhales. In either case, such uneven movement indicates a loss of normal chest wall function.

Breathing rate and pattern

Assess your patient's respiratory function by determining the rate, rhythm, and quality of respirations.

Count on it

To find the patient's respiratory rate, count for a full minute or longer, if you note abnormalities. Don't tell the patient what you're doing or he might alter his natural breathing pattern. Adults normally breathe at a rate of 12 to 20 breaths per minute.

The respiratory pattern should be even, coordinated and regular, with occasional sighs. The normal ratio of inspiration to expiration (I:E ratio) is about 1:2.

Abnormal respiratory patterns

Identifying abnormal respiratory patterns can be a great help in understanding the patient's respiratory status and overall condition.

Tachypnea

Tachypnea is a respiratory rate greater than 20 breaths/minute; usually the breaths are shallow. It's commonly seen in patients with restrictive lung disease, pain, sepsis, obesity, anxiety, and respiratory distress. Fever is another possible cause. The respiratory rate may increase by 4 breaths/minute for every 1° F (0.6° C) increase in body temperature.

Bradypnea

Bradypnea is a respiratory rate below 10 breaths/minute. It's commonly noted just before a period of apnea or full respiratory arrest.

The rate, rhythm, and quality of respirations are key indicators of respiratory function.

As your patient's body temperature increases with fever, respiratory rate also increases.

Depressed CNS

Patients with bradypnea might have central nervous system (CNS) depression as a result of excessive sedation, tissue damage, diabetic coma, or any situation in which the brain's respiratory center is depressed. Note that respiratory rate is usually slower during sleep.

Apnea

Apnea is the absence of breathing. Periods of apnea may be short and occur sporadically, such as in Cheyne-Stokes respirations or other abnormal respiratory patterns. This condition may be life-threatening if periods of apnea last long enough and should be addressed immediately.

Hyperpnea

Hyperpnea is characterized by deep breathing. It occurs in patients who exercise, patients who have metabolic acidosis, and patients who are highly anxious or are experiencing pain.

Kussmaul's respirations

Kussmaul's respirations are rapid and deep, with sighing breaths. This type of breathing occurs in patients with metabolic acidosis, especially when associated with diabetic ketoacidosis, as the respiratory system tries to lower the carbon dioxide level in the blood and restore it to normal pH.

Cheyne-Stokes respirations

Cheyne-Stokes respirations have a regular cycle of change in the rate and depth of breathing. Respirations are initially shallow but gradually become deeper and deeper; then a period of apnea follows, lasting up to 20 seconds, and the cycle starts again. This respiratory pattern is seen in patients with heart failure, kidney failure, or CNS damage. Cheyne-Stokes respirations can be a normal breathing pattern during sleep in elderly patients.

Biot's respirations

Biot's respirations involve rapid deep breaths that alternate with abrupt periods of apnea. It's an ominous sign of severe CNS damage.

Inspecting related structures

Inspect the patient's skin for pallor, cyanosis, or diaphoresis.

Don't be blue

Skin color varies considerably among patients, but a patient with a bluish tint to his skin, nail beds, and mucous membranes is con-

Address long periods of apnea immediately! They may be life-threatening.

EMERGENCY

sidered cyanotic. Cyanosis, which occurs when oxygenation to the tissues is poor, is a late sign of hypoxemia.

Finger findings

When you inspect the fingers, assess for clubbing, a sign of long-standing respiratory or cardiac disease. The fingernail normally enters the skin at an angle of less than 180 degrees. When clubbing occurs, the angle is greater than or equal to 180 degrees.

Palpation

Palpation of the chest provides some important information about the respiratory system and the processes involved in breathing. (See *Palpating the chest*, page 302.)

Leaky lungs

The chest wall should feel smooth, warm, and dry. Crepitus, which feels like puffed-rice cereal crackling under the skin, indicates that air is leaking from the airways or lungs.

If a patient has a chest tube, you may find a small amount of subcutaneous air around the insertion site. If the patient has no chest tube, or the area of crepitus is getting larger, alert the doctor right away.

Probing palpation pain

Gentle palpation shouldn't cause the patient pain. If the patient complains of chest pain, try to find a painful area on the chest wall. Here's a guide to assessing some types of chest pain:
• Painful costochondral joints are typically located at the mid-clavicular line or next to the sternum.
• A rib or vertebral fracture is quite painful over the fracture.
• Sore muscles may result from protracted coughing.
• A collapsed lung can cause pain in addition to dyspnea.

Feeling for fremitus

Palpate for tactile fremitus (palpable vibrations caused by the transmission of air through the bronchopulmonary system). Fremitus is decreased over areas where pleural fluid collects, when the patient speaks softly, and with pneumothorax, atelectasis, and emphysema.

Fremitus is increased normally over the large bronchial tubes and abnormally over areas in which alveoli are filled with fluid or exudates, as happens in pneumonia. (See *Checking for tactile fremitus*, page 303.)

Cyanosis occurs when tissue oxygenation is poor. It's a late sign of hypoxemia.

Assess your patient's pain to find clues to its cause.

Palpating the chest

To palpate the chest, place the palm of your hand (or hands) lightly over the thorax, as shown below left. Palpate for tenderness, alignment, bulging, and retractions of the chest and intercostal spaces. Assess the patient for crepitus, especially around drainage sites. Repeat this procedure on the patient's back.

Next, use the pads of your fingers, as shown below right, to palpate the front and back of the thorax. Pass your fingers over the ribs and any scars, lumps, lesions or ulcerations. Note the skin temperature, turgor, and moisture. Also note tenderness and bony or subcutaneous crepitus. The muscles should feel firm and smooth.

Evaluating symmetry

To evaluate your patient's chest wall symmetry and expansion, place your hands on the front of the chest wall with your thumbs touching each other at the second intercostal space. As the patient inhales deeply, watch your thumbs. They should separate simultaneously and equally to a distance several centimeters away from the sternum.

Repeat the measurement at the fifth intercostal space. You may make the same measurement on the back of the chest near the 10th rib.

Warning signs

The patient's chest may expand asymmetrically if he has:
- pleural effusion
- atelectasis
- pneumonia
- pneumothorax.

Asymmetry or abnormal chest expansion may be warning signs of diseases and disorders.

Checking for tactile fremitus

When you check the back of the thorax for tactile fremitus, ask the patient to fold his arms across his chest, as shown at right. This movement shifts the scapulae out of the way.

What to do
Check for tactile fremitus by lightly placing your open palms on both sides of the patient's back without touching his back with your fingers, as shown at right. Ask the patient to repeat the phrase "ninety-nine" loud enough to produce palpable vibrations. Then palpate the front of the chest using the same hand positions.

What the results mean
Vibrations that feel more intense on one side than the other indicate tissue consolidation on that side. Less intense vibrations may indicate emphysema, pneumothorax, or pleural effusion. Faint or no vibrations in the upper posterior thorax may indicate bronchial obstruction or a fluid-filled pleural space.

Chest expansion may be decreased at the level of the diaphragm if the patient has:
- emphysema
- respiratory depression
- diaphragm paralysis
- atelectasis
- obesity
- ascites.

Percussion

Percuss the chest to:
- find the boundaries of the lungs
- determine whether the lungs are filled with air or fluid or solid material
- evaluate the distance the diaphragm travels between the patient's inhalation and exhalation. (See *Percussing the chest*, page 304.)

Sites and sounds

Listen for normal, resonant sounds over most of the chest. In the left front chest wall from the third or fourth intercostal space at the sternum to the third or fourth intercostal space at the midclavicular line listen for a dull sound because that's the space occu-

Percussing the chest

To percuss the chest, hyperextend the middle finger of your left hand if you're right-handed or the middle finger of your right hand if you're left-handed. Place your hand firmly on the patient's chest. Use the tip of the middle finger of your dominant hand—your right hand if you're right-handed, left hand if you're left-handed—to tap on the middle finger of your other hand just below the distal joint (as shown at right).

The movement should come from the wrist of your dominant hand, not your elbow or upper arm. Keep the fingernail you use for tapping short so you don't hurt yourself. Follow the standard percussion sequence over the front and back chest walls.

pied by the heart. With careful percussion, you can identify the borders of the heart when lung tissue is normal. Resonance resumes at the sixth intercostal space. The sequence of sounds in the back is slightly different. (See *Percussion sequences.*)

Warning sounds

When you hear hyperresonance during percussion, it means you've found an area of increased air in the lung or pleural space. Expect to hear hyperresonance in your patients with:
• pneumothorax
• acute asthma
• bullous emphysema (large holes in the lungs from alveolar destruction).

When you hear abnormal dullness, it means you've found areas of decreased air in the lungs. Expect abnormal dullness in the presence of:
• pleural fluid
• consolidation atelectasis
• tumor.

Detecting diaphragm movement

Percussion also allows you to assess how much the diaphragm moves during inspiration and expiration. The normal diaphragm descends 1⅛″ to 1⅞″ (3 to 5 cm) when the patient inhales. The diaphragm doesn't move as far in patients with emphysema, respiratory depression, diaphragm paralysis, atelectasis, obesity, or ascites.

> Hyperresonance indicates increased air in the lung or pleural space; dullness is a sign of decreased air in the lungs. I hear that!

Percussion sequences

Follow these percussion sequences to distinguish between normal and abnormal sounds in the patient's lungs. Compare sound variations from one side with the other as you proceed. Carefully describe abnormal sounds you hear and note their locations. (Follow the same sequence for auscultation.)

Anterior

Posterior

Auscultation

As air moves through the bronchi, it creates sound waves that travel to the chest wall. The sound produced by breathing changes as air moves from larger to smaller airways. Sounds also change if they pass through fluid, mucus, or narrowed airways.

Auscultation preparation

Auscultation sites are the same as percussion sites. Listen to a full cycle of inspiration and expiration at each site, using the diaphragm of the stethoscope. Ask the patient to breathe through his mouth if it doesn't cause discomfort; nose breathing alters the pitch of breath sounds.

When things get hairy

If the patient has abundant chest hair, mat it down with a damp washcloth so the hair doesn't make sounds that can be mistaken for crackles.

> To auscultate breath sounds, press the diaphragm side of the stethoscope firmly against the patient's skin.

Be firm

To auscultate for breath sounds, press the diaphragm side of the stethoscope firmly against the skin. Remember that if you listen through clothing or chest hair, breath sounds won't be heard clearly, and you may hear unusual and deceptive sounds.

Normal breath sounds

During auscultation, listen for four types of breath sounds over normal lungs. (See *Locations of normal breath sounds.*)

Here's a rundown of the normal breath sounds and their characteristics:
• Tracheal breath sounds, heard over the trachea, are harsh and discontinuous. They occur when the patient inhales or exhales.
• Bronchial breath sounds, usually heard next to the trachea just above or below the clavicle, are loud, high-pitched, and discontinuous. They're loudest when the patient exhales.
• Bronchovesicular sounds are medium-pitched and continuous. They're best heard over the upper third of the sternum and between the scapulae when the patient inhales or exhales.
• Vesicular sounds, heard over the rest of the lungs, are soft and low-pitched. They're prolonged during inhalation and shortened during exhalation. (See *Qualities of normal breath sounds.*)

Locations of normal breath sounds

These photographs show the normal locations of different types of breath sounds.

Qualities of normal breath sounds

Use this chart as a quick reference for the qualities of normal breath sounds.

Breath sound	Quality	Inspiration-expiration ratio	Location
Tracheal	Harsh, high-pitched	I < E	Over trachea
Bronchial	Loud, high-pitched	I > E	Next to trachea
Bronchovesicular	Medium in loudness and pitch	I = E	Next to sternum, between scapula
Vesicular	Soft, low-pitched	I > E	Remainder of lungs

Interpreting breath sounds

Classify each breath sound you auscultate by its intensity, pitch, duration, characteristic, and location. Note whether it occurs during inspiration, expiration, or both.

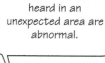

Breath sounds heard in an unexpected area are abnormal.

Inspect the unexpected

Breath sounds heard in an unexpected area are abnormal. For instance, if you hear bronchial sounds where you expect to hear vesicular sounds, the area you're auscultating might be filled with fluid or exudates, as in pneumonia. The vesicular sounds you expect to hear in those areas are absent because no air is moving through the small airways.

Vocal fremitus

Vocal fremitus is the sound produced by chest vibrations as the patient speaks. Abnormal transmission of voice sounds can occur over consolidated areas because sound travels well through fluid. There are three common abnormal voice sounds:
• *Bronchophony* — Ask the patient to say "ninety-nine" or "blue moon." Over normal tissue, the words sound muffled, but over consolidated areas, the words sound unusually loud.
• *Egophony* — Ask the patient to say "E." Over normal lung tissue, the sound is muffled, but over consolidated areas, it sounds like the letter A.
• *Whispered pectoriloquy* — Ask the patient to whisper "1, 2, 3." Over normal lung tissue, the numbers are almost indistinguishable. Over consolidated tissue, the numbers sound loud and clear.

Abnormal breath sounds

Because solid tissue transmits sound better than air or fluid, breath sounds (as well as spoken or whispered words) are louder than normal over areas of consolidation. If pus, fluid, or air fills the pleural space, breath sounds are quieter than normal. If a foreign body or secretions obstruct a bronchus, breath sounds are diminished or absent over lung tissue distal to the obstruction.

Adventitious sounds

Adventitious sounds are abnormal no matter where you hear them in the lungs. (See *Abnormal breath sounds*, page 308.)

There are five types of adventitious breath sounds:

Crackles are intermittent, nonmusical, and brief crackling sounds caused by collapsed or fluid-filled alveoli popping open that are heard primarily when the patient inhales. They're classified as either fine or coarse and usually don't clear with coughing.

If they do, they're most likely caused by secretions. (See *Types of crackles*.)

Wheezes are high-pitched sounds heard first when a patient exhales. They're caused by narrowed airways. As the severity of the block increases, they may also be heard on inspiration. Patients may wheeze as a result of asthma infection, heart failure, or airway obstruction from a tumor or foreign body. (See *When wheezing stops*.)

Rhonchi are low-pitched, snoring, rattling sounds that occur primarily when a patient exhales, although they may also be heard when the patient inhales. Rhonchi usually change or disappear with coughing. The sounds occur when fluid partially blocks the large airways.

Stridor is a loud, high-pitched crowing sound that's heard, usually without a stethoscope, during inspiration. It's caused by an obstruction in the upper airway and requires immediately attention.

Pleural friction rub is a low-pitched, grating, rubbing sound heard when the patient inhales and exhales. Pleural inflammation causes the two layers of pleura to rub together. The patient may complain of pain in areas where the rub is heard.

Diagnostic tests

If your patient's history and the physical examination findings reveal evidence of pulmonary dysfunction, diagnostic testing is done to identify and evaluate the dysfunction. These tests include:

- blood and sputum studies
- endoscopy and imaging
- pulmonary angiography
- bedside testing procedures.

Prepping the patient

Diagnostic testing may be routine for you, but it can be frightening to the patient. Take steps to prepare the patient and his family for each procedure and monitor the patient during and after the procedure.

Some tests can be performed at the bedside in the critical care unit. Many others, however, must be performed in the imaging department; in these cases, you may need to accompany unstable patients who require monitoring.

Abnormal breath sounds

Here's a quick guide to assessing abnormal breath sounds:

- *crackles*—intermittent, nonmusical, crackling sounds heard during inspiration; classified as fine or coarse; common in elderly people when small sections of the alveoli don't fully aerate and secretions accumulate during sleep; alveoli reexpand or pop open when the patient takes deep breaths upon awakening
- w*heezes*—high-pitched sounds caused by blocked airflow, heard on exhalation
- *rhonchi*—low-pitched snoring or rattling sounds; heard primarily on exhalation
- *stridor*—loud, high-pitched sound heard during inspiration
- *pleural friction rub*—low-pitched, grating sound heard during inspiration and expiration; accompanied by pain.

Types of crackles

Here's how to differentiate fine crackles from coarse crackles, a critical distinction when assessing the lungs.

Fine crackles

These characteristics distinguish fine crackles:
- They occur when the patient stops inhaling.
- They're usually heard in lung bases.
- They sound like a piece of hair being rubbed between the fingers or like Velcro being pulled apart.
- They occur in restrictive diseases, such as pulmonary fibrosis, asbestosis, silicosis, atelectasis, heart failure, and pneumonia.

Coarse crackles

These characteristics distinguish coarse crackles:
- They occur when the patient starts to inhale and may be present when the patient exhales.
- They may be heard through the lungs and even at the mouth.
- They sound more like bubbling or gurgling as air moves through secretions in the larger airways.
- They occur in chronic obstructive pulmonary disease, bronchiectasis, pulmonary edema, and in severely ill patients who can't cough; also called the "death rattle."

Advice from the experts

When wheezing stops

If you no longer hear wheezing in a patient having an acute asthma attack, the attack may be far from over. When bronchospasm and mucosal swelling become severe, little air can move through the airways. As a result, wheezing stops.

If all other assessment criteria—labored breathing, prolonged expiratory time, and accessory muscle use— point to acute bronchial obstruction (a medical emergency), maintain the patient's airway and give oxygen and medications as ordered to relieve the obstruction. The patient may begin to wheeze again when the airways open more.

Blood and sputum studies

Blood and sputum studies include arterial blood gas (ABG) analysis and sputum analysis.

ABG analysis

ABG analysis enables evaluation of gas exchange in the lungs by measuring the partial pressures of gases dissolved in arterial blood.

The ABCs of ABGs

Arterial blood is used because it reflects how much oxygen is available to peripheral tissues. Together, ABG values tell the story of how well oxygenated a patient is and whether he's developing acidosis or alkalosis.

Here's a summary of commonly assessed ABG values and what the findings indicate:
- pH measurement of the hydrogen ion (H^+) concentration is an indication of the blood's acidity or alkalinity.
- Partial pressure of arterial carbon dioxide ($PaCO_2$) reflects the adequacy of ventilation of the lungs.
- PaO_2 reflects the body's ability to pick up oxygen from the lungs.

• Bicarbonate (HCO_3^-) level reflects the activity of the kidneys in retaining or excreting bicarbonate.
• Oxygen saturation (SaO_2) is the ratio of actual hemoglobin oxygen content to potential maximum oxygen carrying capacity of the hemoglobin. (See *Normal ABG values.*)

Interpreting ABG values

Here's an interpretation of possible ABG values:
• A PaO_2 value greater than 100 mm Hg reflects more-than-adequate supplemental oxygen administration. A value less than 80 mm Hg indicates hypoxemia.
• An SaO_2 value less than 95% represents decreased saturation and may contribute to a low PaO_2 value.
• A pH value above 7.45 (alkalosis) reflects an H^+ deficit; a value below 7.35 (acidosis) reflects an H^+ excess.

A sample scenario

Suppose you find a pH value greater than 7.45, indicating alkalosis. Investigate further by checking the $PaCO_2$ value, which is known as the respiratory parameter. This value reflects how efficiently the lungs eliminate carbon dioxide. A $PaCO_2$ value below 35 mm Hg indicates respiratory alkalosis and hyperventilation.

Next, check the HCO_3^- value, called the metabolic parameter. An HCO_3^- value greater than 26 mEq/L indicates metabolic alkalosis.

Likewise, a pH value below 7.35 indicates acidosis. A $PaCO_2$ value above 45 mm Hg indicates respiratory acidosis; an HCO_3^- value below 22 mEq/L indicates metabolic acidosis.

See-saw systems

The respiratory and metabolic systems work together to keep the body's acid-base balance within normal limits. If respiratory acidosis develops, for example, the kidneys compensate by conserving HCO_3^-. That's why you expect to see an above-normal HCO_3^- value.

Similarly, if metabolic acidosis develops, the lungs compensate by increasing the respiratory rate and depth to eliminate carbon dioxide. (See *Understanding acid-base disorders.*)

Nursing considerations

• In most critical care units, a doctor, respiratory therapist, or specially trained critical care nurse draws ABG samples, usually from an arterial line if the patient has one. If a percutaneous puncture must be done, the site must be chosen carefully. The most common site is the radial artery but the brachial or femoral arteries can be used. When a radial artery is used, an Allen's test is done before drawing the sample to determine that the ulnar artery

---

Normal ABG values

Arterial blood gas (ABG) values provide information about the blood's acid-base balance and oxygenation.

Normal values are:
• pH—7.35 to 7.45
• $PaCO_2$—35 to 45 mm Hg
• PaO_2—80 to 100 mm Hg
• HCO_3^-—22 to 26 mEq/L
• SaO_2—95% to 100%.

The respiratory and metabolic systems work together to maintain acid-base balance.

Understanding acid-base disorders

This chart provides an overview of selected acid-base disorders.

Disorder and ABG findings	Possible causes	Signs and symptoms
Respiratory acidosis (excess carbon dioxide retention) pH < 7.35 HCO_3^- > 26 mEq/L (if compensating) $Paco_2$ > 45 mm Hg	• Central nervous system depression from drugs, injury, or disease • Asphyxia • Hypoventilation from pulmonary, cardiac, musculoskeletal, or neuromuscular disease	Diaphoresis, headache, tachycardia, confusion, restlessness, apprehension, flushed face
Respiratory alkalosis (excess carbon dioxide excretion) pH > 7.45 HCO_3^- < 22 mEq/L (if compensating) $Paco_2$ < 35 mm Hg	• Hyperventilation from anxiety, pain, or improper ventilator settings • Respiratory stimulation by drugs, disease, hypoxia, fever, or high room temperature • Gram-negative bacteremia	Rapid, deep respirations; paresthesias; light-headedness; twitching; anxiety; fear
Metabolic acidosis (bicarbonate loss, acid retention) pH < 7.35 HCO_3^- < 22 mEq/L $Paco_2$ < 35 mm Hg (if compensating)	• Bicarbonate depletion from diarrhea • Excessive production of organic acids from hepatic disease, endocrine disorders, shock, or drug intoxication • Inadequate excretion of acids from renal disease	Rapid, deep breathing; fruity breath; fatigue; headache; lethargy; drowsiness; nausea; vomiting; coma (if severe); abdominal pain
Metabolic alkalosis (bicarbonate retention, acid loss) pH > 7.45 HCO_3^- > 26 mEq/L $Paco_2$ > 45 mm Hg (if compensating)	• Loss of hydrochloric acid from prolonged vomiting or gastric suctioning • Loss of potassium from increased renal excretion (as in diuretic therapy) or steroids • Excessive alkali ingestion	Slow, shallow breathing; hypertonic muscles; restlessness; twitching; confusion; irritability; apathy; tetany; convulsions; coma (if severe)

can provide adequate circulation to the hand, in case the radial artery is damaged. (See *Performing Allen's test*, page 312.)

• After obtaining the sample, apply pressure to the puncture site for 5 minutes and tape a gauze pad firmly in place. Regularly monitor the site for bleeding and check the arm for signs of complications, such as swelling, discoloration, pain, numbness, and tingling. (See *Obtaining an ABG sample*, page 313.)

• Note whether the patient is breathing room air or oxygen. If the patient is on oxygen, document the number of liters. If the patient is receiving mechanical ventilation, document the fraction of inspired oxygen.

• Examples of conditions that can interfere with test results are failure to properly heparinize the syringe before drawing a blood sample or exposing the sample to air. Venous blood in the sample may lower Pao_2 levels and elevate $Paco_2$ levels. Make sure you re-

Performing Allen's test

Before obtaining an arterial blood gas sample from the radial artery, make sure you perform Allen's test to assess the patient's collateral arterial blood supply:

- Direct the patient to close his hand while you occlude the radial and ulnar arteries for 10 to 30 seconds, watching for the hand to blanch.

- Tell the patient to open his hand.

- Release pressure on the ulnar artery. Color should return to the patient's hand in 15 seconds. If the color doesn't return, select another site for an arterial puncture.

move all air bubbles in the sample syringe because air bubbles also alter results.

- Make sure the sample of arterial blood is kept cold, preferably on ice, and delivered as soon as possible to the laboratory for analysis. Some chemical reactions that alter findings continue to take place after the blood is drawn; rapid cooling and analysis of the sample minimizes this.

Sputum analysis

Sputum analysis assesses sputum specimens (the material expectorated from a patient's lungs and bronchi during deep coughing) to diagnose respiratory disease, identify the cause of pulmonary infection (including viral and bacterial causes), identify abnormal lung cells, and manage lung disease.

Under the microscope

Sputum specimens are stained and examined under a microscope and, depending on the patient's condition, sometimes cultured. Culture and sensitivity testing is used to identify a specific microorganism and its antibiotic sensitivities. A negative culture may suggest a viral infection.

Keep it cold and be quick! Deliver the chilled arterial blood sample ASAP for analysis.

Obtaining an ABG sample

Follow the steps below to obtain a sample for arterial blood gas (ABG) analysis:
• After performing Allen's test, perform a cutaneous arterial puncture (or, if an arterial line is in place, draw blood from the arterial line).
• Use a heparinized blood gas syringe to draw the sample.
• Eliminate all air from the sample, place it on ice immediately, and transport it for analysis.
• Apply pressure to the puncture site for 3 to 5 minutes. If the patient is receiving anticoagulants or has a coagulopathy, hold the puncture site longer than 5 minutes if necessary.
• Tape a gauze pad firmly over the puncture site. If the puncture site is on the arm, don't tape the entire circumference because this may restrict circulation.

Nursing considerations
• If the patient's condition permits and he isn't on fluid restriction, increase fluid intake the night before sputum collection to aid expectoration.
• To prevent foreign particles from contaminating the specimen, instruct the patient not to eat, brush his teeth, or use mouthwash before expectorating. He may rinse his mouth with water.
• When he's ready to expectorate, instruct the patient to take three deep breaths and force a deep cough.
• Before sending the specimen to the laboratory, make sure it's sputum, not saliva. Saliva has a thinner consistency and more bubbles (froth) than sputum.

Instruct your patient not to eat, brush his teeth, or use mouthwash before sputum collection.

Endoscopy and imaging

Endoscopy and imaging tests include bronchoscopy, chest X-ray, magnetic resonance imaging (MRI), thoracic computed tomography (CT) scan, and $\dot{V}/\dot{Q}$ scan.

Bronchoscopy

Bronchoscopy allows direct visualization of the larynx, trachea, and bronchi through a fiber-optic bronchoscope, a slender flexible tube with mirrors and a light at its distal end. The flexible fiber-optic bronchoscope is preferred to metal because it's smaller, allows a better view of the bronchi, and carries less risk of trauma.

To remove and evaluate

The purpose of a bronchoscopy is to:

• remove foreign bodies, malignant or benign tumors, mucus plugs, or excessive secretions from the tracheobronchial tree and control massive hemoptysis

• pass brush biopsy forceps or a catheter through the broncho-scope to obtain specimens for cytologic evaluation.

Nursing considerations

• Before bronchoscopy, collect the patient's history. A physical examination is performed; preprocedure studies may include a chest X-ray, ABG analysis, and clotting studies.

• The patient usually goes to a procedure suite for the bronchoscopy. In some cases — such as when the patient is on a ventilator — it may be performed at the bedside. Explain the procedure to the patient and his family and answer their questions.

• The patient may be premedicated with atropine to dry secretions and a mild sedative or antianxiety agent such as midazolam (Versed) to help him relax. Before insertion of the bronchoscope, a topical anesthetic is applied to the oropharynx, nasopharynx, larynx, vocal cords, and trachea to suppress the cough reflex and prevent gagging.

• The doctor introduces the bronchoscope tube through the patient's nose or mouth into the airway. Various ports on the bronchoscope allow for suctioning, oxygen administration, and biopsies during the procedure. Monitor vital signs, oxygen saturation levels with pulse oximetry, and heart rhythm throughout the procedure.

• After the procedure, the patient is positioned on his side or may have the head of the bed elevated 30 degrees until the gag reflex returns. Assess respiratory status and monitor vital signs, oxygen saturation levels, and heart rhythm. Report signs and symptoms of respiratory distress, such as dyspnea, laryngospasm, or hypoxemia.

• Monitor cardiac status frequently for changes in heart rate or rhythm. Report any tachycardia or evidence of arrhythmia.

• If the patient isn't intubated, assess for return of the gag, cough, and swallow reflexes. Maintain nothing-by-mouth status until these reflexes return. Explain to the patient that temporary hoarseness or sore throat may occur after the procedure and that gargle or lozenges may be ordered to ease discomfort.

• Obtain a chest X-ray as ordered, to detect pneumothorax and evaluate lung status.

• Keep resuscitative equipment available during the test and for 24 hours afterward.

> Bronchoscopy allows removal of tissue or foreign bodies from the tracheobronchial tree.

(Text continues on page 315.)

Pulmonary artery catheterization

Pulmonary artery catheterization can give you information about a patient's cardiovascular and pulmonary status. With a basic pulmonary artery catheter, you can measure intracardiac pressure, pulmonary artery wedge pressure (PAWP), and cardiac output.

    When your patient requires a pulmonary artery catheter, your responsibilities include assisting with insertion, caring for the insertion site and catheter, and hemodynamic monitoring. Before you care for a patient who requires pulmonary artery catheterization, familiarize yourself with a basic catheter.

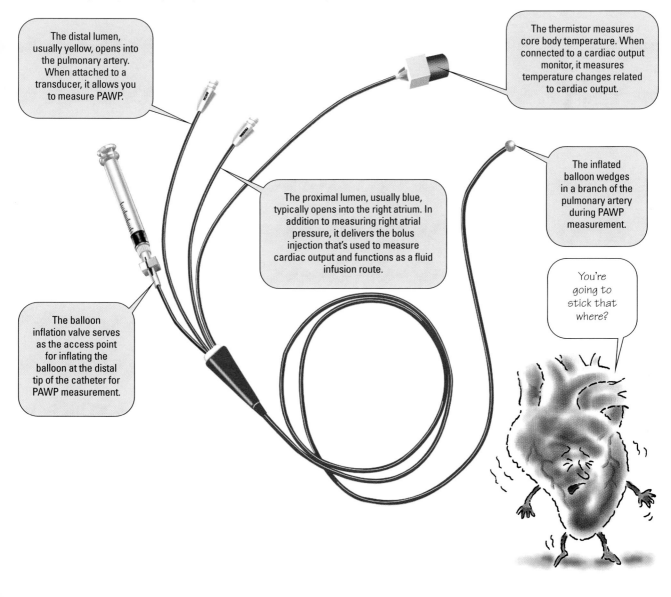

The distal lumen, usually yellow, opens into the pulmonary artery. When attached to a transducer, it allows you to measure PAWP.

The thermistor measures core body temperature. When connected to a cardiac output monitor, it measures temperature changes related to cardiac output.

The proximal lumen, usually blue, typically opens into the right atrium. In addition to measuring right atrial pressure, it delivers the bolus injection that's used to measure cardiac output and functions as a fluid infusion route.

The inflated balloon wedges in a branch of the pulmonary artery during PAWP measurement.

The balloon inflation valve serves as the access point for inflating the balloon at the distal tip of the catheter for PAWP measurement.

You're going to stick that where?

Normal pulmonary artery waveforms

After insertion into a large vein (usually the subclavian, jugular, or femoral vein), a pulmonary artery catheter is advanced through the vena cava into the right atrium, through the right ventricle and into a branch of the pulmonary artery. During insertion, the monitor shows various waveforms as the catheter advances through the heart chambers.

The catheter tip enters the right atrium.

When the catheter tip enters the right atrium, this waveform appears on the monitor, representing right atrial pressure.

Watch the patient's ECG monitor closely. Ventricular arrhythmias can occur as the catheter passes through the right ventricle.

Next, the catheter tip reaches the right ventricle.

As the catheter tip reaches the right ventricle, you'll see a waveform with sharp systolic upstrokes and lower diastolic dips.

The catheter floats into the pulmonary artery.

As the catheter reaches the pulmonary artery, the upstroke of the waveform becomes smoother than that of the right ventricular waveform.

The dicrotic notch indicates closure of the pulmonic valve.

The catheter's balloon floats into a distal branch of the pulmonary artery. The balloon wedges where the vessel becomes too narrow for it to pass.

The monitor now shows a pulmonary artery wedge pressure waveform with two small uprises. The balloon is then deflated and the catheter is left in the pulmonary artery.

Measuring cardiac output

Measuring cardiac output—the volume of blood ejected from the heart in 1 minute—helps evaluate cardiac function. Normally, cardiac output ranges from 4 to 8 L/minute. To measure cardiac output at the bedside, a pulmonary artery catheter containing a thermistor is inserted. The thermistor detects blood temperature changes and transmits information to a monitoring computer, which calculates and displays cardiac output.

The injection should take no longer than 4 seconds to complete.

When measuring cardiac output, inject the specified amount of injectant into the proximal port of the pulmonary artery catheter during end expiration.

Repeat the injection procedure at least three times to obtain a mean cardiac output value.

Check the thermodilution curve on the patient's monitor to make sure the injection was properly performed. You should see a smooth, sharp rise in the curve.

Chest X-ray

During chest radiography (commonly known as chest X-ray), X-ray beams penetrate the chest and react on specially sensitized film. Because normal pulmonary tissue is radiolucent, such abnormalities as infiltrates, foreign bodies, fluid, and tumors appear dense on the film.

More is better

A chest X-ray is most useful when compared with the patient's previous films, allowing the radiologist to detect changes.

By themselves, chest X-rays may not provide definitive diagnostic information. For example, they may not reveal mild to moderate obstructive pulmonary disease. However, they can show the location and size of lesions and can also be used to identify structural abnormalities that influence ventilation and diffusion.

X-ray vision

A chest X-ray is most useful when it's compared with previous films, allowing changes to be detected.

Examples of abnormalities visible on X-ray include:
• pneumothorax
• fibrosis
• atelectasis
• infiltrates.

Nursing considerations

• When a patient in the critical care unit can't be moved, chest X-ray is commonly performed at the bedside. Explain to the patient that someone will help him to a sitting position while a cold, hard film plate is placed behind his back. If testing is done in the radiology department, you may need to accompany the patient. The patient usually lies on a stretcher or X-ray table and is asked to take a deep breath and to hold it for a few seconds while the X-ray is taken. Instruct the patient to remain still for those few seconds.

Minimal exposure

• Provide reassurance that the amount of radiation exposure is minimal. Facility personnel leave the area when the technician takes the X-ray because they're potentially exposed to radiation many times per day.
• Make sure that female patients of childbearing age wear a lead apron. Males should have protection for the testes.

Provide reassurance that the amount of radiation exposure during chest X-ray is minimal.

Magnetic resonance imaging

MRI is a noninvasive test that employs a powerful magnet, radio waves, and a computer. It's used to diagnose respiratory disorders by providing high-resolution, cross-sectional images of lung structures and by tracing blood flow.

A view that's see-through

The greatest advantage of MRI is that it enables one to "see through" bone and delineate fluid-filled soft tissue in great detail, without using ionizing radiation or contrast media. It's used to distinguish tumors from other structures such as blood vessels.

Nursing considerations

• All metal objects must be removed from the patient before entering the scanning room. (See *MRI and metals don't mix.*)
• If the patient is claustrophobic, sedation may be ordered before the test. You or another nurse generally accompanies the patient to the MRI suite.
• Tell the patient that he'll be asked to lie on a table that slides into an 8′ (2.4 m) tunnel inside the magnet. Some facilities can perform open MRIs, which are more tolerable for patients who are claustrophobic. The test usually takes 15 to 30 minutes.
• Instruct the patient to breathe normally but not to talk or move during the test, to avoid distorting the results.
• Explain that the machinery is noisy, with sounds ranging from an incessant ping to a loud bang. The patient may feel claustrophobic or bored. Encourage him to relax and to concentrate on breathing or a favorite subject or image.

Thoracic computed tomography scans

Thoracic CT scan provides cross-sectional views of the chest by passing an X-ray beam from a computerized scanner through the body at different angles and depths. A contrast agent is sometimes used to highlight blood vessels and allow greater visual discrimination.

CT in 3-D

Thoracic CT scan provides a three-dimensional image of the lung, allowing the doctor to assess abnormalities in the configuration of the trachea or major bronchi and evaluate masses or lesions, such as tumors and abscesses, and abnormal lung shadows.

MRI and metals don't mix

Before your patient undergoes magnetic resonance imaging (MRI) make sure he doesn't have a pacemaker or surgically implanted joint, pin, clip, valve, or pump containing metal. Such objects could be attracted to the strong MRI magnet.

Ask your patient whether he's ever worked with metals or has metal in his eyes. (Some facilities have a checklist that covers all pertinent questions regarding metals, clips, pins, pacemakers, and other devices). If he has such a device, the test can't be done.

Three cheers for thoracic CT scanning! It allows 3-D imaging of the lungs.

Nursing considerations

• Confirm that the patient isn't allergic to iodine or shellfish. A patient with these allergies may have an adverse reaction to the contrast medium.
• If a contrast medium is used, explain that it's injected into the existing I.V. line or that a new line may be inserted.
• Explain to the patient that he may feel flushed or notice a metallic or salty taste in his mouth when the contrast medium is injected.
• Explain that the CT scanner circles around the patient for 10 to 30 minutes, depending on the procedure, and that the equipment may make him feel claustrophobic.
• Instruct the patient to lie still during the test.
• Inform the patient that the contrast medium may discolor his urine for 24 hours.
• Encourage oral fluid intake to flush the contrast medium out of the patient's system, unless it's contraindicated or the patient is on nothing-by-mouth status. The doctor may write an order to increase the rate of I.V. fluid infusion.

> Encourage fluid intake to flush the contrast medium from your patient's system, unless it's contraindicated.

Ventilation-perfusion scan

A V̇/Q̇ scan is used to:
• evaluate V̇/Q̇ mismatch
• detect pulmonary emboli
• evaluate pulmonary function, especially in patients with marginal lung reserves.

Although it's less reliable than pulmonary angiography, V̇/Q̇ scanning carries fewer risks.

Two-tined test

A V̇/Q̇ scan has two parts:

During the ventilation portion of the test, the patient inhales the contrast medium gas; ventilation patterns and adequacy of ventilation are noted on the scan.

During the perfusion scan, the contrast medium is injected I.V. and the pulmonary blood flow to the lungs is visualized.

> Take two! A V̇/Q̇ scan is a two-part test.

A caveat

V̇/Q̇ scans aren't commonly used for patients on mechanical ventilators because the ventilation portion of the test is difficult to perform. (Pulmonary angiography is the preferred test for a critically ill patient with a suspected pulmonary embolus.)

Nursing considerations

• Explain the test to the patient and his family, telling them who performs the test and where it's done.
• Like pulmonary angiography, a V̇/Q̇ scan requires the injection of a contrast medium. Confirm that the patient doesn't have an allergy to the contrast material.
• Explain to the patient that the test has two parts. During the ventilation portion, a mask is placed over his mouth and nose and the patient breathes in the contrast medium gas mixed with air while the scanner takes pictures of his lungs. For the perfusion portion, the patient is placed in a supine position on a movable table as the contrast medium is injected into the I.V. line while the scanner again takes pictures of the lungs.
• After the procedure, maintain bed rest as ordered and monitor the patient's vital signs, oxygen saturation levels, and heart rhythm.
• Monitor for adverse reactions to the contrast medium, which may include restlessness, tachypnea and respiratory distress, tachycardia, urticaria, and nausea and vomiting. Keep emergency equipment nearby in case of a reaction.

Pulmonary angiography

Pulmonary angiography, also called *pulmonary arteriography*, allows radiographic examination of the pulmonary circulation.

After injecting a radioactive contrast dye through a catheter inserted into the pulmonary artery or one of its branches, a series of X-rays is taken to detect blood flow abnormalities, possibly caused by emboli or pulmonary infarction.

More reliable, more risks

Pulmonary angiography yields more reliable results than a V̇/Q̇ scan, but carries higher risks for certain conditions, such as cardiac arrhythmias (especially ventricular arrhythmias due to myocardial irritation from passage of the catheter through the heart chambers). It may be the preferred test, especially if the patient is on a ventilator.

Nursing considerations

• Explain the procedure to the patient and his family and answer their questions. Tell him who performs the test, where it's done, and how long it takes.

Preprocedure patient preparation

• Confirm that the patient isn't allergic to shellfish or iodine. Notify the doctor if the patient has such an allergy because the patient

Pulmonary angiography may be preferred over V̇/Q̇ scanning, especially if your patient is on a ventilator.

may have an adverse reaction to the contrast medium. Diphenhydramine (Benadryl) and prednisone (Deltasone) may be administered, as ordered, before the test to reduce the risk of a reaction to the dye.

• Preprocedure testing should include evaluation of renal function (by serum creatinine levels and blood urea nitrogen [BUN] levels) and potential risk of bleeding (by prothrombin time, partial thromboplastin time (PTT), and platelet count). Notify the doctor of abnormal results.

• Instruct the patient to lie still for the procedure.

• Explain that he'll probably feel a flushed sensation in his face as the dye is injected.

Postprocedure procedures

• Maintain bed rest, as ordered, and monitor the patient's vital signs, oxygen saturation levels, and heart rhythm.

• Keep a sandbag or femoral compression device over the injection site as ordered.

• After the procedure, check the pressure dressing for signs of bleeding. Monitor the patient's peripheral pulse in the arm or leg used for catheter insertion (mark the site), check the temperature, color and sensation of the extremity, and compare with the opposite side.

• Unless contraindicated, encourage the patient to drink more fluids to flush the dye or contrast medium from his system, or increase the I.V. flow rate as ordered.

• Check serum creatinine and BUN levels after the procedure because the contrast medium can cause acute renal failure.

• Monitor for adverse reactions to the contrast medium, which may include restlessness, tachypnea and respiratory distress, tachycardia, facial flushing, urticaria, and nausea and vomiting. Keep emergency equipment nearby in case of a reaction.

Check serum creatinine and BUN levels because the contrast medium can cause acute renal failure.

Bedside testing procedures

Diagnostic tests used at the bedside to evaluate respiratory function include pulse oximetry, mixed venous oxygen saturation, and end-tidal carbon dioxide monitoring.

Pulse oximetry

Pulse oximetry is a relatively simple procedure used to monitor arterial oxygen saturation noninvasively. It's performed either intermittently or continuously.

Shedding light on the subject

In this procedure, two diodes send red and infrared light through a pulsating arterial vascular bed such as the one in the fingertip.

A photodetector (also called a *sensor* or *transducer*) slipped over the finger measures the transmitted light as it passes through the vascular bed, detects the relative amount of color absorbed by arterial blood, and calculates the saturation without interference from the venous blood, skin, or connective tissue. The percentage expressed is the ratio of oxygen to hemoglobin. (See *A closer look at pulse oximetry*.)

Note denotation

In pulse oximetry, arterial oxygen saturation values are usually denoted with the symbol SpO_2. Arterial oxygen saturation values, which are measured invasively via ABG analysis, are denoted by the symbol SaO_2.

Nursing considerations

• Place the sensor over the finger or other site, such as the toe, bridge of the nose, or earlobe, so that the light beams and sensors are opposite each other.
• Protect the sensor from exposure to strong light, such as fluorescent lighting, because it interferes with results. Check the sen-

Place the sensor over a finger or other site so that the light beams and sensors are opposite each other.

A closer look at pulse oximetry

Oximetry may be intermittent or continuous and is used to monitor arterial oxygen saturation. Normal oxygen saturation levels are 95% to 100% for adults. Lower levels may indicate hypoxemia and warrant intervention.

Interfering factors
Certain factors can interfere with the accuracy of oximetry readings. For example, an elevated bilirubin level may falsely lower oxygen saturation readings, whereas elevated carboxyhemoglobin or methemoglobin levels can falsely elevate oxygen saturation readings.

Certain intravascular substances, such as lipid emulsions and dyes, can also prevent accurate readings. Other interfering factors include excessive light (such as from phototherapy or direct sunlight), excessive patient movement, excessive ear pigment, hypothermia, hypotension, and vasoconstriction.

Some acrylic nails and certain colors of nail polish (blue, green, black, and brown-red) may also interfere with readings.

sor site frequently to make sure the device is in place and to examine the skin for abrasion and circulatory impairment.
• The pulse oximeter displays the patient's pulse rate and oxygen saturation reading. The pulse rate on the oximeter must correspond to the patient's actual pulse. If the rates don't correspond, the saturation reading can't be considered accurate. You may need to reposition the sensor to obtain an accurate reading.
• Rotate the sensor site at least every 4 hours, following the manufacturer's instructions and your facility's policy for site rotation, to avoid skin irritation and circulatory impairment.
• If oximetry is done properly, the oxygen saturation readings are usually within 2% of ABG values. A normal reading is 95% to 100%.

Poisoning precludes pulse oximetry

• Pulse oximetry isn't used when carbon monoxide poisoning is suspected because the oximeter doesn't differentiate between oxygen and carbon monoxide bound to hemoglobin. An ABG analysis should be performed in such cases.

Mixed venous oxygen saturation monitoring

Mixed venous oxygen saturation ($S\bar{v}o_2$) reflects the oxygen saturation level of venous blood. It's determined by measuring the amount of oxygen extracted and used or consumed by the body's tissues.

$S\bar{v}o_2$ indications

In a healthy adult, an $S\bar{v}o_2$ level between 60% and 80% indicates adequate tissue perfusion.

Decreased values less than 60% indicate increased oxygen extraction by the tissues. A decrease in oxygen delivery or an increase in tissue demands can cause this.

Increased values greater than 80% may occur in states of increased oxygen delivery or may indicate decreased oxygen extraction by the tissues (when tissue hypoxia exists despite the availability of oxygen).

Drawing from the right location

Ideally, the $S\bar{v}o_2$ sample is obtained from the most distal port of the pulmonary artery (PA) catheter, which contains the ideal mix of all venous blood in the heart. Samples may be drawn from a central catheter if a PA catheter isn't available.

A calculating catheter

Continuous $S\bar{v}o_2$ monitoring is done using the $S\bar{v}o_2$ or oximetric PA catheter. This specialized PA catheter calculates oxygen satu-

The patient's $S\bar{v}o_2$ level reflects the amount of oxygen extracted by the body's tissues.

ration of hemoglobin by measuring the wavelengths of reflected light through fiber-optic bundles.

The information is exhibited on a bedside computer and may be displayed numerically and graphically. The manufacturer's instructions for catheter calibration must be followed to ensure accurate readings.

Follow the manufacturer's instructions for catheter calibration to ensure accurate readings.

Nursing considerations

• Explain the procedure to the patient and his family. Make sure they understand the expected outcomes and risks of the procedure related to catheter placement, pneumothorax, cardiac arrhythmias, and infection.

• If you assist with catheter insertion, monitor the patient's vital signs and heart rhythm as you assess for changes in ventilatory function.

• Apply a sterile dressing or sterile transparent dressing over the catheter insertion site. Follow your facility's policy for changing the dressing and pulmonary artery monitoring system (tubing and solution).

• Document the date and time of catheter insertion, initial $S\bar{v}o_2$ readings, and any changes in the patient's condition. Monitor the pulmonary artery pressure (PAP) and $S\bar{v}o_2$ readings, and document hourly or according to your facility's policy.

• Closely monitor the patient's hemodynamic status. Troubleshoot the catheter for problems that can interfere with accurate testing, such as loose connections, balloon rupture, or clot formation on the tip of the catheter.

End-tidal carbon dioxide monitoring

End-tidal carbon dioxide monitoring ($ETco_2$) is used to measure the carbon dioxide concentration at end expiration. An $ETco_2$ monitor may be a separate monitor or part of the patient's bedside hemodynamic monitoring system.

Indications for $ETco_2$ monitoring include:

• monitoring patency of the airway in acute airway obstruction and apnea and respiratory function

• early detection of changes in carbon dioxide production and elimination with hyperventilation therapy, or hypercapnia or hyperthermia states

• assessing effectiveness of interventions such as mechanical ventilation or neuromuscular blockade used with mechanical ventilation, and prone positioning.

In-lightened

In ETCO$_2$ monitoring, a photodetector measures the amount of infrared light absorbed by the airway during inspiration and expiration. (Light absorption increases along with the carbon dioxide concentration.) The monitor converts these data to a carbon dioxide value and a corresponding waveform, or capnogram if capnography is used. (See *Understanding ETCO$_2$ monitoring*, page 324.)

Crunching the numbers

Values are obtained by monitoring samples of expired gas from an endotracheal (ET) tube or an oral or nasopharyngeal airway. Although the values are similar, the ETCO$_2$ values are usually 2 to 5 mm Hg lower than the PaCO$_2$ value.

Capnograms and ETCO$_2$ monitoring reduce the need for frequent ABG sampling.

Nursing considerations

• Explain the procedure to the patient and his family.
• Assess the patient's respiratory status, vital signs, oxygen saturation, and ETCO$_2$ readings. Observe waveform quality and trends of ETCO$_2$ readings and observe for suddenly increased readings (which may indicate hypoventilation, partial airway obstruction, or respiratory depressant effects from drugs), or decreased readings (due to complete airway obstruction, dislodged ET tube, or ventilator malfunction). Notify the doctor of a 10% increase or decrease in readings.

> Notify the doctor if there's a 10% increase or decrease in ETCO$_2$ readings.

Treatments

Respiratory disorders interfere with airway clearance, breathing patterns, and gas exchange. If not corrected, they can adversely affect many other body systems and can be life-threatening.

Treatments for patients with respiratory disorders include drug therapy, surgery, and inhalation therapy.

> Drugs are used for airway management in patients with some respiratory disorders.

Drug therapy

Drugs are used for airway management in patients with such disorders as acute respiratory failure, ARDS, asthma, emphysema, and chronic bronchitis. Some types of drugs commonly seen in the critical care environment include anti-inflammatory agents, bronchodilators, neuromuscular blocking agents, and sedatives.

Understanding ETco$_2$ monitoring

The optical portion of an end-tidal carbon dioxide (ETco$_2$) monitor contains an infrared light source, a sample chamber, a special carbon dioxide (CO$_2$) filter, and a photodetector.

In ETco$_2$ monitoring, the infrared light passes through the sample chamber and is absorbed in varying amounts, depending on the amount of CO$_2$ the patient just exhaled. The photodetector measures CO$_2$ content and relays this information to the microprocessor in the monitor, which displays the CO$_2$ value and waveform.

Capnogram reading

The CO$_2$ waveform, or capnogram, produced in ETco$_2$ monitoring reflects the course of CO$_2$ elimination during exhalation. A normal capnogram (shown below) consists of several segments, which reflect the various stages of exhalation and inhalation.

Normally, any gas eliminated from the airway during early exhalation is dead-space gas that hasn't undergone exchange at the alveolocapillary membrane. Measurements taken during this period contain no CO$_2$. As exhalation continues, CO$_2$ concentration increases sharply and rapidly. The sensor now detects gas that has undergone exchange, producing measurable quantities of CO$_2$.

The final stages of alveolar emptying occur during late exhalation. During the alveolar plateau phase, CO$_2$ concentration increases gradually because alveolar emptying is relatively constant.

The point at which the ETco$_2$ value is derived is the end of exhalation, when CO$_2$ concentration peaks. However, this value doesn't accurately reflect alveolar CO$_2$ if no alveolar plateau is present. During inhalation, the CO$_2$ concentration declines sharply to zero.

ETco$_2$ monitor

Exhaled CO$_2$

Infrared light source

Sample chamber

CO$_2$ filter

Photodetector

This peak that occurs during the end of exhalation indicates the point at which the ETco$_2$ value is derived.

Alveolar plateau

mm Hg

Early exhalation of dead-space gas

Rise of CO$_2$ concentration

End of exhalation

Decline of CO$_2$ concentration

Anti-inflammatory agents

Anti-inflammatory agents (corticosteroids) are used to reduce bronchial inflammation.

Reversing obstruction

Corticosteroids are the most effective anti-inflammatory agents used to treat patients with reversible airflow obstruction. They work by suppressing immune responses and reducing inflammation.

Systemic drugs, such as dexamethasone (Decadron), methylprednisolone (Medrol), and prednisone (Deltasone) are given to manage an acute respiratory event such as acute respiratory failure or exacerbation of COPD. These drugs are initially given I.V. and, when the patient stabilizes, the dosage is tapered and oral dosing may be substituted.

Patients with asthma commonly use inhaled steroids, such as beclomethasone (Qvar), budesonide (Pulmicort Turbuhaler), flunisolide (AeroBid), fluticasone (Flovent) and triamcinolone (Azmacort). These agents, too, work by suppressing the immune response and reducing airway inflammation (See *Understanding corticosteroids.*)

> Systemic drugs are given I.V. at first, then tapered and delivered orally when the patient stabilizes.

Understanding corticosteroids

Use this table to learn about the indications, adverse reactions, and practice pointers associated with corticosteroids.

Drugs	Indications	Adverse reactions	Practice pointers
Systemic steroids Dexamethasone Methylprednisolone Prednisone	• Anti-inflammatory for acute respiratory failure, acute respiratory distress syndrome, and chronic obstructive pulmonary disease • Anti-inflammatory and immunosuppressor for asthma	• Heart failure • Arrhythmias • Edema, • Circulatory collapse, • Thromboembolism • Pancreatitis • Peptic ulcer	• Use cautiously in patients with recent myocardial infarction, hypertension, renal disease, and GI ulcer. • Monitor blood pressure and blood glucose levels.
Inhaled steroids Beclomethasone Budesonide Flunisolide Fluticasone Triamcinolone	• Long-term asthma control	• Hoarseness • Dry mouth • Wheezing • Bronchospasm • Oral candidiasis	• Don't use for treatment of acute asthma attack. • Use a spacer to reduce adverse effects. • Rinse the patient's mouth after use to prevent oral fungal infection.

Bronchodilators

Bronchodilators relax bronchial smooth muscles and are used to treat patients with bronchospasms. Here's how some types of bronchodilators are used:

- Short-acting inhaled beta$_2$-adrenergic agonists, such as albuterol (Proventil) and pirbuterol (Maxair), are used to relieve acute symptoms in asthma and bronchospasm.
- Epinephrine acts on both alpha- and beta-adrenergic receptors. It's used to relieve anaphylactic, allergic, and other hypersensitivity reactions. Its beta-adrenergic effects relax bronchial smooth muscle and relieve bronchospasm.
- Anticholinergic agents, such as ipratropium (Atrovent), act by inhibiting the action of acetylcholine at bronchial smooth-muscle receptor sites and thus produce bronchodilation. (See *Understanding bronchodilators.*)

Epinephrine is used to relieve anaphylactic, allergic, and other hypersensitivity reactions.

Neuromuscular blocking agents

Patients on mechanical ventilation may require neuromuscular blocking agents to eliminate spontaneous breathing efforts that can interfere with the ventilator's function. Neuromuscular blocking agents cause paralysis without altering the patient's level of consciousness (LOC). (See *Understanding neuromuscular blocking agents,* pages 328 and 329.)

Sedatives

Benzodiazepines, such as midazolam and lorazepam (Ativan), are used for conscious sedation and preoperative sedation to reduce anxiety in patients undergoing diagnostic or surgical procedures.

These drugs are also used to relieve anxiety and promote sedation in patients on mechanical ventilators, especially those receiving neuromuscular blocking agents. Such agents cause paralysis without altering the patient's LOC, which—without sedation—is frightening for the patient. (See *Understanding sedatives,* pages 330 and 331.)

Surgery may be necessary if drugs or other treatment measures fail.

Surgery

If drugs or other therapeutic modes fail to maintain the patient's airway patency and protect healthy tissues from disease, surgery may be necessary. Some types of respiratory surgeries are tracheotomy, chest tube insertion, thoracotomy, and lung transplant.

Understanding bronchodilators

Use this table to learn about the indications, adverse reactions, and practice pointers associated with bronchodilators.

Drugs	Indications	Adverse reactions	Practice pointers
Beta₂-adrenergic agonists			
Albuterol	• Short-acting relief of acute symptoms with asthma and bronchospasm	• Paradoxical bronchospasm • Tachycardia • Palpitations • Tremor • Hyperactivity	• Warn patient about possibility of paradoxical bronchospasm. If it occurs, stop drug and seek medical treatment. • Elderly patient may require a lower dose. • Monitor respiratory status, vital signs and heart rhythm.
Epinephrine	• Relax bronchial smooth muscle by stimulating beta₂-adrenergic receptors; used for bronchospasm, hypersensitivity reaction, anaphylaxis, asthma	• Ventricular fibrillation • Palpitations • Tachycardia • Cerebral hemorrhage	• Use cautiously in elderly patients and those with long-standing asthma and emphysema with degenerative heart disease. • Monitor respiratory status, vital signs, and heart rhythm. • Contraindicated in patients with angle-closure glaucoma, coronary insufficiency, and cerebral arteriosclerosis.
Pirbuterol	• Relief of acute symptoms with asthma and bronchospasm	• Palpitations • Tachycardia • Tremor • Paradoxical bronchospasm	• Warn patient about possibility of paradoxical bronchospasm. If it occurs, stop drug and seek medical treatment. • Elderly patient may require a lower dose. • Monitor respiratory status, vital signs, and heart rhythm.
Anticholinergic agents			
Ipratropium	• Bronchospasm associated with chronic bronchitis and emphysema	• Bronchospasm • Chest pain • Palpitations • Nervousness	• Because of delayed onset of bronchodilation, drug isn't recommended for acute respiratory distress. • Use cautiously in patients with angle-closure glaucoma, bladder neck obstruction, and prostatic hypertrophy. • Monitor respiratory status, vital signs, and heart rhythm.

Tracheotomy

A tracheotomy is a surgical procedure to create an opening into the trachea, called a *tracheostomy,* which allows insertion of an indwelling tube to keep the patient's airway open.

(Text continues on page 331.)

Understanding neuromuscular blocking agents

Use this table to learn about the indications, adverse reactions, and practice pointers associated with neuromuscular blocking agents.

Drugs	Indications	Adverse reactions	Practice pointers
Depolarizing			
Succinylcholine	• Adjunct to general anesthesia to aid endotracheal (ET) intubation • Induction of skeletal muscle paralysis during surgery or mechanical ventilation	• Bradycardia, arrhythmias, cardiac arrest • Postoperative muscle pain • Respiratory depression, apnea, bronchoconstriction • Malignant hyperthermia, increased intraocular pressure, flushing	• Contraindicated in patients with history of malignant hyperthermia, myopathies associated with creatinine phosphokinase, acute angle-closure glaucoma, and penetrating eye injuries. • Monitor the patient for histamine release and resulting hypotension and flushing.
Nondepolarizing			
Atracurium	• Adjunct to general anesthesia, to facilitate ET intubation, and to provide skeletal muscle relaxation during surgery or mechanical ventilation	• Flushing, bradycardia • Prolonged dose-related apnea, bronchospasm, laryngospasm • Anaphylaxis	• Drug doesn't affect consciousness or relieve pain. Be sure to keep the patient sedated. Have emergency respiratory support readily available. • Drug has little or no effect on heart rate and doesn't counteract or reverse the bradycardia caused by anesthetics or vagal stimulation. Thus, bradycardia is seen more frequently with atracurium than with other neuromuscular blocking agents. Pretreatment with anticholinergics (atropine or glycopyrrolate) is advised. • Use drug only if ET intubation, administration of oxygen under positive pressure, artificial respiration, and assisted or controlled ventilation are immediately available. • Use a peripheral nerve stimulator to monitor responses during critical care unit administration; it may be used to detect residual paralysis during recovery and to avoid atracurium overdose.
Cisatracurium	• Adjunct to general anesthesia, to facilitate ET intubation, and to provide skeletal muscle relaxation during surgery or mechanical ventilation in the CCU	• Hypotension • Flushing	• Drug isn't compatible with propofol injection or ketorolac injection for Y-site administration. Drug is acidic and also may not be compatible with an alkaline solution having a pH greater than 8.5, such as barbiturate solutions for Y-site administration. Don't

Understanding neuromuscular blocking agents (continued)

Drugs	Indications	Adverse reactions	Practice pointers
Nondepolarizing *(continued)*			
Cisatracurium *(continued)*	• Maintenance of neuro-muscular blockade in the CCU		dilute in lactated Ringer's injection because of chemical instability. • Drug isn't recommended for rapid sequence ET intubation because of its intermediate onset of action. • In patients with neuromuscular disease (myasthenia gravis and myasthenic syndrome), watch for possible prolonged neuromuscular block. • Monitor the patient's acid-base balance and electrolyte levels.
Pancuronium	• Adjunct to anesthesia to induce skeletal muscle relaxation, facilitate intubation and ventilation, and weaken muscle contractions in induced seizures	• Residual muscle weakness • Prolonged, dose-related respiratory insufficiency or apnea • Allergic or idiosyncratic hypersensitivity reactions	• If using succinylcholine, allow its effects to subside before giving pancuronium. • Don't mix in same syringe or give through same needle with barbiturates or other alkaline solutions. • Large doses may increase frequency and severity of tachycardia.
Tubocurarine	• Adjunct to general anesthesia to induce skeletal muscle relaxation, facilitate intubation, and reduce fractures and dislocations • Assistance with mechanical ventilation	• Arrhythmias, cardiac arrest, bradycardia • Respiratory depression or apnea, bronchospasm • Hypersensitivity reactions	• The margin of safety between a therapeutic dose and a dose causing respiratory paralysis is small. • Assess baseline tests of renal function and serum electrolyte levels before drug administration. Electrolyte imbalance, particularly of potassium and magnesium, can potentiate effects of drug.
Vecuronium	• Adjunct to anesthesia, to facilitate intubation, and to provide skeletal muscle relaxation during surgery or mechanical ventilation	• Prolonged, dose-related respiratory insufficiency or apnea	• Administer by rapid I.V. injection or I.V. infusion. Don't give I.M. • Recovery time may double in patients with cirrhosis or cholestasis. • Assess baseline serum electrolyte levels, acid-base balance, and renal and hepatic function before administration.

Understanding sedatives

Use this table to learn about the indications, adverse reactions, and practice pointers associated with sedatives.

Drugs	Indications	Adverse reactions	Practice pointers
Lorazepam	• Anxiety, tension, agitation, irritability, especially in anxiety neuroses or organic (especially GI or cardiovascular) disorders • Status epilepticus	• Drowsiness, sedation • Acute withdrawal syndrome (after sudden discontinuation in physically dependent patients)	• Contraindicated in patients with acute angle-closure glaucoma. • Use cautiously in patients with pulmonary, renal, or hepatic impairment and in elderly, acutely ill, or debilitated patients. • Parenteral lorazepam appears to possess potent amnesic effects. • For I.V. administration, dilute lorazepam with an equal volume of a compatible diluent, such as D_5W, sterile water for injection, or normal saline solution. • Inject the drug directly into a vein or into the tubing of a compatible I.V. infusion, such as normal saline solution or D_5W solution. The rate of lorazepam I.V. injection shouldn't exceed 2 mg/minute. Have emergency resuscitative equipment available when administering I.V. • Monitor liver function studies to prevent cumulative effects and to ensure adequate drug metabolism. • Parenteral administration of drug is more likely to cause apnea, hypotension, bradycardia, and cardiac arrest in elderly patients.
Midazolam	• Preoperative sedation (to induce sleepiness or drowsiness and relieve apprehension) • Conscious sedation • Continuous infusion for sedation of intubated and mechanically ventilated patients as a component of anesthesia or during treatment in a critical care setting • Sedation, anxiolysis, and amnesia before diagnostic, therapeutic, or endoscopic procedures or before induction of anesthesia	• Pain • Cardiac arrest • Nausea • Hiccups • Decreased respiratory rate • Apnea • Respiratory arrest	• Contraindicated in patients with acute angle-closure glaucoma and in those experiencing shock, coma, or acute alcohol intoxication. • Use cautiously in patients with uncompensated acute illnesses, in elderly or debilitated patients, and in patients with myasthenia gravis or neuromuscular disorders and pulmonary disease. • Closely monitor cardiopulmonary function; continuously monitor patients who have received midazolam to detect potentially life-threatening respiratory depression. • Have emergency respiratory equipment readily available. Laryngospasm and bronchospasm, although rare, may occur. • Solutions compatible with midazolam include D_5W, normal saline solution, and lactated Ringer's solution.

Understanding sedatives *(continued)*

Drugs	Indications	Adverse reactions	Practice pointers
Propofol	• Induction and maintenance of sedation in mechanically ventilated patients	• Hypotension • Bradycardia • Hyperlipidemia • Apnea	• Contraindicated in patients hypersensitive to propofol or components of the emulsion, including soybean oil, egg lecithin, and glycerol. Because drug is administered as an emulsion, administer cautiously to patients with a disorder of lipid metabolism (such as pancreatitis, primary hyperlipoproteinemia, and diabetic hyperlipidemia). Use cautiously if the patient is receiving lipids as part of a total parenteral nutrition infusion; I.V. lipid dose may need to be reduced. Use cautiously in elderly or debilitated patients and in those with circulatory disorders. • Although the hemodynamic effects of drug can vary, its major effect in patients maintaining spontaneous ventilation is arterial hypotension (arterial pressure can decrease as much as 30%) with little or no change in heart rate and cardiac output. However, significant depression of cardiac output may occur in patients undergoing assisted or controlled positive pressure ventilation. • Don't mix propofol with other drugs or blood products. If it's to be diluted before infusion, use only D_5W and don't dilute to a concentration of less than 2 mg/ml. After dilution, drug appears to be more stable in glass containers than in plastic.

The tracheostomy tube may be made of plastic, polyvinyl chloride, or metal and comes in various sizes, lengths, and styles depending on the patient's needs. A patient receiving mechanical ventilation needs a cuffed tube to prevent backflow of air around the tube. A cuffed tracheostomy tube also prevents an unconscious or a paralyzed patient from aspirating food or secretions.

Emergency or planned procedure

In emergency situations, such as laryngeal edema with anaphylactic shock or foreign body obstruction, tracheotomy may be done at the bedside. More commonly, it's a planned procedure that's done in an operating room when a patient is likely to need prolonged mechanical ventilation.

Nursing considerations

- Before an emergency tracheotomy, briefly explain the procedure to the patient as time permits and quickly obtain supplies or a tracheotomy tray.
- Before a scheduled tracheotomy, explain the procedure and the need for anesthesia to the patient and his family. If possible, mention whether the tracheostomy is permanent or temporary. Tell them the patient is monitored in the critical care unit before and after the procedure.
- Ensure that samples for ABG analysis and other diagnostic tests have been collected and that the patient or a responsible family member has signed a consent form.

Afterward ward

- After the procedure, assess the patient's respiratory status, breath sounds, oxygen saturation level, vital signs, and heart rhythm. Note any crackles, rhonchi, wheezes, or diminished breath sounds.
- Assess the patient for complications that can occur within the first 48 hours after tracheostomy tube insertion, including hemorrhage, edema into tracheal tissue causing airway obstruction, aspiration of secretions, hypoxemia, and introduction of air into surrounding tissue causing subcutaneous emphysema.
- Keep appropriate equipment at the bedside for immediate use in an emergency. (See *Emergency tracheostomy equipment.*)
- Perform tracheostomy care at least every 8 hours or as needed. Change the dressing as often as needed because a wet dressing with exudate or secretions predisposes the patient to skin excoriation, breakdown, and infection.

> In an emergency, tracheotomy may be performed at the patient's bedside rather than in an operating room.

EMERGENCY

Advice from the experts

Emergency tracheostomy equipment

Make sure you keep emergency tracheostomy equipment at the patient's bedside, including:
- sterile tracheal dilator or sterile hemostat
- sterile obturator that fits the tracheostomy tube
- extra sterile tracheostomy tube and obturator in the appropriate size
- suction equipment and supplies.

Keep the emergency equipment in full view in the patient's room at all times for easy access in case of emergency. Consider taping a wrapped, sterile tracheostomy tube to the head of the bed for easy access. If your patient coughs or pulls the tracheostomy tube out, you may use a sterile tracheal dilator to keep the stoma open and the airway patent until a new tube can be inserted.

Deflating and inflating a tracheostomy cuff

During tracheostomy care, you may need to deflate and inflate a tracheostomy cuff. If so, gather a 5-ml or 10-ml syringe, padded hemostat, and stethoscope and follow these steps:

1. Read the cuff manufacturer's instructions because cuff types and procedures vary.

2. Assess the patient's condition, explain the procedure to him, and reassure him. Wash your hands thoroughly.

3. Help the patient into semi-Fowler's position if possible, or place him in a supine position so secretions above the cuff site will be pushed up into his mouth if he's receiving positive-pressure ventilation.

4. Suction the oropharyngeal cavity to prevent pooled secretions from descending into the trachea after cuff deflation.

5. Release the padded hemostat clamping the cuff inflation tubing, if a hemostat is present.

6. Insert a 5-ml or 10-ml syringe into the cuff pilot balloon and very slowly withdraw all air from the cuff. Leave the syringe attached to the tubing for later reinflation of the cuff.

7. Remove any ventilation device. Suction the lower airway through any existing tube to remove all secretions, and then reconnect the patient to the ventilation device.

8. Maintain cuff deflation for the prescribed time. Observe the patient for adequate ventilation, and suction as necessary. If the patient has difficulty breathing, reinflate the cuff immediately by depressing the syringe plunger very slowly. Use a stethoscope to listen over the trachea for the air leak, then inject the least amount of air needed to achieve an adequate tracheal seal.

9. When inflating the cuff, you may use the minimal-leak technique or the minimal occlusive-volume technique to help gauge the proper inflation point.

10. If you're inflating the cuff using cuff pressure measurement, be careful not to exceed 25 mm Hg.

11. After you've inflated the cuff, if the tubing doesn't have a one-way valve at the end, clamp the inflation line with a padded hemostat (to protect the tubing) and remove the syringe.

12. Check for a minimal-leak cuff seal. You shouldn't feel air coming from the patient's mouth, nose, or tracheostomy site, and a conscious patient shouldn't be able to speak. Be alert for air leaks from the cuff itself.

13. Note the exact amount of air used to inflate the cuff to detect tracheal malacia if more air is consistently needed.

14. Make sure the patient is comfortable and can easily reach the call bell and communication aids.

15. Properly clean or dispose of equipment, supplies, and trash according to your facility's policy. Replenish used supplies and make sure necessary emergency supplies are at the bedside.

To avoid dislodging the tube, don't change your patient's tracheostomy ties unnecessarily.

CAUTION!

• Don't change the tracheostomy ties unnecessarily during the immediate postoperative period (usually 4 days) to avoid accidentally dislodging the tube.

• Document the procedure, the amount, color, and consistency of secretions, stoma and skin conditions, the patient's respiratory status, the duration of any cuff deflation, and cuff pressure readings with inflation. (See *Deflating and inflating a tracheostomy cuff.*)

Chest tube insertion

Chest tube insertion may be needed when treating patients with pneumothorax, hemothorax, empyema, pleural effusion, or chylothorax. The tube, which is inserted into the pleural space, allows blood, fluid, pus, or air to drain and allows the lung to reinflate.

Gotta have some negative pressure

The tube restores negative pressure to the pleural space through an underwater-seal drainage system. The water in the system prevents air from being sucked back into the pleural space during inspiration. If a leak occurs through the bronchi and can't be sealed, suction applied to the underwater-seal system removes air from the pleural space faster than it can collect.

Put a valve on it

A one-way flutter valve, such as the Heimlich valve, is sometimes used instead of an underwater-seal drainage system. The one-way valve is connected to the end of the chest tube and allows accumulated air to escape, but not enter. This type of valve allows portability for patients who need long-term chest tube placement.

Nursing considerations

• Assess respiratory function and obtain vital signs and oxygen saturation levels immediately after insertion. Routinely assess chest tube function. Describe and record the amount of drainage at least every 8 hours. Notify the doctor immediately if the amount of drainage is greater than 200 ml in 1 hour (indicates bleeding).
• The fluid in the water-seal chamber typically rises on inspiration and decreases on expiration. If the patient is receiving positive-pressure ventilation, the opposite is normal.
• Avoid creating dependent loops, kinks, or pressure in the tubing. Don't lift the drainage system above the patient's chest because fluid may flow back into the pleural space. Keep two rubber-tipped clamps at the bedside to clamp the chest tube if the system cracks, or to locate an air leak in the system. (See *Checking for chest tube leaks.*)
• If the drainage collection chamber fills, replace it according to your facility's policy. To do so, double-clamp the chest tube close to the insertion site (using two clamps facing in opposite directions), exchange the system, remove the clamps, and retape the connection.
• To prevent a tension pneumothorax (which can occur when clamping stops air and fluid from escaping), never leave the chest tube clamped for more than 1 minute.

Checking for chest tube leaks

When trying to locate a leak in your patient's chest tube system, try:
• briefly clamping the tube at various points along its length, beginning at the tube's proximal end and working down toward the drainage system
• paying special attention to the seal around the connections
• pushing any loose connections back together and taping them securely.

Bubble may mean trouble

The bubbling of the system stops when a clamp is placed between an air leak and the water seal. If you clamp along the tube's entire length and the bubbling doesn't stop, you probably need to replace the drainage unit because it may be cracked.

• Notify the doctor immediately if the patient develops cyanosis, rapid or shallow breathing, subcutaneous emphysema, chest pain, or excessive bleeding.

Thoracotomy

Thoracotomy is usually used to remove part or all of a lung.

Thoracotomy, a surgical incision into the thoracic cavity, is done to locate and examine abnormalities, such as tumors, bleeding sites, or thoracic injuries; to perform a biopsy; or to remove diseased lung tissue. It's most commonly used to remove part or all of a lung to spare healthy lung tissue from disease.

Lung excisions

Types of lung excisions include pneumonectomy, lobectomy, segmental resection, and wedge resection:

Bye-bye lung

A *pneumonectomy* is the excision of an entire lung. It's usually performed to treat patients with bronchogenic cancer, but may be used to treat those with TB, bronchiectasis, or lung abscess. Pneumonectomy is used only when a less radical approach would fail to remove all diseased tissue. After pneumonectomy, chest cavity pressures stabilize and, over time, fluid fills the cavity where lung tissue was removed, preventing significant mediastinal shift.

One out of five lobes

A *lobectomy* is the removal of one of the five lung lobes. It's used to treat patients with bronchogenic cancer, TB, lung abscess, emphysematous blebs, benign tumors, or localized fungal infections. After this surgery, the remaining lobes expand to fill the entire pleural cavity.

How do you like your resection?

A *segmental resection* is the removal of one or more lung segments. This procedure preserves more functional tissue than lobectomy; it's commonly used to treat patients with bronchiectasis.

A *wedge resection* is removal of a small portion of the lung without regard to segments. It preserves the most functional tissue of all the surgeries but is used only when the patient has a small, well-circumscribed lesion. Remaining lung tissue should be reexpanded.

Other thoracic surgeries

Here are some other types of thoracic surgeries:
• Exploratory thoracotomy is used to examine the chest and pleural space in evaluating chest trauma and tumors.

- Decortication is used to help reexpand the lung in a patient with empyema. It involves removing or stripping the thick, fibrous membrane covering the visceral pleura.
- Thoracoplasty is performed to remove part or all of one rib and to reduce the size of the chest cavity. It decreases the risk of mediastinal shift when TB has reduced lung volume.
- Bronchoplastic (sleeve) reduction involves the excision of one lobar bronchus along with part of the right or left bronchus. The distal bronchus is then reanastomosed to the proximal bronchus or trachea.
- Lung reduction surgery is used to treat patients with emphysema. Giant bullae are excised, thereby reducing lung volume and allowing compressed alveoli to reexpand.
- Video-assisted thoracic surgery is a minimally invasive technique used to treat patients with some pulmonary conditions, perform open lung biopsies, and to stage and diagnose some lung cancers.

Nursing considerations

- Explain the procedure to the patient and his family. Tell them that, after surgery, the patient may have a chest tube and oxygen delivery system in place.
- After thoracic surgery, assess vital signs, oxygen saturation levels, breath sounds, and cardiopulmonary and hemodynamic status. Monitor for cardiac arrhythmias. Atrial arrhythmias, especially atrial fibrillation, commonly occur after pneumonectomy due to pulmonary vasculature blood flow changes and atrial enlargement; patients may be treated prophylactically with cardiac glycosides.
- Monitor the chest tube insertion site and assess and record the amount and characteristics of drainage. Suction isn't used after a pneumonectomy and the chest tube is attached to gravity drainage only.
- If the patient underwent a pneumonectomy, position him only on his operative side or his back until stabilized. This prevents fluid from draining into the unaffected lung if the sutured bronchus opens.
- Monitor for complications of thoracotomy, including hemorrhage, infection, tension pneumothorax, bronchopleural fistula, and empyema.

Lung transplantation

Lung transplantation involves the replacement of one or both lungs with that from a donor. Cystic fibrosis is the most common underlying disease that necessitates lung transplantation; others

In thoracoplasty, part or all of a rib is removed to reduce the size of the chest cavity.

include bronchopulmonary dysplasia, pulmonary hypertension, and pulmonary fibrosis.

In some cases, only one lobe may be involved in transplantation. Single lung transplantation is considered for patients with end-stage COPD. Typically, the patient has a life expectancy of less than 2 years. One-year survival rates after transplantation range from 75% to 85%, decreasing to 50% after 5 years.

Must-haves

To be a candidate for lung transplantation, a patient must:
- have forced vital capacity less than 40%
- have forced expiratory volume (FEV_1) less than 30% of predicted value
- have PaO_2 less than 60 mm Hg on room air at rest
- exhibit evidence of major pulmonary complications
- demonstrate increased antibiotic resistance.

Not gonna happen

Lung transplantation is absolutely contraindicated in cases of:
- major organ dysfunction, especially involving the renal or cardiovascular system
- human immunodeficiency virus infection
- active malignancy
- hepatitis C with positive biopsy for liver damage
- progressive neuromuscular disease.
    Relative contraindications include symptomatic osteoporosis.

Cardiopulmonary bypass is common during lung transplantation.

TKO for transplant

Lung transplantation is performed under general anesthesia. Bilateral anterior thoracotomy incisions and a transverse sternotomy provide access to the thoracic cavity. After removal of the patient's lungs, the donor lungs are implanted with anastomoses to the patient's bronchus.

Cardiopulmonary bypass is commonly used during the transplantation procedure.

Complications

The major complication after lung transplantation is organ rejection, which occurs because the recipient's body responds to the implanted tissue as a foreign body and triggers an immune response. This leads to fibrosis and scar formation.

Secondary snags

Another major complication after lung transplantation is infection due to immunosuppressive therapy.

Other possible complications include hemorrhage and reperfusion edema. Long-term complications (typically occurring after 3 years) include obliterative bronchiolitis and posttransplant lymphoproliferative disorder. Either may be fatal.

Nursing considerations

Provide care before and after transplantation.

Educate and administer

- Answer all questions about the transplantation and what the patient can expect. Explain postoperative care (intubation, for example), equipment used in the acute postoperative phase, and availability of analgesics for pain.
- Administer medications and obtain laboratory testing as ordered.

Keep on assessing

- Assess cardiopulmonary status frequently (every 5 to 15 minutes in the immediate postoperative period) until the patient is stabilized. Be alert for cardiac index less than 2.2, hypotension, fever higher than 99.5° F (37.5° C), crackles or rhonchi, and decreased oxygen saturation.
- Assess respiratory status and ventilatory equipment frequently and suction secretions as necessary. Expect frequent ABG analyses and daily chest X-rays to evaluate the patient's readiness to wean from the ventilator.
- Assess chest tube drainage for amount, color, and characteristics. Assess for bleeding. Notify the doctor according to the hospital's and surgeon's parameters for normal drainage.
- Closely monitor fluid intake and output. If the patient becomes hemodynamically unstable, administer vasoactive and inotropic agents as ordered and titrate the dose to achieve the desired response.
- After extubation, assess the patient often for shortness of breath, tachypnea, dyspnea, malaise, and increased sputum production; these suggest acute rejection.
- After a single-lung transplantation, the newly implanted lung is denervated, but the patient's remaining lung continues to send messages to the brain indicating poor oxygenation. The patient may complain of shortness of breath and dyspnea even with oxygen saturation levels greater than 90%.
- Maintain strict infection control precautions such as meticulous hand washing.
- Inspect surgical dressings for bleeding in the early postoperative phase. Inspect the surgical incisions later for redness, swelling, and other signs of infection.

Check the patient's ABG levels and chest X-rays daily to decide whether he can be weaned from the ventilator.

After a single-lung transplantation, the remaining lung tells me it's oxygen-starved, even though oxygen saturation is over 90%.

Inhalation therapy

Inhalation therapy involves carefully controlled ventilation techniques to help the patient maintain optimal ventilation in case of respiratory failure. Techniques include ET intubation and mechanical ventilation. Proper weaning from ventilation techniques is also a part of inhalation therapy.

ET intubation

ET intubation involves insertion of a tube into the trachea through the mouth or nose to establish a patent airway. It protects patients from aspiration by sealing off the trachea from the digestive tract and permits removal of tracheobronchial secretions in patients who can't cough effectively. ET intubation also provides a route for mechanical ventilation.

Too good to be true?

Drawbacks of ET intubation are that it bypasses normal respiratory defenses against infection, reduces cough effectiveness, may be uncomfortable, and prevents verbal communication.

Potential complications of ET intubation include:
• bronchospasm or laryngospasm
• aspiration of blood, secretions, or gastric contents
• tooth damage or loss
• injury to the lips, mouth, pharynx, or vocal cords
• hypoxemia (if attempts at intubation are prolonged or oxygen delivery interrupted)
• tracheal stenosis, erosion, and necrosis
• cardiac arrhythmias.

Orotracheal intubation

In orotracheal intubation, the oral cavity is used as the route of insertion. It's preferred in emergency situations because it's easier and faster. However, maintaining exact tube placement is more difficult because the tube must be well secured to avoid kinking and prevent bronchial obstruction or accidental extubation. It's also uncomfortable for conscious patients because it stimulates salivation, coughing, and retching.

The right size

The typical size for an oral ET tube is 7.5 mm (indicates the size of the lumen) for women and 8 mm for men.

ET intubation bypasses normal respiratory defenses against infection. That's good news for me, but bad news for the patient!

Not for everyone

Orotracheal intubation is contraindicated in patients with orofacial injuries, acute cervical spinal injury, and degenerative spinal disorders.

Nasal intubation

In nasal intubation, a nasal passage is used as the route of insertion. Nasal intubation is preferred for elective insertion when the patient is capable of spontaneous ventilation for a short period.

A conscious choice

Nasal intubation is more comfortable than oral intubation and is typically used in conscious patients who are at risk for imminent respiratory arrest or who have cervical spinal injuries. It's contraindicated in patients with facial or basilar skull fractures.

Difficult and damaging

Although it's more comfortable than oral intubation, nasal intubation is more difficult to perform. Because the tube passes blindly through the nasal cavity, it causes more tissue damage, increases the risk of infection by nasal bacteria introduced into the trachea, and increases the risk of pressure necrosis of the nasal mucosa.

Nursing considerations

• After securing the ET tube, reconfirm tube placement by noting bilateral breath sounds and ETco$_2$ readings. (See *Securing an ET tube.*)
• Auscultate breath sounds and watch for chest movement to ensure correct tube placement and full lung ventilation.
• A chest X-ray may be ordered to confirm tube placement.
• Disposable ETco$_2$ detectors are commonly used to confirm tube placement in emergency departments, postanesthesia care units, and critical care units that don't use continual ETco$_2$ monitoring. Follow the manufacturer's instructions for proper use of the device. Don't use the detector with a heated humidifier or nebulizer because humidity, heat, and moisture can interfere with the device. (See *Analyzing carbon dioxide levels,* page 342.)
• Follow standard precautions, and suction through the ET tube as the patient's condition indicates, to clear secretions and prevent mucus plugs from obstructing the tube. After suctioning, hyperoxygenate the patient being maintained on a ventilator with the handheld resuscitation bag. If available, use a closed tracheal suctioning system, which permits the ventilated patient to remain on the ventilator during suctioning. (See *Closed tracheal suctioning,* page 343.)

Nasal intubation is preferred when the patient can breathe spontaneously for a short period.

On the downside, nasal intubation is more difficult to do than oral intubation and causes more tissue damage.

Securing an ET tube

When securing an endotracheal (ET) tube, use either tape or ties and make sure the tube is immobile.

When you're using tape
• Tear about 2′ (60 cm) of tape, split both ends in half about 4″ (10 cm), and place the tape adhesive-side up on a flat surface.
• Tear another piece of tape about 10″ (25 cm) long and place it adhesive-side down in the center of the 2′ piece.
• Slide the tape under the patient's neck and center it.
• Bring the right side of the tape up and wrap the top split end counter-clockwise around the tube; secure the bottom split end beneath the patient's lower lip.
• Bring the left side of the tape up and wrap the bottom split piece clockwise around the tube; secure the top split above the patient's upper lip.

When you're using ties
• Cut about 2′ of a tracheostomy tie and place it under the patient's neck.
• Bring both ends up to the tube and cross them at the bottom of the tube near the patient's lips.
• Bring the ends to the top of the tube and tie them in an overhand knot.
• Bring the ends back to the bottom of the tube, tie another overhand knot, and then secure the ties with a square knot (right over left and then left over right).

Mechanical ventilation

Mechanical ventilation involves the use of a machine to move air into a patient's lungs. Mechanical ventilators use either positive or negative pressure to ventilate patients.

When to ventilate

Indications for mechanical ventilation include:
• acute respiratory failure due to ARDS, pneumonia, acute exacerbations of COPD, pulmonary embolism, heart failure, trauma, tumors, or drug overdose
• respiratory center depression due to stroke, brain injury, or trauma
• neuromuscular disturbances caused by neuromuscular diseases, such as Guillain-Barré syndrome, multiple sclerosis, and myasthenia gravis; trauma, including spinal cord injury; or CNS depression.

Accentuate the positive

Positive pressure ventilators exert a positive pressure on the airway, which causes inspiration while increasing tidal volume (V_T).

Mechanical ventilation uses a machine to move air into my lungs.

Analyzing carbon dioxide levels

Depending on which end-tidal carbon dioxide ($ETCO_2$) detector you use, the meaning of color changes within the detector dome may differ. Here's a description of one type of detector, the Easy Cap detector, and what color changes mean:

• The rim of the Easy Cap is divided into four segments (clockwise from the top): CHECK, A, B, and C. The CHECK segment is solid purple, signifying the absence of carbon dioxide.

• The numbers in the other sections range from 0.03 to 5, indicating the percentage of exhaled carbon dioxide. The color should fluctuate during ventilation from purple (section A) during inspiration to yellow (section C) at the end of expiration. This indicates that the $ETCO_2$ levels are adequate (above 2%).

• An end-expiratory color change from C to the B range may be the first sign of hemodynamic instability.

• During cardiopulmonary resuscitation (CPR), an end-expiratory color change from the A or B range to the C range may mean the return of spontaneous ventilation.

• During prolonged cardiac arrest, inadequate pulmonary perfusion leads to inadequate gas exchange. The patient exhales little or no carbon dioxide, so the color stays in the purple range even with proper intubation. Ineffective CPR also leads to inadequate pulmonary perfusion.

Color indications on detector dome

A high-frequency ventilator uses high respiratory rates and low V_T to maintain alveolar ventilation.

The inspiratory cycles of these ventilators may be adjusted for volume, pressure, or time:

• A volume-cycled ventilator, the type used most commonly, delivers a preset volume of air each time, regardless of the amount of lung resistance.

• A pressure-cycled ventilator generates flow until the machine reaches a preset pressure, regardless of the volume delivered or the time required to achieve the pressure.

Closed tracheal suctioning

The closed tracheal suction system can ease removal of secretions and reduce patient complications. The system consists of a sterile suction catheter in a clear plastic sleeve. It permits the patient to remain connected to the ventilator during suctioning.

Catheter sleeve

T-piece

Suction catheter

As a result, the patient can maintain the tidal volume, oxygen concentration, and positive end-expiratory pressure delivered by the ventilator while being suctioned. In turn, this reduces the occurrence of suction-induced hypoxemia.

Another advantage of this system is a reduced risk of infection, even when the same catheter is used many times. The caregiver doesn't need to touch the catheter and the ventilator circuit remains closed.

Performing the procedure

To perform the procedure, gather a closed suction control valve, a T-piece to connect the artificial airway to the ventilator breathing circuit, and a catheter sleeve that encloses the catheter and has connections at each end for the control valve and the T-piece. Then follow these steps:
• Remove the closed suction system from its wrapping. Attach the control valve to the connecting tubing.
• Depress the thumb suction control valve, and keep it depressed while setting the suction pressure to the desired level.
• Connect the T-piece to the ventilator breathing circuit, making sure that the irrigation port is closed; then connect the T-piece to the patient's endotracheal or tracheostomy tube (as shown above right).
• With one hand keeping the T-piece parallel to the patient's chin, use the thumb and index finger of the other hand to ad-

vance the catheter through the tube and into the patient's tracheobronchial tree (as shown below).

• If necessary, gently retract the catheter sleeve as you advance the catheter.
• While continuing to hold the T-piece and control valve, apply intermittent suction and withdraw the catheter until it reaches its fully extended length in the sleeve. Repeat the procedure as necessary.
• After you finish suctioning, flush the catheter by maintaining suction while slowly introducing normal saline solution or sterile water into the irrigation port.
• Place the thumb control valve in the off position.
• Dispose of and replace the suction equipment and supplies according to your facility's policy.
• Change the closed suction system every 24 hours to minimize the risk of infection.

Ventilator modes

Positive pressure ventilators are categorized as volume or pressure ventilators and have various modes and options.

Volume modes

Volume modes include controlled ventilation (CV) or controlled mandatory ventilation (CMV), assist-control (A/C) or assisted mandatory ventilation (AMV), and intermittent mandatory ventilation (IMV) and synchronized intermittent mandatory ventilation (SIMV).

CV or CMV

In the CV or CMV mode, the ventilator supplies all ventilation for the patient. The respiratory rate, tidal volume (V_T), inspiratory time, and positive end expiratory pressure (PEEP) are preset. This mode is usually used when a patient can't initiate spontaneous breaths, such as when he's paralyzed from a spinal cord injury or neuromuscular disease, or chemically paralyzed with neuromuscular blocking agents.

A/C or AMV

In the A/C or AMV mode, the basic respiratory rate is set along with the V_T, inspiratory time, and PEEP, but the patient is allowed to breathe faster than the preset rate. The sensitivity is set so that when the patient initiates a spontaneous breath, a full V_T is delivered, so that all breaths are the same V_T, whether triggered by the patient or delivered at the set rate. If the patient tires and his drive to breathe is negated, the ventilator continues to deliver breaths at the preset rate.

IMV or SIMV

IMV and SIMV modes require preset respiratory rate, V_T, inspiratory time, sensitivity, and PEEP. Mandatory breaths are delivered at a set rate and V_T. In between the mandatory breaths, the patient can breathe spontaneously at his own rate and V_T. The V_T of these spontaneous breaths can vary because the breaths are determined by the patient's ability to generate negative pressure in his chest. With SIMV, the ventilator synchronizes the mandatory breaths with the patient's own inspirations.

Pressure modes

Pressure modes include pressure support ventilation (PSV), pressure controlled ventilation (PCV), and pressure-controlled/inverse ratio ventilation (PC/IRV).

PSV

The PSV mode augments inspiration for a spontaneously breathing patient. The inspiratory pressure level, PEEP, and sensitivity are preset. When the patient initiates a breath, the breath is delivered at the preset pressure level and is maintained throughout inspiration. The patient determines the V_T, respiratory rate, and inspiratory time.

PCV

In PCV mode, inspiratory pressure, inspiratory time, respiratory rate, and PEEP are preset. V_T varies with the patient's airway pressure and compliance.

PC/IVR

PC/IVR combines pressure-limited ventilation with an inverse ratio of inspiration to expiration. In this mode, the inspiratory pressure, respiratory rate, inspiratory time (1:1, 2:1, 3:1, or 4:1), and PEEP are preset. PCV and PC/IRV modes may be used in patients with acute respiratory distress syndrome.

• A time-cycled ventilator generates flow for a preset amount of time.

Several different modes of ventilatory control are found on the ventilator. The choice of mode depends on the patient's respiratory condition. (See *Ventilator modes*.)

Out goes the thorax, in flows the air

Negative-pressure ventilators work by creating negative pressure, which pulls the thorax outward and allows air to flow into the lungs. They're used primarily to treat patients with neuromuscular disorders. Examples of such ventilators include the iron lung, the cuirass (chest shell), and the body wrap.

Nursing considerations

• Provide emotional support to the patient during all phases of mechanical ventilation to reduce anxiety and promote successful treatment. Even if the patient is unresponsive, continue to explain all procedures and treatments.

Be alarmed

• Make sure the ventilator alarms are on at all times to alert you to potentially hazardous conditions and changes in the patient's status. If an alarm sounds and the problem can't be easily identified, disconnect the patient from the ventilator and use a handheld resuscitation bag to ventilate him. (See *Responding to ventilator alarms*, page 346.)
• Assess cardiopulmonary status frequently, at least every 2 to 4 hours or more often, if indicated. Assess vital signs and auscultate breath sounds. Monitor pulse oximetry or $ETco_2$ levels and hemodynamic parameters as ordered. Monitor intake and output and assess for fluid volume excess or dehydration.
• Unless contraindicated, turn the patient from side to side every 1 to 2 hours to aid lung expansion and removal of secretions. Perform active or passive range-of-motion (ROM) exercises for all extremities to reduce the hazards of immobility.
• Place the call bell within the patient's reach and establish a method of communication (such as a communication board) because intubation and mechanical ventilation impair the patient's ability to speak.
• Administer a sedative or neuromuscular blocking agent, as ordered, to relax the patient or eliminate spontaneous breathing efforts that can interfere with the ventilator's action.

Be extra vigilant

• Remember that the patient receiving a neuromuscular blocking agent requires close observation because he can't breathe or communicate. In addition, if the patient is receiving a neuromuscular blocking agent, make sure he also receives a sedative. Neuromuscular blocking agents cause paralysis without altering the patient's LOC. Reassure the patient and his family that the paralysis is temporary. Provide routine eye care and instill artificial tears because the patient can't blink.
• Make sure emergency equipment is readily available in case the ventilator malfunctions or the patient is extubated accidentally. If there's a problem with the ventilator, disconnect the patient from the ventilator and manually ventilate with 100% oxygen; use a

Negative-pressure ventilators include the iron lung, the cuirass, and the body wrap.

Pay attention! Your patient receiving a neuromuscular blocking agent requires close observation because of his inability to breathe or communicate.

Responding to ventilator alarms

This chart outlines the possible causes and the nursing interventions needed if a ventilator alarm sounds.

Signal	Possible cause	Interventions
Low-pressure alarm	• Tube disconnected from ventilator • Endotracheal (ET) tube displaced above vocal cords or tracheostomy tube extubated • Leaking tidal volume from low cuff pressure (from an underinflated or ruptured cuff or a leak in the cuff or one-way valve) • Ventilator malfunction • Leak in ventilator circuitry (from loose connection or hole in tubing, loss of temperature-sensitive device, or cracked humidification jar)	• Reconnect the tube to the ventilator. • Check the tube placement and reposition, if needed. If extubation or displacement has occurred, ventilate the patient manually and call the doctor immediately. • Listen for a whooshing sound around the tube, indicating an air leak. If you hear one, check the cuff pressure. If you can't maintain pressure, call the doctor; he may need to insert a new tube. • Disconnect the patient from the ventilator and ventilate him manually, if necessary. Obtain another ventilator. • Make sure all connections are intact. Check for holes or leaks in the tubing and replace, if necessary. Check the humidification jar and replace, if cracked.
High-pressure alarm	• Increased airway pressure or decreased lung compliance caused by worsening disease • Patient biting on oral ET tube • Secretions in airway • Condensate in large-bore tubing • Intubation of right mainstem bronchus • Patient coughing, gagging, or attempting to talk • Chest wall resistance • Failure of high-pressure relief valve • Bronchospasm	• Auscultate the lungs for evidence of increasing lung consolidation, barotrauma, or wheezing. Call the doctor if indicated. • Insert a bite block if needed. • Look for secretions in the airway. To remove them, suction the patient or have him cough. • Check tubing for condensate and remove any fluid. • Check tube position. If it has slipped, call the doctor, who may need to reposition it. • If the patient fights the ventilator, the doctor may order a sedative or neuromuscular blocking agent. • Reposition the patient to see if doing so improves chest expansion. If repositioning doesn't help, administer the prescribed analgesic. • Have the faulty equipment replaced. • Assess the patient for the cause. Report to the doctor and treat the patient, as ordered.

handheld resuscitation bag connected to the ET or tracheostomy tube, troubleshoot the ventilator, and correct the problem. If you can't determine the cause, call for help and have the respiratory therapist evaluate the problem. (See *Understanding manual ventilation.*)

Understanding manual ventilation

A handheld resuscitation bag is an inflatable device that can be attached to a face mask or directly to a tracheostomy or an endotracheal (ET) tube to allow manual delivery of oxygen or room air to the lungs of a patient who can't breathe by himself.

Although usually used in an emergency, manual ventilation can also be performed while the patient is disconnected temporarily from a mechanical ventilator, such as during a tubing change, during transport, or before suctioning. In such instances, the use of the handheld resuscitation bag maintains ventilation. Oxygen administration with a resuscitation bag can help improve a compromised cardiorespiratory system.

Ventilation guidelines

To manually ventilate a patient with an ET or tracheostomy tube, follow these guidelines:
• If oxygen is readily available, connect the handheld resuscitation bag to the oxygen. Attach one end of the tubing to the bottom of the bag and the other end to the nipple adapter on the flowmeter of the oxygen source.
• Turn on the oxygen and adjust the flow rate according to the patient's condition.
• Before attaching the handheld resuscitation bag, suction the ET or tracheostomy tube to remove any secretions that may obstruct the airway.
• Remove the mask from the ventilation bag and attach the handheld resuscitation bag directly to the tube.
• Keeping your nondominant hand on the connection of the bag to the tube, exert downward pressure to seal the mask against his face. For an adult patient, use your dominant hand to compress the bag every 5 seconds to deliver approximately 1 L of air.

• Deliver breaths with the patient's own inspiratory effort if any is present. Don't attempt to deliver a breath as the patient exhales.

• Observe the patient's chest to ensure that it rises and falls with each compression. If ventilation fails to occur, check the connection and the patency of the patient's airway; if necessary, reposition his head and suction.
• Be alert for possible underventilation, which commonly occurs because the handheld resuscitation bag is difficult to keep positioned while ensuring an open airway. In addition, the volume of air delivered to the patient varies with the type of bag used and the hand size of the person compressing the bag. An adult with a small- or medium-sized hand may not consistently deliver 1 L of air. For these reasons, have someone assist with the procedure if possible.
• Keep in mind that air is forced into the patient's stomach with manual ventilation, placing the patient at risk for aspiration of vomitus (possibly resulting in pneumonia) and gastric distention.
• Record the date and time of the procedure, reason and length of time the patient was disconnected from mechanical ventilation and received manual ventilation, any complications and the nursing action taken, and the patient's tolerance of the procedure.

Weaning

The patient's body quickly comes to depend on artificial ventilation and must gradually be reintroduced to normal breathing.

Spontaneous strength

Successful weaning depends on a strong spontaneous respiratory effort, a stable cardiovascular system, sufficient respiratory muscle strength and LOC to sustain spontaneous breathing. Certain criteria must be met before weaning can begin. (See *Criteria for weaning.*)

Weaning methods

Several weaning methods are used:
• In *intermittent mandatory ventilation* (IMV), the number of breaths produced by the ventilator is gradually reduced, allowing the patient to breathe independently. Decreasing the number of breaths allows the patient to gradually increase his respiratory muscle strength and endurance.
• *Pressure support ventilation* (PSV) may be used alone or as an adjunct to IMV in the weaning process. In this procedure, a set burst of pressure is applied during inspiration with the patient's normal breathing pattern, allowing the patient to build respiratory muscle strength.

Criteria for weaning

Successful weaning from a ventilator depends on the patient's ability to breathe independently. This means the patient must have a spontaneous respiratory effort that can maintain ventilation, a stable cardiovascular system, and sufficient respiratory muscle strength and level of consciousness to sustain spontaneous breathing.

Pulmonary function criteria

Pulmonary function criteria include:
• minute ventilation less than or equal to 10 L/minute, indicating that the patient is breathing at a stable rate with adequate tidal volume
• negative inspiratory force greater than or equal to –20 cm H_2O, indicating the patient's ability to initiate respirations independently
• maximum voluntary ventilation greater than or equal to twice the resting minute volume, indicating the patient's ability to sustain maximal respiratory effort
• tidal volume of 5 to 10 ml/kg, indicating the patient's ability to ventilate lungs adequately
• partial pressure of arterial oxygen (PaO_2) greater than or equal to 60 mm Hg (if the patient has chronic lung disease, 50 mm Hg or the ability to maintain baseline levels)
• partial pressure of arterial carbon dioxide ($PaCO_2$) less than or equal to 45 mm Hg (or normal for the patient)

• arterial pH ranging from 7.35 to 7.45 (or normal for the patient)
• fractional concentration of inspired oxygen less than or equal to 0.4.

Other criteria

Other criteria include:
• adequate natural airway or functioning tracheostomy
• ability to cough and mobilize secretions
• successful withdrawal of any neuromuscular blocker such as pancuronium bromide or vecuronium
• clear or clearing chest X-ray
• absence of infection, acid-base or electrolyte imbalance, hyperglycemia, arrhythmia, renal failure, anemia, fever, or excessive fatigue.

After weaning

After being weaned, the patient should ultimately demonstrate:
• respiratory rate less than 24 breaths/minute
• heart rate and blood pressure within 15% of his baseline
• tidal volume of at least 3 to 5 ml/kg
• arterial pH greater than 7.35
• PaO_2 maintained at greater than 60 mm Hg
• $PaCO_2$ maintained at less then 45 mm Hg
• oxygen saturation maintained at greater than 90%
• absence of cardiac arrhythmias
• absence of accessory muscle use.

• *Spontaneous breathing trials* are the next step in weaning. In this procedure, a T-piece is attached to the end of the ET tube or a trach collar is attached to the tracheostomy tube. The ventilator is then disconnected and the patient is allowed to breathe on his own through the ET or tracheostomy tube. The amount of time spent off the ventilator is initially short, 1 to 2 minutes, then gradually increased as the patient can tolerate it.

Nursing considerations

• When weaning the patient, continue to observe for respiratory distress, fatigue, hypoxemia or cardiac arrhythmias.
• Schedule weaning to comfortably and realistically fit into the patient's daily regimen, avoiding weaning during such times as meals, baths, or lengthy therapeutic procedures.
• Document the length of the weaning trial and the patient's toleration of the procedure.
• After the patient is successfully weaned and extubated, place him on the appropriate oxygen therapy. (See *Types of oxygen therapy*, pages 350 and 351.)

Is your patient ready for weaning? If so, several methods are available.

Disorders

Common respiratory disorders you encounter in the critical care unit include:
• ARDS
• acute respiratory failure
• COPD
• pneumonia
• pneumothorax
• pulmonary embolism
• pulmonary hypertension
• status asthmaticus.

ARDS can quickly lead to acute respiratory failure.

Acute respiratory distress syndrome

ARDS is a type of pulmonary edema not related to heart failure. It's also known as shock, white, wet, or Da Nang lung. ARDS may follow direct or indirect lung injury and can quickly lead to acute respiratory failure.

The three hallmark features of ARDS are:

bilateral patchy infiltrates on chest X-ray

no signs or symptoms of heart failure

(Text continues on page 352.)

Types of oxygen therapy

Various types of devices are used to deliver oxygen therapy. Regardless of the type, always assess the patient closely and check the results of pulse oximetry or arterial blood gas analysis 20 to 30 minutes after adjusting the flow rate.

Delivery device	Oxygen concentration administered	Administration guidelines
Nasal cannula	Low flow, 1 to 6 L/minute (24% to 40% fraction of inspired oxygen [FIO_2])	• Ensure patency of nostrils with flashlight. • Hook the cannula tubing behind the patient's ears and under his chin, sliding the adjuster upward under the chin to secure. • Alternatively, position elastic strap over the patient's ears and around the back of his head; avoid applying too tightly, which can cause pressure on the facial structures and occlude the cannula. • With this device, oral breathers achieve the same oxygen delivery as nasal breathers. • Headache may occur if flow rate is greater than 6 L/minute.
Simple mask	Oxygen at 5 to 8 L/minute (40% to 60% FIO_2)	• Ensure proper fitting mask for the patient. • Place mask over the patient's nose, mouth, and chin, molding the flexible metal edge to the bridge of his nose. • Adjust elastic band around the patient's head to hold the mask firmly but comfortably in place. • If necessary, tape gauze pads to the mask over the patient's cheek area to make an airtight seal. • If the mask doesn't fit snugly, room air will dilute the oxygen, interfering with the delivery of the prescribed concentration. • A minimum of 5 L/minute is required in all masks to flush carbon dioxide from it so that the patient doesn't rebreathe it.
Partial rebreather mask	Oxygen at 6 to 10 L/minute (40% to 60% FIO_2)	• Follow the measures as for a simple mask with these additions: – Monitor the reservoir bag collapse; if it collapses more than slightly during inspiration, raise the flow rate until only a slight deflation is seen. – Marked or complete deflation indicates insufficient oxygen flow, which could possibly lead to carbon dioxide accumulation in the mask. – Keep the reservoir bag from twisting or kinking. – Ensure free expansion of the bag by keeping it outside of the patient's gown and bedcovers.
Nonrebreather mask	Oxygen at 6 to 8 L/minute (60% to 80% FIO_2)	• This type of mask delivers the highest percentage of oxygen without intubation and mechanical ventilation. • Follow the measures as for a simple mask with these additions: – Make sure the mask fits snugly and the one-way valves are secure and functioning. – Watch for possible signs of carbon dioxide buildup due to a malfunctioning valve.

Types of oxygen therapy *(continued)*

Delivery device	Oxygen concentration administered	Administration guidelines
Nonrebreather mask *(continued)*		– Monitor the deflation of the reservoir bag; if it collapses more than slightly during inspiration, raise the flow rate until only a slight deflation is seen. – Marked or complete deflation indicates insufficient oxygen flow, which could possibly lead to carbon dioxide accumulation in the mask. – Keep the reservoir bag from twisting or kinking. – Ensure free expansion of the bag by keeping it outside of the patient's gown and bedcovers.
Venturi mask	Oxygen at 4 to 10 L/minute (24% to 55% FIO_2)	• Follow the measures as for a simple mask with these additions:. – Ensure that the proper device is used and that the oxygen flow rate is set at the amount specified on each mask. – Make sure that the Venturi valve is set for the desired FIO_2. – Ensure a snug but comfortably fitting mask; a loose fit or twisting, kinking, or blocked oxygen ports may alter the oxygen concentration being given.
Continuous positive airway pressure (CPAP) mask	Variable	• This system allows the spontaneously breathing patient to receive CPAP with or without an artificial airway. • This type of mask is contraindicated in patients with chronic obstructive pulmonary disease, bullous lung disease, low cardiac output, or tension pneumothorax. • Place one strap behind the patient's head and the other strap over it to ensure a snug fit. • Assess the patient's respiratory, cardiac, circulatory, and GI function hourly.
Transtracheal oxygen	Variable	• This catheter device supplies oxygen throughout the respiratory cycle. • After insertion, obtain a chest X-ray as ordered to confirm placement of the catheter. • Assess the patient for bleeding, respiratory distress, pneumothorax, pain, coughing, or hoarseness. • Don't use the catheter for approximately 1 week after insertion to reduce the risk of subcutaneous emphysema.
Aerosols	Variable; high-humidity oxygen that can be heated or cooled delivered by a jet nebulizer	• Be alert for condensation buildup in the tubing; empty the tubing at frequent intervals. • Ensure that condensate doesn't enter the trachea. • Monitor the tracheostomy tube site (if the patient has one) for signs of irritation and pressure. • When using a high-output nebulizer, watch for signs of overhydration, pulmonary edema, crackles, and electrolyte imbalances.

no improvement in PaO_2 despite increasing oxygen delivery.

The prognosis for patients with ARDS varies depending on the cause and the patient's age and health status before developing ARDS.

What causes it

Some of the most common predisposing factors for ARDS are:
- sepsis
- lung injury from trauma such as airway contusion
- trauma related factors such as fat emboli, multiple blood transfusions, and shock
- shock (any type)
- disseminated intravascular coagulation
- pancreatitis
- massive blood transfusions
- burns
- cardiopulmonary bypass
- drug overdose
- aspiration of stomach contents
- pneumonitis
- near drowning
- pneumonia
- inhalation of noxious gases (such as ammonia or chlorine).

Pathophysiology

In ARDS, the tissues lining the alveoli and the pulmonary capillaries are injured, either directly by aspiration of gastric contents or inhalation of noxious gases, or indirectly, by chemical mediators released into the bloodstream in response to systemic disease.

Inflammation follows injury

The injured tissues release cytokines and other molecules that cause inflammation as white blood cells (WBCs) collect at the site and swelling occurs. The tissues become more permeable to fluid and proteins, and the hydrostatic pressure gradient between the alveoli and the capillaries is reversed.

Impaired exchange

Proteins and fluid begin to move from the capillaries into the alveoli. When this happens, gas exchange is impaired in the affected alveoli. As the process continues, the alveoli collapse (atelectasis), and gas exchange becomes impossible.

Ventilation prevention

The fluid that accumulates in the interstitial spaces, alveolar spaces, and small airways causes the lungs to stiffen, preventing air from moving into the lungs (ventilation).

Shunt stunts

As alveoli fill with fluid or collapse, the capillaries surrounding the alveoli fail to absorb oxygen. The body responds by shunting blood away from these alveoli, a process called right-to-left shunting.

Responses to the big buildup

As fluid builds up in the alveoli, the patient develops thick, frothy sputum and marked hypoxemia with increasing respiratory distress. As pulmonary edema worsens, inflammation leads to fibrosis, further impeding gas exchange.

Fluid in the interstitial spaces, alveolar spaces, and small airways prevents air from moving into the lungs.

Off-line alkaline

Tachypnea due to respiratory distress causes alkalosis as carbon dioxide levels decrease. The body tries to compensate and to bring the blood pH back into the normal range through metabolic acidosis. The lack of oxygen also forces the body into anaerobic metabolism, which adds to the acidosis.

Unless gas exchange is restored and this process is reversed, acidosis worsens until all organ systems are affected and fail.

What to look for

ARDS occurs in four stages, each with these typical signs and symptoms:

Stage I involves dyspnea, especially on exertion. Respiratory and heart rates are normal to high. Auscultation may reveal diminished breath sounds, particularly when the patient is tachypneic. Stage I develops hours to days after the initial injury in response to decreasing oxygen levels in the blood.

Stage II is marked by greater respiratory distress. Respiratory rate is high, and the patient may use accessory muscles to breathe. He may appear restless, apprehensive, and mentally sluggish, or agitated. He may have a dry cough or frothy sputum. The heart rate is elevated and the skin is cool and clammy. Lung auscultation may reveal basilar crackles. The symptoms at this stage are sometimes incorrectly attributed to trauma.

Stage III involves obvious respiratory distress, with tachypnea, use of accessory breathing muscles, and decreased mental

Uh-oh! Unless gas exchange is restored, increasing acidosis could be the downfall of all the organ systems.

acuity. The patient exhibits tachycardia with arrhythmias (usually premature ventricular contractions) and labile blood pressure. The skin is pale and cyanotic. Auscultation may disclose diminished breath sounds, basilar crackles, and rhonchi. This stage generally requires ET intubation and mechanical ventilation.

Stage IV is characterized by decreasing respiratory and heart rates. The patient's mental status nears loss of consciousness. The skin is cool and cyanotic. Breath sounds are severely diminished to absent. (See *Understanding ARDS*.)

> Patients with stage III ARDS generally require ET intubation and mechanical ventilation.

What tests tell you

These test results are used to diagnose ARDS:
- ABG analysis initially shows decreased PaO_2 despite oxygen supplementation. Because of tachypnea, $PaCO_2$ is also decreased, causing an increase in blood pH (respiratory alkalosis).
- As ARDS worsens, $PaCO_2$ increases and pH decreases as the patient becomes acidotic. This is worsened by metabolic acidosis caused by a lack of oxygen that forces the body to switch to anaerobic metabolism.
- Initially, chest X-rays may be normal. Basilar infiltrates begin to appear in about 24 hours. In later stages, lung fields have a ground glass appearance and, eventually, as fluid fills the alveoli, white patches appear. These may eventually cover both lung fields entirely in later stages of ARDS.
- PA catheterization may be used to identify the cause of pulmonary edema through pulmonary artery wedge pressure (PAWP) measurement. PAWP is 18 mm Hg or lower in patients with ARDS.
- A differential diagnosis must be done to rule out cardiogenic pulmonary edema, pulmonary vasculitis, and diffuse pulmonary hemorrhage. Tests used to determine the causative agent may include sputum analysis, blood cultures, toxicology tests, and serum amylase levels (to rule out pancreatitis).

> Chest X-rays may be normal early in ARDS; however, that changes as ARDS progresses.

How it's treated

The goal of therapy is to correct the original cause, if possible, and provide enough oxygen to allow normal body processes to continue until the lungs begin to heal.
- Antibiotics and steroids may be administered to fight infection and minimize inflammation.
- Diuretics may be needed to reduce interstitial and pulmonary edema. In later stages of ARDS, however, vasopressors are usually prescribed to maintain blood pressure and blood supply to critical tissues.

Understanding ARDS

Here's how acute respiratory distress syndrome (ARDS) progresses:

1. Injury reduces normal blood flow to the lungs. Platelets aggregate and release histamine (H), serotonin (S), and bradykinin (B).

2. The released substances inflame and damage the alveolar capillary membrane, increasing capillary permeability. Fluids then shift into the interstitial space.

3. Capillary permeability increases and proteins and fluids leak out, increasing interstitial osmotic pressure and causing pulmonary edema.

4. Decreased blood flow and fluids in the alveoli damage surfactant and impair the cell's ability to produce more. The alveoli then collapse, thus impairing gas exchange.

5. Oxygenation is impaired, but carbon dioxide (CO_2) easily crosses the alveolar capillary membrane and is expired. Blood oxygen (O_2) and CO_2 levels are low.

6. Pulmonary edema worsens and inflammation leads to fibrosis. Gas exchange is further impeded.

• Respiratory support is most important. Humidified oxygen delivery through a tight-fitting mask and using continuous positive airway pressure may be adequate. ET intubation and mechanical ventilation are commonly required. Positive end-expiratory pressure (PEEP) may prevent alveolar collapse. High-frequency jet ventilation is sometimes used. Suctioning as necessary removes accumulated secretions from the tracheobronchial tree.

• Prone positioning may improve the patient's oxygenation. (See *Prone positioning.*)

More meds

Additional medications are generally required when intubation and mechanical ventilation are instituted. Sedatives, including opioids and, sometimes, neuromuscular blocking agents, minimize restlessness and allow ventilation.

What to do

ARDS requires careful monitoring and supportive care. When your patient isn't intubated, watch carefully for signs of respiratory failure, which can happen quickly and necessitate intubation and mechanical ventilation.

• Assess the patient's respiratory status at least every 2 hours or more often, if indicated. Note respiratory rate, rhythm, and depth.

Prone positioning

Prone positioning (also known as *proning*) is a therapeutic maneuver to improve oxygenation and pulmonary function in patients with acute lung injury or acute respiratory distress syndrome (ARDS). It involves physically turning a patient facedown, which shifts blood flow to regions of the lung that are better ventilated.

The criteria for prone positioning commonly include:
• acute onset of acute respiratory failure
• hypoxemia, specifically a partial pressure of arterial oxygen/fraction of inspired oxygen (PaO_2/FIO_2) ratio of 300 or less for acute lung injury or a PaO_2/FIO_2 ratio of 200 or less for ARDS
• radiological evidence of diffuse bilateral pulmonary infiltrates.

Equipment innovations
Innovative equipment, such as a lightweight, cushioned frame that straps to the front of the patient before turning, minimizes the risks associated with moving patients and keeping them prone for several hours at a time.

With the right equipment, prone positioning may aid movement of the diaphragm by allowing the abdomen to expand more fully. It's usually used for 6 or more hours per day, for up to 10 days, until the patient's need for a high concentration of inspired oxygen resolves. Patients with extrapulmonary ARDS (such as ARDS due to multiple traumas) respond well to prone positioning.

Pro-prone positioning
Prone positioning is indicated to support mechanically ventilated patients with ARDS, who require high concentrations of inspired oxygen. In patients who respond, prone positioning may correct severe hypoxemia and aid maintenance of adequate oxygenation (PaO_2 greater than 60%) in patients with acute lung injury, while avoiding ventilator-induced lung injury. It isn't clear whether patients' survival rates are increased.

No prone positioning
Prone positioning is contraindicated in patients whose heads can't be supported in a facedown position or who can't tolerate a headdown position. Relative contraindications include increased intracranial pressure, spinal instability, unstable bone fractures, multiple trauma, left-sided heart failure (nonpulmonary respiratory failure), shock, abdominal compartment syndrome, abdominal surgery, extreme obesity (weight greater than 300 lb [136.1 kg]) and pregnancy. Hemodynamically unstable patients (systolic blood pressure less than 90 mm Hg) despite aggressive fluid resuscitation and vasopressors should be thoroughly evaluated before being placed in the prone position.

Report the presence of dyspnea and accessory muscle use. Be alert for inspiratory retractions.

• Administer oxygen as ordered. Monitor fraction of inspired oxygen levels.

• Auscultate lungs bilaterally for adventitious or diminished breath sounds. Inspect the color and character of sputum; clear, frothy sputum indicates pulmonary edema. To maintain PEEP, suction only as needed.

• Check ventilator settings often. Assess oxygen saturation continuously by pulse oximetry or SvO_2 by PA catheter. Monitor serial ABG levels; document and report changes in oxygen saturation as well as metabolic and respiratory acidosis and PaO_2 changes.

• Monitor vital signs. Institute cardiac monitoring and observe for arrhythmias that may result from hypoxemia, acid-base disturbances, or electrolyte imbalance.

• Monitor the patient's LOC, noting confusion or mental sluggishness.

• Be alert for signs of treatment-induced complications, including arrhythmias, disseminated intravascular coagulation, GI bleeding, infection, malnutrition, paralytic ileus, pneumothorax, pulmonary fibrosis, renal failure, thrombocytopenia, and tracheal stenosis.

• Give sedatives as ordered to reduce restlessness. Administer sedatives and analgesics at regular intervals if the patient on mechanical ventilation is receiving neuromuscular blocking agents.

• Provide routine eye care and instill artificial tears to prevent corneal drying and abrasion from the loss of the blink reflex in mechanically ventilated patients receiving neuromuscular blocking agents.

• Administer anti-infective agents as ordered if the underlying cause is sepsis or an infection.

• Place the patient in a comfortable position that maximizes air exchange, such as semi-Fowler's or high Fowler's position. A continuous rotation bed or prone positioning may be needed.

• Allow for periods of rest to prevent fatigue and reduce oxygen demand.

• If your patient has a PA catheter in place, know the desired PAWP level and check readings as indicated. Watch for decreasing SvO_2. Because PEEP may reduce cardiac output, check for hypotension, tachycardia, and decreased urine output.

• Evaluate the patient's serum electrolyte levels frequently as ordered. Monitor urine output hourly to ensure adequate renal function. Measure intake and output. Weigh the patient daily.

Institute cardiac monitoring to observe for arrhythmias caused by hypoxemia, acid-base disturbances, or electrolyte imbalance.

Place the patient in a comfortable position that maximizes air exchange, such as semi-Fowler's or high Fowler's position.

- Record caloric intake. Administer tube feedings and parenteral nutrition as ordered.
- Perform passive ROM exercises to maintain joint mobility. Provide meticulous skin care to prevent breakdown.

Acute respiratory failure

Acute respiratory failure results when the lungs can't adequately oxygenate blood or eliminate carbon dioxide.

In patients with normal lung tissue, respiratory failure is indicated by a $Paco_2$ above 50 mm Hg and a Pao_2 below 50 mm Hg. These limits don't apply to patients with chronic lung disease, such as COPD, who typically have consistently high carbon dioxide levels and low Pao_2.

> Uh-oh! When I can't oxygenate blood or remove carbon dioxide, acute respiratory failure results.

What causes it

Conditions that cause alveolar hypoventilation, $\dot{V}/\dot{Q}$ mismatch, or right-to-left shunting can lead to respiratory failure. These include:
- COPD
- bronchitis
- pneumonia
- bronchospasm
- ventilatory failure
- pneumothorax
- atelectasis
- cor pulmonale
- pulmonary edema
- pulmonary emboli
- CNS disease
- CNS depression due to head trauma or misuse of opioids, sedatives, or tranquilizers.

Pathophysiology

Respiratory failure results from impaired gas exchange. Any condition associated with $\dot{V}/\dot{Q}$ mismatch caused by alveolar hypoventilation or intrapulmonary shunting can lead to acute respiratory failure if left untreated.

Poor ventilation

Alveolar hypoventilation occurs when respiratory effort is diminished or when airway obstruction leads to decreased airflow in the alveoli. This can occur with neuromuscular diseases or conditions that interfere with respiration.

The most common cause of alveolar hypoventilation is airway obstruction, commonly seen with emphysema or bronchitis.

Poor oxygenation

Blood that passes through the lungs but isn't oxygenated due to alveolar hypoventilation is known as shunted blood. Blood flow in the lung can be impaired by obstruction or hypovolemia. Obstruction is the most acute form, and is most commonly caused by pulmonary emboli.

The rise and fall of partial pressures

When $Paco_2$ levels rise above normal and pH drops below normal, respiratory acidosis develops. (Pao_2 levels also drop below normal in acute respiratory failure.) Other organ systems respond with compensatory responses. For example, the sympathetic nervous system triggers vasoconstriction, increases peripheral resistance, and increases the heart rate.

Lots of lactic acid

As tissue hypoxemia develops, tissues resort to anaerobic metabolism, which results in a buildup of lactic acid (a by-product of anaerobic metabolism) and thus metabolic acidosis. This takes longer to develop than respiratory acidosis, but the result is increasing acidity of the blood, which interferes with normal metabolism of all body systems.

What to look for

Your patient's history may reveal an underlying respiratory condition or an acute process leading to respiratory failure (such as asphyxia, drug overdose, or trauma).

Got no time

There's usually little time to collect a thorough history and the patient typically can't give the history himself. His family members or medical records may be the main sources of such information.

Time is of the essence

Physical assessment findings vary, depending on the duration of the condition. Initially, the body responds with secretion of epinephrine. Eventually, as the patient's condition worsens, epinephrine secretion has less effect.

On inspection, note nasal flaring due to hypoxemia, ashen skin, and cyanosis of the oral mucosa, lips, and nail beds. The patient may use accessory muscles of respiration to breathe and sit bolt upright or slightly hunched over. He may be agitated or highly anxious. In later stages, as the patient's level of mentation decreases due to hypoxemia, he may lie down and appear confused and disoriented.

If pneumothorax is present, you may observe asymmetrical chest movement. Tactile fremitus may be present as well.

Finding failure

Look for these physical signs of respiratory failure:
• Tachypnea increases the patient's respiratory rate so it's greater than the normal range of 16 to 20 breaths per minute.
• Tachycardia is a heart rate greater than 100 beats per minute. You may not see this in patients with heart disease who are taking medications that prevent tachycardia. The pulse may be strong and rapid initially, but thready and irregular in later stages.
• Cold, clammy skin and frank diaphoresis are apparent, especially around the forehead and face.
• Percussion reveals hyperresonance in patients with COPD. In patients with atelectasis or pneumonia, percussion sounds are dull or flat.
• Lung auscultation usually reveals diminished breath sounds. In patients with pneumothorax, breath sounds are absent over the affected lung tissue. In other cases of respiratory failure, adventitious breath sounds, such as wheezes (in asthma) and rhonchi (in bronchitis), may be heard. If you auscultate crackles, suspect pulmonary edema as the cause of respiratory failure.

What tests tell you

• ABG analysis indicates early respiratory failure when PaO_2 is low (usually less than 60 mm Hg) and $PaCO_2$ is high (greater than 45 mm Hg) and the HCO_3^- level is normal. The pH is also low. ABG levels in patients with COPD may be difficult to interpret, so compare them with earlier ABG values.
• Chest X-ray is used to identify pulmonary diseases, such as emphysema, atelectasis, pneumothorax, infiltrates, and effusions.
• Electrocardiogram (ECG) can demonstrate arrhythmias, commonly found with cor pulmonale and myocardial hypoxia.
• Pulse oximetry reveals a decreasing oxygen saturation level. SvO_2 levels less than 50% indicate impaired tissue oxygenation.
• WBC count aids detection of an underlying infection. Blood cultures, sputum cultures, and Gram stain may also be used to identify pathogens.
• Abnormally low hemoglobin and hematocrit levels signal blood loss, indicating decreased oxygen carrying capacity.
• PA catheterization is used to distinguish pulmonary causes from cardiovascular causes of acute respiratory failure, and to monitor the effects of treatment.

If you note asymmetrical chest movement and tactile fremitus, your patient has pneumothorax.

If you auscultate crackles, pulmonary edema is the suspected cause of respiratory failure.

How it's treated

The primary goal of treatment is to restore adequate gas exchange. The secondary goal is to correct the underlying cause and development of respiratory failure.

Go to the O₂

Oxygen therapy is initiated immediately to optimize oxygenation of pulmonary blood. You may instruct the patient to try pursed-lip breathing to prevent alveolar collapse. If the patient can't breathe on his own, ET intubation and mechanical ventilation are instituted. High-frequency or pressure ventilation is sometimes used to force airways open.

Oh, and drug therapy, too

Various drug therapies may be ordered:
• Reversal agents such a naloxone (Narcan) are given if drug overdose is suspected.
• Bronchodilators are given to open airways.
• Antibiotics are given to combat infection.
• Corticosteroids may be given to reduce inflammation.
• Continuous I.V. solutions of positive inotropic agents may be given to increase cardiac output, and vasopressors may be given to induce vasoconstriction to maintain blood pressure. Fluids are generally restricted to reduce cardiac workload and edema.
• Diuretics may be given to reduce fluid overload and edema.

What to do

• Assess the patient's respiratory status at least every 2 hours or more often, as indicated. Observe for a positive response to oxygen therapy, such as improved breathing, color, and oximetry and ABG values.
• Position the patient for optimal breathing effort when he isn't intubated. Put the call bell within easy reach to reassure the patient and prevent unnecessary exertion when he needs to call the nurse.
• Maintain a normothermic environment to reduce the patient's oxygen demand.
• Monitor vital signs, heart rhythm, and fluid intake and output, including daily weights, to identify fluid overload (from I.V. fluids and medications) or impending dehydration (from aggressive diuretic therapy).
• After intubation, auscultate the lungs to check for accidental intubation of the esophagus or the mainstem bronchus. Be alert for aspiration, broken teeth, nosebleeds, and vagal reflexes causing bradycardia, arrhythmias, and hypotension.

• Don't suction too often without identifying the underlying cause of an equipment alarm. Use strict sterile technique during suctioning. ET intubation bypasses many of the body's normal barriers to infection, so the patient is at high risk during this procedure.

• Watch oximetry and capnography values because these are important indicators of changes in the patient's condition.

• Note the amount and quality of lung secretions and look for changes in the patient's status.

• Check cuff pressure on the ET tube to prevent erosion from an overinflated cuff. Normal cuff pressure is about 20 mm Hg.

• Implement measures to prevent nasal tissue necrosis. Position and maintain the nasotracheal tube midline in the nostrils and reposition daily. Tape the tube securely but use skin protection measures and nonirritating tape to prevent skin breakdown.

• Be alert for GI bleeding. Inspect gastric sections for blood, especially if the patient has a nasogastric (NG) tube or reports or shows evidence of epigastric or abdominal tenderness. Decreasing hemoglobin level and hematocrit and occult blood in the stools are other indicators of GI bleeding.

• Provide a means of communication for patients who are intubated and alert. Institutions use different approaches, based on signs and signals, or communication boards. Explain all procedures to the patient and his family.

> Be sure to provide a means of communication for patients who are intubated and alert.

Chronic obstructive pulmonary disease

COPD (also called chronic obstructive lung disease) results from emphysema, chronic bronchitis, asthma, or a combination of these disorders. It's the most common chronic lung disease in the United States.

Out...

COPD is a chronic condition that can usually be managed on an outpatient basis even in advanced disease, when a patient may require continuous oxygen therapy.

...or in

Exacerbations of COPD that necessitate hospitalization are caused by various factors that place additional demand on the respiratory system, such as infection, heart failure, and exposure to allergens.

What causes it

Common causes of COPD include:

- cigarette smoking or exposure to cigarette smoke
- recurrent or chronic respiratory tract infections
- air pollution
- allergies.

Familial and hereditary factors, such as alpha$_1$-antitrypsin deficiency paired with cigarette smoking, may also be responsible for emphysema.

Pathophysiology

Patients with COPD have decreased gas exchange ability due to alveolar damage caused by exposure to smoke or chemical irritants over a long period.

Quit it!

Smoke inhalation impairs ciliary action and macrophage function and causes inflammation in the airways and increased mucus production. Early inflammatory changes may be reversed if the patient stops smoking before lung disease becomes extensive.

Air trap

In chronic bronchitis, mucus plugs and narrowed airways cause air trapping. Air trapping also occurs with asthma and emphysema. In emphysema, permanent enlargement of the acini is accompanied by destruction of the alveolar walls. Obstruction and air trapping result from tissue changes rather than mucus production.

Here's what happens in air trapping: Hyperinflation of the alveoli occurs on expiration. On inspiration, airways enlarge, allowing air to pass beyond the obstruction; on expiration, airways narrow and prevent gas flow.

Pressure pockets

As the alveolar walls are destroyed, they're no longer separate, but coalesce into large air pockets that put additional pressure on surrounding tissues. This affects the lung's blood supply as well, because it increases the pressure needed to push blood through the lungs. This form of high blood pressure is known as pulmonary hypertension.

Overwhelming work

Eventually, the high workload overwhelms the right side of the heart and hypertrophy and right-sided failure (cor pulmonale) result. Patients commonly have supraventricular arrhythmias such as atrial fibrillation, which increase the danger of thrombus formation.

Because gas exchange is impaired, hypercapnia ($PaCO_2$ above 40 mm Hg) becomes the norm for these patients. The respiratory center of the brain, which stimulates breathing when $PaCO_2$ rises, becomes dependent instead on low PaO_2. This is an important consideration when oxygen is given for hypoxemia.

What to look for

Your patient usually has a history of COPD and may be able to identify the precipitating cause (exposure to an allergen, for example).

In COPD, your patient usually has a history of the disorder and may know the precipitating cause.

Tachy and not-so-tachy finds

Your patient is likely to have tachycardia and an irregular heart rhythm as well as tachypnea and dyspnea on exertion. Fever may be present in the case of infection, but if the patient takes steroids regularly, the immune response is suppressed.

When you inspect the chest, you may notice that the anterolateral diameter is increased (barrel chest), and the patient may appear generally cachectic. He may be coughing, with copious sputum production, if he has chronic bronchitis, or he may be wheezing.

When you listen to breath sounds, listen for a prolonged expiratory phase, perhaps crackles or rhonchi, and generally some decreased air movement.

Time will tell

Patients with COPD have abnormal breath sounds to begin with, and it may be hard to tell at first what's baseline and what's newly abnormal. As you listen over several hours or days abnormal breath sounds eventually become apparent.

Your patient with COPD may have abnormal baseline breath sounds.

What tests tell you

Stable COPD patients exhibit these abnormal diagnostic test results, which may be considered their baseline values:
• Pulmonary function tests show increased residual volume, with decreased vital capacity and FEV_1.
• Chest X-ray shows increased bronchovascular markings and overaeration of lungs. In advanced disease, the diaphragm is flattened and bronchovascular markings may be reduced.
• ABG analysis may show reduced PaO_2 and normal or increased $PaCO_2$. In advanced COPD, it isn't uncommon for baseline $PaCO_2$ levels to be 50 mm Hg or higher.

• ECG may show atrial arrhythmias and, in advanced disease, right ventricular hypertrophy.
• Blood count reveals elevated hemoglobin levels.

When it worsens

During an exacerbation, diagnostic tests may yield these additional results:
• ABG analysis shows Pao_2 below the patient's baseline. $Paco_2$ may be low, normal, or high, depending on the patient's baseline.
• Chest X-ray may show infiltrates if pneumonia is present.
• ECG may show sinus tachycardia with supraventricular and, sometimes, ventricular arrhythmias.

How it's treated

Provide supportive treatments for your patients with COPD. Bronchodilators and membrane stabilizing aerosols are useful in maintaining open airways. Steroids may be given to reduce inflammation if necessary. In some cases, continuous oxygen supplementation is needed.

Address the effects, then treat the cause

During exacerbations, management is twofold. First, respiratory support is given to avoid respiratory failure and cardiac arrest. Equally important is treatment addressing the underlying cause of the exacerbation.
• Your patient may receive oxygen supplementation. Care must be taken when the baseline $Paco_2$ level is high. The patient's respiratory center relies on low oxygen levels to stimulate breathing. Administer controlled oxygen therapy by monitoring ABG levels and patient assessments.
• If respiratory failure is imminent, ET intubation and mechanical ventilation are needed.
• Aerosolized bronchodilators, such as albuterol, are given to open airways.
• Epinephrine, a potent bronchodilator, may be given.
• Corticosteroids, usually by I.V., are given to reduce inflammation.
• Diuretic agents may be given to reduce edema and cardiac workload.
• Antiarrhythmic medications may be given. The patient is usually put on continuous ECG monitoring to observe the heart rate and any arrhythmias.
• Antibiotics are given to treat or prevent infection.
• If pneumothorax is present, a chest tube may be inserted.

I.V. corticosteroids are given to reduce inflammation when COPD is exacerbated.

What to do

• Assess respiratory status, auscultate breath sounds, monitor oxygen saturation and ABG values, and observe for a positive response to oxygen therapy, such as improved breathing, color, or oximetry and ABG values. Anticipate the need for intubation and mechanical ventilation.

• Frequent and careful assessment is key. Changes can be subtle and rapid. Be sure to assess mental status because it's an early and sensitive indicator of respiratory status. New onset of confusion and agitation are red flags, as is lethargy.

• Monitor vital signs and heart rhythm and observe for arrhythmias, which may indicate hypoxemia, right-sided heart failure, or an adverse effect of bronchodilator use.

• Obtain laboratory tests as ordered and report results promptly.

• Offer emotional support. Keep the environment as calm as possible and the air temperature warm. The patient may not be able to speak easily because of shortness of breath, so explain what's happening and try to anticipate his needs.

> Frequent and careful assessment is the key to care because changes can be subtle and develop rapidly.

Pneumonia

Pneumonia is an acute infection of the lung parenchyma that commonly impairs gas exchange. More than 3 million cases of pneumonia are diagnosed yearly in the United States.

Those at risk

The prognosis is good for patients with pneumonia who are otherwise healthy. Debilitated patients are at much greater risk; bacterial pneumonia is a leading cause of death among such individuals. Pneumonia occurs in both sexes and in all ages, but older adults are at greater risk for developing it. (See *Pneumonia in older adults.*)

What starts it

Infectious agents may be bacterial, viral, mycoplasmal, rickettsial, fungal, protozoal, or mycobacterial.

Where it infects

Types of pneumonia based on location of the infection include:
• bronchopneumonia, involving distal airways and alveoli
• lobular pneumonia, involving part of a lobe
• lobar pneumonia, involving an entire lobe.

Senior moment

Pneumonia in older adults

Older adults are at greater risk for developing pneumonia because their weakened chest musculature reduces their ability to clear secretions. Those in long-term care facilities are especially susceptible.

Bacterial pneumonia is the most common type found in older adults; viral pneumonia is the second most common type. Aspiration pneumonia occurs from impaired swallowing ability and a diminished gag reflex due to stroke or prolonged illness.

And presenting...
An older adult with pneumonia may present with fatigue, slight cough, and a rapid respiratory rate. Pleuritic pain and fever may be present. An absence of fever doesn't mean absence of infection in an older adult. Many older adults develop a subnormal body temperature in response to infection.

Get it here, there, or anywhere

Pneumonia may be classified as community-acquired, hospital-acquired (nosocomial), or aspiration pneumonia. (See *Types of pneumonia*, pages 368 and 369.)

Shared with the community

As the name implies, community-acquired pneumonia occurs in the community setting or within the first 48 hours of admission to a health care facility because of community exposure.

Not-so-comical pneumonia

Nosocomial pneumonia refers to the development of pneumonia 48 hours after admission to a health care facility. For example, development of pneumonia after ET intubation and placement on a ventilator can be a type of nosocomial pneumonia.

When location doesn't matter

Aspiration pneumonia can occur in the community or health care facility setting.

What causes it

Primary pneumonia results from inhalation of a pathogen, such as bacteria or virus. Examples are pneumococcal and viral pneumonia.

Pneumonia is classified according to the infectious agent, location, or other factors.

Types of pneumonia

Here's an overview of the various types of pneumonia, including their causative agents and common assessment findings.

Type	Causative agent	Assessment findings
Aspiration pneumonia	Aspiration of gastric or oropharyngeal contents into trachea or lungs	• Fever • Crackles • Dyspnea • Hypotension • Tachycardia • Cyanosis • Chest X-ray with infiltrates
Community-acquired pneumonias		
Streptococcal pneumonia (pneumococcal pneumonia)	*Streptococcus pneumoniae*	• Sudden onset of single shaking chill • Fever 102° to 104° F (38.9° to 40° C) • History of previous upper respiratory infection • Pleuritic chest pain • Severe cough • Rust-colored sputum • Areas of consolidation on chest X-ray (usually lobar) • Elevated white blood cell (WBC) count • Sputum culture possibly positive for gram-positive *S. pneumoniae*
Hemophilus influenza	*Haemophilus influenzae*	• Insidious onset • History of upper respiratory tract infection 2 to 6 weeks earlier • Fever • Chills • Dyspnea • Productive cough • Nausea and vomiting • Chest X-ray with infiltrates in one or more lobes

Type	Causative agent	Assessment findings
Community-acquired pneumonias (continued)		
Mycoplasma pneumonia	*Mycoplasma pneumoniae*	• Insidious onset • Sore throat • Nasal congestion • Ear pain • Headache • Low-grade fever • Pleuritic pain • Erythema rash • Pharyngitis
Viral pneumonia	Influenza virus, type A	• Initially beginning as upper respiratory infection • Cough (initially nonproductive; later purulent sputum) • High fever • Chills • Malaise • Dyspnea • Substernal pain • Moist crackles • Cyanosis • Frontal headache • Chest X-ray with diffuse bilateral bronchopneumonia radiating from hilus • Normal to slightly elevated WBC
Legionnaires' disease	*Legionella pneumophila*	• Flulike symptoms • Malaise • Headache within 24 hours • Fever • Shaking chills • Progressive dyspnea • Mental confusion • Anorexia

Types of pneumonia (continued)

Type	Causative agent	Assessment findings	Type	Causative agent	Assessment findings
Community-acquired pneumonias *(continued)*			**Hospital-acquired pneumonias** *(continued)*		
Legionnaires' disease *(continued)*		• Nausea, vomiting • Myalgia • Chest X-ray with patchy infiltrates, consolidation, and possible effusion	Pseudomonas pneumonia	*Pseudomonas aeruginosa*	• Fever • Chills • Confusion • Delirium • Green foul-smelling sputum • Chest X-ray with diffuse consolidation
Hospital-acquired pneumonias					
Klebsiella pneumonia	*Klebsiella pneumoniae*	• Fever • Recurrent chills • Rusty, bloody viscous sputum • Cyanosis of lips and nail beds • Shallow grunting respirations • Severe pleuritic chest pain • Chest X-ray typically with consolidation in upper lobe • Elevated WBC • Sputum culture and Gram stain possibly positive for gram-negative cocci, *Klebsiella*	Staphylococcal pneumonia (may also be community acquired)	*Staphylococcus aureus*	• Cough • Chills • High fever 102° to 104° F (38.9° to 40° C) • Pleuritic pain • Progressive dyspnea • Bloody sputum • Tachypnea • Hypoxemia • Chest X-ray with multiple abscesses and infiltrate; empyema • Elevated WBC • Sputum culture and Gram stain possibly positive for gram-positive staphylocci

Secondary pneumonia may follow initial lung damage from a noxious chemical or other insult (superinfection) or may result from hematogenous spread of bacteria from a distant area.

Aspiration pneumonia results from inhalation of foreign matter, such as vomitus or food particles, into the bronchi. It's more common in elderly or debilitated patients; those receiving NG tube feedings; and those with an impaired gag reflex, poor oral hygiene, or a decreased LOC.

Pathophysiology

The disease process varies among bacterial, viral, and aspiration pneumonia.
• In bacterial pneumonia, which can affect any part of the lungs, an infection initially triggers alveolar inflammation and edema. Capillaries become engorged with blood, causing stasis. As the alveolocapillary membrane breaks down, the alveoli fill with blood and inflammatory exudates, resulting in atelectasis.
• Viral pneumonia more commonly attacks bronchiolar epithelial cells, causing interstitial inflammation and desquamation. It then spreads to the alveoli. In advanced infection, a hyaline membrane may form, further compromising gas exchange.
• Aspiration pneumonia triggers similar inflammatory changes in the affected area, and also inactivates surfactant over a large area, leading to alveolar collapse. Acidic gastric contents may directly damage the airways and alveoli, and small particles may cause obstruction. The resulting inflammation makes the lungs susceptible to secondary bacterial pneumonia.

We get around! Bacterial pneumonia can move through the bloodstream to the lungs.

What to look for

Signs and symptoms of pneumonia include pleuritic chest pain, cough, and fever.

Sounds, sights, and sensations

Your patient's cough may be dry, as in mycoplasma pneumonia, or very productive. The sputum may be creamy yellow, green, or rust-colored.

In advanced cases of all types of pneumonia, percussion reveals dullness over the affected area of the lung. Auscultation may disclose crackles, wheezes, or rhonchi over the affected areas as well as decreased breath sounds and decreased tactile fremitus.

Percussion performed. Dullness revealed. Advanced pneumonia is what I feel.

What tests tell you

• Chest X-rays disclose infiltrates, confirming the diagnosis.
• Sputum specimen for Gram stain and culture and sensitivity testing may reveal inflammatory cells as well as bacterial cells.
• WBC count and differential may indicate the presence and type of infection. Elevated polymorphonucleocytes may indicate bacterial infection; in viral or mycoplasmal pneumonia, though, WBC count may not be elevated at all.
• ABG analysis is done to determine the extent of respiratory compromise due to alveolar inflammation.

• Bronchoscopy or transtracheal aspiration allows the collection of material for cultures to identify the specific infectious organism. Pleural fluid may also be sampled for culture and Gram stain.
• Pulse oximetry may show a reduced oxygen saturation level and indicate the need for oxygen supplementation.

How it's treated

Because the cause is commonly infectious and, in cases of secondary and aspiration pneumonia, bacterial secondary infections are a risk, antimicrobial therapy is started immediately. The type of antibiotic used depends on the infectious agent.

More oxygen, please

Your patient may receive oxygen supplementation, including ET intubation and mechanical ventilation in severe cases when respiratory arrest is imminent. In severe cases, PEEP may be needed to prevent alveolar collapse.

Add-ons

Other treatment measures include:
• bronchodilator therapy
• antitussives for cough
• high-calorie diet and adequate fluid intake
• bed rest
• analgesics to relieve pleuritic chest pain.

In severe cases, PEEP may be needed to prevent alveolar collapse.

What to do

• Maintain a patent airway and oxygenation. Place the patient in Fowler's position to maximize chest expansion and give supplemental oxygen as ordered. Monitor oxygen saturation and ABG levels as ordered.
• Assess respiratory status often, at least every 2 hours. Auscultate the lungs for abnormal breath sounds, such as crackles, wheezes, or rhonchi. Encourage coughing and deep breathing.
• If your patient's respiratory status deteriorates, anticipate the need for intubation and mechanical ventilation.
• Adhere to standard precautions and institute appropriate transmission-based precautions, depending on the causative organism.
• Institute cardiac monitoring to detect the development of arrhythmias secondary to hypoxemia.
• Reposition your patient to maximize chest expansion, allow rest, and reduce discomfort and anxiety.
• Obtain ordered diagnostic tests and report results promptly.
• Administer drug therapy as ordered.

Adhere to standard precautions and other appropriate safety measures, depending on the causative organism.

• Carefully monitor your patient's intake and output to allow early identification of dehydration, fluid overload, and accurate tracking of nutritional status.

Pneumothorax

Pneumothorax is an accumulation of air in the pleural cavity that leads to partial or complete lung collapse. The amount of air trapped in the intrapleural space determines the degree of lung collapse. In some cases, venous return to the heart is impeded, causing a life-threatening condition called *tension pneumothorax*.

Pneumothorax can be classified as either traumatic or spontaneous. *Traumatic pneumothorax* may be further classified as open or closed. (Note that an open [penetrating] wound may cause closed pneumothorax.) *Spontaneous pneumothorax*, which is also considered closed, is most common in older patients with COPD but can occur in young, healthy patients as well.

What causes it

The causes of pneumothorax vary according to classification.

Traumatic pneumothorax

Causes of open pneumothorax include:
• penetrating chest injury (stab or gunshot wound)
• insertion of a central venous catheter
• chest surgery
• transbronchial biopsy
• thoracentesis or closed pleural biopsy.
    Causes of closed pneumothorax include:
• blunt chest trauma
• air leakage from ruptured blebs
• rupture resulting from barotrauma caused by high intrathoracic pressures during mechanical ventilation
• tubercular or cancerous lesions that erode into the pleural space
• interstitial lung disease such as eosinophilic granuloma.

Spontaneous pneumothorax

Spontaneous pneumothorax is usually caused by the rupture of a subpleural bleb (a small cystic space) at the surface of a lung.

Tension pneumothorax

Causes of pneumothorax include:
• penetrating chest wound treated with an airtight dressing
• fractured ribs

Yikes! An accumulation of air in the pleural cavity causes partial or complete lung collapse.

- mechanical ventilation
- high-level PEEP that causes alveolar blebs to rupture
- chest tube occlusion or malfunction.

Pathophysiology

The pathophysiology of pneumothorax also varies according to classification.

Traumatic pneumothorax

Open pneumothorax occurs when atmospheric air flows directly into the pleural cavity (under negative pressure). As the air pressure in the pleural cavity becomes positive, the lung on the affected side collapses, causing decreased total lung capacity. As a result, the patient develops a $\dot{V}/\dot{Q}$ imbalance that leads to hypoxia.

Closed pneumothorax occurs when an opening is created between the intrapleural space and the parenchyma of the lung. Air enters the pleural space from within the lung, causing increased pleural pressure and preventing lung expansion during inspiration.

Spontaneous pneumothorax

In spontaneous pneumothorax, the rupture of a subpleural bleb causes air leakage into the pleural spaces, which causes the lung to collapse. Hypoxia results from decreased total lung capacity, vital capacity, and lung compliance.

Tension pneumothorax

Tension pneumothorax results when air in the pleural space is under higher pressure than air in the adjacent lung. Here's what happens:
- Air enters the pleural space from the site of pleural rupture, which acts as a one-way valve. Thus, air enters the pleural space on inspiration but can't escape as the rupture site closes on expiration.
- More air enters with each inspiration and air pressure begins to exceed barometric pressure.
- The air pushes against the recoiled lung, causing compression atelectasis, and pushes against the mediastinum, compressing and displacing the heart and great vessels.
- The mediastinum eventually shifts away from the affected side, affecting venous return, and putting ever-greater pressure on the heart, great vessels, trachea and contralateral lung.

Without immediate treatment, this emergency can rapidly become fatal. (See *Understanding tension pneumothorax*, page 374.)

Hurry! Without immediate treatment, tension pneumothorax can rapidly become fatal.

EMERGENCY

Understanding tension pneumothorax

In tension pneumothorax, air accumulates intrapleurally and can't escape. As intrapleural pressure increases, the lung on the affected side collapses.

On inspiration, the mediastinum shifts toward the unaffected lung, impairing ventilation.

On expiration, the mediastinal shift distorts the vena cava and reduces venous return.

What to look for

Assessment findings depend on the severity of the pneumothorax. Spontaneous pneumothorax that releases a small amount of air into the pleural space may cause no signs and symptoms. Generally, tension pneumothorax causes the most severe respiratory signs and symptoms.

Every breath hurts

Your patient's history reveals sudden, sharp, pleuritic chest pain. The patient may report that chest movement, breathing, and coughing exacerbate the pain. He may also report shortness of breath.

Further findings

Inspection reveals asymmetric chest wall movement with overexpansion and rigidity on the affected side. The skin may be cool and clammy and cyanotic. Palpation of the chest wall may reveal crackling beneath the skin (subcutaneous emphysema) and decreased vocal fremitus.

In addition, percussion may reveal hyperresonance on the affected side, auscultation may disclose decreased or absent breath sounds on the affected side,

Listen up! Auscultation may disclose decreased or absent breath sounds on the affected side.

and vital signs may follow the pattern of respiratory distress seen with respiratory failure.

Did we mention the tension?

Tension pneumothorax also causes:
- hypotension and tachycardia due to decreased cardiac output
- tracheal deviation to the opposite side (a late sign)
- distended jugular veins due to high intrapleural pressure, mediastinal shift, and increased cardiovascular pressure.

What tests tell you

- Chest X-rays reveal air in the pleural space and a mediastinal shift that confirm pneumothorax.
- ABG analysis reveals hypoxemia, usually with elevated $PaCO_2$ and normal bicarbonate ion levels in the early stages.
- ECG may reveal decreased QRS amplitude, precordial T-wave inversion, rightward shift of frontal QRS axis, and small precordial R voltage.

How it's treated

Treatment of pneumothorax depends on the cause and severity.

With trauma

Open or traumatic pneumothorax may necessitate surgical repair of affected tissues, followed by chest tube placement with an underwater seal.

With less lung collapse

Spontaneous pneumothorax with less than 30% lung collapse, no signs of increased pleural pressure, and no dyspnea or indications of physiologic compromise, may be corrected with:
- bed rest to preserve energy
- monitoring of vital signs to detect physiologic compromise
- oxygen administration to improve hypoxia
- aspiration of air from the intrapleural space with a large-bore needle attached to a syringe to restore negative pressure within the pleural space.

With more lung collapse

Greater than 30% lung collapse may necessitate other measures, such as:
- placing a chest tube in the second or third intercostal space in the midclavicular line to reexpand the lung by restoring negative intrapleural pressure

Your patient's treatment depends on the cause and severity of pneumothorax.

• connecting the chest tube to underwater seal or low-pressure suction to reexpand the lung.

With tension

Treatment for your patient with tension pneumothorax typically involves:
• immediate large-bore needle insertion into the pleural space through the second intercostal space to reexpand the lung, followed by insertion of a chest tube if large amounts of air escape through the needle after insertion
• analgesics to promote comfort and encourage deep breathing and coughing.

What to do

• Assess the patient's respiratory status, including auscultation of bilateral breath sounds, at least every 1 to 2 hours. Monitor oxygen saturation levels closely for changes; obtain ABG analysis as ordered.
• Monitor hemodynamic parameters frequently as appropriate and indicated; anticipate the need for cardiac monitoring because hypoxemia can predispose the patient to arrhythmias.
• Watch for complications, signaled by pallor, gasping respirations, and sudden chest pain. Carefully monitor vital signs at least every hour for indications of shock, increasing respiratory distress, or mediastinal shift. If your patient's respiratory status deteriorates, anticipate the need for ET intubation and mechanical ventilation and assist as necessary.
• Assist with the chest tube insertion and connect to suction, as ordered. Monitor your patient for possible complications associated with chest tube insertion.
• Check chest tube devices frequently for drainage and proper functioning.
• Reposition your patient to promote comfort and drainage.

Anticipate the need for cardiac monitoring because hypoxemia can predispose your patient to arrhythmias.

Pulmonary embolism causes a $\dot{V}/\dot{Q}$ mismatch that results in hypoxemia and intrapulmonary shunting.

Pulmonary embolism

Pulmonary embolism is an obstruction of the pulmonary arterial bed. It occurs when a mass lodges in a pulmonary artery branch, partially or completely obstructing blood flow distal to it. This causes a $\dot{V}/\dot{Q}$ mismatch, resulting in hypoxemia and intrapulmonary shunting.

What causes it

The most common source of pulmonary embolism is a dislodged thrombus that originated in the deep veins of the leg, or, less commonly, in the pelvic, renal, or hepatic veins, or right side of the heart. Other emboli arise from fat, air, amniotic fluid, tumor cells, or a foreign object, such as a needle, catheter part, or talc (from drugs intended for oral administration that are injected I.V. by addicts).

Fixins for increased risk

Risk factors for developing pulmonary embolism include:
• predisposing disorders, including lung disorders, cardiac disorders (valvular disease and arrhythmias, such as atrial fibrillation), infection, diabetes, history of thromboembolism, sickle cell disease, and polycythemia
• venous stasis in those who are on prolonged bed rest, immobile, obese, burn victims, older than age 40, or in orthopedic casts.
• venous injury caused by surgery (especially of the legs, pelvis, abdomen, and thorax), long-bone or pelvic fractures, I.V. drug abuse, I.V. therapy, or manipulation or disconnection of central lines
• increased blood coagulability resulting from cancer, high-estrogen hormonal contraceptive use (particularly in women older than age 40 who smoke cigarettes), or pregnancy (which involves hypercoagulability, decreased mobility, edema, and decreased venous return).

Pathophysiology

Here's what happens when pulmonary embolism develops:
• A thrombus forms as a result of trauma to the vascular wall, venous stasis, or hypercoagulability of the blood.
• Further trauma, clot dissolution, sudden muscle spasm, pressure changes, or a change in peripheral blood flow can cause the thrombus to loosen or fragment.
• After it's dislodged, the thrombus becomes an embolus and floats through the venous system to the right side of the heart and on to the pulmonary vasculature, where it lodges in a small vessel and occludes blood flow beyond the occlusion.
• A $\dot{V}/\dot{Q}$ mismatch results in hypoxemia that's commonly irreversible.

After it's dislodged, a thrombus becomes an embolus, which can float through the venous system to the heart and lungs.

What to look for

Your patient's history may reveal a predisposing condition or other risk factor for pulmonary embolism.

Symptoms may include acute shortness of breath and pleuritic or anginal pain. The patient may verbalize a sense of impending doom. Severity of the symptoms depends on the area of lung affected.

Low O$_2$ signs

Look for signs of hypoxemia, such as tachypnea, tachycardia, and a weak, irregular pulse. Your patient may have a productive cough, possibly producing blood-tinged sputum. Less common signs include chest splinting, massive hemoptysis, leg edema and, with a large embolus, cyanosis, syncope, and distended jugular veins.

Swelling, crackling, and rubbing

Palpation of the lower extremities may reveal a warm and tender area of localized swelling. Auscultation may reveal crackles or a pleural friction rub at the embolus site.

What tests tell you

- $\dot{V}/\dot{Q}$ scan demonstrates a mismatch, indicating abnormal perfusion.
- Pulmonary angiography may reveal a pulmonary vessel filling defect or an abrupt vessel ending, indicating pulmonary embolism. Angiography is the definitive test for pulmonary embolus, even though the risk of test-related complications, such as cardiac arrhythmias, is high.
- ECG results distinguish pulmonary embolism from myocardial infarct and show right axis deviation, right bundle-branch block, tall, peaked P waves, depressed ST segments, T-wave inversions, and supraventricular arrhythmias.
- Chest X-ray is used to rule out other pulmonary diseases, but it's inconclusive within 1 to 2 hours of the embolic event. It may also indicate areas of atelectasis, an elevated diaphragm, pleural effusion, a prominent pulmonary artery and, occasionally, the characteristic wedge-shaped infiltrate that suggests pulmonary infarction.
- ABG analysis reveals hypoxemia and possibly hypocapnia due to tachypnea.
- PA catheterization may reveal an elevated PAP.
- MRI is used to identify the embolus or blood flow changes indicating an embolus.

> Angiography is the definitive test for pulmonary embolus...

> ...but the risk of test-related complications, such as cardiac arrhythmias, is high.

How it's treated

The goal of treatment is to allow adequate gas exchange until the obstruction can be removed or resolves on its own. Oxygen therapy is the primary treatment.

In addition to oxygen therapy, these treatment measures may be indicated:
• For patients with blood clots, anticoagulation with heparin inhibits the formation of more thrombi. It's followed by warfarin (Coumadin) for 3 to 6 months, depending on risk factors.
• Patients with massive pulmonary embolism and shock may need fibrinolytic therapy with streptokinase (Streptase) or alteplase (Activase) to enhance fibrinolysis of the pulmonary emboli and remaining thrombi.
• Embolism from other sources may necessitate other therapy to dissolve the embolus, depending on its nature. Septic embolism, for example, calls for antibiotic therapy rather than anticoagulation.
• If hypotension occurs, vasopressors may be required to maintain blood pressure.

Surgical salvation

• Surgery is indicated for patients who can't take anticoagulants because of recent surgery or blood dyscrasia, or who have recurrent emboli during anticoagulant therapy. Surgery, which shouldn't be performed without angiographic evidence of pulmonary embolism, consists of vena caval ligation, plication, or insertion of a device (umbrella filter) to filter blood returning to the heart and lungs.

What to do

• Monitor your patient's respiratory status, oxygen saturation, and breath sounds, and administer oxygen therapy as ordered. If breathing is severely compromised, anticipate the need for ET intubation and mechanical ventilation.
• Monitor vital signs and heart rhythm to detect arrhythmias secondary to hypoxemia. Because many signs and symptoms of pulmonary embolism mimic those of myocardial infarction (MI), obtain a 12-lead ECG to rule out MI.
• Obtain laboratory tests as ordered and report results promptly.
• Monitor PTT regularly for patients on anticoagulation therapy. Effective heparin therapy increases PTT to about 2 to 2½ times normal.
• Keep antidotes for anticoagulants readily available. These include protamine sulfate for heparin and vitamin K for warfarin. Blood products may be needed in case of life-threatening bleeding.

If your patient's breathing is severely affected, he may need ET intubation and mechanical ventilation.

• During anticoagulant therapy, assess your patient for epistaxis, petechiae, and other signs of abnormal bleeding. Apply pressure over venous puncture sites for 5 to 10 minutes and 15 to 20 minutes for arterial sites, until bleeding stops. Avoid giving I.M. injections.
• Avoid giving aspirin and other nonsteroidal anti-inflammatory drugs (NSAIDs) if the patient is taking anticoagulants.
• Promote your patient's comfort by repositioning him often and administering analgesics for pain. Encourage leg movement if the patient is alert. Never vigorously massage the lower extremities.
• Monitor nutritional intake to ensure adequate calorie and fluid intake.
• Explain all procedures to the patient, even if his mentation is altered, and to the patient's family when present.

Avoid giving aspirin and other NSAIDs if your patient is taking anticoagulants.

Pulmonary hypertension

Pulmonary hypertension refers to chronically elevated PAP, over 30 mm Hg, and a mean PAP over 18 mm Hg.

What causes it

Primary, or idiopathic, pulmonary hypertension has no known cause. It's most common in women between ages 20 and 40 and is usually fatal within 3 to 4 years. Mortality is highest in pregnant women.

Prefaced with heart or lung disease

Secondary pulmonary hypertension results from existing cardiac or pulmonary disease, or both. Cardiac causes include:
• left-sided heart failure
• ventricular septal defect
• patent ductus arteriosus.
   Pulmonary causes include COPD and vasoconstriction of the arterial bed due to hypoxemia and acidosis.

Pathophysiology

In primary pulmonary hypertension, the intimal lining of the pulmonary arteries thickens, narrowing the lumen of the artery, impairing distensibility, and increasing vascular resistance.
   Alveolar hypoventilation can result from diseases causing alveolar destruction or diseases that prevent the chest wall from expanding sufficiently to allow air into the alveoli. The resulting decreased ventilation increases pulmonary vascular resistance.

Hypoxemia resulting from the $\dot{V}/\dot{Q}$ mismatch causes vasoconstriction, further increasing vascular resistance and resulting in pulmonary hypertension.

Sans treatment

If a patient with pulmonary hypertension doesn't receive treatment, here's what happens:
• Hypertrophy occurs in the medial smooth-muscle layer of the arterioles, worsening nondistensibility.
• Increased pressure in the lungs is transmitted to the right ventricle (which supplies the pulmonary artery).
• The ventricle becomes hypertrophic and eventually fails (cor pulmonale).
• Impaired distensibility due to hypertrophy can cause arrhythmias.

What to look for

Patients with pulmonary hypertension typically report increasing dyspnea on exertion, weakness, syncope, and fatigue.

Look, touch, and listen

Look for the signs of pulmonary hypertension, including:
• tachycardia
• tachypnea with mild exertion
• decreased blood pressure
• changes in mental status, from restlessness to agitation or confusion
• signs of right-sided heart failure, such as ascites and jugular vein distention
• an easily palpable right ventricular lift and a reduced carotid pulse
• possible peripheral edema
• decreased diaphragmatic excursion and respiration
• point of maximal impulse displaced beyond the mid-clavicular line.
• systolic ejection murmur; a widely split S_2, and an S_3 or S_4 sound; or decreased breath sounds and loud, turbulent sounds heard on auscultation.

What tests tell you

• ABG analysis reveals hypoxemia.
• ECG changes commensurate with right ventricular hypertrophy include right axis deviation and tall or peaked P waves in inferior leads.
• PA catheterization reveals increased PAP, with systolic pressure above 30 mm Hg. It may also show an increased PAWP if the un-

> Simply put, hypoxemia causes vasoconstriction, which causes pulmonary hypertension.

> Don't forget me! Check ECG readings for changes that indicate right ventricular hypertrophy.

derlying cause is left atrial myxoma, mitral stenosis, or left-sided heart failure; otherwise, PAWP is normal.

• Pulmonary angiography is used to detect filling defects in pulmonary vasculature.

• Pulmonary function studies may show decreased flow rates and increased residual volume in underlying obstructive disease. In underlying restrictive disease, they may show reduced total lung capacity.

• Radionuclide imaging reveals abnormal right and left ventricular function.

• Echocardiography allows assessment of ventricular wall motion and possible valvular dysfunction. It's also used to identify right ventricular enlargement, abnormal septal configuration, and reduced left ventricular cavity size.

• Perfusion lung scanning may yield normal results or multiple patchy and diffuse filling defects not consistent with pulmonary embolism.

How it's treated

Treatment measures include:

• oxygen therapy to correct hypoxemia

• fluid restriction to decrease preload and minimize workload of the right ventricle.

In severe cases with irreversible changes, heart-lung transplantation may be necessary.

In severe cases with irreversible changes, heart-lung transplantation may be necessary.

Diverse drugs

Your patient may receive:

• inotropic medications such as digoxin to increase cardiac output

• diuretics to decrease intravascular volume and venous return

• calcium channel blockers and other vasodilators (possibly including continuous vasodilator infusion therapy) to reduce myocardial workload and oxygen consumption

• bronchodilators to relax smooth muscles and increase airway patency

• beta-adrenergic blockers to reduce cardiac workload and improve oxygenation

• anticoagulant therapy in case of concurrent hypercoagulability.

What to do

• Assess cardiopulmonary status. Auscultate heart and breath sounds, being alert for S_3 heart sounds, murmurs, or crackles indicative of heart failure. Monitor vital signs, oxygen saturation, and heart rhythm.

- Assess hemodynamic status, including PAP and PAWP every 2 hours or more often, depending on the patient's condition, and report any changes.
- Monitor intake and output closely and obtain daily weights. Institute fluid restriction as ordered.
- Administer medications as ordered to promote adequate heart and lung function. Assess for potential adverse reactions, such as postural hypotension with diuretics and beta-adrenergic blockers.
- Administer supplemental oxygen as ordered and organize care to allow rest periods.

Administer drugs as ordered to promote adequate heart and lung function.

Status asthmaticus

Status asthmaticus is a life-threatening situation resulting from an acute asthma attack. It begins with impaired gas exchange and—without rapid intervention—may lead to respiratory failure and, eventually, death.

Asthma overview

Asthma is a chronic inflammatory airway disorder that causes episodic airway obstruction and hyperresponsiveness of the airway to multiple stimuli. It results from bronchospasms, increased mucus secretion, and mucosal edema. If left untreated or if the patient doesn't respond to drug therapy after 24 hours, status asthmaticus is diagnosed.

Making things worse

Asthma exacerbations are acute or subacute episodes of worsening shortness of breath, coughing, and wheezing, with measurable decreases in expiratory airflow.

What causes it

Many asthmatics, especially children, have intrinsic and extrinsic asthma.

Extrinsic allergens, such as pollen and pet dander, can trigger an asthma attack.

Outside factors

Extrinsic, or *atopic*, asthma begins in childhood. Patients are typically sensitive to specific external allergens. Extrinsic allergens that can trigger an asthma attack include such elements as pollen, animal dander, house dust or mold, kapok or feather pillows, food additives containing sulfites, and other sensitizing substances.

Extrinsic asthma in childhood is commonly accompanied by other hereditary allergies, such as eczema and allergic rhinitis.

Factors within

Patients with *intrinsic*, or *nonatopic*, asthma react to internal, nonallergenic factors. Intrinsic factors that can trigger an asthma attack include irritants, emotional stress, fatigue, endocrine changes, temperature variations, humidity variations, exposure to noxious fumes, anxiety, coughing or laughing, and genetic factors.

Most episodes occur after a severe respiratory tract infection, especially in adults.

Irritants in the workplace

Many adults acquire an allergic form of asthma or exacerbation of existing asthma from exposure to agents in the workplace. Such irritants as chemicals in flour, acid anhydrides, and excreta of dust mites in carpet are a few such agents that trigger asthma.

Genetic messes

Asthma is associated with two genetic influences, including:
• the ability to develop asthma because of an abnormal gene (atopy)
• the tendency to develop hyperresponsive airways (without atopy).

A potent mix

Environmental factors interact with inherited factors to cause asthmatic reactions with associated bronchospasms.

Pathophysiology

Status asthmaticus begins with an asthma attack. In asthma, bronchial linings overreact to various stimuli, causing episodic smooth-muscle spasms that severely constrict the airways. (See *Understanding asthma.*)
Here's how asthma develops into status asthmaticus:
• Immunoglobulin (Ig) E antibodies attached to histamine-containing mast cells and receptors on cell membranes initiate
intrinsic asthma attacks.
• When exposed to an antigen, such as pollen, the IgE antibody combines with the antigen.
• On subsequent exposure to the antigen, mast cells degranulate and release mediators.
• Mast cells in the lung are stimulated to release histamine and the slow-reacting substance of anaphylaxis.
• Histamine attaches to receptor sites in the larger bronchi, where it causes swelling in smooth muscles.

Hah! Most intrinsic asthma attacks in adults follow severe respiratory tract infection.

When exposed to antigens such as pollen, mast cells in the lung release histamine, which causes swelling in smooth muscles.

Understanding asthma

Asthma is an inflammatory disease of the airways. The inflammation causes hyperresponsive-ness (to various stimuli) and bronchospasms occur. Here's how an asthma attack progresses:

Histamine attaches to receptor sites in larger bronchi, causing swelling of the smooth muscles.

Histamine

Leukotrienes attach to receptor sites in the smaller bronchi and cause swelling of smooth muscle there. Leukotrienes also cause prostaglandins to travel via the bloodstream to the lungs, where they enhance histamine's effects.

Leukotrienes

Histamine stimulates the mucous membranes to secrete excessive mucus, further narrowing the bronchial lumen. On inhalation, the narrowed bronchial lumen can still expand slightly; however, on exhalation, the increased intrathoracic pressure closes the bronchial lumen completely.

Bronchial lumen on inhalation

Bronchial lumen on exhalation

Mucus fills lung bases, inhibiting alveolar ventilation. Blood is shunted to alveoli in other parts of the lungs, but it still can't compensate for diminished ventilation.

• Mucous membranes become inflamed, irritated, and swollen. The patient may experience dyspnea, prolonged expiration, and an increased respiratory rate.
• Leukotrienes attach to receptor sites in the smaller bronchi and cause local swelling of the smooth muscle.

• Leukotrienes also cause prostaglandins to travel by way of the bloodstream to the lungs, where they enhance the effect of histamine. A wheeze may be audible during coughing; the higher the pitch, the narrower is the bronchial lumen.

• Histamine stimulates the mucous membranes to secrete excessive mucus, further narrowing the bronchial lumen.

• Goblet cells secrete viscous mucus that's difficult to cough up, resulting in coughing, rhonchi, increased-pitch wheezing, and increased respiratory distress. Mucosal edema and thickened secretions further block the airways.

• On inhalation, the narrowed bronchial lumen can still expand slightly, allowing air to reach the alveoli. On exhalation, increased intrathoracic pressure closes the bronchial lumen completely. Air enters but can't escape.

• When status asthmaticus occurs, hypoxemia worsens and expiratory rate and volume decrease even further.

• Obstructed airways impede gas exchange and increase airway resistance. The patient labors to breathe.

• As breathing and hypoxemia tire the patient, respiratory rate drops to normal, $Paco_2$ levels rise and the patient hypoventilates from exhaustion.

• Respiratory acidosis develops as $Paco_2$ increases.

• The situation becomes life-threatening when no air is audible on auscultation (a silent chest) and $Paco_2$ rises to over 70 mm Hg.

• Without treatment, the patient experiences acute respiratory failure.

What to look for

An asthma attack may begin slowly or dramatically. Progressive cyanosis, confusion, and lethargy may indicate that the acute asthma attack has progressed to status asthmaticus.

What the patient reports

Typically, the patient reports exposure to a particular allergen followed by a sudden onset of dyspnea, wheezing, and tightness in the chest accompanied by a cough that produces thick clear or yellow sputum.

The patient may complain of feeling suffocated, appear visibly dyspneic, and be able to speak only a few words before pausing to catch his breath.

What you may find

Mental status is a sensitive indicator of oxygen deprivation, and the patient may initially be irritable or anxious. As hypoxemia progresses, the patient becomes confused and increasingly lethargic, a sign of impending respiratory failure.

Your patient's mental status is a sensitive indicator of oxygen deprivation that may signal impending respiratory failure.

The patient's heart rate is elevated and commonly irregular. Respiratory rate is also well above normal. When the patient begins to tire, his respiratory rate begins to slow, which may be another sign of impending respiratory failure if the patient is also confused and lethargic.

On inspection, you may see a barrel chest if the patient has chronic asthma. During an attack, the patient's face may appear pale and diaphoretic and he may use accessory muscles of respiration. The patient generally sits bolt upright or leans forward slightly.

On percussing the chest wall, you may find hyperresonance; palpation may reveal vocal fremitus.

Listen to the lungs

When you listen to the lungs, you may hear harsh respirations with inspiratory and expiratory wheezes and, possibly, reduced breath sounds over some areas of the lung. The expiratory phase of respiration is prolonged. Marked wheezing may develop due to increased edema and mucus in the lower airways.

Breath sounds and wheezing may suddenly stop (status) because of severe bronchoconstriction and edema.

What tests tell you

These tests are used to establish the diagnosis:
• Pulmonary function tests reveal decreased vital capacity and increased total lung and residual capacities during an acute attack. Peak and expiratory flow rate measurements are less than 60% of baseline.
• Pulse oximetry commonly shows that oxygen saturation is less than 90%.
• Chest X-ray may show hyperinflation with areas of atelectasis and flat diaphragm due to increased intrathoracic volume.
• ABG analysis reveals decreasing Pao_2 and increasing $Paco_2$.
• ECG shows sinus tachycardia during an attack.
• Sputum analysis may indicate increased viscosity, mucus plugs, presence of Curschmann's spirals (casts of airways), Charcot-Leyden crystals, and eosinophils; culture may disclose causative organisms if infection is the trigger.
• A complete blood count with differential shows an increased eosinophil count secondary to inflammation and an elevated WBC count and granulocyte count if an acute infection is present.

How it's treated

In acute status asthmaticus, the patient is monitored closely for respiratory failure. Oxygen, bronchodilators, epinephrine, corticosteroids, and nebulizer therapies may be ordered. The patient may be intubated and placed on mechanical ventilation if $Paco_2$ increases or if respiratory arrest occurs.

Addressing asthma

Correcting asthma typically involves:
• prevention by identifying and avoiding precipitating factors, such as environmental allergens or irritants
• desensitization to specific antigens if the stimuli can't be removed entirely, which decreases the severity of asthma attacks with future exposure
• bronchodilators (such as epinephrine, albuterol) to decrease bronchoconstriction, reduce bronchial airway edema, and increase pulmonary ventilation
• anticholinergics to increase the effects of bronchodilators
• corticosteroids (such as methylprednisolone) to decrease bronchoconstriction, reduce bronchial airway edema, and increase pulmonary ventilation
• subcutaneous epinephrine to counteract the effects of mediators of an asthma attack
• mast cell stabilizers (cromolyn [Intal] and nedocromil [Tilade] in patients with atopic asthma who have seasonal disease; when given prophylactically, they block the acute obstructive effects of antigen exposure by inhibiting the degranulation of mast cells, thereby preventing the release of chemical mediators responsible for anaphylaxis
• humidified oxygen to correct dyspnea, cyanosis, and hypoxemia and to maintain an oxygen saturation greater than 90%
• mechanical ventilation, which is necessary if the patient doesn't respond to initial ventilatory support and drugs or develops respiratory failure
• relaxation exercises to increase circulation and aid recovery from an asthma attack.

> Listen up! If your patient suddenly stops wheezing, respiratory collapse may be imminent.

What to do

• Conduct careful and frequent assessment of the patient's respiratory status, especially if the patient isn't intubated. Check the respiratory rate, auscultate breath sounds, and monitor oxygen saturation.
• Be alert for a patient who was wheezing but suddenly stops wheezing and continues to show signs of respiratory distress. In this case the absence of wheezing may be due to severe bronchial constriction that narrows the airways severely during inhalation and exhalation. As a result, so little air passes through the narrowed airways that no sound is made. This is a sign of

imminent respiratory collapse; the patient needs intubation and mechanical ventilation. Reassure the patient and stay with him. Help him to relax as much as possible.

• Assess the patient's mental status for confusion, agitation, or lethargy.

• Assess the patient's heart rate and rhythm. Be alert for cardiac arrhythmias related to bronchodilator therapy or hypoxemia.

• Obtain ordered tests and report results promptly.

• Administer medications as ordered. I.V. fluids are commonly ordered to replace insensible fluid loss from hyperventilation.

• When the acute phase is over, position the patient for maximum comfort, usually in semi-Fowler's position. Encourage coughing to clear secretions. Offer emotional support and reassurance.

Quick quiz

1. When auscultating a patient's lungs, you hear crackles. These are caused by:

    A.   secretions blocking the bronchial airways.

    B.   collapsed or fluid-filled alveoli snapping open.

    C.   a foreign body obstructing the trachea.

    D.   consolidation.

Answer: B. Crackles are caused by alveoli opening and are usually associated with fluid in the alveolar space.

2. Which ABG analysis results would you expect to find in a patient with acute respiratory failure?

    A.   pH 7.25, Pao_2 48, $Paco_2$ 55

    B.   pH 7.40, Pao_2 82, $Paco_2$ 45

    C.   pH 7.50, Pao_2 60, $Paco_2$ 30

    D.   pH 7.30, Pao_2 85, $Paco_2$ 48

Answer: A. The patient with a Pao_2 less than 50, a decreased pH, and elevated $Paco_2$ is hypoxemic and in respiratory acidosis.

3. Which option isn't a method of weaning a patient from mechanical ventilation?

    A.   Intermittent mandatory ventilation

    B.   Pressure support ventilation

    C.   Spontaneous breathing trials with T-piece

    D.   Controlled mandatory ventilation

Answer: D. Controlled mandatory ventilation is used when the patient can't initiate spontaneous breaths, such as a patient paralyzed because of a spinal cord injury. It isn't an acceptable weaning method.

4. ET tubes have inflatable cuffs to:
A. measure pressure on tracheal tissues.
B. drain gastric contents.
C. prevent backflow of oxygen.
D. treat laryngeal edema.

Answer: C. ET tube cuffs prevent backflow of oxygen so that it's delivered fully to the lungs.

5. A patient diagnosed with status asthmaticus who was previously wheezing suddenly stops wheezing and continues to show signs of respiratory distress. Your assessment findings would indicate that:
A his condition is slowly improving.
B. he's in imminent danger of respiratory collapse.
C. he isn't as sick as you thought because he stopped wheezing.
D. you need more information because wheezing isn't a sensitive indicator of asthma.

Answer: B. Wheezing that stops suddenly when signs of respiratory distress continue indicates severe bronchial constriction with little air movement during inspiration and expiration. This is a dangerous event, requiring immediate intervention to prevent respiratory collapse.

Scoring

☆☆☆ If you answered all five questions correctly, breathe a big sigh of relief. You're a respiratory mastermind!

☆☆ If you answered four questions correctly, don't wait to exhale. You're an inspiration!

☆ If you answered fewer than four questions correctly, you're on the verge of expiration. Take a deep breath and dive back into the chapter.

Guess what the next chapter is about...That's right! It's the GI system!

Gastrointestinal system

Just the facts

In this chapter, you'll learn:

♦ structure and function of the GI system
♦ assessment of the GI system
♦ diagnostic tests and treatments
♦ GI disorders and related nursing care.

Understanding the GI system

The GI system has two major components: the alimentary canal (also called the *GI tract*) and accessory organs of digestion.

GI function

The two major functions of the GI tract are:
• digestion, or breaking down food and fluid into simple chemicals that can be absorbed into the blood-stream and transported through the body
• elimination of wastes through excretion of stool.

GI failure

The GI system has a profound effect on a person's overall health. When a GI process malfunctions, the patient can experience problems ranging from loss of appetite to acid-base imbalance.

> The GI system has a profound effect on overall health.

Alimentary canal

The alimentary canal is a hollow muscular tube that begins in the mouth and extends to the anus. It includes the pharynx, esophagus, stomach, and small and large intestines. (See *Structures of the GI system*, page 392.)

Structures of the GI system

The GI system includes the alimentary canal (pharynx, esophagus, stomach, and small and large intestines) and the accessory organs (liver, biliary duct system, and pancreas). These structures are illustrated below.

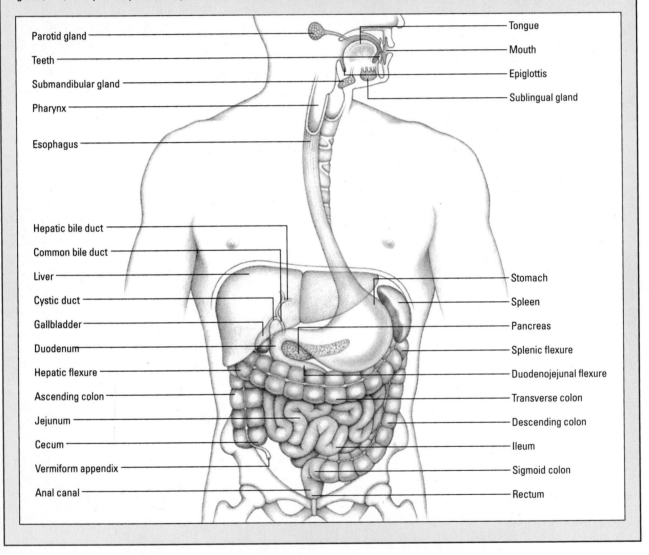

Mouth

Digestion begins in the mouth with chewing, salivating, and swallowing. The tongue provides a person's sense of taste. Saliva moistens food during chewing and is produced by three pairs of glands:

1. parotid

2. submandibular

3. sublingual.

Pharynx

The pharynx, or throat, is a cavity that extends from the oral cavity to the esophagus. The pharynx assists in swallowing by grasping food and propelling it toward the esophagus.

Esophagus

The esophagus is a muscular tube that extends from the pharynx through the mediastinum to the stomach. When food is swallowed, the cricopharyngeal sphincter — a sphincter at the upper border of the esophagus — relaxes for food to enter the esophagus. Peristalsis propels liquids and solids through the esophagus into the stomach.

How perfect! Peristalsis propels liquids and solids through the esophagus into me!

Stomach

The stomach, a reservoir for food, is a collapsible, pouchlike structure in the left upper part of the abdominal cavity, just below the diaphragm. Its upper border is attached to the lower end of the esophagus. The lateral surface of the stomach is called the *greater curvature;* the medial surface, the *lesser curvature.*

Distinctive sphincters

The stomach contains two important sphincters:

1. the cardiac sphincter, which protects the entrance to the stomach

2. the pyloric sphincter, which guards the exit.

Food processor

The stomach has several major functions. It:
- serves as a temporary storage area for food
- begins digestion
- breaks down food into chyme, a semifluid substance
- moves the gastric contents into the small intestine.

Small intestine

The small intestine is about 20′ (6 m) long and is named for its diameter, not its length. Nearly all digestion and nutrient absorption takes place in the small intestine.

There are three major divisions of the small intestine:

- duodenum, the longest and most superior division

- jejunum, the middle and shortest segment

- ileum, the most inferior portion.

Absorptive wall

The intestinal wall has several structural features that increase its absorptive surface area, including:
• plicae circulares, which are circular folds of the intestinal mucosa
• villi, which are fingerlike projections on the mucosa
• microvilli, which are tiny cytoplasmic projections on the surface of epithelial cells.

The small intestines also contain:
• intestinal crypts of Lieberkühn, which are simple glands lodged in the grooves separating villi
• Peyer's patches, which are collections of lymphatic tissue within the submucosa
• Brunner's glands, which secrete mucus.

Small intestine functions, no small feat

The small intestine functions by:
• completing food digestion
• absorbing food molecules, water, and vitamins through its wall into the circulatory system, which then delivers them to cells throughout the body
• secreting hormones that control the secretion of bile, pancreatic juices, and intestinal juice.

Large intestine

The large intestine, or colon, has six segments:

The cecum, a saclike structure, makes up the first few inches. It's connected to the ileum of the small intestine by the ileocecal pouch.

The ascending colon rises on the right posterior abdominal wall and then turns sharply under the liver at the hepatic flexure.

There's nothing small about the job of the small intestine. It does most of the digesting and absorbing!

The transverse colon is situated above the small intestine, passing horizontally across the abdomen and below the liver, stomach, and spleen. At the left colic flexure, it turns downward.

The descending colon starts near the spleen and extends down the left side of the abdomen into the pelvic cavity.

The sigmoid colon descends through the pelvic cavity, where it becomes the rectum.

The rectum, the last few inches of the large intestine, terminates at the anus.

Food's finale

The functions of the large intestine include absorbing excess water and electrolytes, storing food residue, and eliminating waste products in the form of feces.

The large intestine, or colon, consists of six segments.

Accessory organs of digestion

The accessory organs of the GI tract are the liver, gallbladder, and pancreas. They contribute hormones, enzymes, and bile, which are vital to digestion.

Liver

The liver is located in the right upper quadrant under the diaphragm. It has four lobes:
- left lobe
- right lobe
- caudate lobe (behind the right lobe)
- quadrate lobe (behind the left lobe).

Liver's lobule

The liver's functional unit is called the *lobule*. It consists of hepatic cells, or hepatocytes, that encircle a central vein and radiate outward.

Separating the hepatocytes' plates from each other are sinusoids, the liver's capillary system. Reticuloendothelial macrophages (Kupffer's cells) that line the sinusoids remove bacteria and toxins that enter the blood through the intestinal capillaries.

Liver at work

The liver's functions include:
- metabolizing carbohydrates, fats, and proteins

I may be considered an accessory, but my role is important.

- detoxifying various endogenous and exogenous toxins in plasma
- converting ammonia to urea for excretion
- synthesizing plasma proteins, nonessential amino acids, and vitamin A
- storing essential nutrients, such as iron and vitamins D, K, and B_{12}
- regulating blood glucose levels
- secreting bile.

Gallbladder

The gallbladder is a small, pear-shaped organ that lies halfway under the right lobe of the liver. It stores and concentrates bile produced by the liver and then releases bile into the common bile duct for delivery to the duodenum in response to the contraction and relaxation of the sphincter of Oddi.

Bile talk

Bile is a greenish liquid composed of water, cholesterol, bile salts, and phospholipids. It has several functions, including emulsifying (breaking down) fat and promoting intestinal absorption of fatty acids, cholesterol, and other lipids.

Pancreas

The pancreas lies horizontally in the abdomen behind the stomach. Its head and neck extend into the curve of the duodenum and its tail lies against the spleen. The pancreas performs exocrine and endocrine functions. (See *A look at the biliary tract.*)

Exocrine function and enzymes

The pancreas's exocrine function involves scattered cells that secrete more than 1,000 ml of digestive enzymes every day. Vagal stimulation and release of the hormones secretin and cholecystokinin control the rate and amount of pancreatic secretion.

Clustered lobules and lobes (acini) of enzyme-producing cells release their secretions into the pancreatic duct. The pancreatic duct runs the length of the pancreas and joins the bile duct from the gallbladder before entering the duodenum.

I'm a multifunctional little organ! I perform exocrine and endocrine functions.

Endocrine function and hormones

The endocrine function of the pancreas involves the islets of Langerhans, located between the acinar cells. Over 1 million of these islets house two cell types:

A look at the biliary tract

Together, the gallbladder and pancreas constitute the biliary tract. The illustration below shows the parts of the biliary tract.

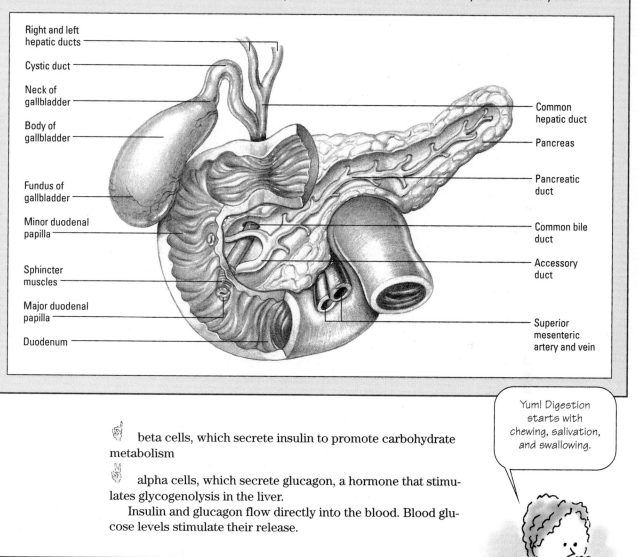

Right and left hepatic ducts

Cystic duct

Neck of gallbladder

Body of gallbladder

Fundus of gallbladder

Minor duodenal papilla

Sphincter muscles

Major duodenal papilla

Duodenum

Common hepatic duct

Pancreas

Pancreatic duct

Common bile duct

Accessory duct

Superior mesenteric artery and vein

beta cells, which secrete insulin to promote carbohydrate metabolism

alpha cells, which secrete glucagon, a hormone that stimulates glycogenolysis in the liver.

Insulin and glucagon flow directly into the blood. Blood glucose levels stimulate their release.

Digestion and elimination

Digestion starts in the oral cavity, where chewing (mastication), salivating (the beginning of starch digestion), and swallowing (deglutition) all take place.

Yum! Digestion starts with chewing, salivation, and swallowing.

Down it goes!

When a person swallows, the hypopharyngeal sphincter in the upper esophagus relaxes, allowing food to enter the esophagus. In the esophagus, the glossopharyngeal nerve activates peristalsis, which moves the food down toward the stomach. As food passes through the esophagus, glands secrete mucus, which lubricates the bolus.

Gotta get gastrin

As the food bolus reaches the stomach, digestive juices (hydrochloric acid and pepsin) are secreted. When the food enters the stomach through the cardiac sphincter, the stomach wall stretches. This distention of the stomach wall stimulates the stomach to release gastrin.

Gastrin stimulates the stomach's motor functions and secretion of gastric juices by the gastric gland. These digestive secretions consist mainly of:

- pepsin
- hydrochloric acid
- intrinsic factor
- proteolytic enzymes.

Not much for absorption

Little food absorption, except for alcohol, occurs in the stomach. Peristaltic contractions churn the food into tiny particles and mix it with gastric juices, forming chyme. Peristaltic waves move the chyme into the antrum of the stomach, where it backs up against the pyloric sphincter before being released into the duodenum.

> By the time chyme enters the large intestine, it's mostly indigestible.

Digestion and absorption powerhouse

The small intestine performs most of the work of digestion and absorption. Intestinal contractions and various digestive secretions break down carbohydrates, proteins, and fats, actions that enable the intestinal mucosa to absorb these nutrients into the bloodstream (along with water and electrolytes).

Small to large

By the time chyme passes through the small intestine and enters the ascending colon of the large intestine, it has been reduced to mostly indigestible substances.

Journey through the large intestine

The food bolus begins its journey through the large intestine where the ileum and cecum join with the ileocecal pouch. Then the bolus moves up the ascending colon, past the right abdominal cavity, to the liver's lower border. It crosses horizontally below the liver and stomach by way of the transverse colon and descends through the left abdominal cavity to the iliac fossa through the descending colon.

From there, the bolus travels through the sigmoid colon to the lower midline of the abdominal cavity, then to the rectum, and finally to the anal canal. The anus opens to the exterior through two sphincters:
• The internal sphincter contains thick, circular smooth muscle under autonomic control.
• The external sphincter contains skeletal muscle under voluntary control.

All about the absorption

The large intestine produces no hormones or digestive enzymes; it continues the absorptive process. Through blood and lymph vessels in the submucosa, the proximal half of the large intestine absorbs all but about 100 ml of the remaining water in the colon. It also absorbs large amounts of sodium and chloride.

Harboring the enemy?

The large intestine harbors the bacteria *Escherichia coli*, *Enterobacter aerogenes*, *Clostridium perfringens*, and *Lactobacillus bifidus*. All of these bacteria aid in synthesizing vitamin K and breaking down cellulose into a usable carbohydrate. Bacterial action also produces flatus, which helps propel stool toward the rectum.

We're not all bad! Some bacteria help break down cellulose into a usable carbohydrate.

Lube job

In addition, the mucosa of the large intestine produces alkaline secretions. This alkaline mucus lubricates the intestinal walls and protects the mucosa from acidic bacterial action.

Elimination round

In the lower colon, long and relatively sluggish contractions cause propulsive waves. Normally occurring several times per day, these movements propel intestinal contents into the rectum and produce the urge to defecate. Defecation normally results from the defecation reflex, a sensory and parasympathetic nerve-mediated response, along with the voluntary relaxation of the external anal sphincter.

GI assessment

Being able to identify subtle changes in a patient's GI system can mean all the difference between effective and ineffective care. GI signs and symptoms can have many baffling causes. When your patient is critically ill, your GI assessment can be used to determine whether the patient's signs and symptoms are related to his current medical problem or indicate a new problem.

Unless the critically ill patient requires immediate stabilizing treatment, begin by taking a thorough patient history. Then probe further by conducting a thorough physical examination, using inspection, auscultation, palpation, and percussion.

History

In the health history, include information about the patient's chief complaint, medications used, family history, and social history. Conduct this part of the assessment as privately as possible because the patient may feel embarrassment when talking about GI functions.

> Listen up! Your patient is likely to report pain, heartburn, and other GI-related signs and symptoms.

Current health status

The patient with a GI problem usually complains of:
• pain
• heartburn
• nausea
• vomiting
• altered bowel habits.

To investigate these and other signs and symptoms, ask about the onset, duration, and severity of each. Also, inquire about the location of the pain, precipitating factors, alleviating factors, and associated symptoms. (See *Asking the right questions*.)

Previous health status

To determine if the patient's problem is new or recurring, ask about GI illnesses, such as an ulcer, gallbladder disease, inflammatory bowel disease, or GI bleeding. Also, ask if he has had abdominal surgery or trauma.

Further questions

Ask the patient additional questions, such as:
• Are you allergic to any foods or medications?

Asking the right questions

When assessing a patient with GI-related signs and symptoms, be sure to ask the right questions. To establish a baseline for comparison, ask about the patient's current state of health, including questions about the onset, duration, quality, severity, and location of problems as well as precipitating factors, alleviating factors, and associated symptoms.

Onset

How did the problem start? Was it gradual or sudden and with or without previous symptoms? What was the patient doing when he noticed it? If he has diarrhea, has he been traveling? If so, when and where?

Duration

When did the problem start? Has the patient had the problem before? Has he had any abdominal surgery. If yes, when? If he's in pain, find out when the problem began. Is the pain continuous, intermittent, or colicky (cramplike)?

Quality

Ask the patient to describe the problem. Has he ever had it before? Was it diagnosed? If he's in pain, find out whether the pain feels sharp, dull, aching, or burning.

Severity

Ask the patient to describe how badly the problem bothers him — for example, have him rate it on a pain scale of 0 to 10. Does it keep him from his normal activities? Has it improved or worsened since he first noticed it? Does it wake him at night? If he's in pain, does he double over from it?

Location

Where does the patient feel the problem? Does it spread, radiate, or shift? Ask him to point to where he feels it the most.

Precipitating factors

Does anything seem to bring on the problem? What makes it worse? Does it occur at the same time each day or with certain positions? Does the patient notice it after eating or drinking certain foods or after certain activities?

Alleviating factors

Does anything relieve the problem? Does the patient take any prescribed or over-the-counter medications for relief? Has he tried anything else for relief?

Associated symptoms

What else bothers the patient when he has the problem? Has he had nausea, vomiting, dry heaves, diarrhea, constipation, bloating, or flatulence? Has he lost his appetite or lost or gained any weight? If so, how much? When was the patient's last bowel movement? Was it unusual? Has he seen blood in his vomitus or stool? Has his stool changed in size or color or included mucus? Ask the patient whether he can eat normally and hold down foods and liquids. Also, ask about alcohol consumption.

• Have you noticed a change in the color, amount, and appearance of your stool? Have you ever seen blood in your stool?
• Have you recently traveled abroad? (if reason for seeking care is diarrhea because diarrhea, hepatitis, and parasitic infections can result from ingesting contaminated food or water)
• Ask him about his dental history. Poor dentition may impair his ability to chew and swallow food.

Don't forget the drugs

Ask the patient if he's taking medication. Several drugs, including aspirin, sulfonamides, nonsteroidal anti-inflammatory drugs (NSAIDs), analgesics, and some antihypertensives, can cause nausea, vomiting, diarrhea, constipation, and other GI signs and symptoms. Be sure to ask about laxative use because habitual intake can cause constipation.

Family history

Because some GI disorders are hereditary, ask the patient whether anyone in his family has had a GI disorder. Disorders with a familial link include:
- ulcerative colitis
- colon cancer
- stomach ulcers
- diabetes
- alcoholism
- Crohn's disease.

> Family history can be important because some GI disorders are hereditary.

Lifestyle patterns

Psychological and sociologic factors can profoundly affect health. To determine factors that may have contributed to your patient's problem, ask about his occupation, home life, financial situation, stress level, and recent life changes.

Be sure to ask about alcohol, illegal drug, caffeine, and tobacco use as well as food consumption, exercise habits, and oral hygiene. Also ask about sleep patterns, such as hours of sleep and whether sleep is restful.

Cultural factors may affect a patient's dietary habits, so ask about any dietary restrictions the patient has such as following a vegetarian diet.

> You should inspect and palpate your patient's mouth, as part of your physical examination.

Physical examination

Physical examination of the GI system usually includes evaluation of the mouth, abdomen, liver, and rectum. Before beginning your examination, explain the techniques you'll be using and warn the patient that some procedures might be uncomfortable. Perform the examination in a private, quiet, warm, and well-lighted room.

Assessing the mouth

Use inspection and palpation to assess the oral cavity:
- First, inspect the patient's mouth and jaw for asymmetry and swelling. Check his bite, noting

malocclusion from an overbite or underbite. If the patient has dentures, do they fit? Are they intact or broken?
• Inspect the inner and outer lips, teeth, and gums with a penlight. Note bleeding, gum ulcerations, and missing, displaced, or broken teeth. Palpate the gums for tenderness and the inner lips and cheeks for lesions.
• Assess the tongue, checking for coating, tremors, swelling, and ulcerations. Note unusual breath odors.
• Finally, examine the pharynx, looking for uvular deviation, tonsillar abnormalities, lesions, plaques, and exudate.

Assessing the abdomen

When assessing the abdomen, perform the four basic steps in the following sequence: inspection, auscultation, percussion, and palpation. The GI system requires abdominal auscultation before percussion and palpation because the latter can alter intestinal activity and bowel sounds.

Examination preparation

To ensure an accurate assessment, before the examination:
• Ask the patient to empty his bladder, or insert an indwelling urinary catheter as ordered.
• Drape the patient appropriately.
• Place a small pillow under the patient's knees to relax the abdominal muscles.
• Keep the room warm. Chilling can cause abdominal muscles to tense.
• Warm your hands and the stethoscope.
• Speak softly, and encourage the patient to perform breathing exercises or use imagery during uncomfortable procedures.
• Assess painful areas last to avoid the patient becoming tense.

Abdominal inspection

Before inspecting the abdomen, mentally divide it into four quadrants. (See *Identifying abdominal landmarks*, page 404.)

General inspection

Begin by performing a general inspection of the patient:
• Observe the skin, oral mucosa, nail beds, and sclera for jaundice or signs of anemia.
• Stand at the foot of the bed and observe the abdomen for symmetry, checking for bumps, bulges, or masses. A bulge may indicate bladder distention or hernia.
• Note the patient's abdominal shape and contour. The abdomen should be flat to rounded in people of average weight. A protruding abdomen may be caused by obesity, pregnancy, ascites, or ab-

Keep in mind that obesity, pregnancy, ascites, or abdominal distention can make the patient's abdomen protrude.

Identifying abdominal landmarks

To aid accurate abdominal assessment and documentation of findings, you can mentally divide the patient's abdomen into regions. Use the quadrant method—the easiest and most commonly used method—to divide the abdomen into four equal regions using two imaginary perpendicular lines crossing above the umbilicus.

Right upper quadrant
- Liver and gallbladder
- Pylorus
- Duodenum
- Head of pancreas
- Hepatic flexure of colon
- Portions of ascending and transverse colon

Left upper quadrant
- Left liver lobe
- Stomach
- Body of pancreas
- Splenic flexure of colon
- Portions of transverse and descending colon

Right lower quadrant
- Cecum and appendix
- Portion of ascending colon
- Lower portion of right kidney
- Bladder (if distended)

Left lower quadrant
- Sigmoid colon
- Portion of descending colon
- Lower portion of left kidney
- Bladder (if distended)

dominal distention. A slender person may have a slightly concave abdomen.

• Next, inspect the abdominal skin, which normally appears smooth and intact. Striae, or stretch marks, can be caused by pregnancy, excessive weight gain, or ascites. New striae are pink or blue; old striae are silvery white. In patients with darker skin, striae may be dark brown. Note dilated veins. Record the length of any surgical scars on the abdomen.

• Note abdominal movements and pulsations. Usually, waves of peristalsis aren't visible unless the patient is very thin, in which case they may be visible as slight wavelike motions. Marked visible rippling may indicate bowel obstruction; report it immediately. In a thin patient, pulsation of the aorta is visible in the epigastric area. Marked pulsations may occur with hypertension, aortic insufficiency, and other conditions causing widening pulse pressure.

Abdominal auscultation

Auscultation provides information about bowel motility and the underlying vessels and organs.

Follow the clock

Use a stethoscope to auscultate for bowel and vascular sounds. Lightly place the stethoscope diaphragm in the right lower quadrant, slightly below and to the right of the umbilicus. Auscultate in a clockwise fashion in each of the four quadrants, spending at least 2 minutes in each area. Note the character and quality of bowel sounds in each quadrant. In some cases, you may need to auscultate for 5 minutes before you hear sounds. Be sure to allow enough time to listen in each quadrant before you decide that bowel sounds are absent.

Tube tip

Before auscultating the abdomen of a patient with a nasogastric (NG) tube or another abdominal tube connected to suction, briefly clamp the tube or turn off the suction. Suction noises can obscure or mimic actual bowel sounds.

Sound class

Bowel sounds are classified as normal, hypoactive, or hyperactive:
• *Normal* bowel sounds are high-pitched, gurgling noises caused by air mixing with fluid during peristalsis. The noises vary in frequency, pitch, and intensity and occur irregularly from 5 to 34 times per minute. They're loudest before mealtimes. Borborygmus, or stomach growling, is the loud, gurgling, splashing sound heard over the large intestine as gas passes through it.
• *Hypoactive* bowel sounds are heard infrequently. They're associated with ileus, bowel obstruction, or peritonitis and indicate diminished peristalsis. Paralytic ileus, torsion of the bowel, or the use of narcotics and other medications can decrease peristalsis.
• *Hyperactive* bowel sounds are loud, high-pitched, tinkling sounds that occur frequently and may be caused by diarrhea, constipation, or laxative use.

Sound off

Next, use the bell of the stethoscope to auscultate for vascular sounds. Normally, you should detect no vascular sounds. Note a bruit, venous hum, or friction rub. (See *Interpreting abnormal abdominal sounds*, page 406.)

Auscultate for at least 2 minutes in each of the four abdominal quadrants.

Listen for normal, hypoactive, or hyperactive bowel sounds.

Interpreting abnormal abdominal sounds

Sound and description	Location	Possible cause
Abnormal bowel sounds Hyperactive sounds (unrelated to hunger)	Any quadrant	Diarrhea, laxative use, or early intestinal obstruction
Hypoactive, then absent sounds	Any quadrant	Paralytic ileus or peritonitis
High-pitched tinkling sounds	Any quadrant	Intestinal fluid and air under tension in a dilated bowel
High-pitched rushing sounds coinciding with abdominal cramps	Any quadrant	Intestinal obstruction
Systolic bruits Vascular blowing sounds resembling cardiac murmurs	Over abdominal aorta	Partial arterial obstruction or turbulent blood flow
	Over renal artery	Renal artery stenosis
	Over iliac artery	Iliac artery obstruction
Venous hum Continuous, medium-pitched tone created by blood flow in a large engorged vascular organ such as the liver	Epigastric and umbilical regions	Increased collateral circulation between portal and systemic venous systems, such as in cirrhosis
Friction rub Harsh, grating sound like two pieces of sandpaper rubbing together	Over liver and spleen	Inflammation of the peritoneal surface of liver, such as from a tumor

Abdominal percussion

Use abdominal percussion to determine the size and location of abdominal organs and detect excessive accumulation of fluid and air. Begin percussion in the right lower quadrant and proceed clockwise, covering all four quadrants. Keep the approximate locations of the patient's organs in mind as you progress. Use direct or indirect percussion:
• In direct percussion, strike your hand or finger directly over the patient's abdomen.
• With indirect percussion, use the middle finger of your dominant hand or a percussion hammer to strike a finger resting on the patient's abdomen.

Percussion precaution

Don't percuss the abdomen of a patient with an abdominal aortic aneurysm or a transplanted abdominal organ. Doing so can precipitate a rupture or organ rejection.

Tympany and dullness

Normally, you should hear two sounds during percussion of the abdomen: tympany and dullness. When you percuss over hollow organs, such as an empty stomach or bowel, you should hear a clear, hollow sound like a drum beating. This sound, tympany, predominates because air is normally present in the stomach and bowel. The degree of tympany depends on the amount of air and gastric dilation.

When you percuss over solid organs, such as the liver, kidney, or feces-filled intestines, the sound changes to dullness. Note where percussed sounds change from tympany to dullness, which may indicate a solid mass or enlarged organ.

> The degree of tympany you hear depends on the amount of air in the stomach and bowel.

Abdominal palpation

Abdominal palpation includes light and deep touch to determine the size, shape, position, and tenderness of major abdominal organs and to detect masses and fluid accumulation. Palpate all four quadrants, leaving painful and tender areas for last.

Light palpation

Use light palpation to identify muscle resistance and tenderness as well as the location of some superficial organs. To do so, gently press your fingertips ½″ to ¾″ (1.5 to 2 cm) into the abdominal wall. Use the lightest touch possible because too much pressure blunts your sensitivity.

Deep palpation

Use deep palpation by pressing the fingertips of both hands about 1½″ (3.5 cm) into the abdominal wall. Move your hands in a slightly circular fashion so that the abdominal wall moves over the underlying structures.

Deep palpation may evoke rebound tenderness when you suddenly withdraw your fingertips, a possible sign of peritoneal inflammation. (See *Eliciting abdominal pain,* page 408.)

Assessing the liver

You can estimate the size and position of the liver through percussion and palpation.

Eliciting abdominal pain

Rebound tenderness and the iliopsoas and obturator signs can indicate such conditions as appendicitis and peritonitis. You can elicit these signs of abdominal pain, as illustrated below.

Rebound tenderness

Help the patient into a supine position with his knees flexed to relax the abdominal muscles. Place your hands gently on the right lower quadrant at McBurney's point (located about midway between the umbilicus and the anterior superior iliac spine). Slowly and deeply dip your fingers into the area; then release the pressure in a quick, smooth motion. Pain on release—rebound tenderness—is a positive sign. The pain may radiate to the umbilicus.

Caution: To minimize the risk of rupturing an inflamed appendix, don't repeat this maneuver.

Iliopsoas sign

Help the patient into a supine position with his legs straight. Instruct him to raise his right leg upward as you exert slight pressure with your hand. Repeat the maneuver with the left leg. When testing either leg, increased abdominal pain is a positive result, indicating irritation of the psoas muscle.

Obturator sign

Help the patient into a supine position with his right leg flexed 90 degrees at the hip and knee. Hold the leg just above the knee and at the ankle; then rotate the leg laterally and medially. Pain in the hypogastric region is a positive sign, indicating irritation of the obturator muscle.

Percussion discussion

Percussing the liver allows you to estimate its size. Hepatomegaly is commonly associated with hepatitis and other liver disease. Liver borders may be obscured and difficult to assess. (See *Percussing the liver*.)

Palpation problem

It's usually impossible to palpate the liver in an adult patient. If palpable, the liver border feels smooth and firm, with a rounded, regular edge. A palpable liver may indicate hepatomegaly.

To palpate for hepatomegaly:

start at the lower left quadrant

have the patient take a deep breath and hold it while you palpate using the tips of your fingers

slowly move your hand up toward the costal margin and palpate while the patient exhales.

> It's usually impossible to palpate the liver in an adult patient.

Percussing the liver

Begin percussing the abdomen along the right midclavicular line, starting below the level of the umbilicus. Move upward until the percussion notes change from tympany to dullness, usually at or slightly below the costal margin. Mark the point of change with a felt-tip pen.

Then percuss downward along the right midclavicular line, starting above the nipple. Move downward until percussion notes change from normal lung resonance to dullness, usually at the 5th to 7th intercostal space. Again, mark the point of change with a felt-tip pen. Estimate the liver size by measuring the distance between the two marks.

Anatomic landmarks for liver percussion

Hand position for liver percussion

Assessing the rectum

If your patient is age 40 or older, a rectal examination may be part of your GI assessment. Explain the procedure to reassure the patient.

Perianal is primary

To perform a rectal examination, first inspect the perianal area following these steps:
• Put on gloves and spread the buttocks to expose the anus and surrounding tissue, checking for fissures, lesions, scars, inflammation, discharge, rectal prolapse, and external hemorrhoids.
• Ask the patient to strain as if he's having a bowel movement; this may reveal internal hemorrhoids, polyps, or fissures.

Rectum is next

After examining the perianal area, palpate the rectum:
• Apply a water-soluble lubricant to your gloved index finger. Tell the patient to relax and explain to him that he'll feel some pressure.
• Insert your finger into the rectum toward the umbilicus. To palpate, rotate your finger. The walls should feel soft and smooth without masses, fecal impaction, or tenderness.
• Remove your finger from the rectum and inspect the glove for stool, blood, or mucus. Test fecal material adhering to the glove for occult blood using a guaiac test.

Diagnostic tests

Many tests provide information used to guide your care of the patient with a GI problem. Even if you don't participate in testing, you should know why the test was ordered, what the results mean, and what your responsibilities are before, during, and after the test.

Diagnostic tests commonly ordered for patients with known or suspected GI disorders include endoscopy, laboratory tests, nuclear imaging scans, and radiographic tests.

> Know why a test was ordered, what the results mean, and what your responsibilities are before, during, and after testing.

Endoscopy

The doctor can directly view hollow visceral linings by using a fiber-optic endoscope. This test is used to diagnose inflammatory, ulcerative, and infectious diseases; benign and malignant neoplasms; and other esophageal, gastric, and intestinal mucosal lesions. Endoscopy can also be used for therapeutic interventions or to obtain a biopsy.

Bedside or not

The endoscopic procedure is commonly done at the bedside in the critical care unit. However, if it's performed in the procedure suite, you may accompany an unstable patient who requires monitoring.

Colonoscopy

Colonoscopy, also referred to as *lower GI endoscopy,* is used to:
• diagnose inflammatory and ulcerative bowel disease
• pinpoint lower GI bleeding
• detect lower GI abnormalities, such as tumors, polyps, hemorrhoids, and abscesses.

Nursing considerations

• Explain the procedure and its purpose, and tell the patient he'll receive I.V. premedication and conscious sedation for the procedure.
• Make sure that an informed consent form has been signed.
• Withhold all fluids and food for at least 6 to 8 hours before the test.
• Administer bowel preparation, as ordered, such as a clear liquid diet and bowel cleaning solution with electrolyte lavage. If the patient can't swallow or is unconscious, administer electrolyte lavage solution through a feeding tube or an NG tube.
• To decrease the risk of aspiration in a patient receiving electrolyte lavage solution through an NG tube, ensure proper tube placement and elevate the head of the bed or position the patient on his side. Have suction equipment available. (See *Increased risk in elderly patients.*)
• Advise the patient that he may feel the urge to defecate when the scope is inserted; encourage slow, deep breathing through the mouth, as appropriate.
• If the procedure is to be performed at the bedside, have necessary equipment for the procedure available, including emergency equipment and suction.
• Initiate an I.V. line if one isn't already in place for a patient who'll be receiving conscious sedation.
• Obtain the patient's baseline vital signs and oxygen saturation levels. Monitor cardiac rhythm.
• Administer medications, as ordered, such as midazolam (Versed) for sedation. Provide supplemental oxygen, as ordered.

Senior moment

Increased risk in elderly patients

Elderly patients are at increased risk for experiencing adverse effects from the lavage solution, including nausea, vomiting, abdominal cramps, abdominal fullness, dizziness, and fluid and electrolyte imbalances. What's more, elderly patients may have difficulty ingesting the required amount of solution because of these adverse effects.

• During the procedure, monitor the patient's vital signs, airway patency, oxygen saturation, cardiac rhythm, skin color, abdominal distention, level of consciousness (LOC), and pain tolerance.

Assess, administer, document

After colonoscopy:

• Assess your patient's vital signs and cardiopulmonary status, breath sounds, oxygen saturation, and LOC every 15 minutes for the 1st hour, every 30 minutes for the next hour, and then hourly until the patient stabilizes.

• Administer supplemental oxygen, as ordered and as indicated by oxygen saturation levels.

• Watch for adverse effects of sedation, such as respiratory depression, apnea, hypotension, excessive diaphoresis, bradycardia, and laryngospasm. Notify the doctor if any occur.

• Assess the patient's stool for evidence of frank or occult bleeding.

• Monitor the patient for signs and symptoms of perforation, such as vomiting, severe abdominal pain, abdominal distention or rigidity, and fever. Notify the doctor if any occur.

• Document the procedure, interventions, and assessment findings.

EGD

Esophagogastroduodenoscopy (EGD), also called *upper GI endoscopy,* is used to identify abnormalities of the esophagus, stomach, and small intestine, such as esophagitis, inflammatory bowel disease, Mallory-Weiss syndrome, lesions, tumors, gastritis, and polyps.

Bypass surgery

EGD eliminates the need for extensive exploratory surgery and can be used to detect small or surface lesions missed by radiography. It can also be used for sclerotherapy or to remove foreign bodies by suction (for small, soft objects) or electrocautery, snare, or forceps (for large, hard objects).

Nursing considerations

Before endoscopy:

• Explain the procedure and its purpose to the patient.

• Tell him the procedure takes about 30 minutes and that he'll receive I.V. premedication and conscious sedation during the procedure as well as a local anesthetic spray in his mouth and nose.

• Restrict food and fluids for at least 6 hours before the test.

• Make sure that an informed consent form has been signed.

• If the test is an emergency procedure, expect to insert an NG tube to aspirate contents and minimize the risk of aspiration.

EGD is A-OK! It can even eliminate the need for extensive exploratory surgery.

• Make sure that the patient's dentures and eyeglasses are removed before the test.
• If the procedure is to be performed at the bedside, have the necessary equipment available for the procedure, including suction and emergency equipment (medications such as atropine, a monitor defibrillator, and ET intubation equipment), and initiate an I.V. line if one isn't already in place.
• Monitor the patient before and throughout the procedure, including airway patency, vital signs, oxygen saturation, cardiac rhythm, abdominal distention, LOC, and pain tolerance.

After it's over

After endoscopy:
• Monitor your patient's vital signs, oxygen saturation, cardiac rhythm, and LOC every 15 minutes for the 1st hour, every 30 minutes for the next hour, and then hourly until the patient stabilizes.
• Administer oxygen therapy, as ordered.
• Place the patient in a side-lying position with the head of the bed flat until sedation wears off.
• Withhold all food and fluids until your patient's gag reflex returns. After it returns, offer ice chips and sips of water, gradually increasing the patient's intake as tolerated and allowed.
• Observe for adverse effects of sedation, such as respiratory depression, apnea, hypotension, excessive diaphoresis, bradycardia, and laryngospasm. Notify the doctor if any occur.
• Monitor the patient for signs and symptoms of perforation, such as difficulty swallowing, pain, fever, or bleeding as evidenced by black stools or bloody vomitus.
• Document the procedure, interventions, and assessment findings.

> After endoscopy, withhold all food and fluids until your patient's gag reflex returns.

Laboratory tests

Common laboratory tests used to diagnose GI disorders include studies of stool and peritoneal contents. Percutaneous liver biopsy may also be done.

Fecal studies

Normal stool appears brown and formed but soft. These abnormal findings may indicate a problem:
• Narrow, ribbonlike stool signals spastic or irritable bowel, partial bowel obstruction, or rectal obstruction.
• Constipation may be caused by diet or medications.
• Diarrhea may indicate spastic bowel or viral infection.

- Mixed with blood and mucus, soft stool can signal bacterial infection; mixed with blood or pus, colitis.
- Yellow or green stool suggests severe, prolonged diarrhea; black stool suggests GI bleeding or intake of iron supplements or raw-to-rare meat. Tan or white stool shows hepatic duct or gallbladder-duct blockage, hepatitis, or cancer. Red stool may signal colon or rectal bleeding; however, drugs and foods can also cause this coloration.
- Most stool contains 10% to 20% fat. A higher fat content can turn stool pasty or greasy, a possible sign of intestinal malabsorption or pancreatic disease.

Abnormal stool findings might indicate a problem.

Nursing considerations

- Collect the stool specimen in a clean, dry container, and immediately send it to the laboratory.
- Don't use stool that has been in contact with toilet-bowl water or urine.
- Use commercial fecal occult blood slides as a simple method of testing for blood in stool. Follow package directions because certain medications and foods can interfere with test results.

Percutaneous liver biopsy

Percutaneous liver biopsy involves the needle aspiration of a core of liver tissue for histologic analysis. It's done under a local or general anesthetic.

Last resort

Biopsy is used to detect hepatic disorders and cancer after ultrasonography, computed tomography (CT) scans, and radionuclide studies have failed. Because many patients with hepatic disorders have clotting defects, a clotting profile (prothrombin time and partial thromboplastin time) — along with type and crossmatching — should precede liver biopsy.

Nursing considerations

- Explain the procedure to the patient and tell him he'll be awake during the test and that the test may cause discomfort. Reassure him that a medication will be administered to help him relax.
- Restrict food and fluids for at least 4 hours before the test.

After it's over

After the procedure:
- Watch the patient for bleeding and symptoms of bile peritonitis, including tenderness and rigidity around the biopsy site.

• Be alert for symptoms of pneumothorax, such as rising respiratory rate, decreased breath sounds, dyspnea, persistent shoulder pain, and pleuritic chest pain. Report these complications promptly.
• Apply a gauze dressing to the puncture site and reinforce or apply a pressure dressing if needed.
• Maintain the patient in a right side-lying position for several hours; the pressure enhances coagulation at the site.
• Monitor urine output for at least 24 hours and watch for hematuria, which may indicate bladder trauma.

Peritoneal fluid analysis

Peritoneal fluid analysis includes examination of gross appearance, erythrocyte and leukocyte counts, cytologic studies, microbiological studies for bacteria and fungi, and determinations of protein, glucose, amylase, ammonia, and alkaline phosphatase levels.

Peritoneal through paracentesis

Abdominal paracentesis is a bedside procedure involving aspiration of fluid from the peritoneal space through a needle, trocar, or cannula inserted in the abdominal wall.

Paracentesis is used to:
• diagnose and treat massive ascites resistant to other therapy
• detect intra-abdominal bleeding after traumatic injury
• obtain a peritoneal fluid sample for laboratory analysis
• decrease intra-abdominal pressure and alleviate dyspnea.

Nursing considerations
• Explain the procedure to the patient. Make sure an informed consent form has been signed.
• Have the patient empty his bladder. Usually, an indwelling urinary catheter is inserted.
• Record the patient's baseline vital signs, weight, and abdominal girth. Indicate the abdominal area measured with a felt-tipped marking pen.
• The trocar is inserted with the patient supine. After insertion, assist the patient to sit up in bed. (See *Positioning for abdominal paracentesis*, page 416.)
• Remind the patient to remain as still as possible during the procedure.

Abdominal paracentesis is a bedside procedure that's used to aspirate fluid from the peritoneal space.

Positioning for abdominal paracentesis

When positioning a patient for abdominal paracentesis, help him sit up in bed or allow him to sit on the edge of the bed with additional support for his back and arms.

In this position, gravity causes fluid to accumulate in the lower abdominal cavity. The internal organs provide counterresistance and pressure to aid fluid flow.

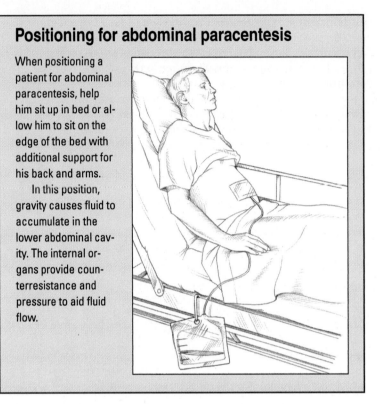

• During the procedure, monitor the patient's vital signs, oxygen saturation, and cardiac rhythm every 15 minutes and observe for tachycardia, hypotension, dizziness, pallor, diaphoresis, and increased anxiety, especially if more than 1,500 ml of peritoneal fluid is aspirated at one time.

• If the patient shows signs of hypovolemic shock, slow the drainage rate by raising the collection container vertically so it's closer to the height of the needle, trocar, or cannula. Stop the drainage if necessary. Limit aspirated fluid to between 1,500 and 2,000 ml.

• After the doctor removes the needle, trocar, or cannula and, if necessary, sutures the incision, apply a dry sterile pressure dressing.

After it's over

After the procedure:

• Monitor the patient's vital signs, oxygen saturation, and cardiac rhythm, and check the dressing for drainage every 15 minutes for the first hour, every 30 minutes for the next 2 hours, every hour for 4 hours, and then every 4 hours for 24 hours.

• Observe the patient for signs of hemorrhage or shock, such as hypotension, tachycardia, pallor, and excessive diaphoresis. These signs may indicate puncture of the inferior epigastric artery, hematoma of the anterior cecal wall, or rupture of the iliac vein or bladder. Observe for hematuria.
• Observe the patient for signs of a perforated intestine, such as increasing pain or abdominal tenderness.
• Document the procedure, and record the patient's daily weight and abdominal girth to detect recurrent ascites.

Nuclear imaging

Nuclear imaging methods are used to study the liver, spleen, and other abdominal organs.

Liver-spleen scan

In a liver-spleen scan, a scanner or gamma camera records the distribution of radioactivity within the liver and spleen after I.V. injection of a radioactive colloid. Kupffer's cells in the liver take up most of this colloid, while smaller amounts lodge in the spleen and bone marrow.

Detective device

By registering the extent of this absorption, the imaging device detects such abnormalities as tumors, cysts, and abscesses. Because the test demonstrates disease nonspecifically (as a cold spot, which is an area that fails to take up the colloid), test results usually require confirmation by ultrasonography, CT or gallium scan, or biopsy.

Ultrasonography, CT or gallium scanning, or biopsy is used to confirm the clues revealed by liver-spleen scanning.

Nursing considerations
• Describe the test to the patient and explain that it's used to examine the liver and spleen through pictures taken with a special scanner or camera.
• Tell the patient he'll receive an injection of a radioactive substance (technetium-99m sulfide) through an I.V. line in his hand or arm to allow better visualization of the liver and spleen.
• Immediately report any adverse reactions, such as flushing, fever, light-headedness, or difficulty breathing.

Magnetic resonance imaging

Magnetic resonance imaging (MRI) is used to examine the liver and abdominal organs. It's useful in evaluating liver disease by characterizing tumors, masses, or cysts found on previous studies. An image is generated by energizing protons in a strong magnetic field. Radio waves emitted as protons return to their former equilibrium and are recorded. No ionizing radiation is transmitted during the scan.

MRI mire

Disadvantages of MRI include the closed tubelike space required for the scan. Newer MRI centers offer a less confining "open-MRI" scan. In addition, the test can't be performed on patients with implanted metal prostheses or devices.

Nursing considerations
• Explain the procedure to the patient and stress the need to remove metal objects, such as jewelry, before the procedure.
• Explain to the patient that he must lie still for 1 to 1½ hours for the procedure.
• Generally, you'll accompany the patient to the MRI suite. If he becomes claustrophobic during the test, administer mild sedation, as ordered.

Stress the need to remove metal objects before MRI scanning.

Radiographic tests

Radiographic tests include abdominal X-rays, various contrast media studies, and CT scans.

Abdominal X-rays

An abdominal X-ray, also called *flat plate of the abdomen* or *kidney-ureter-bladder radiography,* is used to detect and evaluate tumors, kidney stones, abnormal gas collection, and other abdominal disorders. The test consists of two plates: one taken with the patient supine and the other taken while he stands.

Reading the rays

On X-ray, air appears black, fat appears gray, and bone appears white. Although a routine X-ray doesn't reveal most abdominal organs, it does show the contrast between air and fluid. For example, intestinal blockage traps large amounts of detectable fluids and air inside organs. When an intestinal wall tears, air leaks into the abdomen and becomes visible on X-ray.

Nursing considerations
• Explain the procedure to the patient. Radiography requires no special pretest or posttest care. It's usually done at the bedside using portable X-ray equipment.

CT scan

In CT scanning, a computer translates multiple X-ray beams into three-dimensional oscilloscope images of the patient's biliary tract, liver, and pancreas.

Scads of scans

CT scanning is used to:
- distinguish between obstructive and nonobstructive jaundice
- identify abscesses, cysts, hematomas, tumors, and pseudocysts
- evaluate the cause of weight loss and look for occult malignancy
- diagnose and evaluate pancreatitis.

The test can be done with or without a contrast medium, but contrast is preferred unless the patient is allergic to contrast media.

Nursing considerations

- Explain the procedure to the patient and tell him that he should lie still, relax, and breathe normally during the test. Explain that if the doctor orders an I.V. contrast medium, he may experience discomfort from the needle puncture and a localized feeling of warmth on injection.
- Restrict food and fluids after midnight before the test, but continue any drug regimen as ordered.
- Confirm if the patient has an allergy to iodine or shellfish. If he has a seafood or dye allergy, give him a pretest preparation kit containing prednisone and diphenhydramine, as ordered, to reduce the risk of a reaction to the dye. Report immediately any adverse reactions, such as nausea, vomiting, dizziness, headache, and urticaria
- If the patient is on nothing-by-mouth status, increase the I.V. fluid rate as ordered after the procedure to flush the contrast medium from his system. Monitor serum creatinine and BUN levels for signs of acute renal failure, which may be caused by the contrast medium.

Treatments

GI dysfunctions present many treatment challenges because they stem from various mechanisms occurring separately or simultaneously, including tumors, hyperactivity and hypoactivity, malabsorption, infection and inflammation, vascular disorders, intestinal obstruction, and degenerative disease. Treatment options include drug therapy, surgery, GI intubation, and nutritional support.

Treatment measures for GI disorders may include drug therapy, surgery, intubation, and nutritional support.

Drug therapy

Drug therapy may be used for such disorders as acute GI bleeding, peptic ulcer disease, and hepatic failure. Some of the most commonly used drugs in critical care include ammonia detoxicants, antacids, antidiuretic hormone, antiemetics, histamine-2 (H_2) receptor antagonists, and proton pump inhibitors.

How fast?

Some of these drugs, such as antacids and antiemetics, provide relief immediately. Other drugs, such as ammonia detoxicants and H_2-receptor antagonists, may take several days or longer to alleviate the problem. (See *Common GI drugs*.)

Surgery

Surgery may be used to treat the patient with massive bleeding who hasn't responded to medical treatments, such as gastric lavage or sclerotherapy. Be ready to provide special postoperative support for your patient after GI surgery because he may have to make permanent and usually difficult lifestyle changes. Two typical surgical procedures for GI disorders are liver transplantation and LeVeen shunt insertion.

A liver transplant may be the last and best hope for a patient with a life-threatening liver disorder.

Liver transplantation

For a patient with a life-threatening liver disorder who doesn't respond to other treatment, a liver transplant may be the best hope. Candidates include patients with:
• congenital biliary abnormalities
• chronic hepatitis
• inborn errors of metabolism
• end-stage liver disease.

Who's the candidate?

Criteria for referring a patient for transplantation include:
• a patient with advanced hepatic failure with expected survival time less than 2 years
• the unavailability of other medical or surgical therapies that offer long-term survival
• the absence of contraindicated conditions, such as cardiopulmonary disease, metastatic disease, acquired immunodeficiency syndrome, and active alcohol or drug addiction
• the patient and family members who understand all aspects of the transplant process.

Common GI drugs

Drugs	Indications	Adverse reactions	Practice pointers
Ammonia detoxicant			
Lactulose	• To prevent and treat portosystemic enceph-alopathy in patients with severe hepatic disease (increasing clearance of nitrogenous products and decreasing serum ammonia levels through laxative effects) • Laxative to treat consti-pation	Abdominal cramps, diarrhea, flatulence	• After administration through a nasogastric (NG) tube, flush tube with water. • For administration by retention enema, pa-tient should retain drug for 30 to 60 minutes. • Neomycin and other antibiotics may de-crease effectiveness.
Antacids			
Aluminum hydroxide	• Antacid used for heart-burn, acid indigestion, and adjunct therapy with peptic ulcer disease	Constipation, intestinal ob-struction, encephalopathy	• Use cautiously in patients with renal dis-ease. • These drugs may interfere with imaging techniques using sodium pertechnetate Tc 99m. • After administration through an NG tube, flush tube with water.
Aluminum hydroxide and magnesium hydroxide	• Antacid used for heart-burn, acid indigestion, and adjunct therapy with peptic ulcer disease	Diarrhea, hypermagnesemia in patients with severe renal impairment	• These drugs aren't recommended for pa-tients with renal disease. • These drugs may interfere with imaging techniques using sodium pertechnetate Tc 99m. • After administration through an NG tube, flush tube with water.
Calcium carbonate	• Antacid used for heart-burn, acid indigestion, and adjunct therapy with peptic ulcer disease • Calcium supplement	Nausea, vomiting, possibly hypercalcemia (with exces-sive use)	• Use cautiously in patients with renal dis-ease, cardiac disease, or sarcoidosis. • Monitor patients for hypercalcemia.

(continued)

Common GI drugs *(continued)*

Drugs	Indications	Adverse reactions	Practice pointers
Antidiuretic hormone			
Vasopressin	• Injection administered I.V. or intra-arterially into the superior mesenteric artery used as treatment in acute, massive GI hemorrhage (such as peptic ulcer disease, ruptured esophageal varices, and Mallory-Weiss syndrome)	Angina, cardiac arrhythmias (bradycardia, heart block), cardiac arrest, water intoxication, seizures, bronchospasms, coronary thrombosis, possibly mesenteric and small bowel infarction with mesenteric artery intra-arterial infusion	• Intra-arterial infusion requires angiographic catheter placement. • Monitor intake and output closely. • Monitor for water intoxication (drowsiness, headache, confusion, anuria). • Monitor cardiac rhythm. • Use cautiously in patients with coronary artery disease, heart failure, renal disease, asthma, or a seizure disorder. • Use is contraindicated in patients with chronic nephritis. • Use cautiously in elderly, preoperative, or postoperative patients.
Antiemetics			
Dolasetron Ondansetron	• Prevention and treatment of postoperative nausea and vomiting and in conjunction with cancer chemotherapy	Diarrhea, arrhythmias, electrocardiogram changes (prolonged PR and QT intervals and widened QRS complex), liver test abnormalities, pruritus	• Monitor cardiac rhythm. • Use cautiously in patients with prolonged QT intervals or with congenital QT syndrome. • Interacts with cytochrome P-450 drugs. • Monitor liver function.
Metoclopramide	• Prevention and treatment of postoperative nausea and vomiting and in conjunction with cancer chemotherapy • Delayed gastric emptying secondary to diabetic gastroparesis	Restlessness, anxiety, depression, suicidal ideation, seizures, bradycardia, bronchospasm, transient hypertension	• Use cautiously in patients with GI hemorrhage or mechanical obstruction and patients with pheochromocytoma seizures, depression, or hypertension.
Histamine-2 receptor antagonists			
Famotidine	• Treatment of duodenal and gastric ulcers, gastroesophageal reflux disease (GERD), and Zollinger-Ellison syndrome • Prevention of gastric stress ulcers	Headache, palpitations, diarrhea, constipation	• May cause irritation at the I.V. site. • After administration through an NG tube, flush tube with water. • Antacids may be administered concurrently.

Common GI drugs *(continued)*

Drugs	Indications	Adverse reactions	Practice pointers
Histamine-2 receptor antagonists (continued)			
Ranitidine	• Treatment of duodenal and gastric ulcers, GERD, and Zollinger-Ellison syndrome • Prevention of gastric stress ulcers	Malaise, reversible confusion, depression or hallucinations, blurred vision, jaundice, leukopenia, angioedema	• Antacids decrease ranitidine absorption; give 1 hour apart. • Use cautiously in patients with renal disease. • Monitor renal and liver tests.
Proton pump inhibitors			
Lansoprazole Omeprazole Pantoprazole	• Treatment of duodenal and gastric ulcers, erosive esophagitis, GERD, Zollinger-Ellison syndrome, and *Helicobacter pylori* eradication • Prophylaxis for gastric stress ulcer (in critically ill patients)	Diarrhea, abdominal pain, nausea, constipation, chest pain, dizziness, hyperglycemia	• Use cautiously in patients with severe liver disease. • Monitor liver function values and blood glucose.

Teach the patient and his family all about the transplant process, testing, drugs, and risks.

Nursing considerations

When caring for a patient undergoing a liver transplantation, concentrate on preparing the patient and his family physically and emotionally for the procedure, including instructing the patient about the procedure and events after. Also, take steps to prevent postoperative complications. (See *Managing liver transplantation complications*, page 424.)

Before it begins

Before transplantation:
• Instruct the patient and his family about the transplant, necessary diagnostic tests, immunosuppressant medications, and rejection risk.
• Review information about the equipment and procedures, such as cardiac monitoring, endotracheal tube, NG tube, indwelling urinary catheter, and arterial lines. Reassure the patient that discomfort should be minimal and that the equipment will be removed as soon as possible.

Managing liver transplantation complications

Check this table to find possible complications of liver transplantation and assessment and nursing interventions for each complication.

Complication	Assessment and intervention
Hemorrhage and hypovolemic shock	• Assess the patient's vital signs and other indicators of fluid volume hourly and note trends indicating hypovolemia; hypotension; weak, rapid, irregular pulse; oliguria; decreased level of consciousness; and signs of peripheral vasoconstriction. • Monitor the patient's hematocrit and hemoglobin levels daily. • Maintain patency of all I.V. lines, and reserve 2 units of blood in case the patient needs a transfusion.
Vascular obstruction	• Be alert for signs and symptoms of acute vascular obstruction in the right upper quadrant—cramping pain or tenderness, nausea, and vomiting. Notify the doctor immediately if any occur. • As ordered, prepare for emergency thrombectomy. Maintain I.V. infusions, check and document the patient's vital signs, and maintain airway patency.
Wound infection or abscess	• Assess the incision site daily, and report any inflammation, tenderness, drainage, or other signs and symptoms of infection. • Change the dressing daily or as needed. • Note and report any signs or symptoms of peritonitis or abscess, including fever, chills, leukocytosis (or leukopenia with bands), and abdominal pain, tenderness, and rigidity. • Take the patient's rectal temperature every 4 hours. • Collect abdominal drainage for culture and sensitivity studies. Document the color, amount, odor, and consistency of drainage. • Assess the patient for signs of infection in other areas, such as the urinary tract, respiratory system, and skin. Document and report any signs of infection.
Pulmonary insufficiency or failure	• Maintain ventilation at prescribed levels. • Monitor the patient's arterial blood gas levels daily, and change ventilator settings, as ordered. • Auscultate for abnormal breath sounds every 2 to 4 hours. • Suction the patient, as needed.
Effects of immuno-suppressant therapy	• Note any signs or symptoms of opportunistic infection, including fever, tachycardia, chills, leukocytosis, leukopenia, and diaphoresis. • Maintain reverse isolation. • Report adverse reactions to drugs. • Check the patient's weight daily.
Hepatic failure	• Monitor nasogastric tube drainage for upper GI bleeding. • Frequently assess the patient's neurovascular status. • Note development of peripheral edema and ascites. • Monitor the patient's renal function by checking urine output, blood urea nitrogen levels, and serum creatinine and potassium levels. Monitor serum amylase levels daily.

• Administer ordered medications such as immunosuppressant agents.
• Review incentive spirometry and range-of-motion (ROM) exercises with the patient.
• Make sure that an informed consent form has been signed.
• Instruct family members in measures to control infection and minimize rejection after transplantation and advise them to have all their immunizations up-to-date.
• Provide emotional support to the patient and his family.

After it's over

After liver transplantation:
• Assess the patient's cardiopulmonary and hemodynamic status, including vital signs, oxygen saturation, and cardiac rhythm, at least every 15 minutes in the immediate postoperative period and then hourly or as indicated by his condition.
• Monitor the patient's temperature frequently, at least every hour initially and then every 2 to 4 hours. He may be hypothermic in the initial postoperative phase, and it's important to reestablish normal body temperature. Later in the postoperative phase, monitor the patient for fever and signs of infection. (See *What does fever mean?*)
• Monitor laboratory tests, especially liver enzymes, bilirubin, electrolytes, coagulation studies, and complete blood count (CBC).
• Assess insertion sites for indications of bleeding. Assess the incision site closely for oozing or active bleeding. If the patient has an NG tube, assess drainage color at least every 2 hours.
• Institute strict infection control precautions.
• Administer prophylactic antibiotics and postoperative drugs, such as corticosteroids and immunosuppressants, as ordered.
• Assist with extubation as soon as possible (usually within 4 to 6 hours), and administer supplemental oxygen as needed. Encourage coughing, deep breathing, and incentive spirometry.
• Monitor the patient's intake and output at least hourly, and notify the doctor if output is less than 30 ml/hour. Maintain fluids at 2,000 to 3,000 ml/day, or as ordered, to prevent fluid overload.
• Maintain the patient on nothing-by-mouth status with NG decompression, and attach the NG tube to low intermittent suction until bowel sounds return.
• Change the patient's position at least every 2 hours, getting him out of bed and to the chair within 24 hours if his condition is stable.
• Continually assess the patient for signs and symptoms of acute rejection, such as malaise, fever, graft enlargement, and diminished graft function (typically 7 to 14 days after the transplant).

Take charge!

What does fever mean?

A sudden onset of high fever and an increase in liver enzymes suggest hepatic artery thrombosis. If your patient exhibits a fever and infection is suspected, be ready to obtain cultures of all body fluids, X-rays of the chest and abdomen, and a Doppler ultrasound of the hepatic vessels.

Stick with it. Continually assess the patient for signs and symptoms of acute rejection.

• To ease emotional stress, plan care to allow rest and provide as much privacy as possible. Allow family members to visit and comfort the patient as much as possible.
• Teach the patient about danger signs and symptoms and the need to report these immediately.

LeVeen shunt insertion

Ascitic fluid can be drained from the abdominal cavity into the superior vena cava using a LeVeen peritoneovenous shunt. This device is used to control ascites resulting from chronic liver disease. (See *How the LeVeen shunt works*.)

Whys and worries

The LeVeen shunt provides an effective alternative to traditional treatment for ascites such as paracentesis. However, it can cause potentially serious complications, such as:
• ascitic fluid leakage from incisions
• wound infection
• subcutaneous bleeding
• disseminated intravascular coagulation (DIC)
• heart failure.

How the LeVeen shunt works

The LeVeen peritoneovenous shunt consists of a peritoneal tube, a venous tube, and a one-way pressure-sensitive valve that controls fluid flow.

Shunt operation made simple
As the patient inhales, pressure within the abdomen increases while pressure in the superior vena cava decreases. This pressure differential causes the shunt's valve to open, allowing ascitic fluid to drain from the abdominal cavity into the superior vena cava. When the patient exhales, superior vena cava pressure increases and intra-abdominal pressure decreases. This pressure differential forces the valve shut, stopping fluid flow.

The valve's one-way design prevents blood from backing into the tubing, reducing the risk of clotting and shunt occlusion. It also helps prevent the valve from opening if superior vena cava pressure remains higher than intra-abdominal pressure, as commonly occurs in patients with heart failure. This reduces the risk of fluid overload in the vascular system.

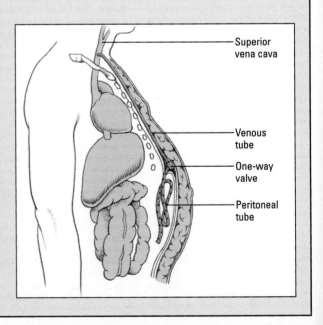

Nursing considerations

Before shunt insertion:
• Show the shunt to the patient and describe how it works.
• Explain that a local anesthetic is administered before the procedure.
• Measure and record the patient's baseline weight and abdominal girth.

After it's over

After shunt insertion:
• Place the patient in low Fowler's or semi-Fowler's position, whichever he prefers, and administer analgesics as ordered.
• Monitor the patient's vital signs, oxygen saturation, cardiac rhythm, and hemodynamic status. Watch for hypervolemia or hypovolemia.
• As ordered, administer diuretics to reduce fluid retention.
• Monitor the patient's intake and output hourly for the first 24 hours, then daily.
• Measure the patient's abdominal girth and weight daily.
• Monitor CBC, serum electrolyte, creatinine, albumin, and blood urea nitrogen (BUN), as ordered.
• Teach the patient to use an incentive spirometer four times daily for at least 15 minutes at a time.
• Apply an abdominal binder, as ordered, for the first 24 hours postoperatively to increase intra-abdominal pressure and enhance ascitic fluid drainage.
• Assess the incision site for bleeding, swelling, inflammation, drainage, and hematoma. Change the patient's dressing, as needed.
• Be alert for signs of heart failure, DIC, and GI bleeding.

> After surgery, place the patient in low Fowler's or semi-Fowler's position.

GI intubation

Nasoenteric, NG, and other specialized tubes may be used in treating the patient with acute intestinal obstruction, bleeding, esophageal varices, or another GI dysfunction.

Gastric lavage

Gastric lavage is an emergency treatment for the patient with GI hemorrhage caused by peptic ulcer disease or ruptured esophageal or gastric varices and as emergency treatment for some drug overdoses.

It involves intubation with a large-bore, single- or double-lumen tube; instillation of irrigating fluid; and aspiration of gastric

Types of nasogastric tubes

There are two common types of nasogastric tubes: Levin and Salem sump.

Levin tube

The Levin tube is a rubber or plastic tube with a single lumen, 42″ to 50″ (106.5 to 127 cm) long, with holes at the tip and along the side.

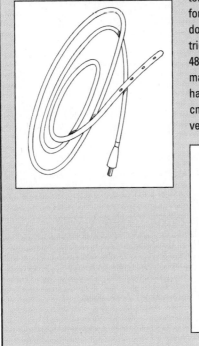

Salem sump tube

The Salem sump tube is a double-lumen tube made of clear plastic. It has a colored sump port (pigtail) that allows atmospheric air to enter the patient's stomach; therefore, the tube floats freely and doesn't adhere to or damage gastric mucosa. The larger port of this 48″ (121.9 cm) tube serves as the main suction conduit. The tube has openings at 45, 55, 65, and 75 cm as well as a radiopaque line to verify placement.

contents. In some cases, a vasoconstrictor, such as norepinephrine, may be added to the irrigating fluid to enhance this action. (See *Types of nasogastric tubes*.)

Rarities

Complications are rare and include:
- vomiting and aspiration
- fluid overload
- electrolyte imbalance or metabolic acidosis
- bradycardia.

Nursing considerations

- Explain the procedure to the patient.
- Determine the length of the tube for insertion. (See *Measuring nasogastric tube length*.)
- Lubricate the end of the tube with a water-soluble lubricant and insert it into the patient's mouth or nostrils, as ordered. Advance the tube through the pharynx and esophagus and into the stomach.
- Check the tube for placement by attaching a piston or bulb syringe, injecting 30 cc of air while auscultating the stomach with a stethoscope. If you can't hear swooshing or gurgling sounds, the tube may be in the bronchus or esophagus. (You can also check the pH of tube aspirate to confirm correct placement of the tube. Gastric aspirate is acidic, with a pH ranging from 0 to 4. An alkaline pH of 7 or greater indicates that the tube is in the respiratory tract.)
- When the tube is in place, lower the head of the bed to 15 degrees and reposition the patient on his left side, if possible.
- Fill the syringe with 30 to 50 ml of irrigating solution and begin instillation. Instill about 250 ml of fluid, wait 30 seconds, and then

If you can't hear swooshing or gurgling sounds, the NG tube may be in the bronchus or esophagus.

Measuring nasogastric tube length

To determine how long the nasogastric tube must be to reach the stomach, hold the end of the tube at the tip of the patient's nose. Extend the tube to the patient's earlobe and then down to the xiphoid process.

Nose

Ear

Xiphoid process

begin to withdraw the fluid into the syringe. If you can't withdraw any fluid, allow the tube to drain into an emesis basin.
• If the doctor orders a vasoconstrictor to be added to the irrigating fluid, wait for the prescribed period before withdrawing fluid to allow absorption of the drug into the gastric mucosa.
• Carefully measure and record fluid return. If the volume of fluid return doesn't at least equal the amount of fluid instilled, abdominal distention and vomiting result.
• Continue lavage until return fluid is clear or as ordered. Remove the tube or secure it, as ordered. If appropriate, send lavage specimens to the laboratory for toxicology studies and gastric contents for pH and guaiac studies.
• Never leave the patient alone during gastric lavage.
• Monitor the patient's cardiac rhythm and observe for possible complications, such as bradycardia, hypovolemia, vomiting, and aspiration.
• Monitor the patient's vital signs and oxygen saturation every 30 minutes until his condition stabilizes.
• Document the procedure and appropriate interventions.

Never leave the patient alone during gastric lavage.

Multilumen esophageal tube placement

In esophagogastric tamponade, an emergency treatment, a multilumen esophageal tube is inserted to control esophageal or gastric hemorrhage resulting from ruptured varices. It's usually a tentative measure until sclerotherapy can be done. (See *Comparing esophageal tubes.*)

How it's done

The tube is inserted through a nostril, or sometimes the mouth, and then passed into the stomach. The tube's esophageal and gastric balloons are inflated to exert pressure on the varices to stop bleeding, while a lumen allows esophageal and gastric contents to be aspirated.

Balloon inflation for longer than 48 hours may cause pressure necrosis, which can lead to further hemorrhage. Follow your facility's policy and procedure for balloon inflation and deflation.

Nursing considerations

Before the procedure:
• Describe the procedure to the patient. Explain that a helmet may be used to apply traction to keep balloon pressure at the gastroesophageal junction. Place the patient in semi-Fowler's position. (If unconscious, place the patient on his left side, with the head of the bed elevated to 15 degrees.) An unresponsive patient may also require endotracheal intubation.

A helmet may be used to keep balloon pressure at the gastroesophageal junction.

Comparing esophageal tubes

Three types of esophageal tubes include the Linton tube, the Minnesota esophagogastric tamponade tube, and the Sengstaken-Blakemore tube.

Linton tube

The Linton tube, a three-lumen, single-balloon device, has ports for esophageal and gastric aspiration. Because the tube doesn't have an esophageal balloon, it isn't used to control bleeding for esophageal varices.

Large-capacity gastric balloon
Esophageal aspiration lumen
Gastric aspiration lumen
Gastric balloon-inflation lumen

Minnesota esophagogastric tamponade tube

The Minnesota esophagogastric tamponade tube has four lumens and two balloons. It has pressure-monitoring ports for both balloons.

Gastric balloon
Esophageal balloon
Gastric balloon-inflation lumen
Gastric balloon pressure-monitoring port
Gastric aspiration lumen
Esophageal aspiration lumen
Esophageal balloon pressure-monitoring port
Esophageal balloon-inflation lumen

Sengstaken-Blakemore tube

The Sengstaken-Blakemore tube, a three-lumen device with esophageal and gastric balloons, has a gastric aspiration port that allows drainage from below the gastric balloon and is also used to instill medication.

Gastric balloon
Esophageal balloon
Gastric balloon-inflation lumen
Gastric aspiration lumen
Esophageal balloon-inflation lumen

• Tape a pair of scissors to the head of the bed in case of acute respiratory distress.
• Check tube balloons for air leaks and patency before insertion.
• Never leave the patient alone during tamponade.

After it's over

After the procedure:
• Closely monitor the patient's condition and lumen pressure. If the pressure changes or decreases, check for bleeding and notify the doctor immediately.
• Monitor the patient's cardiac rhythm, vital signs, and oxygen saturation every 30 to 60 minutes. A change may indicate new bleeding.
• Monitor the patient's respiratory status and observe for respiratory distress. If respiratory distress develops, have someone notify the doctor. If the airway is obstructed, cut both balloon ports and remove the tube. Notify the doctor immediately.
• Maintain suction on the ports. Irrigate the gastric aspiration port to prevent clogging.
• Deflate the esophageal balloon for about 30 minutes every 12 hours or according to your facility's policy and procedure.
• Observe the patient for signs of esophageal rupture, such as shock, increased respiratory difficulty, and increased bleeding. Notify the doctor if such signs are present.
• Keep the patient warm, comfortable, and as still as possible.
• When bleeding has been controlled, assist with tube removal.

Nasoenteric decompression tube

The nasoenteric decompression tube is used to aspirate intestinal contents for analysis and to correct intestinal obstruction. It's inserted nasally and advanced beyond the stomach into the intestinal tract. The tube may also prevent nausea, vomiting, and abdominal distention after GI surgery.

A balloon or rubber bag at one end of the tube holds mercury (or air or water) to stimulate peristalsis and aid the tube's passage through the pylorus and into the intestinal tract. (See *Common nasoenteric decompression tubes.*)

Nursing considerations

The patient with a nasoenteric decompression tube needs special care and continuous monitoring to:
• ensure tube patency
• maintain suction and bowel decompression
• detect such complications as fluid-electrolyte imbalance.

After your patient's bleeding is under control, assist the doctor with tube removal.

Dealing with obstruction

If your patient's tube appears to be obstructed, follow your facility's policy and procedure and notify the doctor if you're unable to restore patency. He may order measures, such as those described here, to restore patency quickly and efficiently:

• First, disconnect the tube from suction and irrigate with normal saline solution. Use gravity flow to help clear the obstruction unless otherwise ordered.

• If irrigation doesn't reestablish patency, the tube may be obstructed by its position against the gastric mucosa. Tug slightly on the tube to move it away from the mucosa.

• If gently tugging doesn't work, the tube may be kinked and need additional manipulation. However, don't reposition or irrigate a tube in a patient who had GI surgery, in one who had the tube inserted during surgery (because this may disturb new sutures), or in a patient who was difficult to intubate.

Common nasoenteric decompression tubes

The type of nasoenteric decompression tube chosen for your patient will depend on the size of the patient and his nostrils, the estimated duration of intubation, and the reason for the procedure.

Most tubes are impregnated with a radiopaque mark so that placement can easily be confirmed by X-ray or another imaging technique. Among the most commonly used types of nasoenteric decompression tubes are the Cantor tube, Miller-Abbott tube, Harris tube, and Dennis tube.

Cantor tube
The Cantor tube is a 10' (3-m) long single-lumen tube and has a balloon that can hold mercury at its distal tip. It may be used to relieve bowel obstructions and to aspirate intestinal contents.

Miller-Abbott tube
The Miller-Abbott tube is 10' long and has two lumens: one for inflating the distal balloon with air and one for instilling mercury or water. It's also used in case of bowel obstruction. This type of tube allows aspiration of intestinal contents.

Harris tube
The single-lumen Harris tube is only 6' (1.8 m) long, also ending with a balloon that holds mercury. Used primarily for treating a bowel obstruction, the Harris tube — usually with a Y tube attached — allows lavage of the intestinal tract.

Dennis tube
The 10' long, three-lumen Dennis sump tube is used to decompress the intestinal tract before or after GI surgery. Each lumen is marked to denote its use: irrigation, drainage, and balloon inflation.

434

Nutritional support

A patient with a GI problem who can't eat or otherwise ingest enough food may require enteral or parenteral nutrition.

Enteral nutrition

Enteral nutrition is used to deliver nutrients to the GI tract using a tube. The upper GI tract is bypassed and pureed food or a special liquid enteral formula is delivered directly into the stomach (gastric gavage), duodenum, or jejunum. It can be administered on an intermittent schedule or as a continuous, slow infusion.

Who needs it?

Enteral nutrition delivery is indicated for the patient with a functional GI tract who can't adequately take food by mouth, such as a patient with:
- Crohn's disease
- ulcerative colitis
- short-bowel syndrome
- head and neck injuries
- neurologic disease
- stroke
- oral cancers
- a psychiatric disorder.

Who can't have it?

Tube feeding is contraindicated in the patient with suspected intestinal obstruction or absent bowel sounds.

Nursing considerations

Before the procedure:
- Explain the procedure to the patient and obtain the necessary formula.
- Assess the patient's abdomen for bowel sounds and distention. Check placement of the feeding tube to ensure it hasn't slipped out since the last feeding. Never give a tube feeding until you're sure the tube is properly positioned in the patient's stomach. Administering a feeding through a misplaced tube can lead to aspiration.
- Check for gastric residual to assess gastric emptying; aspirate and measure gastric residual contents. Withhold feedings if residual volume is more than the amount specified in the doctor's order (usually 50 to 100 ml). Reinstill any aspirate obtained.

> Never give a tube feeding until you're sure the tube is properly positioned in the patient's stomach.

CAUTION!

• When delivering the feeding, elevate the bed to semi-Fowler's or high Fowler's position to prevent aspiration and promote digestion.
• Irrigate the tube, administer the feeding as ordered, and then flush the tube again.

After it's over

After the procedure:
• Record the amount of ingested formula. Note the patient's tolerance of tube feeding.
• Weigh the patient daily and monitor ordered laboratory tests.
• Provide meticulous mouth and tube care.

Parenteral nutrition

When a patient can't meet his nutritional needs by oral or enteral feedings, he may require I.V. nutritional support, or *parenteral nutrition.*

Who needs it?

The patient's diagnosis, history, and prognosis are used to determine the need for parenteral nutrition. Generally, this treatment is prescribed for any patient who can't absorb nutrients through the GI tract for more than 10 days.
    More specific indications include:
• debilitating illness lasting longer than 2 weeks
• loss of 10% or more of pre-illness weight
• serum albumin level below 3.5 g/dl
• excessive nitrogen loss from wound infection, fistulas, or abscesses
• renal or hepatic failure
• severe pancreatitis
• severe burns
• nonfunctioning GI tract for 5 to 7 days in a severely catabolic patient.

Delivery route

Parenteral nutrition may be given through a peripheral or central venous (CV) line. Depending on the solution, parenteral nutrition boosts the patient's calorie intake or surpasses his calorie requirements. There are two types of parenteral nutrition:
• *Total parenteral nutrition* refers to any nutrient solution, including lipids, given through a CV line.
• *Peripheral parenteral nutrition (PPN)* is delivered through a peripheral line. PPN is used to supply the patient's full calorie needs while avoiding the risks that accompany a CV line. (See *Types of parenteral nutrition*, page 436.)

Parenteral nutrition is prescribed for any patient who can't absorb nutrients through the GI tract for more than 10 days.

Types of parenteral nutrition

Type	Solution components per liter	Uses
Total parenteral nutrition by central venous (CV) catheter or peripherally inserted central catheter into the superior vena cava through the infraclavicular vein (most common), supraclavicular vein, internal jugular vein, or antecubital fossa	• $D_{15}W$ to $D_{25}W$ (1 L dextrose 25% = 850 nonprotein calories) • Crystalline amino acids 2.5% to 8.5% • Electrolytes, vitamins, trace elements, and insulin, as ordered • Lipid emulsion 10% to 20% (usually infused as a separate solution)	• When needed for 2 weeks or more • For a patient with large calorie and nutrient needs • Provides calories, restores nitrogen balance, and replaces essential vitamins, electrolytes, minerals, and trace elements • Promotes tissue synthesis, wound healing, and normal metabolic function • Allows bowel rest and healing; reduces activity in the gallbladder, pancreas, and small intestine • Improves tolerance of surgery
Peripheral parenteral nutrition by peripheral catheter	• D_5W to $D_{10}W$ • Crystalline amino acids 2.5% to 5% • Electrolytes, minerals, vitamins, and trace elements, as ordered • Lipid emulsion 10% or 20% (1 L dextrose 10% and amino acids 3.5% infused at the same time as 1 L of lipid emulsion = 1,440 nonprotein calories) • Heparin or hydrocortisone, as ordered	• When needed for 2 weeks or less • Provides up to 2,000 calories/day • Maintains adequate nutritional status in a patient who can tolerate relatively high fluid volume, one who usually resumes bowel function and oral feedings after a few days, and one susceptible to infections associated with the CV catheter

Nursing considerations
• Explain the procedure to the patient.
• Be sure to check the solution against the doctor's order for correct patient name, expiration date, and formula components.
• Throughout the procedure, maintain sterile technique.
• Follow your facility's policy and procedure and administer using an infusion pump with the pump tubing and micron filter. Infuse at a constant rate without interruption to avoid blood glucose fluctuations.
• Monitor the patient's vital signs at least every 2 to 4 hours, or more often if necessary. Watch him for increased temperature, an early sign of catheter sepsis.
• Check the patient's blood glucose level every 6 hours.
• Monitor the patient's intake and output and routine laboratory tests (serum electrolytes, calcium, BUN, creatinine, magnesium, CBC, and albumin).
• Monitor the patient's liver and kidney function.

Special considerations

Basic solution
- Nutritionally complete
- Requires minor surgical procedure for CV line insertion
- Highly hypertonic solution
- May cause pneumothorax (typically during catheter insertion), phlebitis, thrombus formation, air embolus, infection, sepsis, and metabolic complications (glucose intolerance, electrolyte imbalance, essential fatty acid deficiency)
- Must be delivered in a vein with high blood flow rate because glucose content may be increased beyond the level a peripheral vein can handle (commonly six times more concentrated than blood)

I.V. lipid emulsion
- May not be used effectively in a severely stressed patient (especially a patient with burns)
- May interfere with immune mechanisms; in a patient suffering from respiratory compromise, reduces carbon dioxide buildup
- Given by way of CV line

Basic solution
- Nutritionally complete for a short time
- Can't be used in a nutritionally depleted patient
- Can't be used in a volume-restricted patient
- Doesn't cause weight gain
- Avoids insertion and care of the CV line, but requires adequate venous access site; must be changed every 72 hours
- May cause phlebitis and increases risk of metabolic complications
- Less chance of metabolic complications than with CV line
- To avoid venous sclerosis, must contain no more than 10% dextrose, so patient must tolerate large fluid volume to meet nutritional needs

I.V. lipid emulsion
- As effective as dextrose for calorie source
- Diminishes phlebitis if infused at the same time as basic nutrient solution
- Irritates vein in long-term use
- Reduces carbon dioxide buildup when pulmonary compromise is present

- Weigh the patient daily.
- Change the dressing according to your facility's policy. Monitor the catheter site for swelling, which may indicate infiltration.
- Change the solution, tubing, and filter every 24 hours or according to your facility's policy.
- When discontinuing parenteral nutrition, decrease the infusion rate slowly, depending on the patient's current glucose intake, to minimize the risk of hyperinsulinemia and resulting hypoglycemia.

GI disorders

Abdominal disorders commonly encountered in a critical care unit include acute GI bleeding, acute pancreatitis, bowel infarction, cirrhosis, and hepatic failure and hepatic encephalopathy.

Monitor the catheter site for swelling, which may indicate infiltration.

Acute GI bleeding

GI bleeding can occur anywhere along the GI tract. Although GI bleeding stops spontaneously in most patients, acute bleeding accounts for significant morbidity and mortality.

Maybe multiple morbidities

Many patients requiring care in the critical care unit have upper GI bleeding. Additionally, they may have underlying comorbidities that contribute to the risk of upper GI bleeding, such as:
• coronary artery disease
• history of myocardial infarction (MI)
• renal failure
• history of chronic liver damage secondary to alcohol abuse or hepatitis
• history of radiation therapy
• chronic pain condition, such as arthritis, requiring treatment with NSAIDs.

What causes it

Upper GI bleeding includes bleeding in the esophagus, stomach, and duodenum. Bleeding below the Treitz ligament is considered lower GI bleeding; the most common site is in the colon.

Upper causes

The causes of upper GI bleeding include:
• peptic ulcer disease
• rupture of esophageal varices
• esophagitis
• Mallory-Weiss tear
• erosive gastritis
• angiodysplasias
• arteriovenous malformations.

Lower causes

The most common causes of lower GI bleeding include:
• diverticulitis
• inflammatory bowel disease
• polyps
• hemorrhoids
• neoplasm
• arteriovenous malformations.

Pathophysiology

The patient experiences a loss of circulating blood volume, regardless of the cause of bleeding.

What happens

Because the arterial blood supply near the stomach and esophagus is extensive, bleeding can lead to a rapid loss of large amounts of blood, subsequent hypovolemia, and shock. Here's what else happens:
• Loss of circulating blood volume leads to a decreased venous return.
• Cardiac output and blood pressure decrease, causing poor tissue perfusion. In response, the body compensates by shifting interstitial fluid to the intravascular space.
• The sympathetic nervous system is stimulated, resulting in vasoconstriction and increased heart rate.
• The renin-angiotensin-aldosterone system is activated, leading to fluid retention and increasing blood pressure.
• If blood loss continues, cardiac output decreases, leading to cellular hypoxia. Eventually, all organs fail due to hypoperfusion.

What to look for

Because GI bleeding can occur anywhere along the GI tract, assessment is crucial in determining the amount and possible location of bleeding.

Source signs

The appearance of blood in tube drainage, vomitus, and stool indicates the source of GI bleeding:
• Hematemesis—bright red blood in NG tube drainage or vomitus—typically indicates an upper GI source. However, if the blood has spent time in the stomach where it was exposed to gastric acid, the drainage or vomitus resembles coffee grounds.
• Hematochezia—bright red blood from the rectum—typically indicates a lower GI source of bleeding. It also may suggest an upper GI source if the transit time through the bowel was rapid.
• Melena—black, tarry, and sticky stool—usually indicates an upper GI bleeding source. However, it can result from bleeding in the small bowel or proximal colon.

Signs and symptoms

Typically, the patient exhibits signs and symptoms based on the amount and rate of bleeding. With acute GI bleeding and blood loss greater than 30% of the person's blood volume, he exhibits signs and symptoms of hypovolemic shock, including:
• cool, clammy skin

With continued bleeding, all organs eventually fail due to hypoperfusion.

- pallor
- restlessness
- apprehension
- tachycardia
- diaphoresis
- hypotension
- syncope.

Watch for signs and symptoms of hypovolemic shock in patient's with acute GI bleeding.

What tests tell you

These findings aid in diagnosing acute GI bleeding:
- Upper GI endoscopy reveals the source of esophageal or gastric bleeding.
- CBC reveals the amount of blood loss.
- Arterial blood gas (ABG) analysis can indicate metabolic acidosis from hemorrhage and possible hypoxemia.
- 12-lead electrocardiogram (ECG) may reveal evidence of cardiac ischemia secondary to hypoperfusion.
- Abdominal X-ray may indicate air under the diaphragm, suggesting ulcer perforation.
- Angiography may aid in visualizing the bleeding site.

How it's treated

Treatment goals include stopping the bleeding and providing fluid replacement while maintaining the patient's function. Treatment may include:
- fluid volume replacement with crystalloid solutions initially, followed by colloids and blood component therapy
- respiratory support
- gastric intubation with gastric lavage (unless the patient has esophageal varices) and gastric pH monitoring
- drug therapy, such as antacids, H_2-receptor antagonists, and proton pump inhibitors
- endoscopic or surgical repair of bleeding sites.

What to do

- Type and crossmatch at least 2 units of blood.
- Start at least two large-bore I.V. lines (16G or 18G preferred). Assess the patient for blood loss and begin fluid replacement therapy as ordered, initially delivering crystalloid solutions, such as normal saline or lactated Ringer's solution, followed by blood component products.
- Ensure your patient's patent airway. Monitor cardiac and respiratory status and assess LOC at least every 15 minutes until he stabilizes and then every 2 to 4 hours, as indicated by his status. As-

sist with insertion of hemodynamic monitoring devices, and assess hemodynamic parameters.
• Administer supplemental oxygen as ordered. Monitor oxygen saturation levels.
• Monitor the patient's skin color and capillary refill for signs of hypovolemic shock.
• Obtain serial hemoglobin and hematocrit levels. Administer albumin or blood as ordered.
• Monitor the patient's intake and output closely, including all losses from the GI tract. Check all stools and gastric drainage for occult blood.
• Assist with or insert an NG tube and perform lavage using room temperature saline to clear blood and clots from the stomach.
• Assess the patient's abdomen for bowel sounds and gastric pH, as ordered. Expect to resume enteral or oral feedings after bowel function returns and there's no evidence of further bleeding.
• Provide appropriate emotional support to the patient.
• Prepare the patient for endoscopic repair or surgery, if indicated.

Acute pancreatitis

Pancreatitis, inflammation of the pancreas, occurs in acute and chronic forms and may be due to edema, necrosis, or hemorrhage. In men, this disease is commonly associated with alcoholism, trauma, or peptic ulcer; in women, with biliary tract disease.

What causes it

Causes of pancreatitis may include:
• biliary tract disease
• alcoholism
• abnormal organ structure
• metabolic or endocrine disorders, such as high cholesterol levels and hyperparathyroidism
• pancreatic cysts or tumors
• penetrating peptic ulcers
• blunt or surgical trauma
• drugs, such as glucocorticoids, sulfonamides, thiazides, procainamide, tetracycline, and NSAIDs
• kidney failure or transplantation
• endoscopic examination of the bile ducts and pancreas.

Pathophysiology

Acute pancreatitis occurs in two forms:

Pancreatitis occurs in acute and chronic forms. It may be caused by edema, necrosis, or hemorrhage.

 edematous (interstitial) pancreatitis, which causes fluid accumulation and swelling

 necrotizing pancreatitis, which causes cell death and tissue damage.

Damage and destruction

The inflammation that occurs with both types of pancreatitis is caused by premature activation of enzymes, which leads to tissue damage. If pancreatitis damages the islets of Langerhans, diabetes mellitus may result. Sudden severe pancreatitis causes massive hemorrhage and total destruction of the pancreas, manifested as diabetic acidosis, shock, or coma.

Association affects outcome

The prognosis is good for a patient with pancreatitis associated with biliary tract disease but poor when associated with alcoholism. Mortality is as high as 60% when pancreatitis is associated with necrosis and hemorrhage.

Rating mortality

The severity of pancreatitis is predicted using Ranson's criteria. If the patient meets fewer than three of the criteria, the mortality rate is less than 1%. When three or four of the criteria are met, the mortality rate increases to 15% to 20%. With five or six criteria, the mortality rate is 40%. (See *Ranson's criteria.*)

What to look for

Commonly, the patient describes intense epigastric pain centered close to the umbilicus and radiating to the back. He typically reports that the pain is aggravated by:
• eating fatty foods
• consuming alcohol
• lying in a recumbent position.

Take notes

During the physical examination, you may note:
• persistent vomiting (in a severe attack) from hypermotility or paralytic ileus
• abdominal distention (in a severe attack) from bowel hypermotility and fluid accumulation in the peritoneal cavity
• diminished bowel activity (in a severe attack), suggesting altered motility secondary to peritonitis

Good news! The prognosis is good when pancreatitis is associated with biliary tract disease.

Ranson's criteria

The severity of your patient's acute pancreatitis is determined by the existence of certain characteristics. The more criteria met by the patient, the more severe the episode of pancreatitis and, therefore, the greater the risk of mortality.

On admission

Admission criteria include:
• age over 55
• white blood cell count greater than 16,000/µl
• serum glucose greater than 200 mg/dl
• lactate dehydrogenase greater than 350 IU/L
• aspartate aminotransferase greater than 250 U/L.

After admission

During the first 48 hours after admission, criteria include:
• 10% decrease in hematocrit
• blood urea nitrogen increase greater than 5 mg/dl
• serum calcium less than 8 mg/dl
• base deficit greater than 4 mEq/L
• partial pressure of arterial oxygen less than 60 mm Hg
• estimated fluid sequestration greater than 6 L.

• crackles at lung bases (in a severe attack) secondary to heart failure
• left pleural effusion
• mottled skin
• jaundice
• ascites
• tachycardia
• low-grade fever
• cold, sweaty extremities
• restlessness related to pain
• decreased pulmonary artery pressure and cardiac output due to hemorrhage or dehydration; elevated cardiac output and decreased systemic vascular resistance if systemic inflammation or sepsis present.

What tests tell you

Findings that aid in diagnosing acute pancreatitis include:
• serum amylase and lipase levels elevated 3 to 5 times normal
• urine amylase increased for 1 to 2 weeks
• elevated white blood cell (WBC) count; hemoglobin and hematocrit decreased with hemorrhage and increased with dehydration; decreased coagulation
• decreased serum calcium

• other elevated results, including serum bilirubin levels, aspartate aminotransferase (AST), alanine aminotransferase (ALT), lactate dehydrogenase (LD), and alkaline phosphatase
• abdominal and chest X-rays showing pleural effusions and bowel dilation and ileus
• CT scan and ultrasonography showing an enlarged pancreas with fluid collection, cysts, abscess, masses, and pseudocysts
• endoscopic pancreatography showing swelling and ductal system abnormalities
• ABG values that may reveal decreased partial pressure of arterial oxygen, mild respiratory alkalosis, and decreased oxygen saturation
• ECG that may reveal ST-segment depression and T-wave inversion.

Treatment for pancreatitis may include I.V. fluids, drugs, and peritoneal lavage.

How it's treated

Treatment for the patient with acute pancreatitis may include:
• I.V. replacement of fluids, protein, and electrolytes to treat shock
• fluid volume replacement and blood transfusions
• withholding food and fluids to rest the pancreas
• NG tube suctioning
• drugs, such as analgesics, antacids, H_2-receptor antagonists, antibiotics, anticholinergics, and insulin
• peritoneal lavage
• surgical drainage for a pancreatic abscess or pseudocyst
• laparotomy (if biliary tract obstruction causes acute pancreatitis) to remove the obstruction.

What to do

• Ensure a patent airway, and assess the patient's respiratory status at least every hour or more often. Assess oxygen saturation levels and breath sounds for adventitious or diminished breath sounds.
• Closely monitor the patient's cardiac and hemodynamic status at least every hour or more often, as ordered.
• Place the patient in a comfortable position that maximizes air exchange, such as semi-Fowler's or high Fowler's.
• Allow for periods of rest and activity.

Place the patient in a comfortable position that maximizes air exchange.

- If the patient develops acute respiratory distress syndrome, anticipate the need for additional therapies such as prone positioning.
- Initiate I.V. fluid replacement therapy. Monitor serum laboratory values (hematology, coagulation, and chemistry) for changes.
- Be especially alert for signs and symptoms of hypokalemia (hypotension, muscle weakness, apathy, confusion, and cardiac arrhythmias), hypomagnesemia (hypotension, tachycardia, confusion, tremors, twitching, tetany, and hallucinations), and hypocalcemia (positive Chvostek's and Trousseau's signs, seizures, and prolonged QT interval on ECG). Have emergency equipment readily available.
- Monitor the patient's intake and output closely and notify the doctor if urine output is less than 0.5 ml/kg/hour. Weigh the patient daily.
- Monitor the patient's neurologic status, noting confusion or lethargy.
- Maintain your patient in a normothermic state to reduce the body's demand for oxygen.
- Assess the patient's pain level and administer analgesics, as ordered.
- Administer antibiotics, as ordered, and monitor serum peak and trough levels, as appropriate.
- Withhold all oral fluids and food to prevent stimulation of pancreatic enzymes.
- Insert an NG tube, as ordered. Check placement at least every 4 hours. Irrigate with normal saline solution for patency. Monitor drainage for frank bleeding. Monitor vomitus and stool for bleeding.
- Assess the patient's abdomen for distention and bowel sounds; measure his abdominal girth.
- Administer parenteral nutrition therapy, as ordered. Monitor blood glucose levels. Administer insulin, as ordered.
- When bowel sounds become active, anticipate switching to enteral or oral feedings.
- Perform ROM exercises to maintain joint mobility.
- Perform meticulous skin care.
- Provide emotional support to the patient.
- Prepare the patient for surgery, as indicated.

Hold it! Withhold all oral fluids and food to prevent stimulation of pancreatic enzymes.

Infarction leads to vasoconstriction and vasospasm of the bowel.

Bowel infarction

Bowel infarction is a decreased blood flow to the major mesenteric vessels. It leads to vasoconstriction and vasospasm of the bowel and contracted bowel with mucosal ulceration.

What causes it

Bowel infarction can be caused by:
- thrombosis after an MI
- cholesterol plaques in the aorta that become dislodged
- emboli in patients with endocarditis or atrial fibrillation
- arteriosclerosis
- cirrhosis of the liver
- hypercoagulation as seen in polycythemia or after splenectomy
- reduced perfusion from heart failure or shock.

Pathophysiology

Here's what happens with bowel infarction:
- Decreased blood flow to the mesenteric vessels leads to spasms.
- When the spasms subside, the muscles of the bowel are fatigued and unable to receive essential oxygen and nutrients.
- The bowel becomes edematous and cyanotic, and necrosis can occur.
- As pressure in the lumens of the bowel increases, perforation can occur, leading to peritonitis or abscess formation.

What to look for

Look for signs and symptoms that may occur with bowel infarction, including:
- acute abdominal pain
- vomiting
- bloody diarrhea
- weight loss
- abdominal distention with tenderness and guarding
- absent or hypoactive bowel sounds
- signs and symptoms of shock.

> Abdominal distention with tenderness and guarding may indicate bowel infarction.

What tests tell you

These test results may aid in the diagnosis of bowel infarction:
- Abdominal X-rays reveal dilated loops of bowel.
- Barium studies show the infarction location.
- Angiography reveals the infarction location.
- Fecal occult blood test are positive for blood.
- CT scan may reveal the area of infarction.
- Serum phosphate, hematocrit, and serum osmolality levels are elevated.
- Sigmoidoscopy reveals an ischemic bowel.

How it's treated

Treatment for your patient with bowel infarction may include:
• vasodilators for perfusion and pain relief
• angiograms
• anticoagulation
• surgery that may include endarterectomy, thrombectomy, and aortomesenteric bypass grafting.

What to do

• Monitor the patient's vital signs, oxygen saturation, cardiac rhythm, and cardiopulmonary status.
• Assess the patient's abdomen for bowel sounds, and monitor his abdominal girth and weight daily.
• Monitor skin temperature and capillary refill.
• Administer fluid replacement, as ordered.
• Administer vasoactive agents, such as dopamine, as ordered.
• Prepare the patient for surgical repair, as indicated.
• Monitor the patient's intake and output.
• Administer analgesics to control pain and antibiotics, as ordered.
• Observe electrolytes and glucose levels for imbalances.
• Provide nutritional support, as ordered.

Cirrhosis

Cirrhosis is a chronic disorder marked by diffuse destruction and fibrotic regeneration of hepatic cells. As necrotic tissue yields to fibrosis, this disease damages liver tissue and normal vasculature, impairs blood and lymph flow, and ultimately causes hepatic insufficiency.

What causes it

There are several types of cirrhosis, including:
• portal (Laënnec's), caused by malnutrition and chronic alcohol ingestion
• biliary, caused by bile duct disease that suppresses bile flow
• postnecrotic, caused by various types of hepatitis
• pigment, caused by hemochromatosis
• cardiac, caused by liver damage from right-sided heart failure.

There are several types of cirrhosis, including portal, biliary, postnecrotic, pigment, and cardiac.

Pathophysiology

Cirrhosis is characterized by irreversible chronic injury of the liver, extensive fibrosis, and nodular tissue growth. The changes result from liver cell death (hepatocyte necrosis), collapse of the liver's supporting structure (the reticulin network), distortion of the vascular bed, and nodular regeneration of remaining liver tissue.

What to look for

Assess your patient for these signs and symptoms, which are the same regardless of the cause:
• *GI* — anorexia, indigestion, nausea and vomiting, constipation or diarrhea, and dull abdominal ache
• *respiratory* — pleural effusion, limited thoracic expansion
• *central nervous system (CNS)* — lethargy, mental changes, slurred speech, asterixis, peripheral neuritis, hallucinations, coma
• *hematologic* — bleeding tendencies, anemia
• *endocrine* — testicular atrophy, menstrual irregularities, loss of chest and axillary hair
• *skin* — severe pruritus, extreme dryness, poor tissue turgor, abnormal pigmentation, spider angiomas, possible jaundice
• *hepatic* — jaundice, hepatomegaly, ascites, edema of the legs
• *miscellaneous* — musty breath, muscle atrophy, pain in the right upper quadrant, palpable liver or spleen.

The signs and symptoms of cirrhosis are the same regardless of the cause.

What tests tell you

The following findings aid in diagnosing cirrhosis:
• Liver biopsy confirms cirrhosis.
• Liver scan shows abnormal thickening and a liver mass.

These help, too

Other helpful tests include:
• cholecystography and cholangiography to visualize the gallbladder and biliary duct system
• percutaneous transhepatic cholangiography to visualize the portal venous system
• WBC count, hematocrit and hemoglobin, albumin, serum electrolyte, and cholinesterase levels (all decreased)
• globulin, serum ammonia, total bilirubin, alkaline phosphatase, ALT, AST, and LD levels (all increased).

How it's treated

Treatment for your patient with cirrhosis may include:
• high-calorie and moderate- to high-protein diet; restricted protein if hepatic encephalopathy develops

• sodium restricted to 200 to 500 mg/day; fluids to 1,000 to 1,500 ml/day
• possible enteral or parenteral feeding if the patient's condition continues to deteriorate
• drug therapy (requires special caution because the cirrhotic liver can't detoxify harmful substances efficiently; sedatives avoided or prescribed with great care)
• paracentesis and salt-poor albumin infusions to relieve ascites
• surgery (ligation of varices, splenectomy, esophagogastric resection, or liver transplantation).

What to do

• A patient with cirrhosis is generally admitted to the critical care unit because of a complication of cirrhosis, such as hepatic failure or bleeding esophageal varices (See *Managing bleeding from esophageal varices*.)
• Monitor the patient's vital signs, oxygen saturation, cardiac rhythm, and cardiopulmonary status.
• Observe the patient closely for signs of behavioral or personality changes. Report increasing stupor, lethargy, hallucinations, or neuromuscular dysfunction. Watch for asterixis, a sign of developing hepatic encephalopathy.
• Assess the patient for fluid retention, weigh and measure his abdominal girth daily, and inspect his ankles and sacrum for dependent edema.
• Accurately record the patient's intake and output.

> Watch the patient with cirrhosis closely for signs of behavioral or personality changes.

Managing bleeding from esophageal varices

Esophageal varices are dilated, tortuous veins in the submucosa of the lower esophagus resulting from portal hypertension. Varices can go undetected and result in sudden and massive bleeding. Such varices commonly cause massive hematemesis, requiring emergency treatment to control hemorrhage and prevent hypovolemic shock.

Managing bleeding
• Vasopressin infused into the superior mesenteric artery may stop bleeding temporarily. Vasopressin infused by I.V. drip diluted with dextrose 5% in water is less effective.
• Sclerotherapy is done by endoscopy to cause fibrosis and obliteration of the varices.

• A Minnesota or Sengstaken-Blakemore tube is used to control hemorrhage by applying pressure on the bleeding site.
• Iced saline lavage through the tube is used to control bleeding.
• Fresh blood and frozen plasma are given to replace clotting factors.
• Lactulose is administered to promote elimination of old blood from the GI tract and to combat excessive production and accumulation of ammonia.
• Surgical bypass procedures include portosystemic anastomosis, splenorenal shunt, portacaval shunt, and mesocaval shunt.

Viral hepatitis from A to E—plus G

Use this table to compare the features of various types of viral hepatitis characterized to date. Other types are emerging.

Feature	Hepatitis A	Hepatitis B	Hepatitis C	Hepatitis D	Hepatitis E	Hepatitis G
Incubation	15 to 45 days	30 to 180 days	15 to 160 days	14 to 64 days	14 to 60 days	2 to 6 weeks
Onset	Acute	Insidious	Insidious	Acute	Acute	Presumed insidious
Age-group commonly affected	Children, young adults	Any age	More common in adults	Any age	Ages 20 to 40	Any age, primarily adults
Transmission	Fecal-oral, sexual (especially oral-anal contact), non-percutaneous (sexual, maternal-neonatal), percutaneous (rare)	Blood-borne; parenteral route, sexual, maternal-neonatal; virus is shed in all body fluids	Blood-borne; parenteral route	Parenteral route; most people infected with hepatitis D are also infected with hepatitis B	Primarily fecal-oral	Blood-borne; similar to Hepatitis B and C
Severity	Mild	Commonly severe	Moderate	Can be severe and lead to fulminant hepatitis	Highly virulent with common progression to fulminant hepatitis and hepatic failure, especially in pregnant patients	Moderate
Prognosis	Generally good	Worsens with age and debility	Moderate	Fair, worsens in chronic cases; can lead to chronic hepatitis D and chronic liver disease	Good unless pregnant	Generally good; no current treatment recommendations
Progression to chronicity	None	Occasional	10% to 50% of cases	Occasional	None	Not known; no association with chronic liver disease

Hepatic failure and encephalopathy

Hepatic failure is the possible end result of any liver disease. When the liver fails, a complex syndrome involving impairment of many organs and body functions ensues. Failure can be caused by hepatitis, cirrhosis, or liver cancer. (See *Viral hepatitis from A to E—plus G.*)

Ammonia coma

Hepatic encephalopathy, also called *hepatic coma,* is a neurologic syndrome that develops as a manifestation of hepatic failure. It usually reflects ammonia intoxication of the brain.

What causes it

Hepatic encephalopathy is the result of increasing blood ammonia levels, such as from:
- improper shunting of blood from portal hypertension or from surgically created portosystemic shunts
- excessive protein intake
- sepsis
- excessive accumulation of nitrogenous body wastes (caused by constipation or GI bleeding)
- bacterial action on protein and urea to form ammonia.

Pathophysiology

Hepatic encephalopathy—a set of CNS disorders—results when the liver can no longer detoxify the blood. Liver dysfunction and collateral vessels that shunt blood around the liver to the systemic circulation permit toxins absorbed from the GI tract to circulate freely to the brain.

Ammonia's role

Ammonia is one of the main toxins causing hepatic encephalopathy. Ammonia is a by-product of protein metabolism. The liver transforms ammonia to urea, which the kidneys excrete. When the liver fails to do this, ammonia levels increase and ammonia is delivered to the brain.

> When the liver can't transform ammonia to urea, ammonia is delivered to the brain.

What to look for

Signs and symptoms vary, depending on the severity of neurologic involvement. The disorder progresses through these four stages, with symptoms that can fluctuate from one stage to another:

prodromal stage—slight personality changes (disorientation, forgetfulness, and slurred speech) and a slight tremor impending stage—tremor progresses to asterixis (the hallmark of hepatic encephalopathy), characterized by quick irregular extensions and flexions of the wrists and fingers, lethargy, aberrant behavior, and apraxia

stuporous stage—hyperventilation with stupor; noisy and abusive patient when stimulated

comatose stage—includes hyperactive reflexes, a positive Babinski's sign, coma, and a musty, sweet breath odor.

What tests tell you

Tests that aid in diagnosing hepatic encephalopathy include:
• elevated liver function tests
• increased serum albumin and decreased BUN and blood glucose levels
• serum electrolytes that reveal hypokalemia and hyponatremia
• electroencephalogram that's commonly abnormal but with non-specific changes.

How it's treated

Treatment goals for the patient with hepatic failure are correcting the underlying cause and reducing blood ammonia levels. Treatment measures include:
• administration of neomycin to destroy intestinal bacteria that breaks down protein into ammonia
• sorbitol-induced catharsis to produce osmotic diarrhea
• continuous aspiration of blood from the stomach
• reduction of dietary protein
• lactulose administration to reduce blood ammonia levels.

But wait, there's more

Other possible treatments include:
• potassium supplements
• hemodialysis to temporarily clear toxic blood
• exchange transfusions
• salt-poor albumin to maintain fluid and electrolyte balance
• shunt placement or paracentesis if ascites is a problem.

What to do

• Assess the patient's airway and respiratory status frequently, at least every 1 to 2 hours. Maintain a patent airway, and position the patient with the head of the bed elevated.
• Monitor the patient's oxygen saturation levels.

Aim for the treatment targets: correcting the underlying cause and reducing your patient's blood ammonia levels.

• Assess the patient's neurologic status to establish a baseline, and report any changes. Reorient the patient as necessary.
• Monitor the patient's cardiac status and vital signs often, at least every hour.
• Assess the patient's hemodynamic parameters closely, at least every hour. Monitor for indications of fluid volume deficit or excess.
• Assess the patient's urinary output hourly. Notify the doctor if output is less than 0.5 ml/kg/hour.
• Measure the patient's abdominal girth and weight daily.
• Assess the patient for signs and symptoms of fluid excess, including peripheral edema, jugular vein distention, tachypnea, and crackles that don't clear with coughing.
• Monitor laboratory studies, such as renal function, liver enzymes, serum albumin, total protein, and serum electrolytes.
• Monitor the patient's nutritional intake and maintain calorie count.
• Check fingerstick blood glucose levels every 4 hours or as ordered and assess for signs and symptoms of hyperglycemia and hypoglycemia.
• Institute bleeding precautions and monitor the patient for signs and symptoms of bleeding.
• Administer prescribed medications. Check with the doctor to adjust the dose of lactulose to allow for 2 to 3 semiformed stools per day.
• Assist with paracentesis, as indicated.
• Begin emergency treatment to control bleeding if variceal rupture occurs.
• Provide supportive care to the patient and his family.

Quick quiz

1. The stomach's major functions include all of the following actions except:
    A.   moving the gastric contents into the small intestine.
    B.   completing digestion.
    C.   serving as a temporary storage area for food.
    D.   breaking down food into chyme.

Answer: B. The stomach doesn't complete the digestion process.

2. Bowel sounds that are high-pitched and gurgling and occurring 10 times per minute are classified as:
    A.   hypoactive.
    B.   hyperactive.
    C.   dull.
    D.   normal.

Answer: D. Normal bowel sounds are high-pitched, gurgling, and occur irregularly from 5 to 34 times per minute. Hypoactive sounds are heard infrequently. Hyperactive bowel sounds are loud, high-pitched, and occur frequently.

3.   During abdominal paracentesis, the aspirated fluid amount should be limited to:
   A.   1,500 to 2,000 ml.
   B.   2,000 to 3,000 ml.
   C.   1,000 to 2,000 ml.
   D.   1,000 to 1,500 ml.

Answer: A. Removing more than 1,500 to 2,000 ml of peritoneal fluid at one time may lead to hypovolemic shock.

4.   Signs and symptoms of acute rejection after liver transplantation include all of the following findings except:
   A.   malaise.
   B.   fever.
   C.   graft shrinkage.
   D.   diminished graft function.

Answer: C. Graft enlargement is a symptom of acute rejection, which typically occurs 7 to 14 days after the transplant.

5.   Which diagnostic test confirms cirrhosis of the liver?
   A.   Liver biopsy
   B.   Liver scan
   C.   Percutaneous transhepatic cholangiography
   D.   Cholecystography

Answer: A. A liver biopsy allows a definitive diagnosis; the other tests can aid in the diagnosis by allowing visualization of the liver, gallbladder, portal venous system, and biliary duct system.

Scoring

☆☆☆   If you answered all five questions correctly, you deserve a gourmet meal! Clearly, you've digested all the information in this chapter.

☆☆   If you answered four questions correctly, read up and try again! Your hunger for GI information makes it easy to swallow.

☆   If you answered fewer than four questions correctly, you may be fact-starved. Chew over the chapter and then take the test again.

Now that you're full of GI knowledge, I'm passing you on to the renal system.

Renal system

Just the facts

In this chapter, you'll learn:

♦ structure and function of the renal system

♦ assessment of the renal system

♦ diagnostic tests and treatments

♦ common renal disorders and related nursing care.

Understanding the renal system

The renal system is the body's water treatment plant. Its job is to collect waste products and expel them as urine. The structures of the renal system include:
• kidneys
• ureters
• bladder
• urethra.

Kidney siting

The kidneys are located on each side of the abdomen near the lower back. These compact organs contain a filtration system that processes about 45 gallons of fluid each day. The by-product of this process is urine, which contains water and waste products. (See *A close look at a kidney*, page 456.)

It's all downhill from there

After it's produced by the kidneys, urine passes through the urinary system and is expelled from the body. The other structures of the system, extending downward from the kidneys, include the:
• ureters—two 16″ to 18″ (40.5- to 45.5-cm) muscular tubes that contract rhythmically (peristalsis) to transport urine from each kidney to the bladder

> The renal system is the body's water treatment plant; it collects waste products and expels them as urine.

A close look at a kidney

Illustrated below is a kidney along with an enlargement of a nephron, the kidney's functional unit.

Kidney keys

Major structures of the kidney include:
• medulla—inner portion of the kidney, made up of renal pyramids and tubular structures
• renal artery—supplies blood to the kidney
• renal pyramid—channels output to the renal pelvis for excretion
• renal calyx—channels formed urine from the renal pyramids to the renal pelvis
• renal vein—about 99% of filtered blood is circulated through the renal vein back to the general circulation; the remaining 1%, which contains waste products, undergoes further processing in the kidney
• renal pelvis—after blood that contains waste products is processed in the kidney, formed urine is channeled to the renal pelvis
• ureter—a tube that terminates in the urethra; urine enters the urethra for excretion
• cortex—outer layer of the kidney.

Note the nephron

The nephron is the functional and structural unit of the kidney. Each kidney contains about 1 million nephrons. Its two main activities are selective reabsorption and secretion of ions and mechanical filtration of fluids, wastes, electrolytes, and acids and bases.

Components of the nephron include:
• glomerulus—a network of twisted capillaries that acts as a filter for the passage of protein-free and red blood cell–free filtrate to the proximal convoluted tubules
• Bowman's capsule—contains the glomerulus and acts as a filter for urine
• proximal convoluted tubule—the site of reabsorption of glucose, amino acids, metabolites, and electrolytes from filtrate; reabsorbed substances return to the circulation
• loop of Henle—a U-shaped nephron tubule located in the medulla and extending from the proximal convoluted tubule to the distal convoluted tubule; the site for further concentration of filtrate through reabsorption
• distal convoluted tubule—the site from which filtrate enters the collecting tubule
• collecting tubule—releases urine.

Kidney

Renal calyx
Renal pyramid
Medulla
Renal pelvis
Renal artery
Renal vein
Ureter
Cortex

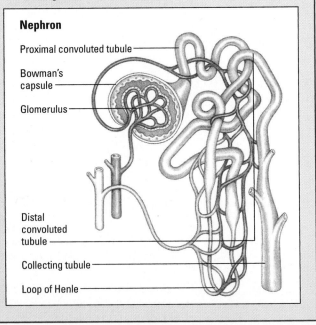

Nephron

Proximal convoluted tubule
Bowman's capsule
Glomerulus
Distal convoluted tubule
Collecting tubule
Loop of Henle

• urinary bladder—a sac with muscular walls that collects and holds urine (300 to 500 ml) expelled from the ureters every few seconds

• urethra—a narrow passageway (surrounded by the prostate gland in men) from the bladder to the outside of the body through which urine is excreted.

That isn't all

The renal system is a major regulatory system as well. Its roles include:
• maintaining fluid and electrolyte balance
• maintaining acid-base balance
• detoxifying the blood and eliminating wastes
• regulating blood pressure
• aiding red blood cell (RBC) production.

I'm a major player in a major regulatory system. Doo-wah-doo, Daddio.

Fluid and electrolyte balance

The kidneys maintain fluid and electrolyte balance in the body by regulating the amount and makeup of the fluid inside and around the cells.

Exchange interchange

The kidneys maintain the volume and composition of extracellular and, to a lesser extent, intracellular fluid. They do so by continuously exchanging water and solutes across their cell membranes. The solutes include electrolytes, such as hydrogen, sodium, potassium, chloride, bicarbonate, sulfate, and phosphate ions.

Hormones and osmoreceptors

Hormones partly control the kidneys' role in fluid balance by regulating the response of specialized sensory nerve endings (osmoreceptors) to changes in osmolality (the ionic concentration of a solution). Problems in hormone concentration can cause fluctuations in sodium and potassium concentrations that, in turn, may lead to hypertension.

The two hormones involved are:

☞   antidiuretic hormone (ADH), produced by the pituitary gland

✌   aldosterone, produced by the adrenal cortex.

Two hormones — ADH and aldosterone — are involved in fluid balance.

The ABCs of ADH

ADH changes the collecting tubules' permeability to water. Here's how:

• When ADH concentration in plasma is high, the tubules are most permeable to water. This condition creates a highly concentrated but small volume of urine.
• When ADH concentration is low, the tubules are less permeable to water. This situation creates a larger volume of less concentrated urine.

Age and ADH

As a person ages, tubular reabsorption and renal concentrating ability decline because the size and number of functioning nephrons decrease.

All about aldosterone and sodium

Aldosterone regulates water reabsorption by the distal tubules and changes urine concentration by increasing sodium reabsorption. Here's how:
• A high plasma aldosterone concentration increases sodium and water reabsorption by the tubules and decreases sodium and water excretion in the urine.
• A low plasma aldosterone concentration promotes sodium and water excretion.

Aldosterone and potassium

Aldosterone also helps control the secretion of potassium by the distal tubules. A high aldosterone concentration increases the excretion of potassium. Other factors that affect potassium secretion include:
• amount of potassium ingested
• number of hydrogen ions secreted
• potassium levels in the cells
• amount of sodium in the distal tubule
• glomerular filtration rate (GFR), which is the rate at which plasma is filtered as it flows through the glomerular capillary filtration membrane.

Aldosterone regulates water reabsorption and changes urine concentration by increasing sodium reabsorption.

Going against the current

The kidneys concentrate urine through the countercurrent exchange system. In this system, fluid flows in opposite directions through parallel tubes, up and down parallel sides of the loops of Henle. A concentration gradient causes fluid exchange; the longer the loop, the greater the concentration gradient.

Acid-base balance

To regulate acid-base balance, the kidneys:
• secrete hydrogen ions

- reabsorb sodium and bicarbonate ions
- acidify phosphate salts
- produce ammonia.

Earning a PhD in pH balance

All of these regulating activities keep the blood at its normal pH of 7.35 to 7.45. Acidosis occurs when the pH falls below 7.35, and alkalosis occurs when the pH rises above 7.45.

Normal blood pH has a narrow range. Acidosis occurs when pH falls below 7.35, and alkalosis occurs when pH rises above 7.45.

Detoxification and waste collection

The kidneys collect and eliminate wastes from the body in a three-step process:

☝ *glomerular filtration*, in which the kidney's blood vessels, or glomeruli, filter blood flowing through them

✌ *tubular reabsorption*, in which the tubules (minute canals that make up the kidney) reabsorb the filtered fluid

🤟 *tubular secretion*, in which the filtered substance is then released by the tubules.

Clear the way

Clearance is the complete removal of a substance from the blood. It's commonly described as the amount of blood that can be cleared in a specific time. For example, creatinine clearance is the volume of blood in milliliters that the kidneys can clear of creatinine in 1 minute.

Some substances are filtered out of the blood by the glomeruli. Dissolved substances that remain in the fluid may be reabsorbed by the renal tubular cells. (See *Understanding GFR*, page 460.)

Nephron compensation

In a patient whose kidneys have atrophied from disease, healthy nephrons (the filtering units of the kidney) enlarge to compensate. As nephron damage progresses, the enlargement no longer adequately compensates, and the patient's GFR slows. (See *Age-related renal changes*.)

Tubular transport-ability

The amount of a substance that's reabsorbed or secreted depends on the substance's maximum tubular transport capacity, or the maximum amount of a substance that can be reabsorbed or secreted in 1 minute without saturating the renal system.

Senior moment

Age-related renal changes

By age 70, a person's blood urea nitrogen levels increase by 21%. Other age-related changes that affect renal function include:
- diminished kidney size
- impaired renal clearance of drugs
- reduced bladder size and capacity
- decreased renal response to sodium intake.

Understanding GFR

Glomerular filtration rate (GFR) is the rate at which the glomeruli filter blood. A normal GFR is about 120 ml/minute. GFR depends on:
• permeability of capillary walls
• vascular pressure
• filtration pressure.

GFR and clearance
Clearance is the complete removal of a substance from the blood. The most accurate measure of glomerular filtration is creatinine clearance because creatinine is filtered by the glomeruli but not reabsorbed by the tubules.

Equal to, greater than, or less than
Here's more about how the GFR affects clearance measurements for a substance in the blood:
• If the tubules neither reabsorb nor secrete the substance—as happens with creatinine—clearance equals the GFR.
• If the tubules reabsorb the substance, clearance is less than the GFR.
• If the tubules secrete the substance, clearance exceeds the GFR.
• If the tubules reabsorb and secrete the substance, clearance may be less than, equal to, or greater than the GFR.

For example, in diabetes mellitus, excess glucose in the blood overwhelms the renal tubules and causes glucose to appear in the urine (glycosuria). In other cases, when glomeruli are damaged, protein appears in the urine (proteinuria) because the large protein molecules pass into the urine instead of being reabsorbed.

Blood pressure regulation

High blood pressure (hypertension) can damage blood vessels as well as cause hardening of the kidneys (nephrosclerosis), a leading cause of chronic renal failure.

Hypertension regulation

Hypertension can stem from renin-angiotensin hyperactivity (as well as from fluid and electrolyte imbalance). The kidneys aid blood pressure regulation by producing and secreting the enzyme renin in response to an actual or perceived decline in extracellular fluid volume. Renin, in turn, forms angiotensin I, which is converted to the more potent angiotensin II.

Simply put, the kidneys secrete renin, which forms angiotensin I, which is converted to angiotensin II.

Pressure promotion

Angiotensin II increases low arterial blood pressure levels by:
• increasing peripheral vasoconstriction
• stimulating aldosterone secretion.

The increase in aldosterone promotes the reabsorption of sodium and water to correct the fluid deficit and inadequate blood flow (renal ischemia).

RBC production

Erythropoietin is a hormone that prompts the bone marrow to increase RBC production (erythropoiesis).

Vitamin D and calcium formation

The kidneys secrete erythropoietin when the oxygen supply in blood for tissues drops. They also produce active vitamin D and help regulate calcium balance and bone metabolism. Loss of renal function results in chronic anemia and insufficient calcium levels (hypocalcemia) because of a decrease in erythropoietin.

Renal assessment

Begin the renal assessment by collecting a patient health history. Next, conduct a thorough physical examination.

History

Collect a thorough health history to gain the information you need to find the cause and severity of the patient's renal disease. The health history includes information about the patient's current and previous illnesses and treatments as well as medication and family and lifestyle factors.

Current health status

Find out how the patient's symptoms developed and progressed. Ask how long he has had the problem, how it affects his daily routine, and when and how it began. Ask about related signs and symptoms, such as nausea and vomiting. If your patient has any pain, ask about its location, radiation, intensity, duration, and what precipitates or relieves it.

Collect clues from the patient's health history to find out about the cause and severity of his renal condition.

Previous health status

For clues about the patient's current condition, explore his past medical problems. Certain systemic diseases, such as diabetes mellitus, systemic lupus erythematosus, hypertension, sickle cell anemia, Goodpasture's syndrome, acute glomerulonephritis, and acute pyelonephritis, may contribute to the development of acute renal failure.

Ask the patient whether he has a history of renal disease or has ever had a kidney or bladder tumor. Find out what treatments he received and the treatment outcomes. Ask about any traumatic injuries, surgery, or conditions that required hospitalization or any recent diagnostic test that involved the use of a contrast medium.

Drug check

Ask your patient if he's now taking any medications and what they are. Ask if he has any known allergies to foods or medications.

Many drugs are eliminated by the kidneys, so the patient with compromised kidney function, such as chronic renal failure, may need to avoid certain drugs or receive reduced dosages to prevent further renal problems. Drugs that may require a reduced dosage include angiotensin-converting enzyme inhibitors, ciprofloxacin, digoxin, histamine-2 receptor antagonists, penicillins, and sulfonamides.

Examples of drugs that impose a risk of nephrotoxicity include aminoglycosides (such as gentamicin, neomycin, and tobramycin), cisplatin, and lithium carbonate.

I do keep busy. Many drugs are eliminated by the kidneys.

Family history

Because some renal disorders are hereditary, ask the patient whether anyone in his family has a history of renal disease. Polycystic kidney disease is one example of an inherited disorder that can lead to renal failure.

Lifestyle patterns

Psychological and sociologic factors can affect the patient's health. To determine how such factors may have contributed to your patient's current problem, ask about his:
- home life
- stress level
- occupation.

Environmental agents that could cause kidney problems might be found in the patient's home or workplace.

At work and play

Ask your patient about possible exposure at work or home to agents that may be nephrotoxic, such as cleaning products, pesticides, lead, or mercury. Also ask about his alcohol, tobacco, caffeine, or illegal drug use as well as his dietary habits, cultural practices that affect diet, and any dietary restrictions, such as a vegetarian or low-potassium diet.

Physical examination

Proceed in an orderly way with the physical examination of your patient's renal system using inspection, auscultation, percussion, and palpation.

Inspection

In a normal adult, the abdomen is smooth, flat or scaphoid (concave), and symmetrical. Abdominal skin should be free from scars, lesions, bruises, and discoloration.

> Compare the left and right sides of the abdomen and note asymmetrical areas.

Disclosing dysfunction

Inspect your patient's abdomen for gross enlargements or fullness by comparing the left and right sides, noting asymmetrical areas. Extremely prominent veins may accompany other vascular signs associated with renal dysfunction, such as hypertension or renal artery bruits.

Distention, skin tightness and glistening, and striae (streaks or linear scars caused by rapidly developing skin tension) may signal fluid retention. If you suspect ascites, perform the fluid wave test. Ascites may suggest nephrotic syndrome.

Urethral meatus inspection

Urethral meatus inspection may reveal several abnormalities. In a male patient, a meatus deviating from the normal central location may represent a congenital defect. In any patient, inflammation and discharge may signal urethral infection. Ulceration usually indicates a sexually transmitted disease.

Assess fluid volume status

Assess fluid volume status by observing for jugular vein distention and peripheral edema, periorbital edema, and sacral edema. Check the skin for turgor and mobility. Inspect the tongue and mucous membranes for moisture.

Skin turgor may be an unreliable sign of hydration in older people because of reduced subcutaneous tissue. Check turgor by pinching the subcutaneous tissue at the forehead or over the xiphoid process and watching for a quick return to baseline.

Auscultation

Auscultate the renal arteries in the left and right upper abdominal quadrants by pressing the stethoscope bell lightly against the abdomen and instructing the patient to exhale deeply. Begin auscultating at the midline and work to the left. Then return to the midline and work to the right.

Whoosh

Systolic bruits (whooshing sounds) or other unusual sounds are potentially significant abnormalities. For example, in a patient with hypertension, systolic bruits suggest renal artery stenosis.

Tube talk

Before auscultating the abdomen of a critically ill patient with a nasogastric (NG) tube or another abdominal tube connected to suction, briefly clamp the tube or turn off the suction. Suction noises can obscure or mimic abdominal sounds.

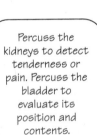

Listen up! Systolic bruits and other unusual sounds can be signs of trouble.

Percussion

After auscultating the renal arteries, percuss the patient's kidneys to detect tenderness or pain, and percuss the bladder to evaluate its position and contents.

How to

To percuss over the kidneys, have the patient sit up. Place your nondominant hand on the patient's back at the costovertebral angle of the 12th rib. Strike that hand with the ulnar surface of your other fist. Use just enough force to cause a painless but perceptible thud.

Percussing problems

Abnormal kidney percussion findings include tenderness and pain, suggesting glomerulonephritis or glomerulonephrosis. A dull sound heard on percussion in a patient who has just urinated may indicate urine retention, reflecting bladder dysfunction or infection.

Palpation

Palpate the kidneys and bladder to detect lumps, masses, or tenderness. To achieve optimal results, ask the patient to relax the

Percuss the kidneys to detect tenderness or pain. Percuss the bladder to evaluate its position and contents.

Palpating the renal organs

In the normal adult, the kidneys usually can't be palpated because of their location deep in the abdomen. However, they may be palpable in a thin patient or in one with reduced abdominal muscle mass. (Because the right kidney is slightly lower than the left, it may be easier to palpate.) Both kidneys descend with deep inhalation. An adult's bladder may not be palpable, either. If palpable, the bladder normally feels firm and relatively smooth. Using bimanual palpation, begin on the patient's right side and proceed with palpating the renal organs as outlined below.

Kidney palpation

Help the patient to a supine position and expose the abdomen from the xiphoid process to the symphysis pubis. Standing at the right side, place your left hand under the back, midway between the lower costal margin and the iliac crest, as shown below.

Next, place your right hand on the patient's abdomen directly above your left hand. Angle this hand slightly toward the costal margin. To palpate the right lower edge of the right kidney, press your right fingertips about 1½" (3.8 cm) above the right iliac crest at the midinguinal line; press your left fingertips upward into the right costovertebral angle.

Instruct the patient to inhale deeply so that the lower portion of the right kidney can move down between your hands. If it does, note the shape and size of the kidney. Normally, it feels smooth, solid, and firm, yet elastic. Ask the patient if palpation causes tenderness. Avoid using excessive pressure to palpate the kidney because this may cause intense pain.

To assess the left kidney, move to the patient's left side and position your hands, as described above, but position your right hand 2" (5 cm) above the left iliac crest. Then apply pressure with both hands as the patient inhales. If the left kidney can be palpated, compare it with the right kidney; it should be the same size.

Bladder palpation

Before palpating the bladder, make sure the patient has voided. Then locate the edge of the bladder by pressing deeply in the midline about 1" to 2" (2.5 to 5 cm) above the symphysis pubis.

As the bladder is palpated, note its size and location and check for lumps, masses, and tenderness. The bladder normally feels firm and relatively smooth. During deep palpation, the patient may report the urge to urinate—a normal response.

abdomen by taking deep breaths through the mouth. (See *Palpating the renal organs*, page 465.)

Peek-a-boo

Because the kidneys lie behind other organs and are protected by muscle, they normally aren't palpable unless they're enlarged. However, in a thin patient, you may be able to feel the lower end of the right kidney as a smooth round mass that drops on inspiration. In an elderly patient, you may be able to palpate both kidneys because of decreased muscle tone and elasticity.

Finding fault

On palpation, a lump, mass, or tenderness may indicate a tumor or cyst. A soft kidney may reflect chronic renal disease; a tender kidney, acute infection. Unequal kidney size may reflect hydronephrosis, a cyst, a tumor, or another disorder. Bilateral enlargement suggests polycystic kidney disease.

Abnormal bladder palpation findings include a lump or mass, possibly signaling a tumor or cyst, and tenderness, which may stem from infection. (See *Interpreting renal findings*.)

Calcium deficiency

When your patient complains of muscle spasms and paresthesia in his limbs, check for signs of calcium deficiency. (See *Checking for hypocalcemia*, page 468.)

In an elderly patient, you may be able to palpate both kidneys because of decreased muscle tone and elasticity.

Diagnostic tests

Diagnostic tests commonly ordered for a patient with known or suspected renal disease may include blood studies, kidney-ureter-bladder (KUB) radiography, renal angiography, and urine studies.

Blood studies

Blood studies used to diagnose and evaluate kidney function include:
• complete blood count (CBC) to evaluate white blood cells, RBCs, hemoglobin (Hb), and hematocrit (HCT)
• blood urea nitrogen (BUN) testing
• electrolyte measurements to evaluate calcium, phosphorus, chloride, potassium, and sodium levels
• serum creatinine, serum osmolality, serum protein, uric acid, creatinine clearance, and urea clearance measurements. (See *Interpreting blood studies in renal disease*, page 469.)

Interpreting renal findings

After completing your assessment, you're ready to form a diagnostic impression of the patient's condition. Check this table to find groupings of significant signs and symptoms, related findings you may discover during the health history and physical assessment, and the possible cause indicated by a cluster of these findings.

Key signs and symptoms	Related findings		Possible cause
• Oliguria, possibly progressing to anuria • Hematuria or coffee-colored urine • Smoky urine	• Poststreptococcal throat or skin infection • Systemic lupus erythematosus, vasculitis, or scleroderma • Pregnancy	• Elevated blood pressure • Periorbital edema progressing to dependent edema • Ascites • Pleural effusion	Acute glomerulonephritis
• Oliguria • Dark, smoky urine • Anorexia and vomiting	• Crush injury or illness associated with shock such as burns • Muscle necrosis • Exposure to nephrotoxic agent such as lead • Excretory urography using dye injection	• Recent aminoglycoside therapy • Oliguria progressing to anuria • Dyspnea • Bibasilar crackles • Dependent edema	Acute tubular necrosis
• Proteinuria, hematuria, vomiting, and pruritus (patient may be asymptomatic until advanced disease stage)	• Primary renal disorder, such as membranoproliferative glomerulonephritis and focal segmental glomerulosclerosis	• Elevated blood pressure • Ascites and dependent edema • Dyspnea • Bibasilar crackles	Chronic glomerulonephritis
• Urinary frequency and urgency • Burning sensation on urination • Nocturia, cloudy hematuria, and dysuria • Lower back or flank pain	• Female patient • Recurrent urinary tract infection • Recent chemotherapy or systemic antibiotic therapy	• Recent vigorous sexual activity • Suprapubic pain on palpation • Fever • Inflamed perineal area	Cystitis
• Severe radiating pain from costovertebral angle to flank and suprapubic region and from external genitalia • Nausea and vomiting • Hematuria	• Strenuous physical activity in hot environment • Previous renal calculi • Recent kidney infection	• Fever and chills • Poor skin turgor, concentrated urine, and dry mucous membranes	Nephrolithiasis
• Abdominal or flank pain • Gross hematuria	• Youth (especially under age 7) • Congenital anomalies • Firm, smooth, palpable abdominal mass in enlarged abdomen	• Fever • Elevated blood pressure • Urine retention	Wilms' tumor

Advice from the experts

Checking for hypocalcemia

Two signs that indicate tetany associated with hypocalcemia are Chvostek's and Trousseau's signs. To elicit these signs, follow the procedures described here. If you detect them, notify the doctor immediately.

While conducting these tests, watch the patient for laryngospasm, monitor his cardiac status, and have resuscitation equipment nearby. Keep in mind the discomfort these tests typically cause.

Chvostek's sign

To elicit this sign, tap the patient's facial nerve just in front of the earlobe and below the zygomatic arch or between the zygomatic arch and the corner of the mouth, as shown below.

A positive response (indicating latent tetany) ranges from simple mouth-corner twitching to twitching of all facial muscles on the side tested. Simple twitching may be normal in some patients. However, a more pronounced response usually confirms Chvostek's sign.

Trousseau's sign

In this test, occlude the brachial artery by inflating a blood pressure cuff on the patient's upper arm to a level between diastolic and systolic blood pressure. Maintain this inflation for 3 minutes while observing the patient for Trousseau's sign, or carpal spasm (shown below).

KUB radiography

KUB radiography, consisting of plain, contrast-free X-rays, shows kidney size, position, and structure. It can also reveal calculi and other lesions. Before performing a renal biopsy, the doctor may

Interpreting blood studies in renal disease

Here's how you may interpret the results of blood studies used in diagnosing renal disease.

Complete blood count

An increased white blood cell count may indicate urinary tract infection, peritonitis (in peritoneal dialysis patients), or kidney transplantation infection and rejection.

Red blood cell (RBC) count, hemoglobin level, and hematocrit (HCT) decrease in a patient with chronic renal insufficiency resulting from decreased erythropoietin production by the kidneys. HCT also provides an index of fluid balance because it indicates the percentage of RBCs in the blood.

Blood urea nitrogen

Increased blood urea nitrogen (BUN) levels may indicate glomerulonephritis, extensive pyogenic infection, oliguria (from mercuric chloride poisoning or posttraumatic renal insufficiency), tubular obstruction, or other obstructive uropathies. Because nonrenal conditions can cause BUN levels to increase, interpret BUN levels in conjunction with serum creatinine levels.

Electrolytes

Because the kidneys regulate fluid and electrolyte balance, a critically ill patient with renal disease may experience significant serum electrolyte imbalances. The most commonly measured electrolytes are:

• *calcium and phosphorus*—Calcium and phosphorus levels have an inverse relationship; when one increases, the other decreases. In renal failure, the kidneys aren't able to excrete phosphorus, resulting in hyperphosphatemia and hypocalcemia.

• *chloride*—Chloride levels relate inversely to bicarbonate levels, reflecting acid-base balance. In renal disease, elevated chloride levels suggest metabolic acidosis. Hyperchloremia occurs in renal tubular necrosis, severe dehydration, and complete renal shutdown. Hypochloremia may occur with pyelonephritis.

• *potassium*—Hyperkalemia occurs with renal insufficiency or acidosis. In renal shutdown, potassium may rapidly increase to life-threatening levels. Hypokalemia may reflect renal tubular disease.

• *sodium*—Sodium helps the kidneys regulate body fluid. Renal disease may result in the loss of sodium through the kidneys.

Serum creatinine

Serum creatinine level reflects the glomerular filtration rate (GFR). Renal damage is indicated more accurately by increases in serum creatinine than by BUN level.

Serum osmolality

An increase in serum osmolality with a simultaneous decrease in urine osmolality indicates diminished distal tubule responsiveness to circulating antidiuretic hormone.

Serum proteins

Levels of the serum protein albumin may decline sharply from loss in the urine during nephritis or nephrosis, which in turn causes edema. Nephrosis may also cause total serum protein levels to decrease.

Uric acid

Because uric acid clears from the body by glomerular filtration and tubular secretion, elevated levels may indicate impaired renal function; below-normal levels may indicate defective tubular absorption.

Creatinine clearance

Creatinine clearance indicates GFR. Typically, high creatinine clearance rates have little diagnostic value. Low creatinine clearance rates may indicate reduced renal blood flow (associated with shock or renal artery obstruction), acute tubular necrosis, acute or chronic glomerulonephritis, advanced bilateral chronic pyelonephritis, advanced bilateral renal lesions, or nephrosclerosis.

Urea clearance

While urea clearance is a less reliable measurement of GFR than creatinine clearance, it still provides a good measure of overall renal function. High urea clearance rates rarely have diagnostic value. Low urea clearance rates may reflect decreased renal blood flow, acute or chronic glomerulonephritis, advanced bilateral chronic pyelonephritis, acute tubular necrosis, nephrosclerosis, advanced bilateral renal lesions, bilateral ureteral obstruction, or dehydration.

use this test to determine kidney placement. For diagnostic purposes, however, the KUB study provides limited information.

Nursing considerations

• KUB radiography requires no special pretest or posttest care. It's commonly a portable X-ray test performed at the bedside in the critical care unit.
• Explain the procedure to the patient.

Renal angiography

Renal angiography is used to visualize the arterial tree, capillaries, and venous drainage of the kidneys. The test involves the use of a contrast medium injected under fluoroscopy into a catheter in the femoral artery or vein.

Angiography of arteries

Renal arteriography (angiography of the arteries) may reveal:
• abnormal renal blood flow
• hypervascular renal tumors
• renal cysts
• renal artery stenosis
• renal artery aneurysms and arteriovenous fistulas
• pyelonephritis
• renal abscesses or inflammatory masses
• renal infarction
• renal trauma.

> Renal arteriography may reveal disorders such as these.

Nursing considerations

• Explain the procedure to the patient and confirm that he isn't allergic to iodine or shellfish. A patient with these allergies may have an adverse reaction to the contrast medium. If he has a seafood or dye allergy, a pretest preparation kit with prednisone and diphenhydramine may be given.
• Preprocedure testing should include evaluation of renal function (serum creatinine and BUN) and potential risk of bleeding (prothrombin time, partial thromboplastin time, and platelet count). Notify the doctor if results are abnormal.
• Report adverse reactions, such as nausea, vomiting, dizziness, headache, and urticaria.
• Depending on the patient's renal status, the doctor may order increased fluids after the procedure or an increased rate of I.V. fluid infusion to flush the contrast medium out of the patient's system.
• After the procedure, check the patient's serum creatinine and BUN levels to evaluate renal function (contrast media can cause acute renal failure).

Urine studies

Urine studies, such as urinalysis and urine osmolality, can indicate acute renal failure, renal trauma, and other disorders. Urinalysis can indicate renal or systemic disorders, warranting further investigation. A random urine specimen is used, preferably the first-voided morning specimen. (See *What urinalysis findings mean*, pages 472 and 473.)

Urine osmolality is used to evaluate the diluting and concentrating ability of the kidneys and varies greatly with diet and hydration status. The ability to concentrate urine is one of the first functions lost in renal failure.

Nursing considerations
• Before urinalysis, collect a random urine specimen from the indwelling urinary catheter or, preferably, the first-voided morning specimen. Send the specimen to the laboratory immediately.
• For urine osmolality testing, collect a random urine sample, preferably the first-voided morning specimen.

A renal disorder can affect every body system of a critically ill patient. It may be fatal without effective treatment.

Treatments

Renal disorders can adversely affect virtually every body system in a critically ill patient and may be fatal without effective treatment. Drug therapy is a treatment option in some cases, and others require dialysis of some kind.

Drug therapy

Drug therapy for renal disorders includes such agents as diuretics, adrenergics (such as dopamine, used for renal perfusion), and sulfonate cation-exchange resins to correct hyperkalemia. (See *Commonly used drugs for renal disorders*, pages 474 and 475.)

Ideally, drug therapy should be effective without impairing renal function. Drugs excreted mainly by the kidneys may require dosage adjustments to prevent nephrotoxicity.

To be effective without impairing renal function, drugs may require dosage adjustments.

Dialysis

A critically ill patient with a renal disorder may need dialysis treatments to remove toxic waste and excess fluid from the body. Depending on the patient's condition, hemodialysis or peritoneal dialysis may be used. In addition, a hemodynamically

(Text continues on page 475.)

What urinalysis findings mean

Test	Normal values or findings	Abnormal findings	Possible causes of abnormal findings
Color and odor	• Straw color	Clear to black	Dietary changes; use of certain drugs; metabolic, inflammatory, or infectious disease
	• Slightly aromatic odor	Fruity odor	Diabetes mellitus, starvation, dehydration
	• Clear appearance	Turbid appearance	Renal infection
Specific gravity	• Between 1.005 and 1.030, with slight variations from one specimen to the next	Below-normal specific gravity	Diabetes insipidus, glomerulonephritis, pyelonephritis, acute renal failure, alkalosis
		Above-normal specific gravity	Dehydration, nephrosis
		Fixed specific gravity	Severe renal damage
pH	• Between 4.5 and 8.0	Alkaline pH (above 8.0)	Fanconi's syndrome (chronic renal disease), urinary tract infection, metabolic or respiratory alkalosis
		Acidic pH (below 4.5)	Renal tuberculosis, phenylketonuria, acidosis
Protein	• No protein	Proteinuria	Renal disease (such as glomerulosclerosis, acute or chronic glomerulonephritis, nephrolithiasis, polycystic kidney disease, and acute or chronic renal failure)
Ketones	• No ketones	Ketonuria	Diabetes mellitus, starvation, conditions causing acutely increased metabolic demands and decreased food intake (such as vomiting and diarrhea)
Glucose	• No glucose	Glycosuria	Diabetes mellitus
Red blood cells (RBCs)	• 0 to 3 RBCs/high-power field	Numerous RBCs	Urinary tract infection, obstruction, inflammation, trauma, or tumor; glomerulonephritis; renal hypertension; lupus nephritis; renal tuberculosis; renal vein thrombosis; hydronephrosis; pyelonephritis; parasitic bladder infection; polyarteritis nodosa; hemorrhagic disorder
Epithelial cells	• Few epithelial cells	Excessive epithelial cells	Renal tubular degeneration

What urinalysis findings mean *(continued)*

Test	Normal values or findings	Abnormal findings	Possible causes of abnormal findings
White blood cells (WBCs)	• 0 to 4 WBCs/high-power field	Numerous WBCs	Urinary tract inflammation, especially cystitis or pyelonephritis
		Numerous WBCs and WBC casts	Renal infection (such as acute pyelonephritis and glomerulonephritis, nephrotic syndrome, pyogenic infection, and lupus nephritis)
Casts	• No casts (except occasional hyaline casts)	Excessive casts	Renal disease
		Excessive hyaline casts	Renal parenchymal disease, inflammation, glomerular capillary membrane trauma
		Epithelial casts	Renal tubular damage, nephrosis, eclampsia, chronic lead intoxication
		Fatty, waxy casts	Nephrotic syndrome, chronic renal disease, diabetes mellitus
		RBC casts	Renal parenchymal disease (especially glomerulonephritis), renal infarction, subacute bacterial endocarditis, sickle cell anemia, blood dyscrasias, malignant hypertension, collagen disease
Crystals	• Some crystals	Numerous calcium oxalate crystals	Hypercalcemia
		Cystine crystals (cystinuria)	Inborn metabolic error
Yeast cells	• No yeast crystals	Yeast cells in sediment	External genitalia contamination, vaginitis, urethritis, prostatovesiculitis
Parasites	• No parasites	Parasites in sediment	External genitalia contamination
Creatinine clearance	• Males (age 20): 90 mg/minute/1.73 m^2 of body surface • Females (age 20): 84 ml/minute/1.73 m^2 of body surface • Older patients: normally decreased concentrations by 6 ml/minute/decade	Above-normal creatinine clearance	Little diagnostic significance
		Below-normal creatinine clearance	Reduced renal blood flow (associated with shock or renal artery obstruction), acute tubular necrosis, acute or chronic glomerulonephritis, advanced bilateral renal lesions (as in polycystic kidney disease, renal tuberculosis, and cancer), nephrosclerosis, heart failure, severe dehydration

Commonly used drugs for renal disorders

Drugs	Indications	Adverse reactions	Practice pointers
Adrenergic agent			
Dopamine	To increase renal and mesenteric perfusion in the patient with renal failure (low dose [less than 5 mcg/kg/minute] dopamine infusions)	Tachycardia, palpitations, angina, conduction abnormalities, ventricular arrhythmias, hypotension, hypertension, nausea and vomiting	• Monitor the patient's cardiac rhythm. • Correct hypovolemia before starting the dopamine infusion. • Administer I.V. infusion with an infusion device to control flow. • Don't mix other drugs with the dopamine infusion. • Administer into a large vein to prevent extravasation. • If extravasation occurs, stop the infusion and infiltrate the site with phentolamine.
Alkalinizing agent			
Sodium bicarbonate	To correct metabolic acidosis in patients with renal failure	Metabolic alkalosis, hypernatremia, local pain and irritation at the injection site	• Use with caution in patients with heart failure or renal insufficiency and patients receiving corticosteroids. • Assess the patient's cardiopulmonary status. • Monitor the patient for metabolic alkalosis and electrolyte imbalance, especially hypocalcemia and hypokalemia. • Monitor the I.V. site for irritation and infiltration. (Extravasation may cause tissue damage and necrosis.)
Loop diuretics			
Bumetanide Furosemide Torsemide	To inhibit sodium reabsorption in the renal tubule, promote diuresis, and manage edema	Dizziness, muscle cramps, hypotension, headache, fluid and electrolyte imbalance (hypokalemia, hypochloremia, and hyponatremia), electrocardiogram (ECG) changes, chest pain, renal failure	• Monitor the patient for fluid and electrolyte imbalance. • Monitor the patient for cardiac arrhythmias, especially ventricular. • Avoid using in the patient with sulfonamide hypersensitivity. • Use is contraindicated in anuria. • Ototoxicity may result with rapid I.V. administration of high dosages.

Commonly used drugs for renal disorders (continued)

Drugs	Indications	Adverse reactions	Practice pointers
Sulfonate cation-exchange resin			
Sodium polystyrene sulfonate	To correct hyperkalemia	GI irritation, anorexia, nausea, vomiting, constipation, hypokalemia, hypocalcemia	• Monitor the patient for electrolyte imbalance, hypokalemia, and hypocalcemia. • Monitor the patient for ECG changes (flat, inverted T wave and prominent U wave) and ventricular arrhythmias. • For oral administration, mix resin with water or sorbitol—never orange juice because of high potassium content. • Monitor elderly patients for constipation and fecal impaction. • Use cautiously in patients who require sodium restriction, such as those with heart failure or hypertension, to prevent risk of sodium overload.

unstable patient may be treated with continuous renal replacement therapy (CRRT).

Continuous renal replacement therapy

CRRT is used to treat a patient with acute renal failure. Unlike the more traditional intermittent hemodialysis (IHD), CRRT is administered around the clock, providing the patient with continuous therapy without the destabilizing hemodynamic and electrolytic changes of IHD.

CRRT for whom?

CRRT is used for a patient who can't tolerate traditional hemodialysis, such as one with hypotension. Also, a patient who has had abdominal surgery and can't receive peritoneal dialysis because of an overwhelming risk of infection is a candidate for CRRT. (See *Understanding CRRT*, page 476.)

CRRT ABCs

CRRT techniques vary in complexity:
• Slow continuous ultrafiltration (SCUF) uses arteriovenous (AV) access and the patient's blood pressure to circulate blood through a hemofilter. Because the goal of this therapy is fluid removal, the patient doesn't receive any replacement fluids.

Because the goal of SCUF therapy is fluid removal, don't administer replacement fluids.

Advice from the experts

Understanding CRRT

Continuous renal replacement therapy (CRRT) filters toxic wastes from a patient's blood and infuses a replacement solution, such as lactated Ringer's solution or a special solution resembling plasma. It's used to correct fluid overload that doesn't respond to diuretics and treat critically ill patients who have acute renal failure, can't tolerate hemodialysis, or have some electrolyte and acid-base disturbances.

Hemofilter how-to

All CRRT equipment is located at the patient's bedside. The procedure doesn't require the immediate supervision of a dialysis nurse. The patient's blood may be accessed by femoral catheter, internal arteriovenous (AV) graft, or AV shunt. The hemofilter is made up of about 5,000 hollow fiber capillaries that filter blood at a rate of about 250 ml/minute, driven by the patient's arterial blood pressure. Because the amount of fluid removed is greater than the amount of replacement solution, the patient gradually loses fluid (12 to 15 L/day).

• Continuous AV hemofiltration (CAVH) uses the patient's blood pressure and AV access to circulate blood through a flow resistance hemofilter. To maintain filter patency and systemic blood pressure, the patient receives replacement fluids.
• Continuous AV hemodialysis (CAVH-D) combines hemodialysis with hemofiltration. In this technique, the infusion pump moves dialysate solution concurrent with blood flow, adding the ability to continuously remove solute while removing fluid. Like CAVH, it can be performed in a patient with hypotension and fluid overload.
• Continuous venovenous hemofiltration (CVVH) combines SCUF and CAVH. A double-lumen catheter provides access to a vein, and a pump moves blood through the hemofilter.
• Continuous venovenous hemodialysis (CVVH-D) is similar to CAVH-D, except that a vein provides the access while a pump is used to move dialysate solution concurrent with blood flow.

Nursing considerations

• If the patient is undergoing CRRT for the first time, explain its purpose and what to expect during treatment.
• Prime the hemofilter and tubing according to the manufacturer's instructions. (See *CAVH and CVVH setups.*)
• Assist with catheter insertion, if necessary, using strict sterile technique.
• If ordered, flush the catheters with a heparin flush solution to prevent clotting.

Flush the catheters with a heparin flush solution to prevent clotting.

CAVH and CVVH setups

The illustrations below show how to set up equipment for continuous arteriovenous hemofiltration (CAVH) and continuous venovenous hemofiltration (CVVH).

CAVH

In CAVH, the doctor inserts two large-bore, single-lumen catheters (depicted below). One catheter is inserted into an artery, most commonly the femoral artery. The other catheter is inserted into a vein, usually the femoral, sub-clavian, or internal jugular vein.

During CAVH, the patient's arterial blood pressure serves as a natural pump, driving blood through the arterial line. A hemofilter removes water and toxic solutes (ultrafiltrate) from the blood. Replacement fluid is infused into a port on the arterial side. This same port can be used to infuse heparin. The venous line carries the replacement fluid and purified blood to the patient.

Replacement solution

Inflow pump

Heparin

Heparin pump

From patient (arterial line)

Hemofilter

Outflow pump

To patient (venous line)

Sampling port

Hemofiltrate collection device

(continued)

CAVH and CVVH setups *(continued)*

CVVH

In CVVH, the doctor inserts a special double-lumen catheter (depicted below) into a large vein, commonly the subclavian, femoral, or internal jugular vein. Because the catheter is in a vein, an external pump is used to move blood through the system. The patient's venous blood moves through the arterial lumen to the pump, which then pushes the blood through the catheter to the hemofilter. Here, water and toxic solutes (ultrafiltrate) are removed from the patient's blood and drain into a collection device. Blood cells aren't removed because they're too large to pass through the filter. As the blood exits the hemofilter, it's then pumped through the venous lumen back to the patient.

Several components of the pump provide safety mechanisms. Pressure monitors on the pump maintain the flow of blood through the circuit at a constant rate. An air detector traps air bubbles before the blood returns to the patient. A venous trap collects blood clots that may be in the blood. A blood-leak detector signals when blood is found in the ultrafiltrate; a venous clamp operates if air is detected in the circuit or if there's a disconnection in the blood line.

Arterial lumen
Heparin solution
Hemofilter
Pressure monitors
Ultrafiltrate collection device

Catheter (double lumen)
Venous lumen
Infusion ports (I.V. solutions)
Replacement fluid
Venous trap
Air detector
Venous clamp

• Apply occlusive dressings to the insertion sites, and mark the dressings with the date and time.
• Before treatment, weigh the patient, take baseline vital signs, and make sure all necessary laboratory studies have been done (usually electrolyte levels, coagulation factors, CBC, BUN, and creatinine studies).
• Monitor the patient's vital signs and oxygen saturation.
• If a pulmonary arterty (PA) catheter has been placed, assess the patient's hemodynamic parameters, including central venous pressure (CVP), pulmonary artery pressure (PAP), and pulmonary artery wedge pressure (PAWP).
• Be alert for indications of hypovolemia (such as decreasing blood pressure and decreases in PAP, CVP, and PAWP) from too rapid removal of ultrafiltrate or hypervolemia due to excessive fluid replacement with a decrease in ultrafiltrate.
• Provide continuous cardiac monitoring because arrhythmias can occur with electrolyte imbalances.
• Monitor the patient's weight and vital signs frequently.
• Inspect the ultrafiltrate during the procedure. It should remain clear yellow, with no gross blood.
• Pink-tinged or bloody ultrafiltrate may signal a membrane leak in the hemofilter, which permits bacterial contamination. With a CVVH system, look for the blood leak detector to signal this. If a leak occurs, notify the doctor so the hemofilter can be replaced.
• Assess the leg used for vascular access for signs of obstructed blood flow, such as coolness, pallor, and weak pulse. Check the groin area on the affected side for signs of hematoma. Ask the patient if he has pain at the insertion sites.
• Calculate the amount of replacement fluid every hour or as ordered, according to your facility's policy. When calculating the amount of replacement fluid, add the amount of fluid in the collection device from the previous hour with any other fluid losses the patient has, such as blood loss, emesis, or NG tube drainage. From this total, subtract the patient's fluid intake for the past hour and the net fluid loss prescribed by the doctor.
• Infuse heparin in low doses (usually starting at 500 units/hour), as ordered, into an infusion port on the arterial side of the setup to prevent blood clotting during CAVH and CVVH.
• Measure thrombin clotting time or activated clotting time (ACT). A normal ACT is 100 seconds; during CRRT, keep it between 100 and 300 seconds, depending on the patient's clotting times.
• Make sure the patient doesn't bend the affected leg more than 30 degrees at the hip, to prevent catheter kinking.

I'm in! A membrane leak in the hemofilter could permit bacterial contamination.

• Obtain serum electrolyte levels every 4 to 6 hours or as ordered; anticipate adjustments in replacement fluid or dialysate based on the results.
• If the patient is receiving CVVH, monitor the arterial and venous pressure alarms.
• Inspect the site dressing for infection and bleeding. Perform skin care at the catheter insertion sites every 48 hours, using sterile technique. Cover the sites with an occlusive dressing.
• If the ultrafiltrate flow rate decreases, raise the bed to increase the distance between the collection device and the hemofilter. Lower the bed to decrease the flow rate.
• Clamping the ultrafiltrate line is contraindicated with some types of hemofilters because pressure may build up in the filter, clotting it and collapsing the blood compartment.
• Record the time the treatment begins, fluid balance figures, vital signs, weight, times of dressing changes, complications, medications given, and the patient's tolerance of the procedure. Document patient assessment parameters when the treatment course has ended.

Hemodialysis

Hemodialysis is used to remove toxic wastes and other impurities from the blood of a patient with renal failure. It's also used to restore or maintain acid-base and electrolyte balance and prevent the complications associated with uremia. To do so, this method extracts the by-products of protein metabolism—notably urea and uric acid—as well as creatinine and excess water from the patient's blood.

Blood, out and back

During hemodialysis, the patient's blood is removed from the body through a surgically created access site, pumped through a dialyzing unit to remove toxins, and then returned to the body.

Osmosis, diffusion, and filtration

The extracorporeal dialyzer works through a combination of osmosis, diffusion, and filtration. (See *How hemodialysis works.*)

Acute use or long-term therapy

Hemodialysis can be done in an emergency in acute renal failure or as regular long-term therapy in end-stage renal disease. In chronic renal failure, the frequency and duration of treatments depend on the patient's condition; up to several treatments per week, each lasting 3 to 4 hours, may be required. Rarely, hemodialysis is done to treat acute poisoning or drug overdose.

Here's how hemodialysis works: Blood is removed from the body, toxins are removed, and then blood is returned to the body.

How hemodialysis works

In hemodialysis, blood flows from the patient to an external dialyzer (or artificial kidney) through an arterial access site.

Inside the dialyzer

Inside the dialyzer, blood and dialysate flow countercurrently, divided by a semipermeable membrane. The composition of the dialysate resembles normal extracellular fluid. The blood contains an excess of specific solutes (such as metabolic waste products and electrolytes), and the dialysate contains electrolytes that may be at abnormal levels in the patient's bloodstream. The dialysate's electrolyte composition can be modified to raise or lower electrolyte levels, depending on the patient's needs.

Diffusion

Excretory function and electrolyte homeostasis are achieved by diffusion—the movement of molecules across the dialyzer's semipermeable membrane—from an area of higher solute concentration to an area of lower concentration.

Ultrafiltration

Water (a solvent) crosses the membrane from the blood into the dialysate by ultrafiltration. Excess water, waste products, and other metabolites are removed through osmotic pressure, the movement of water across the semipermeable membrane from an area of lesser solute concentration to one of greater solute concentration, and hydrostatic pressure, which forces water from the blood compartment into the dialysate compartment.

    After it's cleaned of impurities and excess water, the blood returns to the body through a venous site.

Three systems

Three system types are used to deliver dialysate:

    The proportioning system—the most common type—mixes concentrate with water to form dialysate, which then circulates through the dialyzer and goes down a drain after a single pass, followed by fresh dialysate.

    The batch system uses a reservoir for circulating dialysate.

    The regenerative system uses sorbents to purify and regenerate recirculating dialysate.

Types of dialyzers

There are two types of dialyzers:

    hollow filter

    flat-plate, or parallel flow-plate.

    These dialyzers may be used several times on each patient. Heparin is used to prevent clot formation during hemodialysis.

Hollow-filter dialyzer

The hollow-filter dialyzer, the most common type, contains fine capillaries with a semipermeable membrane enclosed in a plastic chamber. Blood flows through these capillaries as the system pumps dialysate in the opposite direction on the outside of the capillaries.

Blood in

Dialysate out

Hollow fibers

Jacket

Dialysate in

Purified blood out

Flat-plate or parallel flow-plate dialyzer

The flat-plate or parallel flow-plate dialyzer has two or more layers of semipermeable membrane bound by a semirigid or rigid structure. Blood ports are located at both ends, between the membranes. Blood flows between the membranes, and dialysate flows in the opposite direction, along the outside of the membranes.

Dialysate in

Membranes

Purified blood out

Dialysate out

Blood in

Specially trained nurses usually perform the procedure in a hemodialysis unit; in the critically ill patient, it's performed at the bedside using portable equipment.

Nursing considerations

• If the patient is undergoing hemodialysis for the first time, explain its purpose and what to expect during and after treatment. Explain that he'll first undergo a procedure to create a vascular access. (See *Hemodialysis access sites.*)

Access obtained

After vascular access:
• Weigh the patient, take his vital signs, and assess breath and heart sounds. Check for edema and jugular vein distention.
• Use good hand-washing technique and wear protective eyewear, gown, and gloves during the hemodialysis procedure.
• Discard (don't recap) all needles used in the procedure in designated containers.
• Assess the vascular access site for the presence of a bruit and thrill and keep the vascular access site well supported and resting on a sterile drape or sterile barrier shield.
• As ordered, prepare the hemodialysis equipment. Follow the manufacturer's and your facility's protocols and maintain strict aseptic technique to prevent the introduction of pathogens into the patient's bloodstream during treatment.
• Check and record the patient's vital signs every 30 minutes during treatment to detect possible complications. Fever may point to infection from pathogens in the dialysate or equipment; give an antipyretic, an antibiotic, or both, as ordered. Hypotension may indicate hypovolemia or a drop in HCT; give blood or fluid supplements I.V., as ordered. Rapid respirations may signal hypoxemia or fluid overload. Assess breath sounds and oxygen saturation and give supplemental oxygen, as ordered.
• Monitor the patient's cardiac rhythm for arrhythmias that may result from electrolyte and pH changes in the blood due to hemodialysis.
• Periodically check the dialyzer blood lines to make sure all connections are secure. Monitor the lines for clotting.
• Assess the patient for headache, muscle twitching, backache, nausea or vomiting, and seizures, which may indicate disequilibrium syndrome caused by rapid fluid removal and electrolyte changes.
• If disequilibrium syndrome occurs, notify the doctor immediately; he may reduce the blood flow rate or stop dialysis. Muscle cramps also may result from

Assess your patient for headache and other problems caused by rapid fluid removal and electrolyte changes.

Hemodialysis access sites

Hemodialysis requires vascular access through a subclavian or femoral vein or an arteriovenous (AV) fistula, shunt, or graft. The site and type of access used depend on the expected duration of dialysis, the surgeon's preference, and the patient's condition.

Subclavian vein catheterization

Using the Seldinger technique, the doctor or surgeon inserts an introducer needle into the subclavian vein. He then inserts a guide wire through the introducer needle and removes the needle. Using the guide wire, he then threads a 5" to 12" (12.5 to 30.5 cm) plastic or Teflon catheter with a Y-hub into the patient's vein.

Femoral vein catheterization

Using the Seldinger technique, the doctor or surgeon inserts an introducer needle into the right or left femoral vein. He then inserts a guide wire through the introducer needle and removes the needle. Using the guide wire, he then threads a 5" to 12" plastic or Teflon catheter with a Y-hub or two catheters — one for inflow and another, placed about ½" (1.3 cm) distal to the first, for outflow.

AV fistula

To create a fistula, the surgeon makes an incision in the patient's wrist or lower forearm, then a small incision in the side of an artery and another in the side of a vein. He then sutures the edges of the incisions together to make a common opening approximately 1" to 3" (2.5 to 7.5 cm) long.

AV shunt

To create a shunt, the surgeon makes an incision in the patient's wrist, lower forearm, or ankle (rarely). He then inserts a 6" to 10" (15- to 25.5-cm) transparent Silastic cannula into an artery and another into a vein. Finally, he tunnels the cannulas out through incisions and joins them with a piece of Teflon tubing.

AV graft

To create a graft, the surgeon makes an incision in the patient's forearm, upper arm, or thigh. He then tunnels a natural or synthetic graft under the skin and sutures the distal end to an artery and the proximal end to a vein.

rapid fluid and electrolyte shifts. As ordered, relieve cramps by injecting normal saline solution into the venous return line.

• Observe the patient carefully for signs and symptoms of internal bleeding, such as apprehension; restlessness; pale, cold, clammy skin; excessive thirst; hypotension; rapid, weak, thready pulse; increased respirations; and decreased body temperature. Report any of these signs immediately and prepare to decrease heparinization or administer a blood transfusion, as ordered.

• After completion of hemodialysis, monitor the vascular access site for bleeding. If bleeding is excessive, maintain pressure on the site and notify the doctor. If a temporary catheter is used for dialysis, flush the catheter according to your facility's policy.

• Make sure that the arm used for vascular access isn't used for another procedure, including I.V. line insertion, blood pressure monitoring, and venipuncture.

• Assess circulation at the access site by auscultating for the presence of bruits and palpating for thrills. Lack of bruits at a vascular access site for dialysis may indicate a blood clot, requiring immediate surgical attention.

• Keep an accurate record of the patient's food and fluid intake and encourage him to comply with prescribed restrictions, such as increased calorie intake, decreased fluid intake, and limited protein, potassium, and sodium intake.

> Make sure the arm used for vascular access isn't used for another procedure.

Peritoneal dialysis

Like hemodialysis, peritoneal dialysis is used to remove toxins from the blood of a patient with acute or chronic renal failure who doesn't respond to other treatments. Unlike hemodialysis, peritoneal dialysis uses the patient's peritoneal membrane as a semipermeable dialyzing membrane.

How it's done

In peritoneal dialysis, the dialysate (the solution instilled into the peritoneal cavity by catheter) draws waste products, excess fluid, and electrolytes from the blood across the semipermeable peritoneal membrane. (See *Principles of peritoneal dialysis*.) After a prescribed period, the dialysate is drained from the peritoneal cavity, removing impurities with it. The dialysis procedure is then repeated, using a new dialysate each time, until waste removal is complete and fluid, electrolyte, and acid-base balance has been restored.

With special preparation, the critical care nurse may perform peritoneal dialysis using an automatic or semiautomatic cycle machine.

Principles of peritoneal dialysis

Peritoneal dialysis works through a combination of diffusion and osmosis.

Diffusion

In diffusion, particles move through a semipermeable membrane from an area of high-solute concentration to an area of low-solute concentration. In peritoneal dialysis, the water-based dialysate being infused contains glucose, sodium chloride, calcium, magnesium, acetate or lactate, and no waste products. Therefore, waste products and excess electrolytes in the blood cross through the semipermeable peritoneal membrane into the dialysate. Removing the waste-filled dialysate and replacing it with fresh solution keeps the waste concentration low and encourages further diffusion.

Osmosis

In osmosis, fluids move through a semipermeable membrane from an area of low-solute concentration to an area of high-solute concentration. In peritoneal dialysis, dextrose is added to the dialysate to give it a higher solute concentration than the blood, creating a high osmotic gradient. Water migrates from the blood through the membrane at the beginning of each infusion, when the osmotic gradient is highest.

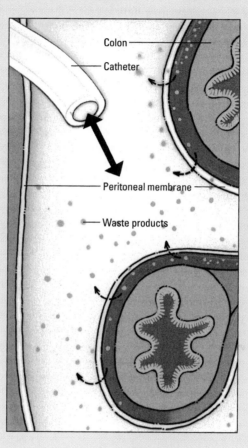

Colon

Catheter

Peritoneal membrane

Waste products

Peritonitis results when bacteria enter the peritoneal cavity through the catheter or insertion site.

Upside

Peritoneal dialysis has several advantages over hemodialysis—it's simpler, less costly, and less stressful. Also, it's nearly as effective as hemodialysis while posing fewer risks.

Downside

Even so, peritoneal dialysis can cause severe complications. The most serious one, peritonitis, results from bacteria entering the peritoneal cavity through the catheter or the insertion site. In addition to causing infection, peritonitis can scar the peritoneum, causing thickening of the membrane and preventing its use as a dialyzing membrane.

Other complications include catheter obstruction from clots, lodging against the abdominal wall, or kinking; hypotension; and hypovolemia from excessive plasma fluid removal.

Nursing considerations

• For the first-time peritoneal dialysis patient, explain the purpose of the treatment and what can be expected during and after the procedure.
• Explain that the doctor first inserts a catheter into the abdomen to allow instillation of dialysate. (See *Comparing peritoneal dialysis catheters.*)
• Before catheter insertion, take and record the patient's baseline vital signs and weight.
• Ask the patient to urinate to reduce the risk of bladder perforation and increase comfort during catheter insertion. If he can't urinate, perform straight catheterization, as ordered, to drain the bladder.
• During dialysis, monitor the patient's vital signs every 10 minutes until they stabilize, then every 2 to 4 hours or as ordered. Report any abrupt or significant changes.
• Periodically check the patient's weight and report any gain.
• Using aseptic technique, change the catheter dressing every 24 hours or whenever it becomes wet or soiled.
• To determine whether a wet abdominal dressing around the catheter site is from leakage of dialysate or wound drainage, use a dextrose test strip. Because of its high dextrose content, dialysate reacts positively while wound drainage doesn't.
• Monitor the patient for signs of infection. (See *Check for signs of peritonitis.*)
• When emptying the collection bag and measuring the solution, wear protective eyewear and gloves.
• Observe the outflow drainage for blood.
• Keep in mind that drainage is commonly blood-tinged after catheter placement but should clear after a few fluid exchanges. Notify the doctor of bright red or persistent bleeding.
• Watch the patient for respiratory distress, which may indicate fluid overload or leakage of dialyzing solution into the pleural space. If it's severe, drain the patient's peritoneal cavity and call the doctor.
• Periodically check the outflow tubing for clots or kinks that may be obstructing drainage.
• Have the patient change position often. Provide passive range-of-motion (ROM) exercises and encourage deep breathing and coughing to improve comfort, reduce the chance of skin breakdown and respiratory problems, and enhance dialysate drainage.

Take charge!

Check for signs of peritonitis

If you detect signs or symptoms of peritonitis, notify the doctor and send a dialysate specimen to the laboratory for smear and culture.

    Watch closely for these signs and symptoms:
• fever
• persistent abdominal pain and cramping
• slow or cloudy dialysis drainage
• swelling and tenderness around the catheter
• increased white blood cell count.

Put me back! The patient loses protein through dialysis and requires protein replacement.

Comparing peritoneal dialysis catheters

The first step in any type of peritoneal dialysis is the insertion of a catheter to allow instillation of dialyzing solution. The doctor may insert a Tenckhoff, flanged collar, or column disk peritoneal catheter.

Tenckhoff catheter

To implant a Tenckhoff catheter, the doctor inserts the first 6¾" (17.1 cm) of the catheter into the patient's abdomen. The next 2¾" (7-cm) segment, which may have a Dacron cuff at one or both ends, is imbedded subcutaneously. Within a few days after insertion, the patient's tissues grow around the cuffs, forming a tight barrier against bacterial infiltration. The remaining 3⅞" (9.8 cm) of the catheter extends outside of the abdomen and is equipped with a metal adapter at the tip that connects to dialyzer tubing.

Flanged collar catheter

To insert a flanged collar catheter, the doctor positions the collar just below the dermis so that the device extends through the abdominal wall. He keeps the distal end of the cuff from extending into the peritoneum, where it could cause adhesions.

Column disk peritoneal catheter (CDPC)

To insert a CDPC, the doctor rolls up the flexible disk section of the implant, inserts it into the peritoneal cavity, and retracts it against the abdominal wall. The implant's first cuff rests just outside the peritoneal membrane and its second cuff rests just under the skin. Because the CDPC doesn't float freely in the peritoneal cavity, it prevents inflowing dialyzing solution from being directed at the sensitive organs, which increases patient comfort during dialysis.

• Maintain adequate nutrition, following any prescribed diet. The patient loses protein through the dialysis procedure and, therefore, requires protein replacement.

• To prevent fluid imbalance, calculate the patient's fluid balance at the end of each dialysis session or after every 8-hour period in a longer session. Include oral and I.V. fluid intake as well as urine output, wound drainage, and perspiration. Record and report any significant imbalance, whether positive or negative.

Renal disorders

The most common renal disorders seen in critical care units include acute renal failure and acute tubular necrosis.

Acute renal failure is sometimes reversible.

Acute renal failure

Acute renal failure is the sudden interruption of renal function resulting from:
• obstruction
• reduced circulation
• renal parenchymal disease.

Acute renal failure is sometimes reversible, but if it's left untreated, permanent damage can lead to chronic renal failure. As a critical care nurse, you play a vital role in assessing and treating patients with acute renal failure.

What causes it

Acute renal failure may be classified as prerenal, intrarenal, or postrenal. Each type has different causes. (See *Causes of acute renal failure.*)

Pathophysiology

Each classification of acute renal failure—prerenal, intrarenal and postrenal—has its own pathophysiology:

• *Prerenal failure* results from conditions that diminish blood flow to the kidneys (hypoperfusion). Examples include hypovolemia, hypotension, vasoconstriction, or inadequate cardiac output. One condition, prerenal azotemia (excess nitrogenous waste products in the blood), accounts for 40% to 80% of all cases of acute renal failure. Azotemia occurs as a response to renal hypoperfusion. Typically, it can be rapidly reversed by restoring renal blood flow and glomerular filtration.

Causes of acute renal failure

Acute renal failure is classified as prerenal, intrarenal, or postrenal. All conditions that lead to prerenal failure impair blood flow to the kidneys (renal perfusion), resulting in decreased glomerular filtration rate and increased tubular reabsorption of sodium and water. Intrarenal failure results from damage to the kidneys. Postrenal failure results from obstructed urine flow. The causes of each type of acute renal failure are listed here.

Prerenal failure	Intrarenal failure	Postrenal failure

Prerenal failure

Cardiovascular disorders
- Arrhythmias
- Cardiac tamponade
- Cardiogenic shock
- Heart failure
- Myocardial infarction

Hypovolemia
- Burns
- Dehydration
- Diuretic overuse
- Hemorrhage
- Hypovolemic shock
- Trauma

Peripheral vasodilation
- Antihypertensive drugs
- Sepsis

Renovascular obstruction
- Arterial embolism
- Arterial or venous thrombosis
- Tumor

Severe vasoconstriction
- Disseminated intravascular coagulation
- Eclampsia
- Malignant hypertension
- Vasculitis

Intrarenal failure

Acute tubular necrosis
- Ischemic damage to renal parenchyma from unrecognized or poorly treated prerenal failure
- Nephrotoxins, including analgesics; anesthetics, such as methoxyflurane; antibiotics, such as gentamicin; heavy metals, such as lead; radiographic contrast media; and organic solvents
- Obstetric complications, such as eclampsia, postpartum renal failure, septic abortion, and uterine hemorrhage
- Myoglobin release, such as crush injury, myopathy, sepsis, and transfusion reaction

Other parenchymal disorders
- Acute glomerulonephritis
- Acute interstitial nephritis
- Acute pyelonephritis
- Bilateral renal vein thrombosis
- Malignant nephrosclerosis
- Papillary necrosis
- Periarteritis nodosa (inflammatory disease of the arteries)
- Renal myeloma
- Sickle cell disease
- Systemic lupus erythematosus
- Vasculitis

Postrenal failure

Bladder obstruction
- Anticholinergic drugs
- Autonomic nerve dysfunction
- Infection
- Tumor

Ureteral obstruction
- Blood clots
- Calculi
- Edema or inflammation
- Necrotic renal papillae
- Retroperitoneal fibrosis or hemorrhage
- Surgery (accidental ligation)
- Tumor
- Uric acid crystals

Urethral obstruction
- Prostatic hyperplasia or tumor
- Strictures

 • *Intrarenal failure,* also called *intrinsic* or *parenchymal* renal failure, results from damage to the filtering structures of the kidneys, usually from acute tubular necrosis, a disorder that causes cell death, or from nephrotoxic substances, such as certain antibiotics or radiologic dyes.

• *Postrenal failure* results from bilateral obstruction of urine outflow, as in prostatic hyperplasia or bladder outlet obstruction.

Going through phases

With treatment, the patient passes through three distinct phases:

- oliguric (decreased urine output)
- diuretic (increased urine output)
- recovery.

Output down

Oliguria is a decreased urine output (less than 400 ml/24 hours). Prerenal oliguria results from decreased blood flow to the kidney. Before damage occurs, the kidney responds to decreased blood flow by conserving sodium and water. Once damage occurs, the kidney's ability to conserve sodium is impaired. Untreated prerenal oliguria may lead to acute tubular necrosis.

During this phase, BUN and creatinine rise, and the ratio of BUN to creatinine falls from 20:1 (normal) to 10:1. Hypervolemia also occurs, causing edema, weight gain, and elevated blood pressure.

After damage occurs, the kidney's ability to conserve sodium is impaired.

Output up

The diuretic phase is marked by urine output that can range from normal (1 to 2 L/day) to as great as 4 to 5 L/day. High urine volume has two causes, including:

- the kidney's inability to conserve sodium and water
- osmotic diuresis produced by high BUN levels.

During the diuretic phase, which lasts several days to 1 week, BUN and creatinine levels slowly increase and hypovolemia and weight loss result. These conditions can lead to deficits of potassium, sodium, and water that can be deadly if left untreated. If the cause of the diuresis is corrected, azotemia gradually disappears and the patient improves greatly — leading to the recovery stage.

When the delicate basement membrane is irreparably damaged, chronic renal failure results.

On the road to recovery...

The recovery phase is reached when BUN and creatinine levels return to normal and urine output is between 1 and 2 L/day.

It gets complicated...

Primary damage to the renal tubules or blood vessels results in kidney failure (intrarenal failure). The causes of intrarenal failure are classified as nephrotoxic, inflammatory, or ischemic.

Irreparable damage

When nephrotoxicity or inflammation causes the damage, the delicate layer under the epithelium (basement membrane) becomes irreparably damaged, commonly proceeding to chronic renal failure.

Severe or prolonged lack of blood flow (ischemia) may lead to renal damage (ischemic parenchymal injury) and excess nitrogen in the blood (intrinsic renal azotemia).

> A change in blood pressure and volume signals prerenal failure.

What to look for

The signs and symptoms of prerenal failure depend on the cause. If the underlying problem is a change in blood pressure and volume, the patient may have:
• oliguria
• tachycardia
• hypotension
• dry mucous membranes
• flat jugular veins
• lethargy progressing to coma
• decreased cardiac output and cool, clammy skin in a patient with heart failure.

Negative progress

As renal failure progresses, the patient may show signs and symptoms of uremia, including:
• confusion
• GI complaints
• fluid in the lungs
• infection.

About 5% of all hospitalized patients develop acute renal failure. The condition is usually reversible with treatment; however, if it isn't treated, it may progress to end-stage renal disease, excess urea in the blood (prerenal azotemia or uremia), and death.

What tests tell you

The following tests are used to diagnose acute renal failure:
• Blood studies reveal elevated BUN, serum creatinine, and potassium levels and decreased blood pH, bicarbonate, HCT, and Hb levels.
• Urine studies show casts, cellular debris, decreased specific gravity and, in glomerular diseases, proteinuria and urine osmolality close to serum osmolality. Urine sodium level is less than 20 mEq/L if oliguria results from decreased perfusion and more than 40 mEq/L if it results from an intrarenal problem.

• Arterial blood gas (ABG) analysis reveals decreased pH and bicarbonate levels, indicating metabolic acidosis.
• Creatinine clearance testing is used to measure the GFR and estimate the number of remaining functioning nephrons.
• Electrocardiogram (ECG) shows tall, peaked T waves, a widening QRS complex, and disappearing P waves if increased blood potassium (hyperkalemia) is present.
• Other studies used to determine the cause of renal failure include kidney ultrasonography, plain films of the abdomen, KUB radiography, excretory urography, renal scan, retrograde pyelography, computed tomography scan, and nephrotomography.

How it's treated

Supportive measures include a diet high in calories and low in protein, sodium, and potassium, with supplemental vitamins and restricted fluids. Meticulous electrolyte monitoring is essential to detect hyperkalemia.

Send in the drugs

Drug therapy for acute renal failure may include:
• sodium bicarbonate and hypertonic glucose and insulin infusions administered I.V. as well as sodium polystyrene sulfonate (Kayexalate) by mouth or by enema and calcium gluconate (in an emergency) to reduce potassium levels
• diuretics to manage hypervolemia
• low-dose dopamine (Intropin) to enhance renal perfusion
• atrial natriuretic peptide to improve perfusion to the glomeruli, by inhibiting sodium and water absorption and dilating the afferent arteriole.

Overload overview

Even with treatment, an elderly patient is susceptible to volume overload, possibly precipitating acute pulmonary edema, hypertensive crisis, hyperkalemia, and infection.

If hyperkalemia can't be reduced with drugs, acute therapy may include dialysis. To control uremic symptoms, hemodialysis or peritoneal dialysis may be necessary. CAVH and CVVH are alternative hemodialysis techniques for treatment of acute renal failure.

What to do

• If the patient is to receive a diuretic, be sure to obtain a urine sample for urine studies before giving the diuretic because these drugs can alter urine results.
• Measure and record the patient's intake and output hourly, including wound drainage, NG tube output, and diarrhea. Insert an

Calcium gluconate may be given in an emergency to reduce your patient's potassium levels.

EMERGENCY

indwelling urinary catheter, if indicated. Assess skin turgor; evidence of peripheral, sacral, or periorbital edema; and degree of pitting, if any. Monitor the patient's daily weight for trends.

• Check urine specific gravity and osmolality, as ordered. With prerenal failure, urine specific gravity is typically greater than 1.020 and urine osmolality is increased up to 500 mOsm; with intrarenal failure, specific gravity is typically less than 1.010 and osmolality is approximately 350 mOsm.

• Anticipate the insertion of a PA catheter to assess the patient's hemodynamic status. Monitor parameters, as ordered.

• Assess Hb levels and HCT and replace blood components, as ordered.

• Don't use whole blood to transfuse the patient if he's prone to heart failure and can't tolerate extra fluid volume. Packed RBCs deliver the necessary blood components without added volume.

• Assess the patient's cardiopulmonary status often, including heart and breath sounds. Monitor his cardiac rhythm. Report any shortness of breath, crackles, gallops, pericardial friction rub, tachycardia, or the presence of S_3 or S_4 heart sounds because these may be signs of fluid overload.

• Monitor the patient's level of consciousness at least every 2 to 4 hours, or more often if indicated.

• Maintain proper electrolyte balance. Strictly monitor the patient's potassium levels, especially during emergency treatment to reduce potassium levels. Avoid administering drugs containing potassium.

• Watch the patient for symptoms of hyperkalemia (malaise, anorexia, paresthesia, or muscle weakness) and ECG changes (tall, peaked T waves; widening QRS complex; and disappearing P waves), and report them immediately.

• Provide a high-calorie, low-protein, low-potassium, low-sodium diet, with vitamin supplements. Give anorectic patients small, frequent meals.

• Use aseptic technique when performing procedures because a critically ill patient with renal failure is highly susceptible to infection.

• Encourage coughing and deep breathing and perform passive ROM exercises to reduce complications of bed rest.

• Use a lubricating lotion to combat dry skin. Provide mouth care frequently because mucous membranes become dry.

• Assess the patient for signs and symptoms of GI bleeding. Administer drugs carefully, especially antacids and stool softeners. Use aluminum-hydroxide-based antacids; magnesium-based antacids can cause serum magnesium levels to increase critically.

• Use appropriate safety measures, such as side rails or assistance with ambulation, because the patient with central nervous

Use aseptic technique when performing procedures on a critically ill patient with renal failure. He's at high risk for infection.

Go team!
You need to
coordinate care
for a patient with
renal failure.

Take charge!

Meet the team

Because acute renal failure affects multiple body systems, a multidisciplinary approach to care is needed, with the critical care nurse coordinating care. Here's how other members of the multidisciplinary team contribute to your patient's care:
• A nephrologist can evaluate and manage the patient's kidney function.
• A respiratory or cardiology specialist may be involved to deal with complications.
• A nutritional therapist may recommend restrictions or supplements.
• A physical or occupational therapist may help the patient with energy conservation and rehabilitation.
• If a prolonged hospital stay is expected and the patient requires long-term care or home care, social services should be consulted early in the patient's care.
• The patient and his family may benefit from spiritual counseling.

system involvement may be dizzy or confused. Institute bleeding precautions to minimize the patient's risk of bleeding.
• Provide appropriate care to a patient receiving hemodialysis, peritoneal dialysis, or CRRT. Provide emotional support to the patient and his family and explain diagnostic tests, treatments, and procedures. Caring for the patient with renal failure requires the involvement of a multidisciplinary team. (See *Meet the team*.)

Acute tubular necrosis

Acute tubular necrosis (also called *acute tubulointerstitial nephritis*) causes 75% of all cases of acute renal failure. This disorder destroys the tubular segment of the nephron, causing renal failure and uremia (excess by-products of protein metabolism in the blood). Because acute tubular necrosis is fatal in 40% to 70% of cases, prevention, prompt recognition, and intervention by the critical care nurse are vital.

What causes it

Acute tubular necrosis may follow two types of kidney injury:
• *Ischemic* injury, the most common cause, interrupts blood flow to the kidneys. The longer the blood flow is interrupted, the worse the kidney damage.
• *Nephrotoxic* injury usually affects debilitated patients, such as the critically ill and those who have undergone extensive surgery.

Blood disruption

In ischemic injury, blood flow to the kidneys may be disrupted by:
- circulatory collapse
- severe hypotension
- trauma
- hemorrhage
- dehydration
- cardiogenic or septic shock
- surgery
- anesthetics
- transfusion reactions.

Toxic talk

Nephrotoxic injury can result from:
- ingesting or inhaling toxic chemicals, such as carbon tetrachloride, heavy metals, and methoxyflurane anesthetics
- a hypersensitivity reaction of the kidneys to such substances as antibiotics and radiographic contrast agents.

Cause and effect

Some specific causes of acute tubular necrosis and their effects include:
- a diseased tubular epithelium that allows glomerular filtrate to leak through the membranes and be reabsorbed into the blood
- obstructed urine flow from the collection of damaged cells, casts, RBCs, and other cellular debris in the tubules
- ischemic injury to glomerular epithelial cells, causing cellular collapse and poor glomerular capillary permeability
- ischemic injury to the vascular endothelium, eventually causing cellular swelling and tubular obstruction.

Nephrotoxic injury can result from ingesting or inhaling toxic chemicals. This looks safe to eat, though.

Pathophysiology

Deep or shallow lesions may occur in acute tubular necrosis.

Lesion lesson

With ischemic injury, necrosis creates deep lesions, destroying the tubular epithelium and basement membrane (the delicate layer underlying the epithelium). Ischemic injury causes patches of necrosis in the tubules. Ischemia can also cause lesions in the connective tissue of the kidney.

With nephrotoxic injury, necrosis occurs only in the epithelium of the tubules, leaving the basement membrane of the nephrons intact. This type of damage may be reversible. (See *A close look at acute tubular necrosis,* page 496.)

A close look at acute tubular necrosis

In acute tubular necrosis caused by ischemia, patches of necrosis occur, usually in the straight portions of the proximal tubules, as depicted below.

In areas without lesions, tubules are usually dilated. In acute tubular necrosis caused by nephrotoxicity, the tubules have a more uniform appearance, as depicted in the second illustration.

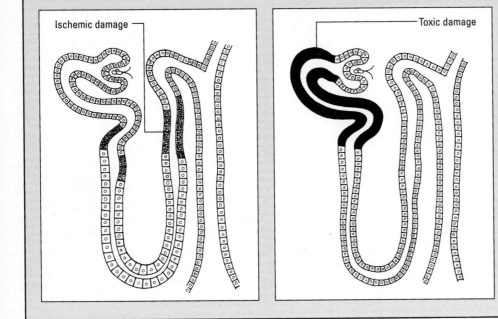

Ischemic damage

Toxic damage

Toll-taking

Toxicity takes a toll on renal structures. Nephrotoxic agents can injure tubular cells by:
- direct cellular toxic effects
- coagulation and destruction (lysis) of RBCs
- oxygen deprivation (hypoxia)
- crystal formation of solutes.

Getting complicated

There are several common complications of acute tubular necrosis:
- Infections (frequently septicemia) complicate up to 70% of all cases and are the leading cause of death.
- GI hemorrhage, fluid and electrolyte imbalance, and cardiovascular dysfunction may occur during the acute or recovery phase.
- Neurologic complications are common in elderly patients and occur occasionally in younger patients.

Common complications of acute tubular necrosis include infections, GI hemorrhage, and hypercalcemia.

• Excess blood calcium (hypercalcemia) may occur during the recovery phase.

What to look for

Early-stage acute tubular necrosis may be hard to spot because the patient's primary disease may obscure the signs and symptoms. The first recognizable sign may be decreased urine output, usually less than 400 ml/24 hours.

Difficult to detect

Acute tubular necrosis is difficult to detect in its early stages, so look closely at members of high-risk populations, such as elderly patients or those with diabetes, and be alert for subtle signs and symptoms during your nursing assessments.

Other signs and symptoms depend on the severity of systemic involvement and may include:
• bleeding abnormalities
• vomiting of blood
• dry skin and mucous membranes
• lethargy
• confusion
• agitation
• edema
• fluid and electrolyte imbalances
• muscle weakness with hyperkalemia
• cardiac arrhythmias.

Mortality can be as high as 70%, depending on complications from underlying diseases. The patient with a nonoliguric form of acute tubular necrosis has a better prognosis.

> Acute tubular necrosis is difficult to detect in its early stages, so look closely at patients who are members of high-risk groups, such as elderly people.

What tests tell you

Acute tubular necrosis is hard to diagnose except in advanced stages. The following tests are commonly performed:
• Urinalysis shows dilute urine, low osmolality, high sodium levels, and urine sediment containing RBCs and casts.
• Blood studies reveal high BUN and serum creatinine levels, low serum protein levels, anemia, platelet adherence defects, metabolic acidosis, and hyperkalemia.
• ECG may show arrhythmias from electrolyte imbalances and, with hyperkalemia, a widening QRS complex, disappearing P waves, and tall, peaked T waves.

How it's treated

The patient with acute tubular necrosis requires vigorous supportive measures during the acute phase until normal kidney function is restored. Therapy may include:
- initially, diuretics and fluids to flush tubules of cellular casts and debris and to replace lost fluids
- low-dose dopamine to improve renal blood flow
- emergency I.V. infusion of 50% glucose, regular insulin, and sodium bicarbonate in case of hyperkalemia
- sodium polystyrene sulfonates given by mouth or by enema to reduce potassium levels
- calcium channel blockers and prostaglandins, which may aid in treating nephrotoxic acute tubular necrosis.

Think of me! ECG may show arrhythmias due to electrolyte imbalances.

Furthermore

Treatment for the patient with acute tubular necrosis may also include:
- daily replacement of projected and calculated fluid losses
- transfusion of packed RBCs for anemia
- non-nephrotoxic antibiotics for infection
- hemodialysis or peritoneal dialysis to prevent severe fluid and electrolyte imbalance and uremia.

What to do

- Take steps to maintain the patient's fluid balance. Accurately record intake and output, including wound drainage, NG tube output, and hemodialysis or peritoneal dialysis balances. Weigh the patient daily.
- Assist with insertion of a central venous or PA catheter to monitor fluid status. Monitor hemodynamic parameters, as indicated.
- Watch the patient for fluid overload, a common complication when infusing large fluid volumes.
- Monitor Hb levels and HCT, and administer blood products, as needed. Use fresh packed cells instead of whole blood to prevent fluid overload and heart failure.
- Maintain electrolyte balance. Monitor laboratory results and report imbalances.
- Monitor the patient's vital signs, oxygen saturation, cardiac rhythm, and cardiopulmonary status. Treat hypotension immediately to avoid renal ischemia. Monitor vital signs closely. Fever and chills may signal the onset of an infection, which is the leading cause of death in acute tubular necrosis. (See *Temperature regulation in elderly patients*.)
- Check for potassium content in prescribed drugs (for example, potassium penicillin). Provide dietary restriction of foods

Watch out for fluid overload! It's a common complication when infusing large fluid volumes.

containing sodium and potassium, such as bananas, orange juice, and baked potatoes.
• Provide adequate calories and essential amino acids while restricting protein intake to maintain an anabolic state. Total parenteral nutrition may be indicated for a critically ill and debilitated or catabolic patient.
• Use aseptic technique, especially when handling catheters, because the critically ill or debilitated patient is vulnerable to infection.
• Administer sodium bicarbonate, as ordered, for acidosis or assist with dialysis in severe cases.
• Provide the patient with reassurance and emotional support. Encourage him and his family to verbalize their concerns. Fully explain each procedure.
• To prevent acute tubular necrosis, make sure the patient is well hydrated before surgery or after X-rays requiring use of a contrast medium. Administer mannitol, as ordered, to the high-risk critically ill patient before and during these procedures. Administer nephrotoxic drugs cautiously and avoid using contrast dyes in the high-risk patient.

Senior moment

Temperature regulation in elderly patients

The aging process changes a person's temperature regulation system, making temperature an unreliable sign of infection. Even with a clinical infection, an older person may register no fever. Furthermore, an older adult is at higher risk for infection because of age-related changes in immunity and increased incidence of hospitalization, which can lead to nosocomial infections.

Quick quiz

1. The kidneys secrete erythropoietin when:
   A.   oxygen supply in tissue decreases.
   B.   calcium levels are insufficient.
   C.   vitamin D becomes inactive.
   D.   pH level drops below 7.35.
Answer: A. The kidneys secrete erythropoietin when the oxygen supply in tissue decreases.

2. In peritoneal dialysis, particles move through a semipermeable membrane from an area of high-solute concentration to an area of low-solute concentration in a process called:
   A.   diffusion.
   B.   active transport.
   C.   passive transport.
   D.   osmosis.
Answer: A. Diffusion is the movement of particles through a semipermeable membrane from an area of high-solute concentration to an area of low-solute concentration. In peritoneal dialysis, waste products and excess electrolytes in the blood cross through

the semipermeable peritoneal membrane into the dialysate through diffusion.

3. Prerenal failure results from:
A. bilateral obstruction of urine outflow.
B. conditions that diminish blood flow to the kidneys.
C. damage to the kidneys.
D. ischemic damage to renal parenchyma.

Answer: B. Prerenal failure is caused by any condition that reduces flood flow to the kidneys, such as hypotension, hypovolemia, vasoconstriction, or inadequate cardiac output.

4. Acute tubular necrosis following ischemic renal injury may be due to:
A. fluid volume overload.
B. inhaling toxic chemicals.
C. a hypersensitivity reaction to radiographic contrast agents.
D. severe hypotension.

Answer: D. Acute tubular necrosis may follow ischemic or nephrotoxic injury to the kidney. Ischemic injury may be caused by severe hypotension as well as circulatory collapse, trauma, hemorrhage, dehydration, surgery, anesthetics, transfusion reactions, and cardiogenic or septic shock.

Scoring

☆☆☆ If you answered all four questions correctly, take a dip in a kidney-shaped pool. Your information-filtering system is intact.

☆☆ If you answered three questions correctly, try to reabsorb what you've read. With a little concentration, you can detoxify your thinking and restore balance through work and play regulation.

☆ If you answered one or two questions correctly, don't expel yourself. Reread the chapter to flush out the facts and then take the test again.

Your future is full of glands and hormones. The endocrine system chapter is near.

Endocrine system

Just the facts

In this chapter, you'll learn:

♦ structure and function of the endocrine system

♦ assessment of the endocrine system

♦ diagnostic tests and treatments for critically ill patients

♦ endocrine system disorders and related nursing care.

Understanding the endocrine system

The endocrine system regulates and integrates the body's metabolic activities and maintains internal homeostasis. It has three major components:

glands, which are specialized organs that secrete hormones and chemical transmitters into the bloodstream to regulate body functions

hormones, which are chemical substances secreted by glands in response to stimulation from the nervous system and other sites

receptors, which are protein molecules that trigger specific physiologic changes in target cells in response to hormonal stimulation.

> Simply put, the endocrine system regulates metabolism and maintains homeostasis.

Glands

The major glands of the endocrine system are the:
• pituitary gland
• thyroid gland
• parathyroid glands
• adrenal glands

Endocrine gland sites

The illustration below shows the location of the major endocrine glands (except the gonads).

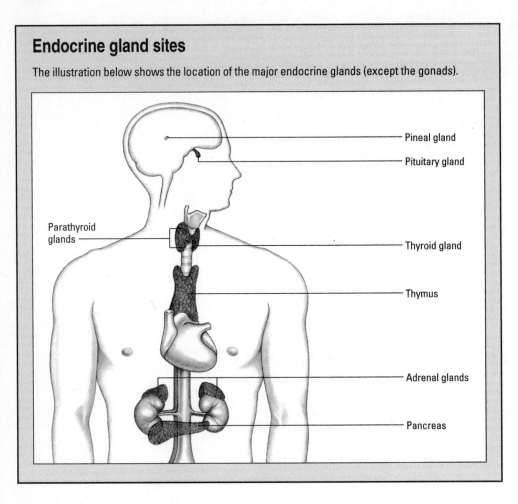

- pancreas
- thymus
- pineal gland
- gonads. (See *Endocrine gland sites*.)

Pituitary gland

The pituitary gland rests in the sella turcica, a depression in the sphenoid bone at the base of the brain. It's connected by the infundibulum to the hypothalamus, from which it receives chemical and nervous stimulation. (See *Understanding the hypothalamus*.)

Powerful pea

The pea-size pituitary gland has two regions, or lobes: posterior and anterior. The posterior pituitary lobe stores and releases oxy-

Understanding the hypothalamus

The hypothalamus integrates the endocrine and autonomic nervous systems. It controls some endocrine gland functions through neural and hormonal stimulation.

Pathways to the posterior pituitary

Neural pathways connect the hypothalamus to the posterior pituitary gland. These neurons stimulate the posterior pituitary gland to secrete two effector hormones—antidiuretic hormone (ADH) and oxytocin—which are stored in the posterior pituitary.

When ADH is secreted, the body retains water. Oxytocin stimulates uterine contractions during labor and milk secretion in lactating women.

Inhibition and stimulation

The hypothalamus produces many other inhibiting and stimulating hormones and other factors that regulate functions of the anterior pituitary.

> The hypothalamus integrates the endocrine and autonomic nervous systems.

tocin and antidiuretic hormone, which are produced by the hypothalamus. The larger anterior pituitary lobe produces at least six hormones:

- growth hormone (GH), or somatotropin
- thyroid-stimulating hormone (TSH), or thyrotropin
- corticotropin
- follicle-stimulating hormone (FSH)
- luteinizing hormone (LH)
- prolactin.

Thyroid gland

The thyroid gland is directly beneath the larynx and partly in front of the trachea. It has two lobes—one on either side of the trachea—connected by a strip of tissue called the isthmus, which gives the gland a butterfly shape. (See *A close look at the thyroid gland,* page 504.)

A close look at the thyroid gland

This illustration shows the structure and location of the thyroid gland.

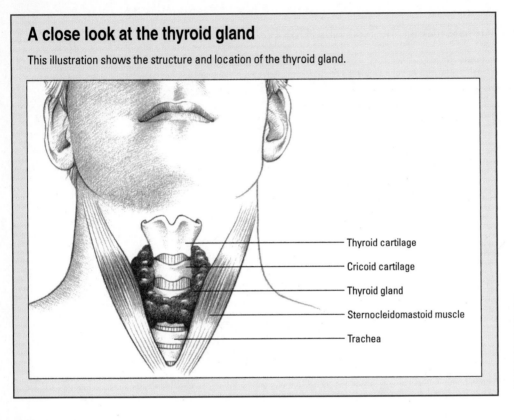

- Thyroid cartilage
- Cricoid cartilage
- Thyroid gland
- Sternocleidomastoid muscle
- Trachea

Three thyroid hormones regulate metabolism and blood calcium levels: T_3, T_4, and calcitonin.

Metabolism master

The thyroid gland regulates the body's metabolism and produces three hormones:

① triiodothyronine (T_3)

② thyroxine (T_4)

③ calcitonin.

T_3 and T_4 work together to regulate cellular metabolism. Calcitonin maintains blood calcium levels by inhibiting calcium release from bone.

Parathyroid glands

There are four parathyroid glands, one in each corner of the thyroid gland. Together, they produce parathyroid hormone (PTH) or parathormone, which maintains the body's calcium levels by traveling to three target tissue types, including:

• bone

- GI tissue
- renal tissue.

Adrenal glands

There are two adrenal glands, one above each kidney. Each adrenal gland has an inner layer (the medulla) and an outer layer (the cortex).

Innie

The adrenal medulla produces catecholamines and is considered a neuroendocrine structure because catecholamines play an important role in the autonomic (involuntary) nervous system.

Outie

The adrenal cortex is the larger, outer layer and has three zones, or cell layers:

zona glomerulosa, the outermost zone, which produces mineralocorticoids, primarily aldosterone

zona fasciculata, the middle and largest zone, which produces the glucocorticoids cortisol (hydrocortisone), cortisone, and corticosterone, and small amounts of the sex hormones androgen and estrogen

zona reticularis, the innermost zone, which produces mainly glucocorticoids and some sex hormones.

Pancreas

The pancreas has endocrine and exocrine functions. It's located behind the stomach, extending to the spleen and within the duodenal curve.

Visit the islets of Langerhans

The islets of Langerhans, which perform the endocrine function of the pancreas, contain alpha, beta, and delta cells. Alpha cells produce glucagon; beta cells, insulin; and delta cells, somatostatin.

Thymus

The thymus is located below the sternum and contains lymphatic tissue. This gland produces hormones

Alpha cells produce glucagon.

Beta cells produce insulin.

Delta cells produce somatostatin.

(thymosin and thymopoietin), but its major role is related to the immune system: It produces T cells, which are involved in cell-mediated immunity.

Pineal gland

The tiny pineal gland lies at the back of the third ventricle of the brain. It produces the hormone melatonin, which regulates a person's sleep-wake cycles and plays a role in mood regulation and the female reproductive cycle.

Gonads

The gonads include the:
- ovaries (in females)
- testes (in males).

Feminine function

The ovaries promote the development and maintenance of female sex-related traits, regulate the menstrual cycle, and maintain the uterus for pregnancy. With the help of other hormones, they also prepare the mammary glands for lactation.

Masculine mode

The testes produce spermatozoa and the male sex hormone testosterone. Testosterone stimulates and maintains male sex-related traits.

Hormones

Hormones can be structurally classified into three types:

✍ amines

✌ polypeptides

🖐 steroids.

Amenable amines

Amines are derived from tyrosine, an essential amino acid found in most proteins. They include the thyroid hormones (T_3 and T_4) and the catecholamines (epinephrine, norepinephrine, and dopamine).

Poly want a peptide?

Polypeptides are protein compounds made of many amino acids connected by peptide bonds. They include:

> The thymus produces T cells, which are involved in cell-mediated immunity.

> Amines are derived from tyrosine, an essential amino acid found in most proteins.

Senior moment

Endocrine changes with aging

A common endocrine change in older adults is a decreased ability to tolerate stress.

Age matters
When stress stimulates an older person's pancreas, the blood glucose concentration increases more and remains elevated longer than in a younger adult. Such diminished glucose tolerance is a normal part of aging. Keep this in mind when evaluating an older person for diabetes.

If coma develops
Older adults rarely become ketoacidotic, even with extremely elevated blood glucose levels. When coma develops, it's usually from hyperosmolar hyperglycemic nonketotic syndrome, which can be triggered by acute illness or surgery in older adults.

Other changes
Other normal variations in endocrine function include a decreased cortisol secretion rate and decline in serum aldosterone levels. Changes in endocrine function during menopause vary from woman to woman, but normally estrogen levels diminish and follicle-stimulating hormone production increases. In men, testosterone levels may decrease.

• anterior pituitary hormones (somatotropin [GH], TSH, corticotropin, FSH, LH, melanocyte-stimulating hormone, and prolactin)
• posterior pituitary hormones (antidiuretic hormone [ADH] and oxytocin)
• PTH
• pancreatic hormones (insulin and glucagon).

Steroidal secretions

Steroids, derived from cholesterol, include:
• adrenocortical hormones (aldosterone and cortisol) secreted by the adrenal cortex
• sex hormones (estrogen and progesterone in females and testosterone in males) secreted by the gonads.

Hormone release and transport

All hormone release results from endocrine gland stimulation, but release patterns vary greatly. For example:
• Corticotropin (secreted by the anterior pituitary lobe) and cortisol (secreted by the adrenal cortex) are released in irregular spurts in response to body rhythm cycles, with levels peaking in the early morning.
• Secretion of PTH (by the parathyroid gland) and prolactin (by the anterior pituitary) occurs fairly evenly throughout the day.
• Secretion of insulin by the pancreas has both steady and sporadic release patterns. (See *Endocrine changes with aging*.)

Hormone function

When a hormone reaches its target site, it binds to a specific receptor on the cell membrane or in the cell:
• Polypeptides and some amines bind to membrane receptor sites.
• Smaller, more lipid-soluble steroids and thyroid hormones diffuse through cell membranes and bind to intracellular receptors.

Right on target!

After binding to the receptor, each hormone produces a unique physiologic change, depending on the target site and the hormone's action at that site. A particular hormone may produce different effects at different target sites.

Hormonal regulation

Hormonal regulation is a complex feedback mechanism involving hormones, the central nervous system, and blood chemicals and metabolites that maintain the body's delicate equilibrium by regulating hormone synthesis and secretion. (Feedback is information sent to endocrine glands that signals the need for changes in hormone levels, either increasing or decreasing hormone production and release.) (See *The feedback loop*.)

Heart and hormones

The heart has a role in endocrine function. In the walls of the atria, there are cells that produce atrial natriuretic hormone (ANH), also referred to as *atrial natriuretic peptide*. The atria secrete ANH in response to increased atrial wall stretching due to increased blood pressure or blood volume. ANH causes increased renal excretion of sodium and water, thus reducing blood volume and blood pressure.

When a hormone reaches its target site, it binds to a receptor on the cell membrane or in the cell.

Endocrine system assessment

To assess the patient's endocrine system, take an accurate health history and conduct a thorough physical examination. When an acutely ill patient with an endocrine disorder arrives in the critical care unit, the information you obtain from the health history, physical examination, and diagnostic tests are used to treat and stabilize the patient. After the patient is stable, you may obtain additional data.

ANH reduces blood volume and pressure by increasing sodium and water excretion by the kidneys.

The feedback loop

This diagram depicts the negative feedback mechanism that regulates the endocrine system.

From simple…

Simple feedback occurs when the level of one substance regulates the secretion of hormones (simple loop). For example, a low serum calcium level stimulates the parathyroid gland to release parathyroid hormone (PTH). PTH, in turn, promotes resorption of calcium. A high serum calcium level inhibits PTH secretion.

…to complex

When the hypothalamus receives negative feedback from target glands, the mechanism is more complicated (complex loop). *Complex feedback* occurs through an axis established between the hypothalamus, pituitary gland, and target organ. For example, secretion of corticotropin-releasing hormone from the hypothalamus stimulates release of corticotropin by the pituitary, which in turn stimulates cortisol secretion by the adrenal gland (the target organ). A rise in serum cortisol levels inhibits corticotropin secretion by decreasing corticotropin-releasing hormone.

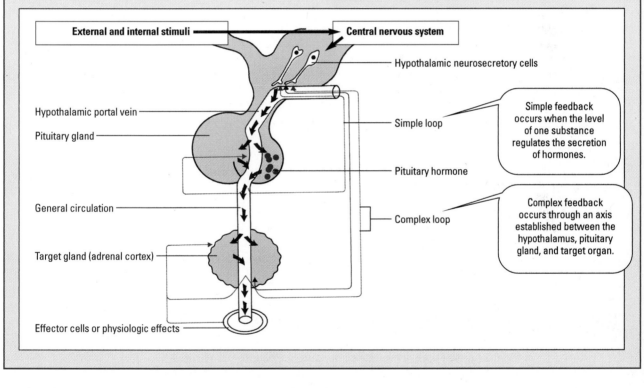

External and internal stimuli — Central nervous system

Hypothalamic neurosecretory cells

Hypothalamic portal vein

Pituitary gland

Simple loop

Simple feedback occurs when the level of one substance regulates the secretion of hormones.

Pituitary hormone

General circulation

Complex loop

Complex feedback occurs through an axis established between the hypothalamus, pituitary gland, and target organ.

Target gland (adrenal cortex)

Effector cells or physiologic effects

Health history

Because the endocrine system interacts with all other systems, conduct a complete body systems review. Ask the patient about overall patterns of health and illness.

Current health status

Ask the patient to describe his chief complaint. Common complaints associated with endocrine disorders include fatigue, weakness, weight changes, mental status changes, polyuria, polydipsia, and abnormalities of sexual maturity and function.

Ask questions

Be sure to ask the patient these questions:
• Have you noticed any changes in your skin?
• Do you bruise more easily than you used to?
• Have you noticed any change in the amount or distribution of your body hair?
• Do your eyes burn or feel gritty when you close them?
• How good is your sense of smell?

Intolerance of cold may indicate hypothyroidism...

Previous health status

Ask about the patient's medical history. You may identify insidious and vague symptoms of endocrine dysfunction if the patient has had a skull fracture, surgery, complications of surgery, or brain infection, such as meningitis or encephalitis.

Family history

Ask about the patient's family history because some endocrine disorders, such as diabetes mellitus and thyroid disease, are inherited or have strong familial tendencies.

Lifestyle patterns

Ask the patient about temperature intolerance, which may indicate certain thyroid disorders. For example, intolerance of cold may indicate hypothyroidism and intolerance of warmth, hyperthyroidism.

...and intolerance of warmth may indicate hyperthyroidism.

Physical assessment

Include a total body evaluation and complete neurologic assessment in the physical examination because the hypothalamus plays an important role in regulating endocrine function.

Permissive condition

If the patient's condition permits, begin by measuring height, weight, and vital signs. Measure blood pressure with the patient lying, sitting, and standing. Compare the findings with normal expected values and the patient's baseline measurements, if available. Then use inspection, palpation, and auscultation to obtain the most objective findings.

Inspection

Systematically inspect the patient's overall appearance and examine all areas of the body.

Outward appearance

Assess the patient's physical appearance and mental and emotional status. Note such factors as affect, speech, level of consciousness (LOC), orientation, appropriateness and neatness of dress and grooming, and activity level. Evaluate general body development, including posture, body build, proportionality of body parts, and distribution of body fat.

Skin deep

Assess the patient's overall skin color and inspect the skin and mucous membranes for lesions or areas of increased, decreased, or absent pigmentation. As you do so, be sure to consider racial and ethnic variations. In a dark-skinned patient, color variations are best assessed in the sclera, conjunctiva, mouth, nail beds, and palms. Next, assess the patient's skin texture and hydration.

Hairy topic

Inspect the hair for amount, distribution, condition, and texture. Observe scalp and body hair for abnormal patterns of growth or hair loss. Remember to consider normal racial, ethnic, and sex-related differences in hair growth and texture.

Nail it

Next, check the patient's fingernails for cracking, peeling, separation from the nail bed (onycholysis), or clubbing; observe the toenails for fungal infection, ingrown nails, discoloration, length, and thickness.

Face it

Assess the patient's face for overall color and the presence of erythematous areas, especially in the cheeks. Note facial expression. Is it pained and anxious, dull and flat, or alert and interested? Note the shape and symmetry of the eyes and look for eyeball protrusion, incomplete eyelid closure, or periorbital edema. Have the patient extend his tongue, and inspect it for color, size, lesions, positioning, and tremors or unusual movements.

Inspect the patient's outward appearance from head to toe.

Neck check

While standing in front of the patient, examine the neck—first with it held straight, then slightly extended. Check for neck symmetry and midline positioning and for symmetry of the trachea.

Use tangential lighting directed downward from the patient's chin to see the thyroid gland. An enlarged thyroid may be diffuse and asymmetrical.

Chest check

Evaluate the overall size, shape, and symmetry of the patient's chest, noting any deformities. In females, assess the breasts for size, shape, symmetry, pigmentation (especially on the nipples and in skin creases), and nipple discharge (galactorrhea). In males, observe for bilateral or unilateral breast enlargement (gynecomastia) and nipple discharge.

Go to extremes

Inspect the patient's extremities. Check the arms and hands for tremors. To do so, have the patient hold both arms outstretched in front with the palms down and fingers separated. Place a sheet of paper on the outstretched fingers and watch for trembling.

Note any muscle wasting, especially in the upper arms. Have the patient grasp your hands to assess the strength and symmetry of his grip.

Next, inspect the legs for muscle development, symmetry, color, and hair distribution. Examine the feet for size and note lesions, corns, calluses, or marks from socks or shoes. Inspect the toes and the spaces between them for maceration and fissures.

Examine the patient's feet for size and other characteristics.

Palpation

Palpate the thyroid gland if possible. When you can palpate it, the gland should be smooth, finely lobulated, nontender, and either soft or firm. You should be able to feel the gland's sections. (See *Palpating the thyroid.*)

A thyroid nodule feels like a knot, protuberance, or swelling; a firm, fixed nodule may be a tumor. Be careful not to confuse thick neck musculature with an enlarged thyroid or a goiter.

Search for signs

Attempt to elicit Chvostek's sign and Trousseau's sign if you suspect a patient has hypocalcemia (low serum calcium levels) related to deficient or ineffective PTH secretion from hypoparathyroidism or surgical removal of the parathyroid glands.

Palpating the thyroid

To palpate the thyroid, follow these steps:
• Stand in front of the patient and place your index and middle fingers below the cricoid cartilage on both sides of the trachea.
• Palpate for the thyroid isthmus as he swallows.
• Then ask the patient to flex his neck toward the side being examined as you gently palpate each lobe.

In most cases, only the isthmus connecting the two lobes is palpable. However, if the patient has a thin neck, you may feel the whole gland. If he has a short, stocky neck, you may have trouble palpating even an enlarged thyroid.

Right and left

To locate the right lobe, follow these steps:
• Use your right hand to displace the thyroid cartilage slightly to your left.
• Hook your left index and middle fingers around the sternocleidomastoid muscle, as shown at right, to palpate for thyroid enlargement.

Then examine the left lobe by using your left hand to displace the thyroid cartilage and your right hand to palpate the lobe.

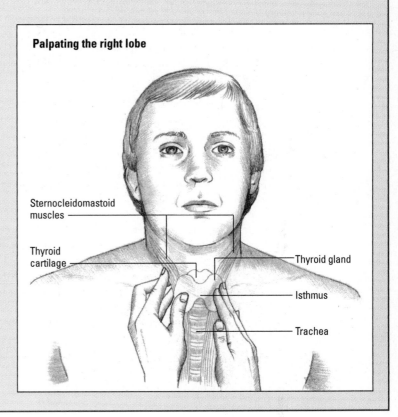

Palpating the right lobe

Sternocleidomastoid muscles

Thyroid cartilage

Thyroid gland

Isthmus

Trachea

To elicit Chvostek's sign, tap the facial nerve in front of the ear with a finger; if the facial muscles contract toward the ear, the test is positive for hypocalcemia.

To elicit Trousseau's sign, place a blood pressure cuff on the arm and inflate it above the patient's systolic pressure. In a positive test, the patient exhibits carpal spasm (ventral contraction of the thumb and digits) within 3 minutes.

Auscultation

If you palpate an enlarged thyroid, auscultate the gland for systolic bruits, a sign of hyperthyroidism. Bruits are heard when accelerated blood flow through the thyroid arteries produces vibrations.

Two techniques

To auscultate for bruits, place the bell of the stethoscope over one of the lateral lobes of the thyroid and then listen carefully for a low, soft, rushing sound. To ensure that tracheal sounds don't obscure bruits, have the patient hold his breath while you auscultate.

To distinguish a bruit from a venous hum, first listen for the rushing sound; then gently occlude the jugular vein with your fingers on the side you're auscultating and listen again. A venous hum (produced by jugular blood flow) disappears during venous compression; a bruit doesn't.

That's amazing! A venous hum disappears during venous compression; a bruit doesn't.

Diagnostic tests

Various tests are used to suggest, confirm, or rule out an endocrine disorder. Some test results also identify a dysfunction as hyperfunction or hypofunction or indicate whether a problem is primary, secondary, or functional. (See *Common endocrine laboratory studies.*) Endocrine function is tested through direct and indirect testing and imaging studies.

Direct and indirect testing

Direct and indirect testing measure hormone levels or substances controlled by hormones. When test results are borderline, provocative testing may be done. (See *Provocative testing*, page 518.)

Direct testing

The most common method, direct testing, is used to measure hormone levels in the blood or urine. Accurate measurement requires special techniques because the body contains only minute amounts of hormones.

Methods of direct testing used to measure hormone levels in the blood and urine are:
• immunoradiometric assays (IRMAs)
• radioimmunoassay (RIA)
• 24-hour urine testing.

IRMA and ICMA

IRMAs measure peptide and protein hormone levels using a receptor antiserum labeled with radioiodine.

(Text continues on page 518.)

Common endocrine laboratory studies

When a patient exhibits signs and symptoms of an endocrine disorder, laboratory studies provide valuable clues to the possible cause, as shown in the table below. (*Note:* Keep in mind that abnormal findings may stem from a problem unrelated to the endocrine system.) Remember that values differ among laboratories; check the normal range for the specific laboratory.

Test and purpose	Normal findings	Abnormal findings	Possible causes of abnormal findings
Blood tests			
Calcium This test is used to detect bone and parathyroid disorders.	9 to 10.5 mg/dl	Above-normal level	Hyperparathyroidism
		Below-normal level	Hypoparathyroidism
Catecholamine This test is used to assess adrenal medulla function.			
Epinephrine, basal supine	30 to 95 pg/ml	Above-normal level	Pheochromocytoma
Epinephrine, standing	0 to 140 pg/ml		
Norepinephrine, basal supine	15 to 475 pg/ml		
Norepinephrine, standing	200 to 1,040 pg/ml		
Cortisol This test is used to evaluate the status of adrenocortical function.	*8 a.m.:* 8 to 24 mcg/dl *4 p.m.:* 2 to 15 mcg /dl (Usually, the 4 p.m. level is half the 8 a.m. level.)	Above-normal level	Cushing's disease, Cushing's syndrome
		Below-normal level	Addison's disease, hypopituitarism
Glucose tolerance test, oral This test is used to detect diabetes mellitus and hypoglycemia.	Normal: 65 to 110 mg/dl Fasting: ≤ 110 mg/dl 30, 60, 90 min: < 200 mg/dl 120 min: < 140 mg/dl	Above-normal level	Diabetes mellitus
		Below-normal level	Hypoglycemia
Glycosylated hemoglobin This test is used to monitor the degree of glucose control in diabetes mellitus over 3 months.	< 6% of total hemoglobin— good control	Above-normal level	Uncontrolled diabetes mellitus

(continued)

Common endocrine laboratory studies *(continued)*

Test and purpose	Normal findings	Abnormal findings	Possible causes of abnormal findings
Blood tests *(continued)*			
Gonadotropin (follicle-stimulating hormone [FSH], luteinizing hormone [LH]) This test is used to distinguish a primary gonadal problem from pituitary insufficiency.	*Males* FSH: 5 to 20 mU/ml LH: 5 to 20 mU/ml	Above-normal level	Primary gonadal failure
		Below-normal level	Pituitary insufficiency
	Females FSH: Follicular phase, 5 to 20 mU/ml Midcycle peak, 2 to 30 mU/ml Luteal phase, 5 to 15 mU/ml Postmenopausal, > 50 mU/ml LH: Follicular phase, 5 to 25 mU/ml Midcycle peak, 25 to 100 mU/ml Luteal phase, 5 to 15 mU/ml Postmenopausal > 50 mU/ml		
Growth hormone (GH) radioimmunoassay This test is used to evaluate GH oversecretion.	*Males:* < 5 ng/ml *Females:* < 10 ng/ml	Above-normal level	Acromegaly
Insulin-induced hypoglycemia This test is used to detect hypopituitarism.	GH increase two to three times greater than baseline	Below-normal level of GH	Hypopituitarism
Parathyroid hormone This test is used to evaluate parathyroid function.	210 to 310 pg/ml	Above-normal level	Hyperparathyroidism
		Below-normal level	Hypoparathyroidism

Common endocrine laboratory studies *(continued)*

Test and purpose	Normal findings	Abnormal findings	Possible causes of abnormal findings
Blood tests *(continued)*			
Phosphorus This test is used to detect parathyroid disorders and renal failure.	3 to 4.5 mg/dl	Above-normal level	Hypoparathyroidism, renal failure
		Below-normal level	Hyperparathyroidism
Thyroid-stimulating hormone This test is used to detect primary hypothyroidism.	0.5 mU/ml 0.5 to 3.5 mU/ml	Above-normal level	Hypothyroidism
		Below-normal level	Hyperthyroidism
Thyroxine (T$_4$) radioimmunoassay This test is used to evaluate thyroid function and monitor iodine or antithyroid therapy.	4 to 11 mcg/dl	Above-normal level	Hyperthyroidism
		Below-normal level	Hypothyroidism
Triiodothyronine radioimmunoassay This test is used to detect hyperthyroidism if T$_4$ levels are normal.	75 to 220 ng/dl	Above-normal level	Hyperthyroidism
		Below-normal level	Hypothyroidism
Urine studies			
Cortisol This test is used to measure free cortisol to evaluate adrenocortical function.	10 to 100 mg/24 hr	Above-normal level	Cushing's disease
17-hydroxycorticosteroid This test is used to evaluate adrenal function.	3 to 15 mg/24 hr	Above-normal level	Hyperadrenalism
		Below-normal level	Hypopituitarism, adrenal disease
17-ketosteroid This test is used to evaluate adrenocortical and gonadal function.	*Males:* 6 to 21 mg/24 hr *Females:* 4 to 17 mg/24 hr	Above-normal level	Congenital adrenal hyperplasia
		Below-normal level	Adrenal insufficiency

Immunochemiluminometric assays (ICMAs) use a chemical reagent that emits a specific light wavelength when activated by a particular substance. IRMA and ICMA tests are more specific, stable, precise, and easier to use than RIAs.

Turn up the radioimmunoassay

RIA determines many hormone levels by incubating blood or urine (or a urine extract) with the hormone's antibody and a radiolabeled hormone tracer (antigen). Antibody-tracer complexes are then measured.

For example, charcoal absorbs and removes a hormone not bound to its antibody-antigen complex. Measuring the remaining radiolabeled complex indicates the extent to which the sample hormone blocks binding, compared with a standard curve showing reactions with known hormone quantities. Although the RIA method provides reliable results, it doesn't measure every hormone.

All-day affair

A 24-hour urine test may be ordered to confirm adrenal, renal, and gonadal disorders. Metabolite measurement is used to evaluate hormones excreted in virtually undetectable amounts.

Nursing considerations

For direct testing, hormone measurement may include serum or urine collection. Provide appropriate teaching:
• Venipuncture will be done to collect blood. Tell the patient when this will be done and who will do it.
• Accurate testing may require several blood samples taken at different times of the day because physiologic factors—such as stress, diet, episodic secretions, and body rhythms—can change circulating hormone levels.
• Urine is collected for 24 hours using the appropriate collection device. If a specimen is accidentally discarded, the collection must be restarted.

Indirect testing

Indirect testing is used to measure the substance controlled by a hormone—not the hormone itself. For example, glucose measurements are used to evaluate insulin levels and calcium measurements are used to assess PTH activity. Although RIAs measure these substances directly, indirect testing is easier and less costly.

Provocative testing

Provocative testing is used to determine an endocrine gland's reserve function when other tests show borderline hormone levels or don't quite pinpoint the site of the abnormality. For instance, an abnormally low cortisol level may indicate adrenal hypofunction or indirectly reflect pituitary hypofunction.

Provocative principle
Provocative testing works on this principle: Stimulate an underactive gland and suppress an overactive gland, depending on the patient's suspected disorder. A hormone level that doesn't increase with stimulation confirms primary hypofunction. Hormone secretion that continues after suppression confirms hyperfunction.

Not so fast

Glucose levels obtained indirectly accurately reflect insulin's effectiveness. Even so, various factors that affect calcium may alter PTH levels and, thus, results of indirect testing.

For example, abnormal protein levels can lead to seemingly abnormal calcium levels because nearly half of calcium binds to plasma proteins. Therefore, other possibilities must be ruled out before assuming that an abnormal calcium level reflects a PTH imbalance.

Rule out other possible causes of abnormal calcium levels before you assume it's PTH imbalance.

Nursing considerations

For indirect testing, hormone measurement may include serum or urine collection. Provide appropriate teaching:
• Venipuncture will be done to collect blood. Tell the patient when this will be done and who will do it.
• Accurate testing may require several blood samples taken at different times of the day because physiologic factors — such as stress, diet, episodic secretions, and body rhythms — can change circulating hormone levels.
• Urine is collected for 24 hours using the appropriate collection device. If a specimen is accidentally discarded, the collection must be restarted.

Imaging studies

Imaging studies are done with or after other tests. Some X-ray studies are performed at the bedside in the critical care unit. Computed tomography (CT) scans, magnetic resonance imaging (MRI), and nuclear medicine scans are done in the department and the nurse accompanies and monitors an unstable patient.

X-rays

Routine X-rays are used to evaluate how an endocrine dysfunction affects body tissues, although they don't reveal endocrine glands. For example, a bone X-ray, routinely ordered for a suspected parathyroid disorder, can show the effects of a calcium imbalance.

Nursing considerations
• Explain the procedure to the patient.
• Radiographic studies require no special pretest or posttest care.

CT scan and MRI

CT scan and MRI are used to assess an endocrine gland by providing high-resolution, tomographic, three-dimensional (3-D) images of the gland's structure, and may be used to identify tumors.

Nursing considerations

- Explain the procedure to the patient.
- Confirm that the patient isn't allergic to iodine or shellfish. A patient with such allergies may have an adverse reaction to the contrast medium. If the patient has an allergy, a pretest allergy preparation may be given.
- If contrast medium is ordered, explain that it's injected into an existing I.V. line or a new line may be inserted.
- Preprocedure testing should include evaluation of renal function (serum creatinine and blood urea nitrogen [BUN] levels) because the contrast medium can cause acute renal failure.
- After the procedure, encourage oral fluid intake to flush the contrast medium out of the patient's body, unless contraindicated or if the patient is on nothing-by-mouth status. The doctor may write an order to increase I.V. fluids.
- Check serum creatinine and BUN levels after the procedure.

Nuclear medicine studies

Nuclear medicine studies include radioactive iodine uptake (RAIU) test and radionuclide thyroid imaging.

One iodine uptake test

The RAIU test is done to evaluate thyroid function and to help distinguish between primary and secondary thyroid disorders.

After ingesting an oral dose of radioactive iodine the patient's thyroid is scanned at 2 hours, 6 hours, and 24 hours using an external single counting probe.

The amount of radioactivity detected by the probe is compared with the amount of radioactivity contained in the original dose to determine the percentage of radioactive iodine retained by the thyroid.

Below-normal iodine uptake may indicate hypothyroidism and above-normal uptake may indicate hyperthyroidism or early Hashimoto's thyroiditis.

Another iodine uptake test

Radionuclide thyroid imaging is done to:
- evaluate thyroid function
- assess size, structure, and position of the thyroid gland.

Such testing typically follows discovery of a palpable mass, enlarged gland, or asymmetrical goiter. After oral administration or I.V. injection of a radioisotope (such as iodine 131 (^{131}I), iodine 123 or technetium 99m pertechnetate) the images are taken of the thyroid gland.

Radionuclide thyroid imaging is ordered after a palpable mass, enlarged gland, or asymmetrical goiter is found.

Hot spots and cold spots

With radionuclide thyroid imaging, hyperfunctioning nodules (areas of excessive iodine uptake) appear as black regions called hot spots. Hypofunctioning nodules (areas of little or no iodine uptake) appear as white or light gray regions called cold spots. Biopsy may be performed on the lesion to rule out malignancy.

Nursing considerations

• Explain the procedure to the patient.
• Confirm that the patient isn't allergic to iodine or shellfish. A patient with such allergies may have an adverse reaction to the contrast medium or radioactive isotope. If the patient has an allergy, a pretest allergy preparation may be given.
• If I.V. radioisotope is ordered, explain that it's injected into an existing I.V. line or a new line may be inserted.
• After the procedure, encourage oral fluid intake to flush the radioisotope out of the patient's body, unless contraindicated or if the patient is on nothing-by-mouth status. The doctor may write an order to increase I.V. fluids.

Endocrine dysfunction can affect all body systems.

Treatments

Endocrine dysfunction can affect all body systems and, if not corrected, can be life-threatening. Treatment of an acutely ill patient with an endocrine disorder is a complex process that may include drug therapy, nonsurgical treatments, and surgical procedures such as pancreas transplantation.

Drug therapy

Drugs are commonly used to treat endocrine disorders, such as adrenal crisis, diabetic ketoacidosis, myxedema coma, and thyrotoxic crisis. Some drug therapies commonly used to treat critical care patients with acute endocrine disorders include:
• insulin therapy
• antithyroid medications
• thyroid replacement medications
• corticosteroids
• antidiuretic hormone. (See *Common endocrine medications*, pages 522 to 524.)

(Text continues on page 524.)

Common endocrine medications

Drugs	Indications	Adverse reactions	Practice pointers
Oral antidiabetics			
Sulfonylureas Glipizide Glyburide	• Type 2 diabetes	• Dizziness • Hypoglycemia • Leukopenia • Nausea • Nervousness • Weight gain	• Check for signs and symptoms of hypoglycemia and hyperglycemia. • Monitor blood glucose levels. An increased risk of hypoglycemia exists when given in combination with insulin.
Biguanides Metformin	• Type 2 diabetes	• Diarrhea • Flatulence • Headache • Hypoglycemia (rare if used as a single agent) • Lactic acidosis • Nausea and vomiting	• Give drug with meals. • Assess renal function. • Monitor for lactic acidosis, especially in patients with renal insufficiency. • Contrast dye may increase risk of lactic acidosis. Stop metformin 48 hours before procedure using contrast dye.
Thiazolidine-diones (TZDs) Pioglitazone Rosiglitazone	• Type 2 diabetes	• Edema • Headache • Hypoglycemia (rare if used as a single agent) • Myalgia • Pharyngitis • Upper respiratory infection • Weight gain	• Monitor liver function studies. • Don't use in patients with active liver disease. • Use cautiously in patients with edema or heart failure.
Alpha-glucosi-dase inhibitors Acarbose	• Type 2 diabetes	• Abdominal pain • Diarrhea • Flatulence	• Acarbose alone doesn't cause hypoglycemia. However, when given with a sulfonylurea or insulin, it may increase the hypoglycemic potential of the sulfonylurea. If hypoglycemia occurs, treat with glucose (dextrose) rather than sucrose because acarbose blocks sucrose uptake.
Insulins			
Rapid-acting: Lispro Short-acting: Regular Intermediate-acting: NPH Long-acting: UltraLente	• All types of diabetes	• Hypoglycemia • Weight gain	• Monitor for hypoglycemia. • Monitor blood glucose levels. • Educate the patient about the symptoms and treatment of hypoglycemia and hyperglycemia. • Use regular humulin insulin only with continuous insulin infusion and administer on I.V. infusion pump.

Common endocrine medications (continued)

Drugs	Indications	Adverse reactions	Practice pointers
Antithyroid medications			
Thyroid hormone antagonist Propylthiouracil	• Hyperthyroidism	• Arthralgia • Constipation • Drowsiness • Edema • Headache • Intolerance to cold • Lethargy • Loss of taste perception • Myxedema coma • Systemic lupus erythematosus–like syndrome • Vertigo • Weakness • Weight gain	• Use cautiously with anticoagulants because bleeding risk is increased. • Instruct the patient to report any signs of bleeding. • Monitor the effects of cardiac medications after hyperthyroidism is corrected; cardiac medication dosages may need to be decreased. • Frequent thyroid tests may be necessary initially to adjust dosing. • Educate the patient about symptoms of hypothyroidism (myxedema coma).
Thyroid replacement medications			
Thyroid hormone Levothyroxine	• Hypothyroidism	• Hypertension • Insomnia • Intolerance to heat • Irritability • Menstrual irregularities • Nervousness • Restlessness • Sleep disturbances • Tachycardia • Thyrotoxicosis • Weight loss	• Avoid aluminum- and magnesium-containing antacids, which decrease thyroxine absorption. • Requirements for antidiabetic medications may change with treatment. • Medications should be taken in the early morning on an empty stomach. • Frequent thyroid tests may be necessary initially to adjust dosing. • Monitor for toxicity. • Teach the patient about symptoms of toxicity (thyrotoxicosis symptoms). • Use cautiously in elderly patients and with those with renal impairment or cardiovascular disorders. • Monitor for cardiac arrhythmias such as tachycardia.

(continued)

Common endocrine medications (continued)

Drugs	Indications	Adverse reactions	Practice pointers
Corticosteroids			
Glucocorticoid Hydrocortisone	• Acute adrenal crisis	• Arthralgia • Cataracts • Delirium and hallucinations • Diabetes mellitus • Epistaxis • Hirsutism • Hypertension • Increased appetite • Insomnia • Muscle wasting • Nervousness • Peptic ulcer • Weight gain	• Avoid abrupt cessation because the adrenal gland is suppressed during steroid use. • Drug-induced diabetes can result. • Use cautiously if the patient is on concomitant anticoagulant use. Prothrombin time results may differ after steroids are initiated. • Use cautiously if potassium-depleting diuretics are used. Steroids can worsen hypokalemia. • Initial signs of infection may be masked due to the drug's anti-inflammatory effects. • Administer with food or milk to avoid GI distress. • Monitor blood pressure, weight, serum glucose level, and serum electrolyte level.

Nonsurgical treatments

Nonsurgical treatments for patients with endocrine disorders include meal planning for patients with diabetes and using a hyperthermia-hypothermia blanket to treat patients with hyperthermia due to an increased hypermetabolic state in thyrotoxic crisis.

Diabetes meal planning

Meal planning is the cornerstone of diabetes care because it directly controls the body's major glucose source. The American Dietetic Association and the American Diabetes Association recommend an individual nutritional assessment to determine appropriate medical nutrition therapy.

Taking control

When the patient's condition is stable, schedule a consultation with the dietitian or diabetes educator. The patient's food intake can be carefully controlled to prevent widely fluctuating blood glucose levels. Adherence to a meal plan to avoid hypoglycemia is even more important if the patient is taking insulin or sulfonylureas.

> Meal planning aids control of the body's major glucose source.

Nursing considerations

• When the patient is stable, explain the need for a special meal plan to control blood glucose levels. Arrange for a dietitian to teach the patient how to plan meals. The dietitian may recommend the food exchange system. This method, based on the carbohydrate, fat, and protein content of six basic food groups, allows greater flexibility in meal planning. Exchange groups include dairy products, vegetables, fruits, breads, meats, and fats.

Hyperthermia-hypothermia blanket

A hyperthermia-hypothermia blanket is used to increase, decrease, or maintain body temperature through conductive heat or cold transfer between the blanket and patient. It can be operated manually or automatically.

Common for cooling

The therapeutic blanket is most commonly used to reduce high fever resulting from infectious and inflammatory processes and hypermetabolic states such as thyrotoxic crisis. The treatment may be initiated when more conservative measures, such as baths, ice packs, and antipyretics, are unsuccessful.

It's also used to:
• maintain normal temperature during surgery or shock
• induce hypothermia during surgery by decreasing metabolic activity, thereby reducing oxygen requirements
• provide warmth in cases of severe hypothermia.

Nursing considerations

• Explain the procedure to the patient. Follow your facility's policy and procedure and the manufacturer's instructions for proper use of the blanket.
• Record baseline vital signs and monitor temperature, pulse, respirations, blood pressure, and cardiac rhythm during the treatment.
• For automatic operation, insert the thermistor probe in the patient's rectum and tape it in place to prevent accidental dislodgment.
• Assess for skin breakdown and reposition the patient every 1 to 2 hours, unless contraindicated. Keep the patient's skin, bedclothes, and blanket free from perspiration and condensation.
• If the patient shivers excessively during hypothermia treatment, discontinue the procedure and notify the doctor immediately. Shivering increases metabolic demand and oxygen consumption and elevates body temperature.

Whew! A hyperthermia-hypothermia blanket is most commonly used to reduce high fever.

If the patient shivers excessively during hypothermia treatment, stop the procedure and tell the doctor immediately.

• To prevent complications, such as premature ventricular contractions, avoid lowering the patient's temperature more than 1 degree every 15 minutes.
• Document the procedure, the patient's tolerance of the treatment, any complications, and interventions.

Surgery

In the critical care unit, you may care for patients with end-stage pancreatic disease requiring transplantation surgery.

Pancreas transplantation

Pancreas transplantation involves the replacement of a person's pancreas with a donor pancreas.

Indications for transplantation

Pancreas transplantation is indicated for patients with end-stage pancreatic disease, primarily type 1 diabetes mellitus. Such patients generally have serious complications of the disease, including neuropathies and macrovascular and microvascular disease.

The risks associated with transplantation surgery and immunosuppressive therapy are less than those associated with the disease complications. The goal of pancreas transplantation is to restore blood glucose levels to normal and limit the progression of complications.

The goals of pancreas transplant are to restore blood glucose levels and limit complications.

Common concurrence

Most commonly, pancreas transplantation is done along with renal transplantation. This procedure is called simultaneous pancreas-kidney, or SPK, transplantation. (See *SPK transplantation.*)

Pancreas transplantation can also be done after renal transplantation using a procedure called pancreas-after-kidney transplantation. In other cases, a single transplant procedure, called pancreas-transplant alone, is done.

It's complicated

Possible surgical complications include:
• graft thrombosis
• infection
• pancreatitis
• intrapancreatic abscess
• leakage at the anastomosis site
• organ rejection.

SPK transplantation

The illustration below depicts simultaneous pancreas-kidney (SPK) transplantation, in which a donor pancreas is anastomosed using the systemic bladder technique.

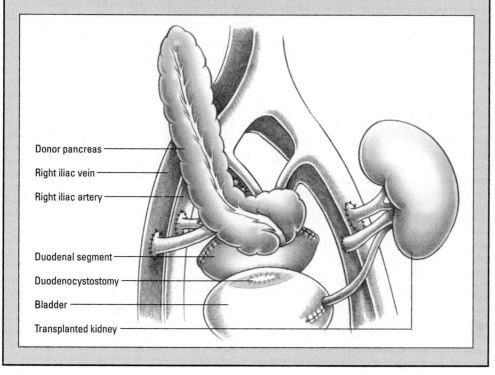

Donor pancreas

Right iliac vein

Right iliac artery

Duodenal segment

Duodenocystostomy

Bladder

Transplanted kidney

When to say no

Contraindications for pancreas transplantation include:
- heart disease that can't be controlled
- active infection
- positive serology for human immunodeficiency virus or hepatitis B surface antigen
- malignancy within the last 3 years
- current and active substance abuse
- history of noncompliance or significant psychiatric illness
- irreversible liver or lung dysfunction
- other systemic illnesses that would delay or prevent recovery.

Nursing considerations

Before surgery:

• Prepare the patient thoroughly for the procedure and prolonged recovery period. Provide emotional support for the patient and his family.
• Review the transplant procedure. If the patient is undergoing SPK transplantation, describe the dialysis procedure that may be required for a short time after transplantation until the new kidney begins to function.
• Discuss the immunosuppressant drugs that are to be taken, and describe potential adverse effects.

> Discuss immunosuppressant drugs and their possible adverse effects with the patient.

The pancreas is in

After surgery:
• Assess vital signs, cardiac rhythm, and cardiopulmonary and hemodynamic status closely at least every 15 minutes in the initial postoperative period and then hourly or as indicated by the patient's condition.
• If the patient is intubated and on a ventilator, assist with extubation as soon as possible, administer supplemental oxygen, and assess respiratory status, including breath sounds and oxygen saturation.
• Monitor hemodynamic parameters, including central venous pressure, pulmonary artery pressure, and pulmonary artery wedge pressure for changes indicating shifts in fluid volume, because the patient is at high risk for fluid and electrolyte imbalance.
• Administer fluid replacement as ordered and carefully monitor intake and output, including urine and nasogastric (NG) tube or wound drainage. Weigh the patient daily and report any rapid gain, which indicates fluid retention.
• In the immediate postoperative period, assess renal and endocrine function and the need for insulin. Monitor laboratory test results, especially BUN, creatinine, serum amylase, and blood glucose levels.
• Because your transplant patient's immune system is suppressed by medications, he's at high risk for infection. Maintain strict infection control precautions, such as meticulous hand washing. Monitor for signs of infection and rejection, including low-grade fever, elevated white blood cell count, swelling of the graft area, and increased serum amylase, lipase, and glucose levels. Administer antibiotics and immunosuppressant medications as ordered.

> Remember, the patient's immune system is suppressed by medications and he's at high risk for infection.

Endocrine system disorders

Some common endocrine disorders you may encounter in the critical care environment are acute adrenal crisis, diabetes mellitus, diabetic ketoacidosis (DKA), diabetes insipidus, hyperosmolar hyperglycemic nonketotic syndrome (HHNS), myxedema coma, syndrome of inappropriate antidiuretic hormone (SIADH), and thyroid storm.

Addison's disease

Addison's disease, also called adrenal hypofunction or adrenal insufficiency, occurs in two forms: primary and secondary. This relatively uncommon disorder occurs in people of all ages and both sexes. Either primary or secondary Addison's disease can progress to adrenal crisis.

Acute adrenal crisis, also called addisonian crisis, is a deficiency of mineralocorticoids and glucocorticoids that requires immediate treatment. (See *Understanding adrenal crisis*, page 530.)

What causes it

Causes of Addison's disease are classified according to whether they result in primary or secondary hypofunction.

Who's on first?

In primary hypofunction, the cause lies with the adrenal glands when approximately 90% of the gland is destroyed, apparently through an autoimmune process.

Other causes of primary hypofunction include:
- tuberculosis
- bilateral adrenalectomy
- hemorrhage into the adrenal glands
- neoplasms
- infections.

What's on second?

In secondary hypofunction, the causes include:
- pituitary gland (decreased function)
- abrupt steroid withdrawal due to adrenal atrophy from long-term therapy (which suppresses corticotropin secretion by the pituitary)
- removal of a corticotropin-secreting tumor.

Possible causes of Addison's disease differ for primary and secondary hypofunction.

Pathophysiology

Addison's disease is characterized by decreased secretion of the adrenal hormones glucocorticoids (cortisol and aldosterone), mineralocorticoids, and androgens. Addisonian crisis can occur with severe stress, such as illness, surgery, sepsis, trauma, and abrupt discontinuation of steroid therapy.

Understanding adrenal crisis

Adrenal crisis (acute adrenal insufficiency) is the most serious complication of Addison's disease. It may occur gradually or suddenly.

Who's at risk

This potentially lethal condition usually develops in patients who:
- don't respond to hormone replacement therapy
- undergo extreme stress without adequate glucocorticoid replacement
- abruptly stop hormone therapy

- undergo trauma
- undergo bilateral adrenalectomy
- develop adrenal gland thrombosis after a severe infection (Waterhouse-Friderichsen syndrome).

What happens

In adrenal crisis, destruction of the adrenal cortex leads to a rapid decline in the steroid hormones cortisol and aldosterone. This directly affects the liver, stomach, and kidneys. The flow-chart below depicts what happens in adrenal crisis.

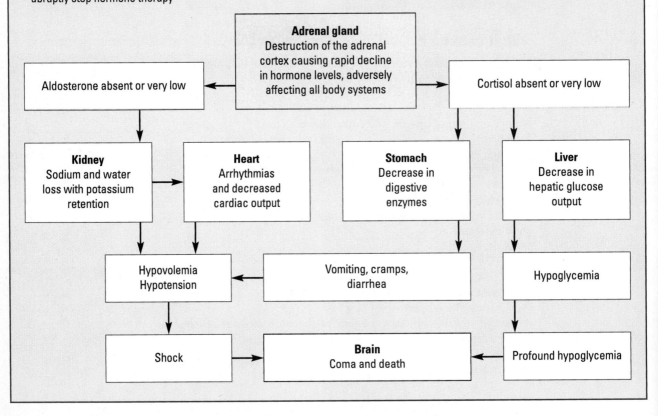

Release the aldosterone!

Aldosterone release occurs in response to hypovolemia as the body attempts to maintain vascular volume. Aldosterone causes the renal tubules to reabsorb sodium. As sodium is reabsorbed, water naturally follows and is reabsorbed. Vascular volume and pressure increase. Cortisol release causes an increase in glucose production as the body attempts to supply the body with this fuel.

Emergency!

In acute addisonian crisis, both hormones are suddenly depleted. Here's what happens:

☝ First, blood pressure drops, due to vascular collapse. Standard pressor therapy is difficult to regulate because the response to catecholamines by the patient is unpredictable.

✌ Second, blood glucose plummets and coma and death ensue if immediate treatment isn't available.

What to look for

Typical clinical features of Addison's disease include:
- profound hypotension
- dehydration
- profound weakness and fatigue
- nausea and vomiting
- hypoglycemia
- neurologic changes
- hyperkalemia
- hyponatremia.

What tests tell you

In a patient with typical addisonian symptoms, findings that strongly suggest acute adrenal insufficiency include:
- decreased plasma cortisol
- decreased serum sodium and fasting blood glucose
- increased corticotropin
- increased serum potassium
- increased serum BUN
- various radiologic tests identifying adrenal gland size such as X-rays showing adrenal calcification.

How it's treated

Treatment for the patient with adrenal crisis is prompt I.V. bolus administration of 100 mg of hydrocortisone, followed by hydrocortisone diluted with dextrose in normal saline given as an I.V. infusion until the patient's condition stabilizes.

Furthermore...

Further treatment includes:

With acute addisonian crisis, coma and death ensue without immediate treatment.

EMERGENCY

Treatment of adrenal crisis begins with prompt I.V. hydrocortisone administration.

• aggressive fluid replacement with up to 5 L I.V. saline and glucose solutions
• vasopressors (if the patient doesn't respond to the initial treatment), such as epinephrine or norepinephrine, titrated to the patient's blood pressure
• blood glucose management with I.V. dextrose solution
• maintenance corticosteroid (hydrocortisone) replacement when the patient's condition is stable.

What to do

• Explain all procedures and tests to the patient and his family.
• Monitor the patient's vital signs and oxygen saturation closely. Assist with insertion of a pulmonary artery catheter as indicated for fluid status evaluation. Assess hemodynamic parameters and monitor for shock.
• Assess the patient's respiratory status and auscultate breath sounds for crackles, which may indicate fluid overload.
• Monitor cardiac rhythm and assess for possible arrhythmias secondary to electrolyte imbalance (evidenced by tall, tented T waves and widening QRS complex associated with hyperkalemia).
• Monitor the patient's intake and output, fluid replacement therapy, and daily weight.
• Monitor the patient's blood glucose levels and administer I.V. glucose if necessary.
• Monitor electrolytes for sodium and potassium imbalances, including hyponatremia and hyperkalemia during crisis.
• Monitor renal function studies and laboratory test results, including hemoglobin and hematocrit, serum electrolyte, and blood glucose levels.
• Monitor the patient's NG tube in case of vomiting.
• Institute emergency measures if needed, such as mechanical ventilation in case of cardiopulmonary arrest.
• Maintain a quiet environment.
• Maintain standard infection control measures.

Monitor the patient's blood glucose levels and administer I.V. glucose if necessary.

Diabetes mellitus

Diabetes mellitus is a chronic disease of absolute or relative insulin deficiency or resistance. It's characterized by disturbances in carbohydrate, protein, or fat metabolism.

Diabetes is the leading cause of blindness in adults. It's also a major risk factor for myocardial infarction (MI), stroke, renal failure, and peripheral vascular disease.

What causes it

Diabetes is classified as type 1 or type 2.

Virus or environment

The cause of type 1 diabetes is thought to be an autoimmune process that's triggered by a virus or environmental factor. However, the cause of the idiopathic form isn't known; patients with this form exhibit no evidence of an autoimmune process.

Lifestyle and heredity

The cause of type 2 diabetes is thought to be beta cell exhaustion due to lifestyle habits and hereditary factors. Risk factors thought to contribute to the development of type 2 diabetes include:
- increased weight
- family history
- Black, Hispanic, or Native American ethnicity
- history of gestational diabetes during pregnancy.

Pathophysiology

When a person is genetically susceptible to type 1 diabetes, a triggering event, possibly a viral infection, causes production of autoantibodies against the beta cells of the pancreas. The resultant destruction of the beta cells leads to a decline and ultimate absence of insulin secretion. After more than 90% of the beta cells are destroyed, hyperglycemia, enhanced lipolysis (decomposition of fat), and protein catabolism result.

Take 2

Genetic factors are significant in type 2 diabetes and obesity and a sedentary lifestyle accelerate its onset. Type 2 diabetes is a chronic disease caused by one or more dysfunctions, including:
- impaired insulin secretion
- inappropriate hepatic glucose production
- peripheral insulin receptor insensitivity

Compliance or resistance

Patients with type 1 diabetes require insulin to prevent death. Type 2 diabetes is sometimes called an insulin-resistant disease. In this type of diabetes, beta cells secrete higher and higher levels of insulin to move glucose into the cell and, over time, the cells become exhausted.

Lifestyle habits and hereditary factors such as these can cause type 2 diabetes.

What to look for

Patients with type 1 diabetes usually report rapid muscle wasting and loss of subcutaneous fat. With type 2 diabetes, symptoms are generally vague, long-standing, and develop gradually.

Similar signs and symptoms

Signs and symptoms of hyperglycemia reported by patients with type 1 or type 2 diabetes include:

- excessive urination (polyuria)
- excessive thirst (polydipsia)
- excessive eating (polyphagia)
- weight loss
- fatigue
- weakness
- vision changes
- frequent skin infections
- dry, itchy skin
- vaginal infections or discomfort.

What tests tell you

Test results that define diabetes when they occur on two separate occasions include:

- fasting serum glucose level greater than 126 mg/dl
- 2-hour oral glucose tolerance test greater than 200 mg/dl with 75-g carbohydrate load
- nonfasting draw of serum glucose greater than 200 mg/dl at any time of the day.

Other results

Other diagnostic tests used to assess and manage diabetes include urinalysis (showing the presence of acetone) and an A_{1c} or glycosylated hemoglobin test, which reflects serum glucose levels over a 3-month period.

When glucose enters the blood, it binds with hemoglobin. The A_{1c} test is used to measure the percent of glucose bound to hemoglobin. People without diabetes average 4% to 6% glucose. For people with diabetes, the goal is to achieve 6% glucose or less. The closer the result is to the normal range, the lower the likelihood of developing complications in the long run.

When glucose enters the blood, it binds with hemoglobin.

How it's treated

The goal of effective treatment for patients with all types of diabetes is to optimize blood glucose control and decrease complications.

Type 1 treatment

Treatment for patients with type 1 diabetes includes:
- insulin replacement
- meal planning
- exercise
- pancreas transplantation.

Type 2 treatment

Treatment for patients with type 2 diabetes includes:
- oral antidiabetic drugs to stimulate endogenous insulin production, increase insulin sensitivity in cells, suppress hepatic gluconeogenesis, and delay GI carbohydrate absorption
- insulin therapy if control isn't achieved with oral agents.

Types 1 and 2 treatment

Treatment for patients with either type 1 or type 2 diabetes includes:
- careful monitoring of blood glucose levels
- individualized meal planning designed to meet nutritional needs, control blood glucose and lipid levels, and reach and maintain appropriate body weight
- weight reduction (for an obese patient with type 2 diabetes) or high caloric allotment depending on the growth stage and activity level (for patients with type 1 diabetes)
- patient and family education about the disease process, possible complications, nutritional management, exercise regimen, blood glucose self-monitoring, and insulin or oral medications.

What to do

In the critical care unit, you may care for patients who have a history of diabetes but are admitted to the unit because of surgery or another medical condition. Some medical conditions, such as stroke or renal failure, result from diabetic effects on the cardiovascular or renal systems.
- Monitor blood glucose levels and assess for acute complications of diabetic therapy, especially diabetic ketoacidosis and hypoglycemia (blood glucose less than 50 mg/dl); signs and symptoms include tachycardia, pallor, diaphoresis, weakness, vagueness, slow cerebration, dizziness, irritability, seizure, and coma. Some medications, such as beta-adrenergic blockers, can mask the symptoms of a hypoglycemic reaction, so more frequent blood glucose monitoring may be necessary.
- Treatment in case of a hypoglycemic reaction is glucose. If the patient is able to swallow, provided oral glucose or a sucrose-

> If type 2 diabetes isn't controllable with oral antidiabetic drugs, insulin therapy is used.

> Patients in critical care units may have diabetes but are usually there because of surgery or another medical condition.

containing drink. If the patient can't drink, give a bolus of 25 g of 50% dextrose. Obtain blood glucose measurements before administering glucose, if possible, to confirm the diagnosis. Document blood glucose levels after treatment as well as the patient's response to treatment.

• Assess for diabetic effects on the cardiovascular system, such as stroke, acute coronary syndromes, peripheral vascular impairment, and peripheral neuropathy. Assess cardiovascular and neurovascular status and fluid balance and monitor for cardiac arrhythmias.

• More frequent blood glucose monitoring and insulin dose adjustments may be necessary during periods of physiologic stress, such as acute illness and surgery, because blood glucose levels increase as result of elevated stress hormones (such as epinephrine and cortisol).

Monitor blood glucose more often and adjust the insulin dose if necessary when the patient is under stress.

Diabetic ketoacidosis

DKA is an acute complication of hyperglycemic crisis in patients with diabetes. It's a life-threatening complication that's most common in patients with type 1 diabetes and is sometimes the first evidence of the disease.

What causes it

DKA may result from:
• infection
• illness
• surgery
• stress
• insufficient or absent insulin.

Pathophysiology

In DKA, production and release of glucose into the blood is increased or uptake of glucose by the cells is decreased.

What happens?

In the absence of endogenous insulin, the body breaks down fats for energy. In the process, fatty acids develop too rapidly and are converted to ketones, resulting in severe metabolic acidosis.

Acidosis also affects potassium levels. For every 0.1 change in pH, there's a reciprocal 0.6 change in potassium. As acidosis worsens, blood glucose levels increase and hyperkalemia worsens. The cycle continues until coma and death occur.

As with diabetes, the liver responds to the lack of fuel (glucose) in cells by converting glycogen to glucose for release into the bloodstream. Excess glucose molecules in the serum trigger osmosis and fluid shifts occur.

When glucose is lacking, the liver converts glycogen to glucose for release into the bloodstream.

What to look for

The patient may have a rapid onset of drowsiness, stupor, and coma. Other assessment findings include:
- severe dehydration
- rapid and deep breathing (Kussmaul's respirations)
- fruity breath odor due to acetone
- polyuria, polydipsia, and polyphagia
- weight loss
- muscle wasting
- vision changes
- recurrent infections
- abdominal cramps
- nausea and vomiting
- leg cramps.

What tests tell you

Findings used to diagnosis DKA include:
- elevated serum glucose of 200 to 800 mg/dl
- increased serum ketone level
- positive urine acetone
- arterial blood gas (ABG) analysis that reveals metabolic acidosis
- initially, normal potassium or hyperkalemia, depending on the level of acidosis, and then hypokalemia
- electrocardiogram (ECG) changes related to hyperkalemia (tall, tented T waves and widened QRS complex); later, with hypokalemia, flattened T wave and presence of U wave
- elevated serum osmolality.

There's a stack of findings used to diagnosis DKA.

How it's treated

Treatment goals for the patient with DKA include rehydration, control of glucose levels, and restoration of electrolyte and acid-base balance. If the patient is comatose, airway support and mechanical ventilation may be indicated.

What to do

- Correct dehydration first, using nondextrose-based I.V. fluids.
- Administer I.V. insulin therapy and fluid and electrolyte replacements based on laboratory test results.

• Monitor blood glucose levels. As blood glucose level nears 250 mg/dl, give dextrose-based I.V. fluid to prevent hypoglycemia.
• Monitor potassium levels. As blood glucose level normalizes, add potassium as ordered to I.V. fluid to prevent hypokalemia.
• Monitor ABG levels. As blood glucose level normalizes, acidosis is corrected.
• Assess the patient's LOC and ability to maintain a patent airway. Monitor respiratory status, including breath sounds and oxygen saturation. Monitor cardiac rhythm for arrhythmias that may result from electrolyte imbalance.
• Monitor the patient's vital signs because changes reflect hydration status.
• Monitor blood glucose and serum electrolyte levels, especially potassium levels and ABG results.
• Administer I.V. fluid replacement initially with 1 to 2 L normal saline and then half-normal saline. When the patient's blood glucose levels reach 250 mg/dl, anticipate the addition of glucose to the fluid replacement to prevent hypoglycemia.
• Administer regular insulin I.V. as ordered, usually as a bolus dose and then by continuous I.V. infusion, using an I.V. infusion pump. Blood glucose levels must be reduced gradually to prevent cerebral fluid shifting and subsequent cerebral edema. Anticipate potassium replacement after insulin therapy is initiated.
• When the patient is stable, consult the diabetes educator to assist with patient teaching.

Monitor the patient's vital signs because changes reflect hydration status.

Diabetes insipidus

Diabetes insipidus is a water metabolism disorder caused by deficiency of ADH. ADH is also called vasopressin. The absence of ADH allows filtered water to be excreted in the urine instead of being reabsorbed. Diabetes insipidus causes excessive urination and excessive thirst and fluid intake.

What causes it

Possible causes of diabetes insipidus include:
• pituitary tumor
• hypothalamic tumor
• cranial trauma (basilar skull fracture)
• cranial surgery
• stroke
• certain medications (lithium, dilantin, and alcohol)
• rare genetic form of an X-linked recessive trait
• other idiopathic, nephrogenic, or neurogenic causes.

Pathophysiology

Diabetes insipidus is a syndrome resulting from a lack of ADH secretion. ADH is a hormone released by the posterior pituitary in response to increased serum osmolality. It controls the body's ability to retain water.

Three forms

There are three forms of diabetes insipidus:

- neurogenic
- nephrogenic
- psychogenic.

Some nerve!

Neurogenic or central diabetes insipidus is caused by inadequate synthesis or release of ADH. It occurs when an organic lesion of the hypothalamus, infundibular stem, or posterior pituitary partially or completely blocks ADH synthesis, transport, or release. Causes of such organic lesions include brain tumors, hypophysectomy, aneurysms, thrombosis, and infection.

The onset of neurogenic diabetes insipidus is acute and involves:
- progressive loss of nerve tissue and increased diuresis
- normal diuresis
- polyuria and polydipsia due to permanent loss of the ability to secrete adequate ADH.

Kidney cause

Nephrogenic diabetes insipidus is caused by inadequate renal response to ADH. It's caused by such conditions as pyelonephritis, polycystic disease, and intrinsic renal disease.

Fluid overflow

Psychogenic diabetes insipidus is caused by extremely large fluid intake, which may be idiopathic or related to psychosis or sarcoidosis. The polydipsia and resultant polyuria wash out ADH more quickly than it can be replaced.

Chronic polyuria can overwhelm the renal medullary concentration gradient, rendering patients partially or totally unable to concentrate urine. Regardless of the cause, insufficient ADH causes the immediate excretion of large volumes of dilute urine and consequent plasma hyperosmolality.

Nephrogenic diabetes insipidus is caused by inadequate renal response to ADH.

What to look for

Your assessment findings in a patient with diabetes insipidus may include:
• abrupt onset of increased urine output (polyuria), sometimes producing 4 to 16 L of dilute urine per day
• extreme thirst (polydipsia) leading to fluid intake of 5 to 20 L/day
• weight loss
• dizziness, weakness
• nocturia leading to sleep disturbance and fatigue
• signs of dehydration, such as fever and dry skin and mucous membranes
• hypotension and tachycardia
• change in LOC.

Most signs and symptoms of diabetes insipidus are related to fluid intake and output.

What tests tell you

Diagnostic test findings may include:
• urinalysis showing almost colorless urine with low urine osmolality (50 to 200 mOsm/kg)
• increased serum osmolality (greater than 300 mOsm/kg)
• decreased urine specific gravity (less than 1.005)
• serum sodium greater than 147 mEq/L
• dehydration test or water deprivation test to identify vasopressin deficiency, which differentiates nephrogenic from pituitary effects.

How it's treated

Until the cause of diabetes insipidus is identified and eliminated, vasopressin or a vasopressin stimulant is given to control fluid balance and prevent dehydration. Treatment measures include:
• hypotonic I.V. solution administration (1 ml for every 1 ml of urine output) to replace free water lost in urine
• medications (subcutaneous [S.C.] or I.M. vasopressin aqueous preparations; S.C., I.V., or nasal spray desmopressin acetate (DDAVP) to maintain volume
• thiazide diuretics for patients with nephrogenic diabetes insipidus
• transphenoidal hypophysectomy for patients with pituitary tumors.

Treatment measures for the patient with diabetes insipidus include controlling fluid balance and preventing dehydration.

What to do

• Vasopressin administration can cause hypertension, angina, and MI due to the vasoconstrictive effects of the drug. Monitor the patient's cardiac status closely, including vital signs, cardiac rhythm, and hemodynamic parameters.
• Monitor urine output and urine specific gravity.

• Monitor other output sources such as drainage tubes.
• Monitor daily weights, serum laboratory test results, and skin turgor.
• Assess the patient's LOC.
• Assess the patient receiving vasopressin for signs of water intoxication, including drowsiness, headache, lightheadedness, seizure, or coma. Notify the doctor immediately if any occurs.

Hyperosmolar hyperglycemic nonketotic syndrome

HHNS is an acute hyperglycemic crisis accompanied by hyperosmolality and severe dehydration without ketoacidosis. If not treated properly, it can cause coma or death.

HHNS is most common in patients with type 2 diabetes (usually middle-aged or older) but can occur in anyone whose insulin tolerance is stressed and in patients who have undergone certain therapeutic procedures, such as peritoneal dialysis, hemodialysis, or total parenteral nutrition.

What causes it

Causes of HHNS include illness, infection, and stress.

Pathophysiology

With HHNS in patients with type 2 diabetes, glucose production and release into the blood is increased or glucose uptake by the cells is decreased. When the cells don't receive fuel (glucose), the liver responds by converting glycogen to glucose for release into the bloodstream. When all excess glucose molecules remain in the serum, osmosis causes fluid shifts. The cycle continues until fluid shifts in the brain cause coma and death.

What to look for

The onset of HHNS is usually gradual and may not be noticed by the patient. The manifestations of HHNS are similar to those of DKA, but there are differences. (See *Comparing HHNS and DKA*, page 542.)

Making progress

As HHNS progresses, assessment findings may include:
• severe dehydration
• hypotension and tachycardia
• diaphoresis
• tachypnea
• polyuria, polydipsia, and polyphagia

> As HHNS progresses, your assessment may turn up these findings.

Comparing HHNS and DKA

Hyperosmolar hyperglycemic nonketotic syndrome (HHNS) and diabetic ketoacidosis (DKA) both are acute complications of diabetes. They share some similarities, but are two distinct conditions. Use the flowchart below to determine which condition your patient has.

- vision changes
- rapid onset of lethargy
- stupor and coma
- neurologic changes.

What tests tell you

These findings may be helpful in diagnosing HHNS:
• Serum glucose level is elevated, sometimes 800 to 2,000 mg/dl.
• Ketones are absent, so there's no acidosis and urine and serum ketone results are negative.
• Urine glucose levels are positive.
• Serum osmolality is increased.
• Serum sodium levels are elevated and serum potassium level is usually normal.
• ABG results are usually normal, without evidence of acidosis.

How it's treated

Treatment for patients with HHNS is focused on correcting fluid volume deficits and electrolyte imbalances and addressing the underlying cause:
• I.V. fluids are given to correct dehydration. Administer isotonic or half-normal saline as ordered. When the patient's blood glucose level approaches 250 mg/dl, add dextrose to the fluid to prevent hypoglycemia.
• I.V. insulin and electrolyte replacement therapy are delivered.
• Blood glucose levels are monitored. As blood glucose levels normalize, so do sodium levels.

What to do

• Assess the patient's LOC and ability to maintain a patent airway. Monitor respiratory status and oxygen saturation.
• Monitor the patient's vital signs. Changes reflect the patient's hydration status.
• Monitor the patient's blood glucose and serum electrolyte levels.
• Administer regular insulin I.V. as ordered, by continuous infusion, and titrate the dosage based on the patient's blood glucose levels.
• Remember, the patient with HHNS has severely elevated glucose levels, but less insulin is usually needed (compared with that required by patients with DKA) to reduce the glucose level because the patient typically secretes some insulin and may be sensitive to additional doses.
• Provide patient and family education to foster prevention of future episodes.

Myxedema coma is a life-threatening form of hypothyroidism.

CAUTION!

Myxedema coma

Myxedema coma is a life-threatening disorder that progresses from hypothyroidism.

What causes it

Causes of hypothyroidism include:
- pituitary failure to produce TSH
- hypothalamic failure
- chronic autoimmune thyroiditis (Hashimoto's disease)
- amyloidosis and sarcoidosis
- inability to synthesize hormones
- use of antithyroid hormones
- postthyroidectomy effects
- postradiation therapy effects.

Pathophysiology

There are two classifications of hypothyroidism: primary and secondary. Primary hypothyroidism originates as a disorder of the thyroid gland. Secondary hypothyroidism is caused by a failure to stimulate normal thyroid function or an inability to synthesize thyroid hormones due to an iodine deficiency (usually dietary) or use of antithyroid medications.

A myx of causes

Myxedema coma can result from either primary or secondary hypothyroidism and progresses slowly and gradually. It's usually precipitated by infection, exposure to cold, or sedative use. Cellular metabolism decreases to a fatal level if the patient with myxedema coma is left untreated.

What to look for

The progression to myxedema coma is usually gradual but may develop abruptly if stress aggravates severe or prolonged hypothyroidism.

Inspect and assess

Periorbital edema, dry flaky skin, thick brittle nails, and sacral or peripheral edema may be present in the patient with myxedema coma. Cardiac assessment may reveal muffled or S_3 heart sounds. In addition, look for changes in the patient's overall appearance and behavior, including:
- decreased mental ability (slight mental slowing to severe obtundation)
- thick and dry tongue
- hoarseness
- slow and slurred speech.

What else?

Assessment findings also include:

- progressive stupor
- significantly depressed respirations and adventitious breath sounds
- hypoglycemia
- hyponatremia
- hypotension and bradycardia
- severe hypothermia without shivering.

What tests tell you

These test findings are used to diagnose myxedema coma:
- Serum levels of T_3 and T_4 are decreased.
- Serum levels of TSH are increased.
- ^{131}I (low serum levels of thyroid hormones) is disclosed.
- Radioisotope scanning of thyroid tissue is used to identify ectopic thyroid tissue.
- A CT scan, MRI, or skull X-ray may disclose an underlying cause, such as pituitary or hypothalamic lesions.
- Chest X-ray may show pleural effusion.

In myxedema coma, a CT scan, MRI, or skull X-ray may disclose an underlying cause, such as pituitary or hypothalamic lesions.

How it's treated

Rapid treatment may be necessary for patients in myxedema coma, including:
- administration of I.V. hydrocortisone and I.V. levothyroxine (a thyroid agent)
- possible ventilatory support if the patient is comatose
- I.V. fluid replacement
- warming devices
- maintenance thyroid replacement.

What to do

- Assess the patient's LOC and ability to maintain a patent airway.
- Monitor the patient's respiratory status, adequacy of ventilation and oxygen saturation, and ABG levels. Administer supplemental oxygen as ordered and anticipate the need for intubation and mechanical ventilation.
- Monitor vital signs and cardiac arrhythmias. Auscultate for muffled heart sounds or changes such as S_3.
- Monitor temperature closely until the patient is stable, and institute warming measures such as applying a warming blanket.
- Administer medications as ordered. Sedatives are contraindicated.
- Administer I.V. fluids as ordered and monitor fluid balance status, serum electrolytes, and blood glucose levels.
- Assess for possible sources of infection—such as blood, sputum, and urine—and provide meticulous skin care.

Syndrome of inappropriate antidiuretic hormone

SIADH is a relatively common complication of surgery or critical illness.

What causes it

The most common cause of SIADH is oat-cell lung cancer, which secretes ADH or a vasopressor-like substance that the body responds to as if ADH were secreted.

Many other possibilities

Other causes include:
• neoplastic diseases (pancreatic, brain, and prostatic tumors; Hodgkin's disease; and thymoma)
• brain abscess
• stroke
• Guillain-Barré syndrome
• pulmonary disorders
• adverse effects of medications (chlorpropamide, tolbutamide, vincristine, cyclophosphamide, haloperidol, carbamazepine, clofibrate, morphine, and thiazides)
• adrenal insufficiency
• anterior pituitary insufficiency.

Pathophysiology

In SIADH, ADH is secreted excessively and the body responds by retaining water. Fluid shifts within compartments cause decreased serum osmolality.

What to look for

Most commonly, a patient with SIADH complains of anorexia, nausea, and vomiting. Despite these symptoms, the patient may report weight gain. Assessment findings also may include:
• thirst
• neurologic changes—such as lethargy, headache, and emotional and behavioral changes—and sluggish deep tendon reflexes
• tachycardia associated with increased fluid volume
• hyponatremia.

What tests tell you

Diagnostic test results may indicate:
• decreased serum osmolality (less than 280 mOsm/kg)
• increased urine sodium (greater than 20 mEq/day)

In SIADH, excessive ADH is secreted and the body responds by retaining water.

- decreased serum sodium level
- elevated serum ADH level.

How it's treated

Treatment is based on the underlying cause and the patient's symptoms.

First thing first

Treatment begins with restricting fluid intake to 500 to 1,000 ml/day. Other measures may include administration of 200 to 300 ml of 3% to 5% sodium chloride solution for patients with severe hyponatremia. A loop diuretic may also be ordered to reduce the risk of heart failure after administration of hypertonic sodium chloride solution.

What to do

- Assess the patient's neurologic, cardiac, and respiratory status.
- Implement seizure and safety precautions if the patient's serum sodium levels are dangerously low. Monitor serum electrolyte levels.
- Monitor the patient's vital signs, oxygen saturation, and cardiac rhythm for potential arrhythmias.
- Administer medications and I.V. fluids as ordered. If hypertonic sodium chloride is ordered, monitor for fluid overload and administer diuretics as ordered.
- Monitor the patient's intake and output and daily weight.
- Enforce fluid restrictions and explain to the patient and his family why this is necessary.

Help me, please! The patient may need a loop diuretic to reduce the risk of heart failure.

Thyroid storm is a life-threatening emergency in a patient with hyperthyroidism.

Thyroid storm

Thyroid storm, also called *thyrotoxic crisis*, is a life-threatening emergency in a patient with hyperthyroidism. Thyroid storm may be the initial symptom in a patient with hyperthyroidism that hasn't been diagnosed.

What causes it

The onset of thyroid storm is almost always abrupt and evoked by a stressful event, such as trauma, surgery, or infection.

Not-so-common causes

Other, less common causes include:
- metastatic carcinoma of the thyroid

- pituitary tumor secreting TSH
- diabetic ketoacidosis.

Pathophysiology

Thyroid storm develops when there's a surge of thyroid hormones. Hyperthyroidism can result from genetic and immunologic factors.

Grave's is grave

Grave's disease — the most common form of hyperthyroidism — is an autoimmune process in which the body makes an antibody similar to TSH and the thyroid responds to it. Overproduction of T_3 and T_4 increases adrenergic activity and severe hypermetabolism results. This can rapidly lead to cardiac, sympathetic nervous system, and GI collapse.

What to look for

A patient in thyroid storm initially shows marked tachycardia, vomiting, and stupor. Other findings may include:
- irritability and restlessness
- vision disturbances such as diplopia
- tremor
- weakness
- heat intolerance
- angina
- shortness of breath
- cough
- swollen extremities.

Raise the flag

On palpation, an enlarged thyroid may be felt. Any change in LOC and increasing temperature in a patient with hyperthyroidism should raise red flags. Fever, typically above 100.4° F (38° C), begins insidiously and rises rapidly to a lethal level. Without treatment, the patient may experience vascular collapse, hypotension, coma, and death.

What tests tell you

These diagnostic test findings may indicate impending thyroid storm:
- Serum T_3 and T_4 levels are elevated.
- TSH level is decreased.
- Radioisotope scanning shows increased uptake.
- CT scan or MRI may disclose an underlying cause such as pituitary lesion.

Without treatment, thyroid storm can lead to vascular collapse, hypotension, coma, and death.

• 12-lead ECG may show atrial fibrillation and supraventricular tachycardia.

Monitor ECG readings because increased adrenergic activity can produce arrhythmias.

How it's treated

Immediate treatment for a patient with thyroid storm is necessary to prevent death and includes:
• beta-adrenergic blockers to block adrenergic effects
• propylthiouracil and methimazole to block thyroid hormone synthesis
• possible corticosteroid administration to block conversion of T_3 and T_4
• avoidance of aspirin because salicylates block binding of T_3 and T_4
• cooling measures such as use of a hyperthermia-hypothermia blanket.

What to do

• Assess the patient's LOC and cardiopulmonary status.
• Monitor the patient's vital signs and core body temperature and institute cooling measures such as use of a hyperthermia-hypothermia blanket.
• Monitor ECG readings. Increased adrenergic activity may produce arrhythmias.
• Monitor the patient for signs of heart failure.
• Monitor I.V. fluids and fluid and electrolyte balance.
• Monitor the patient for high blood glucose levels. Excessive thyroid activity can lead to glycogenolysis.
• Provide a quiet environment.

Quick quiz

1. Pituitary hormones are controlled by the:
   A. hypothalamus.
   B. midbrain.
   C. adrenal glands.
   D. target organs.

Answer: A. The hypothalamus receives, integrates, and directs hormone secretion.

2. Which dysfunction should you address first in a patient with DKA?
- A. Acidosis
- B. Hyperkalemia
- C. Hyperglycemia
- D. Hypovolemia

Answer: D. Hypovolemia may be severe and should be addressed first, followed by hyperglycemia, and then hyperkalemia. Acidosis is corrected by correcting the other imbalances.

3. Which of the following is an appropriate treatment measure for a patient with addisonian crisis?
- A. I.V. fluid replacement
- B. I.V. corticosteroids
- C. Blood glucose management
- D. All of the above

Answer: D. All of the therapies indicated are first-line treatment measures during addisonian crisis.

4. The patient is experiencing thyroid storm. Which of the following drugs is contraindicated?
- A. I.V. beta-adrenergic blockers
- B. Aspirin
- C. Propylthiouracil
- D. Corticosteroids

Answer: B. Aspirin is contraindicated in patients with thyroid storm because it blocks the binding of T_3 and T_4.

5. Which of the following signs is seen in patients with diabetes insipidus?
- A. Decreased urine output
- B. Increased serum osmolality
- C. Increased urine osmolality
- D. Decreased urine specific gravity

Answer: B. Urine output increases with diabetes insipidus; therefore, serum osmolality is increased.

Scoring

☆☆☆   If you answered all five questions correctly, give yourself a gland! Your endocrine energy is practically radioactive.

☆☆   If you answered four questions correctly, don't worry about your target cells. Your knowledge receptors are still uptaking information.

☆   If you answered fewer than four questions correctly, quit the hemming and hormoning and review the chapter.

Hematologic and immune systems

Just the facts

In this chapter, you'll learn:

♦ structure and function of the hematologic and immune systems

♦ assessment of the hematologic and immune systems

♦ diagnostic tests and treatments for critically ill patients

♦ hematologic and immune systems disorders and related nursing care.

Understanding the hematologic and immune systems

The hematologic system consists of the blood and bone marrow. The immune system consists of specialized cells, tissues, and organs found throughout the body.

Transport and delivery

Functions of the hematologic system include:
• transporting blood cells and immunity-related cells, hormones, and gases throughout the body
• delivering oxygen and nutrients to all body tissues
• removing wastes collected from cells and tissues.

Defense! Defense!

The immune system defends the body against invasion by harmful organisms and chemical toxins. The blood plays an important part in this protective system.

Kin systems

The hematologic and immune systems are distinct, yet closely related. Their cells share a common origin in the bone

> Cells of the hematologic and immune systems originate in the same place and travel together.

marrow, and the immune system uses the bloodstream to transport defensive components to the site of an invasion.

Hematologic system

The hematologic system consists of various formed elements, or blood cells, suspended in a fluid called plasma.

Formed elements in the blood include:

- red blood cells (RBCs), or erythrocytes
- platelets
- white blood cells (WBCs), or leukocytes.

RBCs and platelets function entirely within blood vessels. WBCs act mainly in the tissues outside the blood vessels.

Red blood cells

RBCs transport oxygen and carbon dioxide to and from body tissues. They contain hemoglobin (Hb), the oxygen-carrying molecule that gives blood its red color. The RBC surface carries antigens (substances that trigger immune responses), which determine a person's blood group, or blood type.

Days of their lives

RBCs have an average life span of 120 days. Bone marrow releases RBCs into circulation in immature form as reticulocytes. The reticulocytes mature into RBCs in about 1 day. The spleen sequesters, or isolates, old, worn-out RBCs, removing them from circulation.

The rate of reticulocyte release usually equals the rate of old RBC removal. When RBC depletion occurs (for example, with hemorrhage) the bone marrow increases reticulocyte production to maintain the normal RBC count.

Platelets

Platelets are small, colorless, disk-shaped cytoplasmic fragments split from cells in bone marrow called megakaryocytes.

Sticky stabilizers

In the peripheral blood, the sticky platelets contribute to blood clotting in three ways:

They clump together to plug small defects in small blood vessel walls.

They congregate at an injury site in a larger vessel and close the wound so a clot can form.

The rate of reticulocyte release equals the rate of RBC removal. That makes sense!

A granulocyte contains a single multilobed nucleus and granules.

They release substances that stabilize the clot. For example, they release serotonin, which reduces blood flow by vasoconstriction, and thromboplastin, an enzyme essential to clotting.

White blood cells

Five types of WBCs participate in the body's defense and immune systems. They are:
- neutrophils
- eosinophils
- basophils
- monocytes
- lymphocytes.
  The WBCs are classified as either granulocytes or agranulocytes.

Granulocytes

Granulocytes are polymorphonuclear leukocytes. Each contains a single multilobular nucleus and granules in the cytoplasm. Each type of granulocyte exhibits different properties and each is activated by different stimuli. The granulocytes include:
- neutrophils
- eosinophils
- basophils.

Neutrophils engulf, ingest, and digest

The most abundant granulocytes—the neutrophils—account for 47.6% to 76.8% of circulating WBCs. Neutrophils are phagocytic, meaning they engulf, ingest, and digest foreign materials. They leave the bloodstream by passing through the capillary walls into the tissues (a process called diapedesis), then migrate to accumulate at infection sites.

Replacement bands

Worn-out neutrophils form the main component of pus. Bone marrow produces their replacements, which are immature neutrophils called bands. In response to infection, bone marrow produces many immature cells and releases them into circulation, elevating the band count.

Ingestion by eosinophils

Eosinophils account for 0.3% to 7% of circulating WBCs. Eosinophils migrate from the bloodstream by diapedesis in response to an allergic reaction. Eosinophils accumulate in loose connective tissue, where they're involved in ingesting antigen-antibody complexes.

Basophils secrete histamine

The least common granulocyte — basophils — usually make up fewer than 2% of circulating WBCs. They possess little or no phagocytic ability. The basophils' cytoplasmic granules secrete histamine in response to certain inflammatory and immune stimuli. This increases vascular permeability and eases fluid passage from capillaries into body tissues.

Agranulocytes

Agranulocytes have nuclei without lobes and lack specific cytoplasmic granules. They include:
- monocytes
- lymphocytes.

Monstrous monocytes

Monocytes, the largest WBCs, constitute only 0.6% to 9.6% of WBCs in circulation. Like neutrophils, monocytes enlarge and mature, becoming macrophages, or histiocytes. As macrophages, monocytes may roam freely through the body when stimulated by inflammation. Usually, they remain immobile, populating most organs and tissues.

Defense against infection

Monocytes are part of the reticuloendothelial system, which defends the body against infection and disposes of cell breakdown products. Macrophages concentrate in structures that filter large amounts of body fluid, such as the liver, spleen, and lymph nodes, where they defend against invading organisms.

Macrophages are efficient phagocytes (cells that ingest microorganisms, cellular debris such as worn out neutrophils, and necrotic tissue). When mobilized at an infection site, they phagocytize cellular remnants and promote wound healing.

T-lymphocytes attack infected cells directly.

B-lymphocytes produce antibodies against specific antigens.

Lymphocytes: Least but not last

Lymphocytes, the smallest and the second most numerous (16.2% to 43%) of the WBCs, originate from stem cells in the bone marrow. There are two types of lymphocytes:

T-lymphocytes, which attack infected cells directly

B-lymphocytes, which produce molecules called antibodies that attack specific antigens.

Blood clots

Hemostasis (blood clotting) is the complex process by which platelets, plasma, and coagulation factors interact to control bleeding.

Extrinsic coagulation cascade

When a blood vessel ruptures, local vasoconstriction (decrease in the caliber of blood vessels) and platelet clumping (aggregation) at the injury site initially prevent hemorrhage. This initial activation of the coagulation system, called the *extrinsic cascade*, requires the release of tissue thromboplastin from the damaged cells.

Intrinsic clotting cascade

Formation of a more stable clot requires initiation of the complex clotting mechanisms known as the intrinsic cascade system. This clotting system is activated by a protein called factor XII, which is one of 13 substances necessary for coagulation and derived from plasma and tissue.

   The final result of the intrinsic and extrinsic cascade is a fibrin clot, an accumulation of a fibrous, insoluble protein at the injury site. (See *Understanding clotting*, page 556.)

Blood groups

A person's blood is one of four blood types: A, B, AB, and O.

A is for antigen...

In type A blood, A antigens appear on RBCs. Type B blood contains B antigens. Type AB blood contains both antigens. Type O blood has neither antigen.

Testing, testing: A, B, AB, O

Testing for the presence of A and B antigens on RBCs is the most important system for classifying blood. Plasma may contain antibodies that interact with these antigens, causing the cells to agglutinate, or combine into a mass. Plasma can't contain antibodies to its own cell antigen or it would destroy itself. For example, type A blood has A antigens but no A antibodies; however, it does have B antibodies.

Crossmatching for compatibility

Precise blood-typing and crossmatching (mixing and observing for agglutination of donor cells) are essential, especially before blood transfusions. A donor's blood must be compatible with a recipi-

Plasma can't contain antibodies to its own cell antigen or it would destroy itself.

Understanding clotting

When a blood vessel is severed or injured, clotting begins within minutes to stop blood loss. Coagulation factors are essential to normal blood clotting. Absent, decreased, or excess coagulation factors can cause a clotting abnormality. Coagulation factors are commonly designated by Roman numerals.

Two pathways to clotting

Clotting is initiated through two different pathways, the intrinsic pathway or the extrinsic pathway. The intrinsic pathway is activated when plasma comes in contact with damaged vessel surfaces. The extrinsic pathway is activated when tissue thromboplastin, a substance released by damaged endothelial cells, comes in contact with one of the clotting factors.

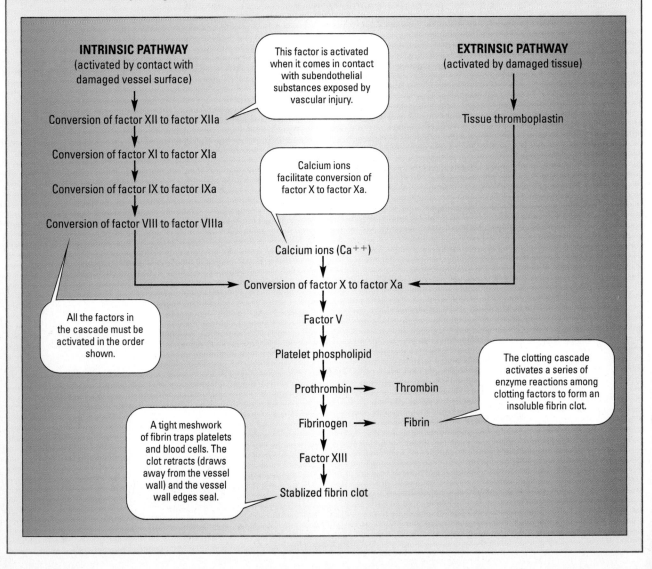

Compatible blood types

Precise blood-typing and crossmatching can prevent the transfusion of incompatible blood, which can be fatal. Usually, typing the recipient's blood and crossmatching it with available donor blood takes less than 1 hour.

Matchmaking

Agglutinogen (an antigen in red blood cells [RBCs]) and agglutinin (an antibody in plasma) distinguish the four ABO blood groups. This table depicts ABO compatibility from the perspectives of recipients and donors.

Blood group	Antibodies in plasma	Compatible RBCs	Compatible plasma
Recipient			
O	Anti-A and anti-B	O	O, A, B, AB
A	Anti-B	A, O	A, AB
B	Anti-A	B, O	B, AB
AB	Neither anti-A nor anti-B	AB, A, B, O	AB
Donor			
O	Anti-A and anti-B	O, A, B, AB	O
A	Anti-B	A, AB	A, O
B	Anti-A	B, AB	B, O
AB	Neither anti-A nor anti-B	AB	AB, A, B, O

ent's or the result can be fatal. The following blood groups are compatible:

- type A with type A or O
- type B with type B or O
- type AB with type A, B, AB, or O
- type O with type O only. (See *Compatible blood types*.)

Factor in Rh

Rh typing is used to determine whether a substance, called an *Rh factor*, is present or absent in a person's blood. Of the eight types of Rh antigens, only C, D, and E are common. The presence or absence of the D antigen determines whether a person has Rh-positive or Rh-negative blood.

Blood typically is Rh-positive, meaning it contains Rh D antigen. Blood without the Rh D antigen is Rh-negative. Anti-Rh antibodies occur only in a person who has become sensitized to the Rh factor.

Anti-Rh antibodies can only appear in the blood of an Rh-negative person after introduction of Rh-positive RBCs into the bloodstream such as from transfusion of Rh-positive blood. An Rh-negative female who carries an Rh-positive fetus may also acquire anti-Rh antibodies.

A person with Rh-negative blood should only receive a transfusion with Rh-negative blood. Repeated transfusions of Rh-positive blood to an Rh-negative patient puts the patient at risk for hemolysis and agglutination.

Anti-Rh antibodies occur in an Rh-negative person after Rh-positive RBCs are introduced into the bloodstream.

Immune system

The organs and tissues of the immune system are involved with the growth, development, and dissemination of lymphocytes. (See *Organs and tissues of the immune system.*)

Immunity divided by 3

The immune system has three major divisions:

- central lymphoid organs and tissues
- peripheral lymphoid organs and tissues
- accessory lymphoid organs and tissues.

Central lymphoid organs and tissues

The bone marrow and thymus play roles in developing B cells and T cells, which are the two major types of lymphocytes.

Bone marrow

The bone marrow contains stem cells, which are multipotential, meaning they may develop into several different cell types. The immune system and blood cells develop from stem cells in a process called hematopoesis.

Stemming from stem cells

Soon after differentiation from the stem cells, some of the cells become part of the immune system and sources of lymphocytes; others develop into phagocytes, which ingest microorganisms and cellular debris.

Organs and tissues of the immune system

The immune system includes cells that circulate in the bloodstream as well as organs and tissues in which lymphocytes predominate. This illustration depicts the central, peripheral, and accessory lymphoid organs and tissue.

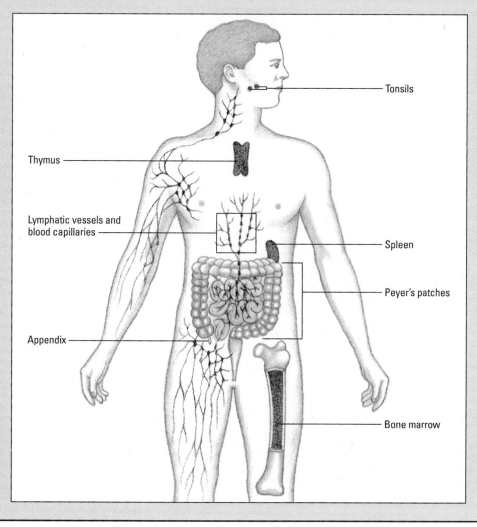

Tonsils

Thymus

Lymphatic vessels and blood capillaries

Spleen

Peyer's patches

Appendix

Bone marrow

To B or to be T

The lymphocytes further differentiate into either B cells (which mature in the bone marrow) or T cells (which travel to the thymus and mature). B cells and T cells are distributed throughout the lymphoid organs, especially the lymph nodes and spleen.

Memory Jogger

To help you remember where lymphocytes mature, remember:

B cells mature in the **B**one marrow

T cells mature in the **T**hymus.

B cells don't attack pathogens themselves but instead produce antibodies, which attack pathogens or direct other cells, such as phagocytes, to attack them. This response is regulated by T cells and their products, lymphokines, which determine the immunoglobulin class a B cell will manufacture.

Thymus

In a fetus or an infant, the thymus is a two-lobed mass of lymphoid tissue located over the base of the heart in the mediastinum. The thymus forms T lymphocytes for several months after birth and gradually atrophies until only a remnant persists in adults.

The thymus forms T lymphocytes until several months after birth and then gradually atrophies.

Teaching T cells

In the thymus, T cells undergo a process called T-cell education, in which the cells "learn" to recognize other cells from the same body (self cells) and distinguish them from all other cells (nonself cells). There are five types of T cells with specific functions:

- memory cells, which are sensitized cells that remain dormant until second exposure to an antigen

- lymphokine-producing cells, which are involved in delayed hypersensitivity reactions

- cytotoxic T cells, which direct destruction of an antigen or the cells carrying the antigen

- helper T cells, also known as T4 cells, which facilitate the humoral and cell-mediated responses

- suppressor T cells, also known as T8 cells, which inhibit humoral and cell-mediated responses.

Peripheral lymphoid organs and tissues

The peripheral lymphoid structures include lymph and the lymphatic vessels, lymph nodes, and spleen.

Lymph

Lymph is a clear fluid that bathes body tissues. It contains a liquid portion that resembles blood plasma.

Lymphatic vessels

The lymphatic vessels form a network of thin-walled channels that drain lymph from body tissues. Lymph seeps into the lymphatic vessels through their thin walls. (See *Lymphatic vessels and lymph nodes.*)

Lymphatic vessels and lymph nodes

The primary lymphatic vessels and structures of a lymph node are depicted below.

Into the nodes

Afferent lymphatic vessels carry lymph into the subcapsular sinus (or cavity) of the lymph node. From there, lymph flows through cortical sinuses and smaller radial medullary sinuses.

Phagocytic cells in the deep cortex and medullary sinuses attack antigens in lymph. Antigens also may be trapped in the follicles of the superficial cortex.

Back into the vessels

Cleansed lymph leaves the node through efferent lymphatic vessels at the hilum (a depression at the exit or entrance of the node). The efferent vessels drain into lymph node chains that, in turn, empty into large lymph vessels, or trunks, that drain into the subclavian vein of the vascular system.

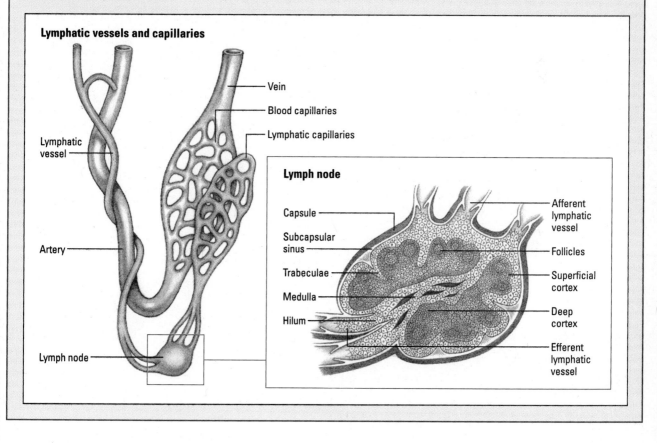

Lymphatic vessels and capillaries

Vein

Blood capillaries

Lymphatic capillaries

Lymphatic vessel

Artery

Lymph node

Lymph node

Capsule

Subcapsular sinus

Trabeculae

Medulla

Hilum

Afferent lymphatic vessel

Follicles

Superficial cortex

Deep cortex

Efferent lymphatic vessel

Fluid enters but can't exit

Lymphatic capillaries are located throughout most of the body. They're wider than blood capillaries and permit interstitial fluid to flow into them but not out.

Lymph nodes

Lymph nodes are small, oval-shaped structures along the lymphatic vessels. They're most abundant in the head, neck, axillae, abdomen, pelvis, and groin. Lymph nodes remove and destroy antigens circulating in the blood and lymph.

From vessels to nodes

Afferent lymphatic vessels, which resemble veins, carry lymph into the lymph nodes; the lymph slowly filters through the node and is collected into efferent lymphatic vessels.

Node-to-node

Lymph usually travels through more than one lymph node because numerous nodes line the lymphatic vessels that drain a region. For example, axillary nodes filter drainage from the arms and femoral nodes filter drainage from the legs. This prevents organisms that enter peripheral areas from entering central areas.

Lymph nodes filter out and destroy circulating antigens.

Spleen

A person's spleen is in the left upper abdominal quadrant beneath the diaphragm. This dark red, oval structure is about the size of a fist. Bands of connective tissue from the dense fibrous capsule surrounding the spleen extend into the spleen's interior.

Red, white, and blood-filled

The interior spleen, called the splenic pulp, contains white and red pulp:
• White pulp contains compact masses of lymphocytes surrounding branches of the splenic artery.
• Red pulp is a network of blood-filled sinusoids supported by a framework of reticular fibers and mononuclear phagocytes, along with some lymphocytes, plasma cells, and monocytes.

Splenic work

The spleen has several functions:
• Its phagocytes engulf and break down worn out RBCs, causing the release of Hb, which then breaks down into its components. These phagocytes also selectively retain and destroy damaged or abnormal RBCs and cells with large amounts of abnormal Hb.
• It filters and removes bacteria and other foreign substances that enter the bloodstream; these substances are promptly removed by splenic phagocytes.
• Splenic phagocytes interact with lymphocytes to initiate an immune response.
• It stores blood and 20% to 30% of platelets.

Accessory lymphoid organs and tissues

The tonsils, adenoids, appendix, and Peyer's patches are the accessory lymphoid organs and tissues. They remove foreign debris in much the same way lymph nodes do. They're located in areas where microbial access is more likely to occur.

Immunity

Immunity is the body's capacity to resist invading organisms and toxins, thereby preventing tissue and organ damage.

Elimination and preservation

The cells and organs of the immune system recognize, respond to, and eliminate foreign substances (antigens), such as bacteria, fungi, viruses, and parasites. They also preserve the body's internal environment by scavenging dead or damaged cells.

The immune system has three basic defensive functions:
• protective surface phenomena
• general host defense
• specific immune responses.

Protective surface phenomena

Protective surface phenomena are physical, chemical, and mechanical barriers that prevent organisms from entering the body. Such phenomena include organs, structures, and processes of many body systems:
• integumentary
• respiratory
• GI
• genitourinary.

Skin-deep defenses

Intact and healing skin and mucous membranes physically defend against microbial invasion by preventing attachment of microorganisms. Skin desquamation (normal cell turnover) and low pH further impede bacterial colonization.

Antibacterial substances, such as the enzyme lysozyme (in tears, saliva, and nasal secretions) chemically protect seromucous surfaces, such as the conjunctiva of the eye and oral mucous membranes.

Defensive breathing

In the respiratory system, turbulent airflow through the nostrils and nasal hairs filters foreign materials. Nasal secretions contain

The skin and mucous membranes prevent microbial invasions.

an immunoglobulin that discourages microbe adherence, and the mucous layer lining the respiratory tract is continually sloughed off and replaced.

GI system GIs

Bacteria that enter the GI system are mechanically removed through salivation, swallowing, peristalsis, and defecation. In addition, the low pH of gastric secretions is bactericidal, making the stomach virtually free from live bacteria. In addition, resident bacteria in the intestines prevent colonization by other microorganisms, protecting the rest of the GI system through a process called *colonization resistance*.

Urinary sterility

The urinary system is sterile except for the distal end of the urethra and the urinary meatus. Urine flow, low urine pH, immunoglobulin, and the bactericidal effects of prostatic fluid impede bacterial colonization. A series of sphincters also inhibits upward bacterial migration into the urinary tract.

Resident bacteria in the intestines protect the GI system through a process called *colonization resistance*.

General host defenses

When an antigen does penetrate the skin or mucous membrane, the immune system launches a nonspecific cellular response to identify and remove the invader.

First response

The first nonspecific response against an antigen, the inflammatory response, involves vascular and cellular changes that eliminate dead tissue, microorganisms, toxins, and inert foreign matter. (See *Understanding inflammation.*)

Next effect

Phagocytosis occurs after inflammation or during chronic infection. In this nonspecific response, neutrophils and macrophages engulf, digest, and dispose of the antigen.

Specific immune responses

All foreign substances elicit the same general host defenses. In addition, particular microorganisms or molecules activate specific immune responses produced by lymphocytes (B cells and T cells) and can initially involve specialized sets of immune cells. Such specific responses are classified as either:
• humoral immunity
• cell-mediated immunity.

Understanding inflammation

The inflammatory response to an antigen involves vascular and cellular changes that eliminate dead tissue, microorganisms, toxins, and inert foreign matter. This nonspecific immune response aids tissue repair in a stepwise fashion.

Soon after microorganisms invade damaged tissue, basophils release heparin, histamine, and kinins.

↓

These substances promote vasodilation and increase capillary permeability.

↓

Blood flow increases to the affected tissues, and fluid collects in them.

↓

Granulocytes—predominantly neutrophils—promptly migrate to the invasion site.

↓

At the invasion site, these cells engulf and destroy the microorganism, foreign materials, and debris from dying cells.

↓

Tissue repair occurs.

Humoral immunity

In humoral immunity, an invading antigen causes B cells to divide and differentiate into plasma cells. Each plasma cell then produces and secretes a large amount of antigen-specific immunoglobulin into the bloodstream.

Each of the five types of immunoglobulins (IgA, IgD, IgE, IgG, and IgM) has a specific function:
- IgA, IgG, and IgM guard against viral and bacterial invasion.
- IgD is an antigen receptor of B cells.
- IgE causes an allergic response.

Defense depends on the antigen

Depending on the antigen, immunoglobulins work in one of several ways:

> B cells and T cells produce humoral and cell-mediated immunity.

• They can disable certain bacteria by linking with toxins that the bacteria produce; these immunoglobulins are called antitoxins.
• They can opsonize (coat) bacteria, making them targets for scavenging by phagocytosis.
• Most commonly, they link to antigens, causing the immune system to produce and circulate enzymes called complements.

Telling time lag

After an initial exposure to an antigen, a time lag occurs during which little or no antibody can be detected in the body. During this time, the B cell recognizes the antigen, and the antigen-antibody complex forms. The complex has several functions:
• A macrophage processes the antigen and presents it to antigen-specific B cells.
• The antibody activates the complement system, causing an enzymatic cascade that destroys the antigen.
• The activated complement system, which bridges humoral and cell-mediated immunity, attracts phagocytic neutrophils and macrophages to the antigen site.

Complement system

The complement system consists of about 25 enzymes that complement the work of antibodies by aiding phagocytosis or destroying bacteria (by puncturing their cell membranes).

Cascading complements

Complement proteins travel in the bloodstream in an inactive form. When the first complement substance is triggered by an antibody interlocked with an antigen, it sets in motion a ripple effect. As each component is activated in turn, it acts on the next component in a controlled sequence called the complement cascade.

Attack complex

The complement cascade leads to formation of the membrane attack complex, which enters the membrane of a target cell and creates a channel through which fluids and molecules flow in and out. The target cell then swells and eventually bursts.

Complementary effects

Effects of the complement cascade also include:
• the inflammatory response (resulting from release of the contents of mast cells and basophils)
• stimulation and attraction of neutrophils (which participate in phagocytosis)
• coating of target cells by C3b (an inactivated fragment of the complement protein C3), making them attractive to phagocytes.

> The complement cascade leads to formation of the membrane attack complex and a ripple of other effects.

Cell-mediated immunity

Cell-mediated immunity protects the body against bacterial, viral, and fungal infections and provides resistance against transplanted cells and tumor cells.

T cells destroy and survey

In cell-mediated immunity, a macrophage processes the antigen, which is then presented to T cells. Some T cells become sensitized and destroy the antigen; others release lymphokines, which activate macrophages that destroy the antigen. Sensitized T cells then travel through the blood and lymphatic systems, providing ongoing surveillance for specific antigens.

Hematologic and immune systems assessment

Many signs and symptoms of hematologic disorders are nonspecific and difficult to assess. Others are more specific; use these to focus on possible disorders. Assess the hematologic system if the patient reports any of these specific signs or symptoms, including:
- abnormal bleeding
- bone and joint pain
- exertional dyspnea
- ecchymoses
- fatigue and weakness
- fever
- lymphadenopathy
- petechiae
- shortness of breath.

If the patient reports these specific signs or symptoms, assess for hematologic disorders.

Immune challenges

Accurately assessing a patient's immune system can likewise challenge your skills. Immune disorders sometimes produce characteristic signs—such as butterfly rash in systemic lupus erythematosus (SLE)—but they usually cause vague symptoms, such as fatigue or dyspnea, which initially seem related to other body systems. For this reason, assess the immune system whenever a patient reports such symptoms as:
- malaise
- fatigue
- frequent or recurrent infections
- slow wound healing.

Health history

Start your assessment by taking a thorough patient history. Gather information about the patient's current and previous illnesses. Also ask about the patient's family and social histories.

Current health status

Ask the patient how long he has had the problem, when it began, and how suddenly or gradually. Ask if it occurs continuously or intermittently. If intermittently, how frequent and how long is each episode?

Next, determine the location and character of the problem and precipitating conditions. Ask if anything makes the problem better or worse. Also ask about other signs and symptoms that occur at the same time as the primary ones.

Previous health status

Examine the patient's medical history for additional clues to his present condition. Look for information about allergies, immunizations, previously diagnosed illnesses (childhood and adult), past hospitalizations and surgeries, and current medications he uses, both prescription and over-the-counter.

Look back

Look at the patient's history for information about past disorders (such as acute leukemia, Hodgkin's disease, sarcoma, and rheumatoid arthritis) that required aggressive immunosuppressant or radiation therapies. Such treatment can diminish blood cell production. Has the patient received any blood products? If so, note when and how often blood product transfusions were used to assess the patient's risk of harboring a blood-borne infection.

Family history

Some hematologic disorders are inherited. Ask about deceased family members; note their ages at death and causes. Note any inheritable hematologic disorders and plot them on a family genogram to determine the patient's inheritance risk.

Lifestyle patterns

The patient may be reluctant to discuss certain habits or lifestyles. Take steps to develop trust between you and the patient to increase cooperation. Inquire about alcohol intake, diet, sexual habits, and possible drug abuse, all of which can impair hematologic or immune function.

Examine the patient's medical history to find clues about the present condition.

Work and service

Make sure you gather a comprehensive occupational and military service history. Exposure to certain hazardous substances can cause bone marrow dysfunction, especially leukemia.

Physical assessment

Because hematologic and immune disorders can involve almost every body system, perform a complete physical examination.

Assessing vital signs

Vital signs can provide important clues about the patient's hematologic and immune system health.

Thermo-measurement

Take the patient's temperature. Frequent fevers can indicate a poorly functioning immune system. Subnormal temperatures usually accompany gram-negative infections.

Heart and BP checks

Note the patient's heart rate. The heart may pump harder or faster to compensate for a decreased oxygen supply resulting from anemia or decreased blood volume from bleeding. This problem can cause tachycardia, palpitations, or arrhythmias.

Measure the patient's blood pressure while lying, sitting, and standing. Check for orthostatic hypotension, which may be caused by septicemia or hypovolemia.

O₂ inquiry

Check the patient's breathing. If he's having difficulty meeting the body's oxygen needs, he may have pronounced tachypnea.

Size up

Next, measure the patient's height and weight. Compare the findings with normal values for the patient's bone structure. Weight loss may result from anorexia or other GI problems related to immune disorders.

Hematologic inspection

Next, concentrate on areas most relevant to a hematologic disorder, including the:
- skin
- mucous membranes
- fingernails

Because hematologic and immune disorders can involve almost every body system, perform a complete physical examination.

- eyes
- lymph nodes
- liver and spleen.

Skin-deep assessment

The patient's skin color directly reflects body fluid composition. Observe for pallor, cyanosis, or jaundice. Check for erythema and plethora (ruddy color), which appear with local inflammation and polycythemia, respectively. Assess the mucous membranes for jaundice, bleeding, redness, swelling, or ulceration.

Examine skin, nails, and eyes

If you suspect a blood-clotting abnormality, check the patient's skin for purpuric lesions, which may vary in size and usually result from thrombocytopenia. Also, inspect for abnormalities, such as telangiectases, and note their locations. Check the patient's skin for dryness and coarseness, which may indicate iron deficiency anemia.

Note abnormalities in the patient's nails. Longitudinal striations can indicate anemia. Spoon-shaped nails characterize iron deficiency anemia. Nail clubbing indicates chronic tissue hypoxia, which can result from such hematologic disorders as anemia.

Inspect the patient's eyes for jaundice, which may occur from excessive hemolysis. Retinal hemorrhages and exudates suggest severe anemia and thrombocytopenia.

Abdominal assessment

Inspect the patient's abdominal area for enlargement, distention, and asymmetry, possibly indicating a tumor. Hepatomegaly and splenomegaly may result from:
- congestion caused by cell overproduction, as in polycythemia or leukemia
- excessive cell destruction, as in hemolytic anemia.

Immune system inspection

An immune disorder can affect the skin and nails as described above. It can also affect the mouth and nose, so assess the nasal cavity for mucous membrane ulceration, which may indicate SLE.

Inspect the oral mucosa. White patches scattered throughout the mouth may indicate candidiasis, and lacy white plaques on the buccal mucosa may be associated with acquired immunodeficiency syndrome (AIDS). Such lesions can occur in a patient with an immunosuppressive disorder or one who receives chemotherapy.

> An immune disorder can affect the skin, nails, mouth, nose, and other body parts.

> Abnormalities in the patient's nails, such as longitudinal striations, spoon shape, and clubbing, can result from anemia.

(Text continues on page 571.)

Acute pancreatitis

Pancreatitis, inflammation of the pancreas, occurs in acute and chronic forms. Acute pancreatitis, a life-threatening emergency, may be either edematous (interstitial) or necrotizing:

• Edematous pancreatitis, the more common type (75% of cases), results in fluid accumulation and swelling. Prognosis for patients with edematous pancreatitis is fairly good (the disease is self-limiting and subsides within 1 week after treatment in about 85% of patients).

• Necrotizing pancreatitis, which occurs in about 25% of pancreatitis cases, causes cell death and tissue damage. Mortality is higher in cases of necrotizing pancreatitis due to cellular necrosis, extensive fat necrosis, and hemorrhage within the pancreas. If infection occurs concomitantly, mortality may be as high as 60%.

How it happens

Normally, the acini in the pancreas secrete inactive enzymes. Inappropriate activation of these enzymes results in autodigestion of the pancreas and tissue necrosis, resulting in acute pancreatitis. The mechanism that triggers this activation is unknown; however, several conditions are associated with it. The most common include biliary tract obstruction by gallstones and alcohol abuse (alcohol increases stimulation of pancreatic secretions).

What to do

Acute pancreatitis requires meticulous supportive care and continuous monitoring of vital systems. Complications of untreated disease include massive hemorrhage, shock, pseudocyst, biliary and duodenal obstruction, portal vein thrombosis, diabetes mellitus, and acute respiratory failure.

Diabetes mellitus

Diabetes is a chronic disease that affects the way the body uses food to make the energy necessary for life. Primarily, diabetes is a disruption of carbohydrate (sugar and starch) metabolism that also affects fats and proteins. There are two main forms of diabetes (type 1 and type 2) as well as conditions of glucose intolerance, gestational diabetes, and diabetes caused by pancreatic disorders. Regardless of the form, metabolic control under the care of a doctor is essential for good health.

What is insulin?
Insulin is an essential hormone that's produced in the pancreas and released into the bloodstream. Insulin attaches itself to cells at places called *insulin receptors.* When attached, insulin allows sugar or glucose from food to enter the body's liver, fat, and muscle cells, where it's used for energy.

Type 1 diabetes mellitus
In type 1 diabetes, the pancreas makes little or no insulin. Without insulin, sugar can't enter cells to be used for energy. The body's tissues are starved and blood glucose levels grow dangerously high. The disorder usually begins in youth, but it may also occur in older adults. Type 1 diabetes occurs in 5% to 10% of patients with diabetes; these patients require insulin therapy for treatment.

Type 2 diabetes mellitus
In type 2 diabetes, the pancreas produces some insulin, but it's either too little or it isn't effective. In addition, insulin receptors that control the transport of sugar into cells may not work properly or are reduced in number. Type 2 diabetes typically develops in people over age 40. Most newly diagnosed patients with type 2 diabetes are overweight but are able to control their diabetes through diet and weight loss. Some patients may require oral medications or insulin injections to achieve glucose control.

Type 1 diabetes

Pancreas with no insulin production

Cell
Glucose
Closed glucose channel
Open glucose channel

Type 2 diabetes

Pancreas producing little or ineffective insulin

Insulin receptor
Insulin

Long-term health problems

High plasma glucose levels caused by diabetes may damage small and large blood vessels and nerves. Diabetes may also reduce the body's ability to fight infection. As a result, people with diabetes are more likely to have serious eye problems, kidney disease, heart attacks, strokes, high blood pressure, poor circulation, tingling in hands and feet, sexual problems, amputations, and infections. Good diabetes control may help prevent these problems or make them less serious.

Loss of vision

Nerve damage

Poor circulation

Good diabetes control may reduce the patient's risk of experiencing these long-term health problems.

Heart disease

Kidney failure

Cirrhosis

Cirrhosis is a chronic liver disease that's characterized by widespread destruction of hepatic cells. The destroyed cells are replaced by fibrotic cells in a process called *fibrotic regeneration.* As necrotic tissue yields to fibrosis, regenerative nodules form and the liver parenchyma undergo extensive and irreversible fibrotic changes. The disease alters normal liver structure and vasculature, impairs blood and lymphatic flow and, ultimately, causes hepatic insufficiency.

   Therapy for cirrhosis aims to remove or alleviate the underlying cause, prevent further liver damage, and prevent or treat complications.

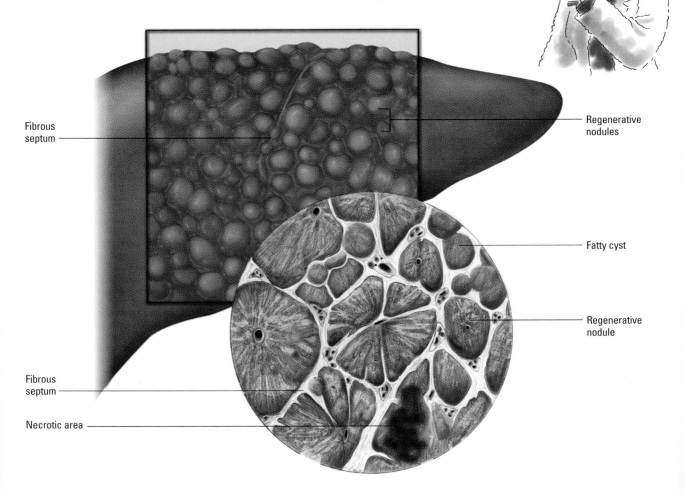

It looks like cirrhosis has already begun to destroy these hepatic cells.

Fibrous septum

Regenerative nodules

Fatty cyst

Regenerative nodule

Fibrous septum

Necrotic area

Eyes, fingers, toes, ears, and nose

Observe the patient's eyelids for signs of infection or inflammation. Assess the fundus of the eye; hemorrhage or infiltration may indicate vasculitis.

Assess the patient's peripheral circulation for Raynaud's phenomenon (intermittent arteriolar vasospasm of the fingers or toes and sometimes of the ears and nose). This phenomena may be caused by SLE or scleroderma.

Urinary system inspection

Because immune dysfunction can affect the urinary system, obtain a urine specimen and evaluate its color, clarity, and odor. Cloudy, malodorous urine may result form a urinary tract infection.

Inspect the urinary meatus. In a patient with WBC deficiency or immunodeficiency, the external genitalia may be focal points for inflammation, which is commonly accompanied by discharge or bleeding related to infection.

LOC signs

Evaluate the patient's level of consciousness (LOC) and mental status. Neurologic effects may provide clues to an underlying disease. A patient with SLE may experience altered mentation, depression, or psychosis.

Look for lumps

Inspect the lymph node areas where the patient reports swollen glands or lumps for color abnormalities and visible lymph node enlargement. Then inspect all other nodal regions. Proceed from head to toe to avoid missing any region. Normally, lymph nodes can't be seen. Visibly enlarged nodes suggest a current or previous inflammation. Nodes covered with red-streaked skin suggest acute lymphadenitis.

Look from head to toe for lumps or visible lymph node enlargement.

Auscultating the abdomen

With the patient lying down, auscultate the abdomen before palpation and percussion to avoid altering bowel sounds. Listen for a loud, high-pitched, tinkling sound, which heralds the early stages of intestinal obstruction. Lymphoma is a hematologic cause of such obstruction.

Listen to the liver

Next, auscultate the liver and spleen. Listen carefully over both organs for friction rubs (grating sounds that fluctuate with respirations). These sounds usually indicate inflammation of the organ's peritoneal covering. Splenic friction rubs also suggest infarction and inflammation.

Percussing the liver and spleen

To determine liver and spleen size, and possibly detect tumors, percuss all four quadrants and compare your findings.

Dullness is normal

The normal liver sounds dull. Establish the organ's approximate size by percussing for its upper and lower borders at the midclavicular line. To determine medial extension, percuss to the midsternal landmark.

The normal spleen also sounds dull. Percuss it from the midaxillary line toward the midline. The average-sized spleen lies near the eighth, ninth, or tenth intercostal space. You might mark the liver and spleen borders with a pen for later reference.

> Percuss all four abdominal quadrants to determine liver and spleen size and to detect tumors.

Palpating lymph nodes, liver, and spleen

Before palpating the lymph nodes, liver, and spleen, make sure the patient is positioned comfortably, draped appropriately, and kept warm. Warm your hands, then palpate using gentle to moderate pressure.

Lymph node palpation

Palpate the patient's neck, axillary, epitrochlear, and inguinal lymph nodes, moving the skin over each area with your finger pads.

Check neck nodes and so on

When palpating nodes in the neck, make sure the patient is sitting.

The patient should remain sitting or should lie down when you palpate the axillary nodes. To check the right axilla, ask the patient to relax the right arm. Use your nondominant hand to support it. Put your other hand as high in the axilla as possible. Palpate against the chest wall for the lateral, anterior, posterior, central, and subclavian nodes. Repeat the procedure for the left axilla.

To assess the epitrochlear nodes, palpate the medial area of the patient's elbow. For the inguinal nodes, palpate below the inguinal ligament and along the upper saphenous vein.

What to look for

As you palpate all nodes, note their location, size, tenderness, texture (hard, soft, or firm), and whether they're movable. For each node group, note current or previous inflammation. Hard or fixed nodes may suggest a tumor. General lymphadenopathy can indicate an inflammation or cancerous condition. (See *Palpating the lymph nodes.*)

Palpating the lymph nodes

When assessing your patient for signs of an immune disorder, palpate the superficial lymph nodes of the head and neck and of the axillary, epitrochlear, inguinal, and popliteal areas, using the pads of your index and middle fingers. Always palpate gently, beginning with light pressure and gradually increasing the pressure.

Head and neck nodes

Head and neck nodes are best palpated with the patient sitting.

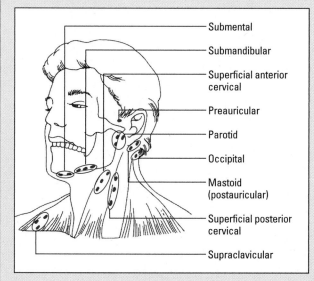

- Submental
- Submandibular
- Superficial anterior cervical
- Preauricular
- Parotid
- Occipital
- Mastoid (postauricular)
- Superficial posterior cervical
- Supraclavicular

Axillary and epitrochlear nodes

Palpate the axillary and epitrochlear nodes with the patient sitting. You can also palpate the axillary nodes with the patient lying in a supine position.

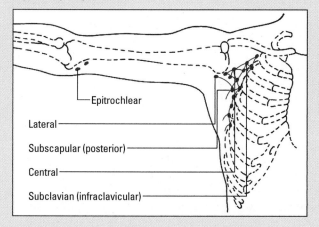

- Epitrochlear
- Lateral
- Subscapular (posterior)
- Central
- Subclavian (infraclavicular)

Inguinal and popliteal nodes

Palpate the inguinal and popliteal nodes with the patient lying in a supine position. You can also palpate the popliteal nodes with the patient sitting or standing.

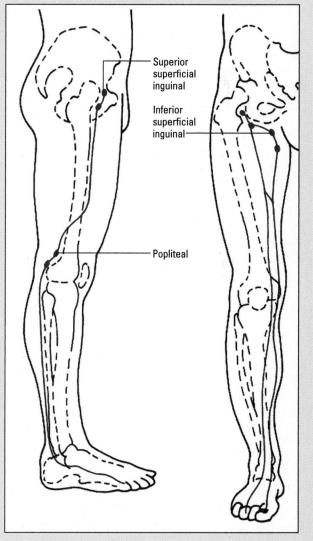

- Superior superficial inguinal
- Inferior superficial inguinal
- Popliteal

Cell-packing problem

As you palpate the patient's nodes, you may discover sternal tenderness. This problem occurs with cell packing in the marrow from anemia, leukemia, and immunoproliferative disorders.

Liver and spleen palpation

Accurate liver palpation is difficult and can depend on the patient's size and comfort level and possible fluid accumulation. Lightly palpate all four abdominal quadrants to distinguish tender sites and muscle guarding. Use deeper palpation to delineate abdominal organs and masses.

If necessary, repeat the procedure, checking your hand position and the pressure you exert. Always palpate tender areas last.

Palpate the spleen to detect tenderness and confirm splenomegaly. The spleen must be enlarged about three times normal size to be palpable. (See *Percussing and palpating the spleen.*)

> Liver palpation can be dicey, depending on the patient's size and comfort level. Always palpate tender areas last.

Diagnostic tests

Various tests may be ordered to diagnose hematologic and immune disorders.

Hematologic system tests

Hematologic diagnostic tests allow direct analysis of the blood, its formed elements (cells), and the bone marrow, where blood cells originate.

ABO blood typing

ABO blood typing is used to classify blood into A, B, AB, and O groups according to the presence of major antigens A and B on RBC surfaces and serum antibodies anti-A and anti-B.

Nursing considerations

• Before the patient receives a transfusion, compare current and past ABO typing and crossmatching to detect possible mistaken identification. Both forward and reverse blood typing are required to prevent a lethal reaction.

• If a patient has received blood in the past 3 months, antibodies to this donor blood may develop and linger, interfering with the patient's compatibility testing.

Advice from the experts

Percussing and palpating the spleen

To assess the spleen, use percussion to estimate its size and palpation to detect tenderness and enlargement. Splenic tenderness may result from infections, which are common in a patient with an immunodeficiency disorder. Splenomegaly may occur with immune disorders that cause congestion by cell overproduction or by excessive demand for cell destruction.

Percussion

To percuss the spleen, follow these steps.

Percuss the lowest intercostal space in the left anterior axillary line; percussion notes should be tympanic.

Ask the patient to take a deep breath, then percuss this area again. If the spleen is normal in size, the area will remain tympanic. If the tympanic percussion note changes on inspiration to dullness, the spleen is probably enlarged.

To estimate spleen size, outline the spleen's edges by percussing in several directions from areas of tympany to areas of dullness.

Palpation

To palpate the spleen, follow these steps.

With the patient in a supine position and you at his right side, reach across him to support the posterior lower left rib cage with your left hand. Place you right hand below the left costal margin and press inward.

Instruct him to take a deep breath. The spleen normally shouldn't descend on deep inspiration below the ninth or tenth intercostal space in the posterior midaxillary line. If the spleen is enlarged, you'll feel its rigid border.

Note: Don't over-palpate the spleen; an enlarged spleen can easily rupture.

Antibody screening test

An antibody screening test—also called *an indirect Coombs' test* and *indirect antiglobulin test*—is used to detect unexpected circulating antibodies to RBC antigens in the recipient's or donor's serum before transfusion. Normally, agglutination doesn't occur, indicating that the patient's serum contains no circulating antibodies (other than anti-A and anti-B).

Positive incompatibility

A positive result reveals the presence of unexpected circulating antibodies to RBC antigens, which indicates donor and recipient incompatibility.

Nursing considerations

• Explain to the patient that the antibody screening test is used to evaluate the possibility of a transfusion reaction.

Antiglobulin test

The direct antiglobulin test, also called the *direct Coombs' test,* is used to detect immunoglobulins (antibodies) on RBC surfaces. These immunoglobulins coat RBCs when they become sensitized to an antigen such as the Rh factor. The test is used to investigate hemolytic transfusion reactions and aid differential diagnosis of anemias, which may result from an autoimmune reaction or a drug's adverse effect.

Nursing considerations

• As ordered, withhold medications that can induce autoimmune hemolytic anemia.

Hold it! Withhold medications that can induce autoimmune hemolytic anemia.

Bleeding time

The bleeding time test is used to measure the duration of bleeding after a standard skin incision. Bleeding time depends on blood vessel wall elasticity, platelet count, and ability to form a hemolytic plug.

Typical testing

Typically, the test is used to evaluate patients whose personal or family history indicates bleeding abnormalities. Along with a platelet count, this test is also used to screen patients scheduled for surgery. It's valuable in detecting vascular abnormalities and other abnormalities or deficiencies.

The bleeding time test is valuable in detecting vascular abnormalities.

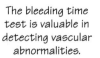

Nursing considerations

• Document any medications the patient has received that may prolong bleeding time, such as anticoagulants, aspirin, nonsteroidal anti-inflammatory drugs, thiazide diuretics, or antineoplastic drugs. If the test is being done to identify a suspected bleeding disorder, stop any medications as ordered, before the test.
• Notify the doctor of abnormal findings.

Coagulation screening tests

Coagulation screening tests are used to detect bleeding disorders and specific coagulation defects.

Nursing considerations

• Explain the test to the patient.
• Allow no more than 4 hours between blood sampling and coagulation testing. Allow only 2 hours between blood centrifugation and coagulation testing because once centrifuged, RBCs lose their buffering effect on the plasma.
• Avoid using hemolyzed plasma, which may cause decreased clotting times. Place the patient's blood sample on ice immediately after it's collected to preserve its labile factors.

Crossmatching

Crossmatching is used to establish the compatibility or incompatibility of donor and recipient blood and is the final check for such compatibility.

Always necessary, except...

Blood is always crossmatched before transfusion, except in extreme emergencies. Because a complete crossmatch may take 45 minutes to 2 hours, an incomplete (10-minute) crossmatch may be acceptable in emergencies. Meanwhile, transfusion can begin with limited amounts of group O packed RBCs. When an emergency transfusion is necessary, proceed with special awareness of the complications that may arise because of incomplete typing and crossmatching.

Nursing considerations

• If more than 48 hours have elapsed since a previous transfusion, previously crossmatched donor blood must be crossmatched with a new recipient serum sample to detect newly acquired incompatibilities before transfusion.
• If the recipient hasn't received a transfusion, donor blood need not be crossmatched again for 72 hours.
• If the patient is scheduled for surgery and has received blood during the previous 3 months, his blood must be crossmatched again to detect recently acquired incompatibilities.

Place the patient's blood sample on ice immediately after it's collected.

Hematocrit

Hematocrit (HCT) test results indicate the percentage of RBCs in whole blood samples. Although normal HCT varies widely, it's roughly three times the person's Hb level and amounts to:

- in men, 42% to 52%
- in women, 36% to 48%
- in children, 30% to 42%.

  Below-normal HCT suggests anemia or hemodilution. Above-normal HCT indicates polycythemia or hemoconcentration due to blood loss.

Nursing considerations
- Explain the purpose of blood studies to the patient.
- Notify the doctor of significant findings and administer blood products as ordered based on test results.

Hemoglobin level (total Hb)

Hb — the main component of RBCs — contains *heme*, a complex molecule of iron and porphyrin that gives blood its color, and globin, a simple protein.

O$_2$ delivery

> HCT test results indicate the percentage of RBCs in whole blood samples.

Hb delivers oxygen from the lungs to the cells and buffers carbon dioxide formed during metabolic activity. A below-normal Hb level may result from anemia, recent hemorrhage, or fluid retention causing hemodilution; an above-normal Hb level from hemoconcentration due to polycythemia or dehydration.

Nursing considerations
- Explain the purpose of blood studies to the patient.
- Notify the doctor of significant findings and administer blood products as ordered based on test results.

Partial thromboplastin time

The partial thromboplastin time (PTT) test is used to evaluate all intrinsic pathway clotting factors (except factors VII and XIII) by measuring the time need for a fibrin clot to form after calcium and phospholipid emulsion is added to a plasma sample.

Normal time

> A low Hb level may result from anemia, hemorrhage, or fluid retention. A high Hb level results from hemoconcentration.

Normally, a fibrin clot forms 25 to 36 seconds after reagent is added. Prolonged times may mean that the plasma sample contains plasma clotting factor deficiencies, heparin, fibrin split products, or circulating anticoagulants that act as antibodies to clotting factors.

Nursing considerations

• Explain to the patient receiving heparin therapy that this test may be repeated at regular intervals to assess his response to treatment.
• Notify the doctor of test results and adjust the heparin infusion dosage as ordered.
• For a patient on anticoagulant therapy, additional pressure may be needed at the venipuncture site to control bleeding.

Plasma thrombin time

The plasma thrombin test—also known as the *thrombin clotting time test*—is used to measure how quickly a clot forms after a standard amount of bovine thrombin is added to a platelet-poor plasma sample from the patient and to a normal plasma control sample. It's used to detect a fibrinogen deficiency or defect, diagnose disseminated intravascular coagulation (DIC) and hepatic disease, and monitor heparin or thrombolytic therapy. Normal plasma thrombin times range from 10 to 15 seconds.

Nursing considerations

• If possible, withhold heparin therapy before the test as ordered. If heparin therapy must be continued, note this on the laboratory request.

Platelet count

Platelet count is used to evaluate platelet (thrombocyte) production, which is necessary for blood clotting. Accurate counts are essential for monitoring chemotherapy and radiation therapy and for assessing the severity of thrombocytosis (abnormally increased platelet count) or thrombocytopenia.

Count down

Normal platelet count varies from 140,000 to 400,000/µl. A platelet count below 50,000/µl can result in spontaneous bleeding; a count below 5,000/µl usually indicates potential for massive hemorrhage.

Count up

Increased platelet count may result from hemorrhage, infectious disorders, cancer, iron deficiency anemia, surgery, pregnancy, splenectomy, or an inflammatory disorder.

Nursing considerations

• Explain the purpose of platelet studies to the patient.

• Notify the doctor of significant findings and administer blood products as ordered based on test results.

Prothrombin time and INR

Prothrombin time (PT) is the time required for a fibrin clot to form in a citrated plasma sample after calcium ion and tissue thromboplastin (factor III) are added. The result is compared to the fibrin clotting time in a control plasma sample.

Indirect test

The PT test is used to measure indirectly prothrombin and is an excellent screening method for evaluating prothrombin, fibrinogen, and extrinsic coagulation factors V, VII, and X. It's the test of choice for monitoring oral anticoagulant therapy. In a patient receiving an oral anticoagulant, PT usually remains between one and one-half and two times the normal control value.

PT testing is best for monitoring oral anticoagulant therapy.

INR standards

The International Normalized Ratio (INR) system is the best means of standardizing measurement of PT to monitor oral anticoagulant therapy. Normal INR for those receiving warfarin therapy is two to three times the control. Increased INR values may indicate:
• DIC
• cirrhosis
• vitamin K deficiency
• uncontrolled oral anticoagulation
• salicylate intoxication
• massive blood transfusion.

Nursing considerations

• Explain to a patient receiving oral anticoagulant therapy that this test may be repeated at regular intervals to assess his response to treatment.
• For a patient on anticoagulant therapy, additional pressure may be needed at the venipuncture site to control bleeding.
• Notify the doctor of test results; oral anticoagulant therapy dosage adjustments are based on test results.

RBC count

RBC count—also known as erythrocyte count—indicates the number of RBCs in whole blood. A depressed RBC count may indicate anemia, fluid overload, recent hemorrhage, or leukemia; an elevated count, dehydration, polycythemia, or acute poisoning.

Nursing considerations

• Explain the purpose of RBC studies to the patient.
• Notify the doctor of significant findings and administer blood products as ordered based on test results.

Rh blood typing

The Rh system is used to classify blood according the presence or absence of antigen D (formerly known as Rho) on RBC surfaces. Rh blood typing is used to determine if donors and recipients are compatible before transfusions and to learn whether the patient needs a RhoGAM (Rho[D] immune globulin) injection.

Nursing considerations

• Before the patient receives a transfusion, the Rh factor must be checked along with ABO typing.

Bone marrow examination yields valuable information about blood disorders.

Biopsy

Biopsy procedures involve removing small samples of tissue for testing.

Bone marrow aspiration and needle biopsy

In aspiration biopsy, a fluid specimen containing bone marrow cells in suspension is collected. Bone marrow aspiration is an important test for evaluating the blood's formed elements.

Needle biopsy is done to remove a marrow core containing cells but no fluid. The best possible marrow specimens are obtained by using both methods.

Aspire to biopsy

Because most hematopoiesis takes place in bone marrow, histologic and hematologic bone marrow examination yields valuable diagnostic information about blood disorders. Bone marrow aspiration and needle biopsy are used to obtain material for that examination.

Bone marrow biopsy is used to diagnose aplastic, hypoplastic, and vitamin B_{12} deficiency anemias; granulomas; leukemias; lymphomas; myelofibrosis; and thrombocytopenia. It's also used to evaluate chemotherapy effectiveness and to monitor myelosuppression.

Nursing considerations

• Describe the procedure and answer the patient's questions. Confirm any medication allergies or past history of hypersensitivity to local anesthetics. Inform the patient that a local anesthetic is used but that he may feel pressure during the biopsy.

• Tell him the test takes 5 to 10 minutes and test results are usually available in 1 day.

• Tell the patient which bone is to be used for the biopsy. (See *Bone marrow aspiration and biopsy sites.*)

• Explain to the patient that he'll receive I.V. sedation before the procedure.

• Monitor vital signs, oxygen saturation, and cardiac rhythm during and after the procedure. After the procedure, check the biopsy site for bleeding and inflammation. Monitor for these signs of bleeding or infection: rapid heart rate, low blood pressure, or fever.

• Change the dressing over the biopsy site every 24 hours to reduce the risk of infection.

Bone marrow aspiration and biopsy sites

The drawings below depict the most common sites for bone marrow aspiration and biopsy. These sites are used because the involved bone structures are relatively accessible and rich in marrow cavities.

Posterior superior iliac crest
The posterior superior iliac crest is the preferred site for aspiration and biopsy because no vital organs or vessels are nearby. The patient lies in a prone or lateral position. The needle is inserted several centimeters lateral to the iliosacral junction and directed downward and toward the anterior inferior spine or entered a few centimeters below the crest at a right angle to the surface of the bone.

Spinous process
The spinous process is preferred if multiple punctures are necessary or if marrow is absent at other sites. The patient sits on the edge of the bed, leaning over the bedside stand. The spinous process of the third or fourth lumbar vertebrae is selected, the needle is inserted at the crest or slightly to one side, and advanced in the direction of the bone plane.

Sternum
The sternum involves the greatest risk but provides the best access. The patient is in a supine position with a small pillow beneath his shoulders to elevate his chest and lower his head. The doctor secures the needle guard 3 to 4 mm from the tip of the needle to avoid accidentally puncturing the heart or a major vessel. Then he inserts the needle at the midline of the sternum at the second intercostal space.

Immune system tests

The doctor may order various tests to evaluate the patient's immune response. Commonly ordered studies include cellular tests, such as T- and B-lymphocyte assays, to detect immunomediated disease.

T- and B- lymphocyte surface marker assays

Surface marker assays are used to identify the specific cells involved in the immune response and to examine the balance between the regulatory activities of several interacting cell types, notably T-helper and T-suppressor cells.

The test involves use of highly specific monoclonal antibodies to define levels of lymphocyte differentiation and to analyze both normal and malignant cells. This information is used to assess immunocompetence in chronic infections, evaluate immunodeficiences, and classify lymphocytic leukemia, lymphoma, and immunodeficiency disease and AIDS.

Surface marker assays are used to analyze both normal and malignant cells.

Nursing considerations

• Explain the test to the patient.
• Send the sample to the laboratory immediately; don't refrigerate or freeze it.

Treatments

Treatments for patients with hematologic and immune disorders may include drug therapy and transfusion therapy.

Drug therapy

Hematologic drugs include hematinics, anticoagulants and heparin agonists, hemostatics, and blood derivatives. (See *Common hematologic medications*, pages 584 and 585.)

For patients with some immune disorders, drugs are the primary treatment. For example, epinephrine is the drug of choice for correcting an anaphylactic reaction.

For patients with other disorders, drugs are prescribed to treat associated symptoms. (See *Drug therapy in immune disorders*, pages 586 and 587.)

Common hematologic medications

Hematologic drugs include hematinics, which help arrest anemia; anticoagulants and heparin antagonists, which impede clotting; hemostatics, which arrest blood flow or reduce capillary bleeding; blood derivatives, which replace blood loss from disease or surgical procedures; and thrombolytic enzymes, which treat thrombotic disorders. The chart below outlines common hemolytic drugs, their indications and adverse effects, and practice considerations.

Drugs	Indications	Adverse effects	Practice pointers
Anticoagulants			
Heparin	• Prevention of pulmonary embolism and deep vein thrombosis (DVT) after hip- or knee-replacement surgery • Continuous I.V. or S.C. therapy for DVT, myocardial infarction (MI), pulmonary embolism	Hemorrhage, thrombocytopenia, chills, fever, pruritis, urticaria, anaphylactoid reactions	• Never administer I.M. • Don't massage the site after subcutaneous (S.C.) injection. Rotate injection sites, keeping a record of sites used. • Monitor platelet count and for signs of bleeding. • Check I.V. infusions regularly for underdosing and overdosing. • Measure partial thromboplastin time (PTT) regularly. Anticoagulation is present when PTT values are one and one-half to two times control values. • Never piggyback other drugs into an infusion line while heparin infusion is running.
Warfarin	• Treatment of pulmonary embolism • Prevention and treatment of DVT, MI, rheumatic heart disease with heart valve damage, atrial arrhythmias	Anorexia, nausea, vomiting, hematuria, hemorrhage, jaundice, urticaria, fever, headache	• Prothrombin time (PT) determinations are essential for proper controls; maintain PT at one and one-half to two times normal. • Give drug at the same time daily. • Regularly inspect for bleeding gums, bruises, petechiae, nosebleeds, melena, hematuria, and hematemesis. • Tell the patient to use an electric razor, avoid scratching the skin, and use a soft toothbrush.
Blood derivatives			
Normal serum albumin 5% Normal serum albumin 25%	• Shock • Hypoproteinemia	Headache, vascular overload after rapid infusion, hypotension, tachycardia, nausea, vomiting, dyspnea, pulmonary edema, chills, fever	• Don't give more than 250 g in 48 hours. • Watch for hemorrhage or shock if used after surgery or injury. • Watch for signs of vascular overload (heart failure or pulmonary edema). • Don't use cloudy solutions or those with sediment.

Common hematologic medications *(continued)*

Drugs	Indications	Adverse effects	Practice pointers
Blood derivatives *(continued)*			
Plasma protein fractions	• Shock • Hypoproteinemia	Headache, hypotension or vascular overload after rapid infusion, tachycardia, nausea, vomiting, dyspnea, pulmonary edema, rash, fever, chills, back pain	• Monitor blood pressure; reduce infusion rate if hypotension occurs. • Watch for signs of vascular overload (heart failure or pulmonary edema). • Monitor intake and output; watch for decreased urine output. • Don't give more than 250 g in 48 hours.
Hematinics			
Ferrous sulfate	• Iron deficiency	Nausea, epigastric pain, vomiting, constipation, black stools, diarrhea, anorexia	• Dilute liquid preparations in orange juice or water, not milk or antacids. Give tablets with orange juice to promote absorption. • Give elixir with a straw to avoid staining teeth. • GI upset is related to dosage; give the drug between meals.
Hemostatics			
Aminocaproic acid	• Excessive bleeding resulting from hyperfibrinolysis	Dizziness, malaise, headache, seizures, arrhythmias, tinnitis, nausea, cramps, diarrhea, generalized thrombosis, rash	• Monitor coagulation studies, heart rhythm, and blood pressure; notify the doctor of changes. • Dilute the solution with sterile water for injection, normal saline solution, dextrose 5% in water, or lactated Ringer's solution.
Heparin antagonist			
Protamine	• Heparin overdose	Bradycardia, circulatory collapse, nausea, vomiting, pulmonary edema, acute pulmonary hypertension, anaphylaxis	• Use cautiously after cardiac surgery. • Give slowly to reduce adverse effects. • Watch for spontaneous bleeding.

Corticosteroid potentials

Corticosteroids are adrenocortical hormones used to treat patients with immune-mediated disorders because of their potent anti-inflammatory and immunosuppressant effects.

Drug therapy in immune disorders

The doctor may order drug therapy to suppress a patient's immune response. Immune serum studies may be ordered after specific antigens are identified. Immunosuppressants may be used to combat tissue rejection or relieve inflammation. Antiviral agents, such as nucleoside reverse transcriptase inhibitors are used to correct human immunodeficiency virus (HIV) infections. Use this table to find information necessary to administer these drugs.

Drugs	Indications	Adverse effects	Practice pointers
Antivirals			
Lamivudine	• Treatment of HIV infection in combination with zidovudine (AZT)	Headache, fatigue, dizziness, insomnia, neutropenia, anemia, thrombocytopenia, cough, fever, chills	• Monitor serum amylase levels. Stop drug if clinical signs and symptoms suggest pancreatitis. • Give with AZT. Not indicated for use alone.
Stavudine	• Treatment of HIV infected patients who have received prolonged zidovudine therapy	Peripheral neuropathy, headache, malaise, insomnia, anxiety, dizziness, chest pain, abdominal pain, diarrhea, nausea, anorexia, weight loss, neutropenia, thrombocytopenia, anemia, rash, hepatotoxicity, chills, fever	• May be taken with or without food. • Teach patient signs and symptoms of peripheral neuropathy, which is the major dose-limiting effect. It may not resolve after drug is discontinued. • Monitor liver function tests.
Zalcitabine	• Treatment of patients with advanced HIV infection who have demonstrated significant clinical or immunology deterioration	Peripheral neuropathy, headache, fatigue, confusion, seizures, heart failure, chest pain, cough, nausea, vomiting, diarrhea, constipation, esophageal ulcer, neutropenia, leukopenia thrombocytopenia, pruritis, night sweats, arthralgia, increased aspartate aminotransferase, alanine aminotransferase, and alkaline phosphate	• Monitor liver function studies and pancreatic enzymes. • Use with extreme caution in patients with peripheral neuropathy. • Use cautiously in patients with a history of pancreatitis.
Zidovudine, AZT	• Symptomatic HIV infection	Headache, seizures, paresthesia, somnolence, anorexia, nausea, vomiting, diarrhea, constipation, severe bone marrow suppression (resulting in anemia), rash, myalgia, fever, increased liver enzymes	• Use cautiously in patients with severe bone marrow depression. • Monitor blood studies every 2 weeks to detect anemia or granulocytopenia. • For I.V. use, dilute before administration. Remove the calculated dose from the vial; add to dextrose 5% in water injection to achieve a concentration not exceeding 4 mg/ml. Infuse over 1 hour at a constant rate. Avoid rapid infusion or bolus injection.

Drug therapy in immune disorders *(continued)*

Drugs	Indications	Adverse effects	Practice pointers
Immune serums			
Hepatitis B immune globulin (H-BIG)	• Hepatitis B exposure	Urticaria, pain and tenderness at injection site, anaphylaxis, angioedema	• Obtain a history of allergies and reactions to immunizations. • Inject the drug into the anterolateral aspect of thigh or deltoid area. • Administer with the hepatitis B vaccine for postexposure prophylaxis (needlestick or direct contact).
Immune globulin	• Bone marrow transplant • Hepatitis exposure	Headache, faintness, nausea, vomiting, hip pain, chest pain, chest tightness, dyspnea, urticaria, muscle stiffness (at injection site), anaphylaxis, fever, chills, malaise	• Have epinephrine available in case of anaphylactic reaction to the medication. • Use cautiously in patients with a history of cardiovascular disease of thrombotic episodes.
Immunosuppressants			
Cyclosporine	Prophylaxis of organ rejection in kidney, liver, bone marrow, and heart transplants	Tremor, headache, seizures, confusion, hypertension, nephrotoxicity, leukopenia, thrombocytopenia, hepatotoxicity, flushing, acne, infections, increased low-density lipoproteins, anaphylaxis	• Measure oral doses carefully in an oral syringe. To increase palatability, mix with whole milk, chocolate milk, or fruit juice. Use a glass container to minimize adherence to container walls. • Give dose once daily in the morning at the same time each day. • Patient may take with meals if drug causes nausea.

Corticosteroids stabilize the vascular membrane, blocking tissue infiltration by neutrophils and monocytes and thus inhibiting inflammation. They also affect T cells in the bone marrow, causing leukopenia. However, because these drugs aren't cytotoxic, lymphocyte concentration can quickly return to normal within 24 hours after they're withdrawn.

Corticosteroid cautions

Steroids should be used cautiously in patients with GI ulceration, renal disease, hypertension, diabetes mellitus, and psychotic tendencies.

Corticosteroids aren't cytotoxic, so lymphocytes can quickly return to normal afterward.

Transfusion therapy

Transfusion procedures allow administration of a wide range of blood products, such as RBCs, which can revive oxygen-starved tissues; leukocytes, which can combat infections beyond the reach of antibiotics; and clotting factors, plasma, and platelets, which can help patients with clotting disorders live virtually normal lives. Common procedures include factor replacement and exchange transfusions.

> Good news! Transfusion can revive oxygen-starved tissues, combat infections, and aid patients with hemophilia.

Factor replacement

I.V. infusion of deficient clotting elements is a major part of treatment for patients with coagulation disorders. Factor replacement typically corrects clotting factor deficiencies, thereby stopping or preventing hemorrhage.

Products depend on disorders

Various blood products are used, depending on the specific disorder being treated:
- Fresh frozen plasma is used to treat clotting disorders with unknown causes, clotting factor deficiencies resulting from hepatic disease or blood dilution, consumed clotting factors secondary to DIC, and deficiencies of clotting factors for which no specific replacement product exists.
- Cryoprecipitate is used to treat von Willebrand's disease, fibrinogen deficiencies, and factor XIII deficiencies.
- Factor VIII (antihemophiliac factor) concentrate serves as the long-term treatment of choice for patients with hemophilia A.
- Prothrombin complex is given to correct hemophilia B, severe liver disease, and acquired deficiencies for the factors it contains (II, VII, IX, and X).

> Administer fresh frozen plasma within 4 hours because it doesn't contain preservatives.

Nursing considerations
- Explain the procedure to the patient and assemble the equipment.
- Verify the doctor's order and make sure that the informed consent form was signed.
- Obtain the blood product from the blood bank or pharmacy.
- Identify the patient. Ask another licensed professional to double-check the patient's name, medical record number, and ABO and Rh status (as well as other compatibility factors). This information should be compared with the identification label on the blood product's bag.
- Check the expiration date, and inspect the plasma fraction for cloudiness or turbidity.

• Administer fresh frozen plasma within 4 hours because it doesn't contain preservatives.
• Administer platelets using a blood component drip administration set; don't use a microaggregate filter. Infuse 100 ml over 15 minutes.
• Take the patient's vital signs, perform a venipuncture if a line isn't in place, and infuse normal saline solution at a keep-vein-open rate.
• During and after administration, monitor vital signs and watch for signs of anaphylaxis and other allergic reactions and fluid overload.
• Monitor for bleeding, increased pain or swelling at the transfusion site, and fever.
• Monitor the patient's PTT.

Hematologic and immune systems disorders

Hematologic and immune systems disorders commonly seen in the critical care environment include acute leukemia, anaphylaxis, DIC, human immunodeficiency virus (HIV) infection, and idiopathic thrombocytopenic purpura.

Acute leukemia

Leukemia is a group of malignant disorders characterized by abnormal proliferation and maturation of lymphocytes and nonlymphocytic cells leading to suppression of normal cells. It's classified as acute or chronic:
• Acute lymphoblastic leukemia involves abnormal growth of lymphoblasts. It accounts for 80% of all childhood leukemias.
• Acute myelogenous leukemia involves rapid accumulation of myeloblasts. It's one of the most common leukemias in adults.
• Chronic myelogenous leukemia is characterized by myeloproliferation in bone marrow. It's common in middle age but may occur in any age group.
• Chronic lymphocytic leukemia is characterized by an increase in well-differentiated lymphocytes in the bone marrow and peripheral blood. It's most common in elderly people.

Age is no object

Acute leukemia ranks 20th as the cause of cancer-related deaths among people of all age-groups. Without treatment, acute leukemia invariably leads to death, usually because of complications that result from leukemic cell infiltration of bone marrow or vital organs. With treatment, the prognosis varies.

Without treatment, acute leukemia is deadly. With treatment, the prognosis varies.

What causes it

The cause of acute leukemia isn't known. Risk factors seem to include some combination of viruses, genetic and immunologic factors, and exposure to radiation and certain chemicals.

Pathophysiology

Malignant WBC precursors (blasts) proliferate in bone marrow or lymph tissue and accumulate in peripheral blood, bone marrow, and body tissues.

What to look for

Typical clinical features include sudden onset of high fever, abnormal bleeding (such as nosebleeds, gingival bleeding, purpura, ecchymoses, and petechiae), easy bruising after minor trauma, and prolonged menses.

Nonspecific signs and symptoms include low-grade fever, pallor, and weakness that may persist for days or months before other symptoms appear.

What tests tell you

• Bone marrow aspiration typically shows a proliferation of immature WBCs and is used to confirm the diagnosis.
• Complete blood count (CBC) shows anemia, thrombocytopenia, and neutropenia.
• Differential leukocyte count is used to determine cell type.

How it's treated

Systemic chemotherapy is used to eradicate leukemic cells and induce remission. Chemotherapy varies with the specific disorder. Bone marrow transplants are an option in some cases.

What to do

• Preventing infection is an important part of care for the patient with acute leukemia. Monitor vital signs every 2 to 4 hours. Assess for bleeding and early signs of infection (fever, chills, tachycardia, and tachypnea). Patients with fever over 101° F (38.3° C) and decreased WBC counts should receive antibiotic therapy promptly.
• Avoid giving aspirin and aspirin-containing drugs.
• Avoid taking rectal temperatures, giving rectal suppositories, and doing digital examinations. Employ measures to prevent constipation.
• Avoid using indwelling catheters and giving I.M. injections.

Preventing infection is an important part of care for the patient with acute leukemia.

• Control mouth ulceration by checking the patient's mouth often and by providing frequent mouth care and saline solution rinses.
• Provide psychological support by establishing a trusting relationship to promote communication.

Anaphylaxis

Anaphylaxis is an exaggerated hypersensitivity reaction to a previously encountered antigen. A severe reaction may precipitate vascular collapse, leading to systemic shock and sometimes death.

What causes it

Causes of anaphylaxis include:
• exposure to sensitizing drugs (such as antibiotics, serums, vaccines, allergen extracts, enzymes, hormones, sulfonamides, local anesthetics, salicylates, polysaccharides, and antineoplastics)
• exposure to diagnostic chemicals (including radiographic contrast media containing iodine)
• foods
• sulfites
• insect venom
• latex.

Pathophysiology

An anaphylactic reaction requires previous sensitization or exposure to the specific antigen. This sensitization causes production of specific IgE antibodies by plasma cells. IgE antibodies then bind to membrane receptors or mast cells and basophils.

Take two

Upon reexposure, the antigens bind to adjacent IgE antibodies or cross-linked IgE receptors, activating a series of reactions that triggers the release of powerful chemical mediators (histamine) from mast cell stores. IgG or IgM enters into the reaction and activates the release of complement fractions.

At the same time, two other chemical mediators, bradykinin and leukotrienes, induce vascular collapse by causing certain smooth muscles to contract and increasing vascular permeability. This collapse leads to decreased peripheral resistance to plasma leakage from the circulation to extravascular tissues. Hypotension ensues, leading to hypovolemic shock and cardiac dysfunction.

Reexposure to a specific antigen triggers the release of histamine.

What to look for

An anaphylactic reaction usually produces sudden distress within seconds or minutes after exposure to an allergen. (A delayed or persistent reaction may occur up to 24 hours later.)

Signs and symptoms from head to toe

Initial signs and symptoms include a feeling of impending doom or fright, weakness, sweating, sneezing, pruritus, urticaria, and angioedema. Cardiovascular signs include hypotension, shock, and arrhythmias. Respiratory signs and symptoms include nasal mucosal edema, profuse watery rhinorrhea, nasal congestion, sudden sneezing attacks, hoarseness, stridor, and dyspnea. GI and genitourinary signs and symptoms include severe stomach cramps, nausea, diarrhea, urinary urgency, and incontinence.

What tests tell you

Anaphylaxis can be diagnosed by the rapid onset of severe respiratory or cardiovascular reactions after exposure to an allergen.

How it's treated

• Anaphylaxis is always an emergency, requiring an immediate injection of epinephrine repeated every 5 to 20 minutes as necessary. With cardiac arrest, initiate cardiopulmonary resuscitation.
• Maintain airway patency. Observe for early signs of laryngeal edema (stridor, hoarseness, and dyspnea), which may necessitate endotracheal (ET) intubation, cricothyrotomy, or a tracheostomy.
• Maintain circulatory volume with volume expanders (plasma, saline solution, and albumin) as needed.
• Watch for hypotension and shock. Stabilize the patient's blood pressure with I.V. vasopressors, such as norepinephrine and dopamine. Monitor the patient's cardiac rhythm, vital signs, oxygen saturation, hemodynamic parameters, and urine output as a response index.

What to do

• After initial emergency measures, administer other medications as ordered, such as subcutaneous epinephrine solution and I.V. corticosteroids or diphenhydramine.
• Closely monitor a patient undergoing diagnostic tests that use radiographic contrast media, such as cardiac catheterization and angiography.

> Rapid onset of severe respiratory or cardiovascular reactions are telltale signs of anaphylaxis. It's always an emergency.

EMERGENCY

Disseminated intravascular coagulation

DIC is a grave coagulopathy that accelerates clotting, causing small blood vessel occlusion, organ necrosis, depletion of circulating clotting factors and platelets, and activation of the fibrinolytic system.

These processes in turn can provoke severe hemorrhage. Clotting in the microcirculation usually affects the kidneys and extremities, but may occur in the brain, lungs, pituitary and adrenal glands, and GI mucosa.

What causes it

Conditions that can cause DIC include:
- infection
- obstetric complications
- neoplastic disease
- disorders that produce necrosis, such as extensive burns, trauma, brain tissue destruction, transplant rejection, and hepatic necrosis
- heat stroke
- shock
- poisonous snakebite
- cirrhosis
- fat embolism
- incompatible blood transfusion
- cardiac arrest
- surgery necessitating cardiopulmonary bypass
- severe venous thrombosis.

Many conditions can cause DIC. Just look at this list!

Pathophysiology

Regardless of how DIC begins, the typical accelerated clotting causes generalized activation of prothrombin and a consequent excess of thrombin.

Clotting and coagulating

Excess thrombin converts fibrinogen to fibrin, producing fibrin clots in the microcirculation. This process consumes large amounts of coagulation factors, causing hypoprothrombinemia, thrombocytopenia, and deficiencies in factors V and VIII.

Circulating thrombin activates the fibrinolytic system, which lyses fibrin clots into fibrin degradation products. Hemorrhage may be the result of the anticoagulant activity of fibrin degradation products as well as depletion of plasma coagulation factors.

What to look for

Abnormal bleeding without a history of serious hemorrhagic disorder can signal DIC.

Blood out of place

Principal signs of such bleeding include cutaneous oozing, petechiae, ecchymoses, hematomas, bleeding from sites of surgical or invasive procedures, and bleeding from the GI tract.

Other signs and symptoms

Also, assess the patient for acrocyanosis. Related or possible signs and symptoms include dyspnea, oliguria, seizures, coma, shock, failure of major organ systems, and severe muscle, back, and abdominal pain.

What tests tell you

Laboratory findings supporting a tentative diagnosis include:
• decreased platelets (less than 100,000/µl)
• decreased fibrinogen level (less than 150 mg/dl)
• increased fibrin degradation products (often greater than 100 mcg/ml).
• prolonged PT (greater than 15 seconds)
• prolonged PTT (greater than 60 seconds)
• decreased urine output (less than 30 ml/hour), elevated blood urea nitrogen level (greater than 25 mg/dl), and elevated serum creatinine level (greater than 1.3 mg/dl).

How it's treated

Effective treatment for patients with DIC requires prompt recognition and adequate attention to the underlying disorder. Treatment may be generally supportive or highly specific.

If the patient isn't actively bleeding, supportive care alone may reverse DIC. However, active bleeding may require I.V. heparin and administration of blood, fresh frozen plasma, platelets, or packed RBCs to support hemostasis. (See *Understanding DIC and its treatment.*)

What to do

• Monitor the patient's cardiac, respiratory, and neurologic status closely, at least every 30 minutes initially. Assess breath sounds and monitor vital signs and cardiac rhythm.
• Assess the patient for signs of hemorrhage and hypovolemic shock. Assist with insertion of a pulmonary artery catheter, if ordered, and monitor hemodynamic parameters, including pulmo-

Assess the patient with DIC for signs of hemorrhage and hypovolemic shock.

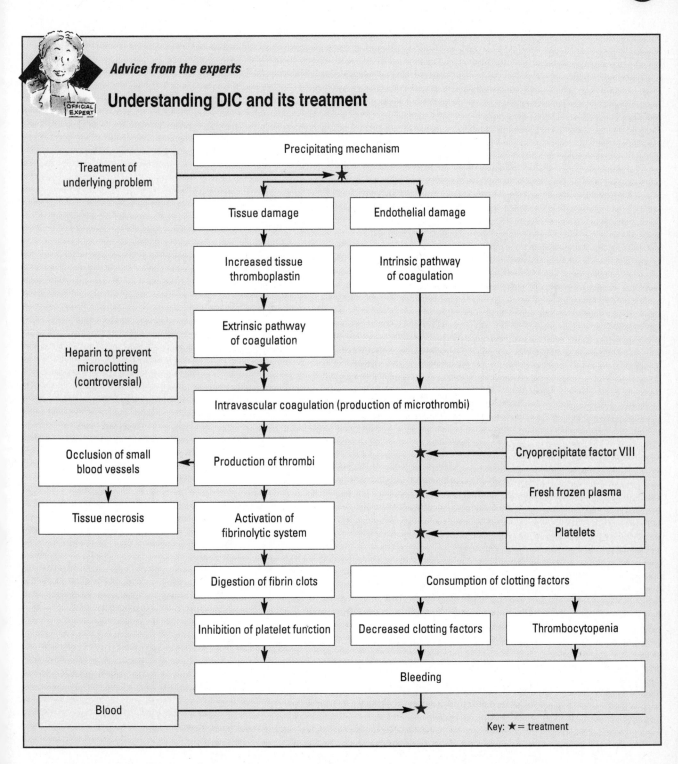

Advice from the experts

Understanding DIC and its treatment

Precipitating mechanism

Treatment of underlying problem

Tissue damage

Endothelial damage

Increased tissue thromboplastin

Intrinsic pathway of coagulation

Extrinsic pathway of coagulation

Heparin to prevent microclotting (controversial)

Intravascular coagulation (production of microthrombi)

Occlusion of small blood vessels

Production of thrombi

Cryoprecipitate factor VIII

Tissue necrosis

Activation of fibrinolytic system

Fresh frozen plasma

Platelets

Digestion of fibrin clots

Consumption of clotting factors

Inhibition of platelet function

Decreased clotting factors

Thrombocytopenia

Bleeding

Blood

Key: ★ = treatment

nary artery pressure, pulmonary artery wedge pressure, and cardiac output. Notify the doctor of a decrease in pulmonary artery pressure readings or blood pressure, an indication of shock and hemorrhage. Observe the patient's skin color and check peripheral circulation and capillary refill. Inspect skin and mucous membranes for signs of bleeding.

• Check all I.V. and venipuncture sites often. Apply pressure to injection sites for at least 15 minutes.

• Administer supplemental oxygen as ordered. Monitor oxygen saturation and blood gas results, assess for signs of hypoxemia, and anticipate the need for ET intubation and mechanical ventilation.

• Keep the patient as quiet and comfortable as possible to minimize oxygen demands. Place the patient in semi-Fowler's position, as tolerated, to maximize chest expansion.

• Monitor the patient's diagnostic laboratory values and administer blood, fresh frozen plasma, or platelets as ordered.

• Monitor the patient's intake and output hourly, especially when administering blood products. Watch for transfusion reactions and signs of fluid overload.

• Assess the patient for potential complications of DIC, including pulmonary emboli due to accelerated clotting, acute tubular necrosis, or multiple organ failure.

• Provide emotional support to the patient and his family.

HIV infection

HIV infection is characterized by progressive decline of immune function that, if left untreated, results in susceptibility to opportunistic infections and malignancies. The most profound state of immunodeficiency caused by HIV is AIDS.

The Centers for Disease Control and Prevention defines AIDS as a confirmed presence of HIV infection, a CD4$^+$ T (helper T) cell count less than 200/μl, or presence of HIV with an opportunistic infection. (See *Conditions associated with AIDS.*)

What causes it

The retrovirus HIV causes AIDS. This virus appears in body fluids, such as blood and semen. Modes of transmission include:

• sexual contact, especially with trauma to the rectal or vaginal mucosa, in patients from any age group (see *HIV in elderly patients*)

• transfusion of contaminated blood or blood products

• use of contaminated needles

• perinatal transmission from mother to fetus.

Senior moment

HIV in elderly patients

HIV infection occurs predominantly in young people (in most cases ages 17 to 55). However, incidence is rapidly increasing in people ages 50 and older. This group may not have benefited from HIV-prevention messages, which are commonly targeted at younger people. Make sure you take a sexual history from older patients or inquire about their sexual activity, which may aid in diagnosing the disease.

Conditions associated with AIDS

The Centers for Disease Control and Prevention (CDC) lists diseases associated with acquired immunodeficiency syndrome (AIDS) under three categories. From time to time, the CDC adds to these lists.

Category A
• Persistent generalized lymph node enlargement
• Acute primary human immunodeficiency virus (HIV) infection with accompanying illness
• History of acute HIV infection

Category B
• Bacillary angiomatosis
• Oropharyngeal or persistent vulvovaginal candidiasis, fever, or diarrhea lasting longer than 1 month
• Idiopathic thrombocytopenic purpura
• Pelvic inflammatory disease, especially with a tubulo-ovarian abscess
• Peripheral neuropathy

Category C
• Candidiasis of the bronchi, trachea, lungs, or esophagus
• Invasive cervical cancer
• Disseminated or extrapulmonary coccidioidomycosis
• Extrapulmonary cryptococcosis
• Chronic interstitial cryptosporidiosis
• Cytomegalovirus (CMV) disease affecting organs other than the liver, spleen, or lymph nodes

• CMV retinitis with vision loss
• Encephalopathy related to HIV
• Herpes simplex infection with chronic ulcers or herpetic bronchitis, pneumonitis, or esophagitis
• Disseminated or extrapulmonary histoplasmosis
• Chronic intestinal isopsoriasis
• Kaposi's sarcoma
• Burkitt's lymphoma or its equivalent
• Immunoblastic lymphoma or its equivalent
• Primary brain lymphoma
• Disseminated or extrapulmonary *Mycobacterium avium-intracellulare* complex or *M. kansasii*
• Pulmonary or extrapulmonary *M. tuberculosis*
• Disseminated or extrapulmonary infection with any other species of *Mycobacterium*
• *Pneumocystis carinii* pneumonia
• Recurrent pneumonia
• Progressive multifocal leukoencephalopathy
• Recurrent *Salmonella* septicemia
• Toxoplasmosis of the brain
• Wasting syndrome caused by HIV

Pathophysiology

For patients with AIDS, the number of CD4+ T cells declines, mainly because HIV selectively binds with and destroys them. A substance called *gp 120* binds HIV to CD4+ T-cell receptor sites.

Enter HIV

After binding to a target cell, HIV enters the cell and sheds its envelope. How the virus enters the cell isn't known. After HIV enters

HIV is picky. It selectively binds with and destroys helper T cells, causing immunodeficiencies.

the cell, the enzyme reverse transcriptase transcribes the genomic ribonucleic acid into deoxyribonucleic acid (DNA).

Afterward, during cell division, a virus-encoded enzyme integrates the DNA into the host genome. At this point, HIV's replication cycle may be suspended until the infected CD4⁺ T cell is activated.

Critical destruction

Because CD4⁺ T cells are critically important in the immune response, destruction of even part of their population can cause immunodeficiencies. These immunodeficiencies leave the patient vulnerable to the potentially fatal opportunistic infections and cancers characteristic of AIDS.

What to look for

Signs and symptoms of AIDS vary widely; nonspecific ones include:
- fatigue
- afternoon fevers
- night sweats
- weight loss
- diarrhea
- cough.

That's all 'til later

Patients may be otherwise asymptomatic until abrupt onset of complications, such as opportunistic infection, Kaposi's sarcoma, and HIV encephalopathy (dementia) marked by confusion, apathy, and paranoia. (See *Opportunistic infections in AIDS.*)

What tests tell you

- Enzyme-linked immunosorbent assay (ELISA) is the most widely used test to determine the presence of antibodies for HIV. If the results are positive, the test is repeated. If the results are still positive, the findings are confirmed by another method, usually the Western blot or an immunofluorescence assay.
- Direct testing is more reliable because it detects HIV itself. Direct testing includes antigen testing, HIV cultures, nucleic acid probes of peripheral blood lymphocytes, and polymerase chain reaction tests.
- CD4⁺ T cell and CD8⁺ T cell subset counts are used to evaluate the severity of immunosuppression. Other useful tests may include erythrocyte sedimentation rate, CBC, and p 24 antigen and anergy testing.

ELISA is the most widely used test to determine the presence of antibodies for HIV, but direct testing is more reliable because it detects HIV itself.

Opportunistic infections in AIDS

The chart below lists microbial forms and specific organisms that cause opportunistic infections in patients with acquired immunodeficiency syndrome (AIDS).

Microbiological agent	Organism	Infection
Protozoa	*Pneumocystis carinii*	Pneumocystosis
	Cryptosporidium	Cryptosporidiosis
	Toxoplasma gondii	Toxoplasmosis
	Histoplasma	Histoplasmosis
Fungi	*Candida albicans*	Candidiasis
	Cryptococcus neoformans	Cryptococcosis
Viruses	Herpes	Herpes simplex 1 and 2
	Cytomegalovirus (CMV)	CMV retinitis
Bacteria	*Mycobacterium tuberculosis*	Tuberculosis
	Mycobacterium avium	*M. avium* complex

Note: Other opportunistic conditions include Kaposi's sarcoma, wasting sydrome, and AIDS dementia complex.

How it's treated

Although no cure has yet been found, signs and symptoms can be managed with treatment. Primary therapy for HIV infection includes three different types of antiretrovirals used in combination. They include:
• protease inhibitors, such as ritonavir, indinavir, nelfinavir, and saquinavir
• nucleoside reverse transcriptase inhibitors, such as zidovudine, didanosine, zalcitabine, lamivudine, and stavudine
• nonnucleoside reverse transcriptase inhibitors, such as nevirapine and delavirdine.

Other options

Other potential therapies include:
• immunomodulatory drugs designed to boost the weakened immune system
• anti-infective and antineoplastic drugs to combat opportunistic infections and associated cancers.

What to do

• Adhere to standard precautions and anticipate the need for transmission-based precautions if the patient develops another infection.
• Assess the patient's cardiopulmonary status — including breath sounds, vital signs, oxygen saturation, and cardiac rhythm — at least every 2 hours or more often, as needed.
• Report any cough, sore throat, or adventitious sounds that may indicate respiratory infection such as pneumonia. Administer supplemental oxygen as ordered. Anticipate the need for ET intubation and mechanical ventilation if the patient's respiratory status deteriorates.
• Monitor the patient for fever, noting its pattern.
• Assess the patient for tender, swollen lymph nodes, and check laboratory values. Watch for signs and symptoms of infection, such as skin breakdown, cough, sore throat, and diarrhea.
• Provide mouth care using normal saline solution or bicarbonate solution. Avoid glycerin swabs that dry mucous membranes.
• Monitor the patient's nutritional status. Although parenteral nutrition may be needed for adequate caloric intake, it provides a potential route for infection.
• For the patient with Kaposi's sarcoma, monitor the progression of lesions and provide meticulous skin care.
• An AIDS diagnosis is profoundly distressing because of the social impact and the discouraging prognosis. Offer support to the patient, his friends, and his family.

Adhere to standard precautions and anticipate the need for transmission-based precautions if the patient develops another infection.

Idiopathic thrombocytopenic purpura

Idiopathic thrombocytopenic purpura (ITP) results from immunologic platelet destruction. It may be acute (postviral thrombocytopenia) or chronic (Werlhof's disease, pupura hemorrhagica, essential thrombocytopenia, and autoimmune thrombocytopenia).

Acute ITP usually affects children. Chronic ITP mainly affects adults under age 50, especially women ages 20 to 40.

What causes it

Acute ITP usually follows a viral infection, such as rubella or chickenpox. Chronic ITP seldom follows infection and is associated with immunologic disorders, such as SLE, or is linked to drug reactions.

Pathophysiology

The platelet membrane is coated with IgG or other antibody and then these sensitized platelets are destroyed. Their destruction is brought about by the reticuloendothelial system of the liver and spleen.

What to look for

Signs and symptoms of ITP include:
• petechiae
• ecchymoses
• mucosal bleeding from the mouth, nose, or GI tract
• purpuric lesions in vital organs (such as the lungs, kidneys, or brain) that may be fatal.

What tests tell you

• A platelet count less than 20,000/µl and prolonged bleeding time suggest ITP.
• Platelets may be abnormal in size and morphologic appearance.
• Anemia may be present.
• Bone marrow studies show an abundance of megakaryocytes and a shortened circulating platelet survival time.

How it's treated

Corticosteroids promote capillary integrity, but are only temporarily effective in chronic ITP. Alternative therapy includes:
• immunosuppression
• high-dose I.V. gamma globulin
• splenectomy for which the patient may require blood, blood products, and vitamin K delivery.

What to do

• Monitor the patient's cardiopulmonary status and assess for signs of bleeding. Monitor laboratory results and administer immunoglobulin as ordered.
• Closely monitor patients receiving immunosuppressants for signs of bone marrow depression, infection, mucositis, GI tract ulceration, and severe diarrhea or vomiting.

Quick quiz

1. The spleen must be enlarged about how many times normal size to be palpable?
  - A.   One
  - B.   Two
  - C.   Three
  - D.   Four

Answer: C. To detect an enlarged spleen on palpation, it must be about three times its normal size.

2. Which is the preferred site for a bone marrow biopsy?
  - A.   Sternum
  - B.   Spinous process
  - C.   Posterior superior iliac crest
  - D.   Anterior superior iliac crest

Answer: C. The posterior superior iliac crest is the preferred site because no vital organs or vessels are nearby.

3. The drug of choice for a patient experiencing anaphylaxis is:
  - A.   epinephrine.
  - B.   aminophylline.
  - C.   dopamine.
  - D.   diphenhydramine.

Answer: A. Epinephrine is a bronchodilator that relaxes bronchial smooth muscle by beta$_2$-adrenergic receptor stimulation.

4. Which of the following blood tests is used first to identify a response to HIV infection?
  - A.   Western blot
  - B.   CD4$^+$ T-cell count
  - C.   Erythrocyte sedimentation
  - D.   ELISA

Answer: D. The ELISA is the first screening test for HIV. A Western blot test confirms a positive ELISA test.

We're next! Read on to learn about multisystem issues.

Scoring

☆☆☆   If you answered all four questions correctly, go have some fun! You're already a bloody genius, Mate!

☆☆   If you answered three questions correctly, don't despair. No one is immune to an occasional information mismatch.

☆   If you answered fewer than three correctly, your oxygen levels may need a boost. Take a break, have a platelet of something nutritious, and get back into circulation as soon as possible.

Multisystem issues

Just the facts

In this chapter, you'll learn:

♦ types of multisystem disorders

♦ indications for blood and fluid replacement

♦ treatments specific to multisystem issues

♦ nursing care of the patient with multisystem issues.

A look at multisystem issues

Multisystem issues result from various disorders. For example, a patient may have a head injury that's accompanied by chest and cardiac trauma.

Prompt, efficient, and organized care of multisystem issues requires a multidisciplinary team approach. Typically, assessment, treatment, and care of multisystem issues occur simultaneously.

Multisystem issues require a multidisciplinary team!

Shock to the multisystem

Multisystem issues commonly develop in patients experiencing septic shock. About two-thirds of septic shock cases occur in hospitalized patients, most of whom have underlying diseases. Patients at high risk for septic shock include those with burns; diabetes mellitus; immunosuppression; malnutrition; stress; chronic cardiac, hepatic, or renal disorders; or a history of excessive antibiotic use. Also at risk are patients who have had invasive diagnostic or therapeutic procedures, surgery, or traumatic wounds.

Assessment

Rapid assessment followed by appropriate interventions influence the outcome of the patient with multisystem issues. General assessment measures should be paired with assessment techniques that are specific to the patient's condition.

History lesson

Begin your assessment by obtaining the patient's history, including:
• chief complaint
• present and previous illnesses
• current medications
• family and social history.
    If the patient is unstable, you may need to wait until he has stabilized to obtain a complete health history.

Is it life-threatening?

Assess the patient for life-threatening problems (such as respiratory distress in the burn victim), and initiate emergency measures such as cardiopulmonary resuscitation (CPR) as appropriate.

The once-over

Your physical examination includes assessment of all body systems, with particular attention to the body systems involved in the multisystem disorder.

Diagnostic tests

Diagnostics studies are performed to help determine the cause or extent of the patient's multisystem issues. Tests may include laboratory studies (such as hematology, coagulation, chemistry, urine studies, and cultures of blood or body fluids), radiographic studies, electrocardiography (ECG), computed tomography (CT) scans, magnetic resonance imaging, ultrasonography, nuclear medicine scans, and interventional radiological studies.

Treatment

Treating multisystem issues is a challenge. At times, the causative factors in a patient's deteriorating condition may not be known. As more organ systems are affected, care becomes more complex.

Yikes! As more organ systems are affected by a patient's deteriorating condition, care becomes more complex.

Supportive measures are a crucial part of treatment; they include drug therapy, blood transfusion, and fluid replacement.

Drug therapy

Drug therapy for multisystem issues varies depending on the patient's underlying condition. For example, antibiotics may be used to treat septic shock or multiple traumas. Vasopressors may be used to treat various types of shock. Corticosteroids and immunosuppressants are used to treat graft-versus-host disease (GVHD). (See *Drug therapy for multisystem disorders*, pages 606 and 607.)

Blood transfusion

Blood transfusions treat decreased hemoglobin (Hb) level and hematocrit (HCT). A whole blood transfusion replenishes the volume and oxygen-carrying capacity of the circulatory system by increasing the mass of circulating red blood cells (RBCs). It's usually used when hemorrhage occurs.

Packing it in

Packed RBCs, a blood component from which 80% of the plasma has been removed, are transfused to restore the circulatory system's oxygen-carrying capacity. Packed RBCs are used when the patient has a normal blood volume to avoid possible fluid and circulatory overload. (See *Transfusing blood and blood components*, pages 608 and 609.)

Perioperative and emergency blood salvage are the most common indications for transfusion in the critical care setting.

Filtered for patient protection

Whole blood and packed RBCs contain cellular debris, requiring in-line filtration during administration. Washed packed RBCs, commonly used for patients previously sensitized to transfusions, are rinsed with a special solution that removes white blood cells (WBCs) and platelets, thus decreasing the chance of transfusion reaction.

Self-supplier

In some cases, the patient may receive his own blood during a transfusion, called *autotransfusion* or *autologous transfusion*. In this process, the patient's own blood is collected, filtrated, and re-

Drug therapy for multisystem disorders

Use the chart below as a guide to drug therapy appropriate for multisystem disorders.

Drugs	Indications	Adverse reactions	Practice pointers
Corticosteroids			
Dexamethasone Prednisone	• Inflammatory conditions • Immunosuppression • Graft-versus-host disease	• Euphoria • Insomnia • Seizures • Heart failure or arrhythmias • Thromboembolism • Peptic ulceration • Pancreatitis • Acute adrenal insufficiency	• Use cautiously in patients with myocardial infarction, hypertension, renal disease, or GI ulcer. • Sudden withdrawal after prolonged use may be fatal. • Administer oral drug with milk or food • Monitor serum electrolytes, blood glucose, and blood levels at onset of therapy.
Vasopressors			
Dopamine Phenylephrine	• Hypotension • Shock	• Restlessness • Anxiety • Headache • Bradycardia, tachycardia, or arrhythmias • Anaphylaxis • Hypotension or hypertension • Tissue necrosis and sloughing (if I.V. drug leaks into surrounding tissue)	• Use a central venous catheter or a large vein, such as in the antecubital fossa, to minimize extravasation. If extravasation occurs, stop infusion and treat with phentolamine infiltrate to prevent tissue necrosis. Use a continuous infusion pump to regulate infusion flow rate. • When discontinuing, taper dosage slowly to evaluate stability of blood pressure.
Immunosupressants			
Cyclosporine Tacrolimus (FK506)	• Prophylaxis of organ rejection	• Headache, tremor, insomnia, paresthesia, delirium, or coma • Peripheral edema • Diarrhea or constipation • Nausea, vomiting, anorexia, abdominal pain, and ascites • Abnormal renal function • Urinary tract infection • Anemia and leukocytosis • Abnormal liver function studies • Electrolyte imbalance • Pleural effusion, atelectasis, and dyspnea • Pruritus and rash • Photosensitivity	• Monitor the patient for signs of neurotoxicity, nephrotoxicity, hyperkalemia, and hypokalemia. • Monitor blood glucose level regularly. • Give drug with adrenal corticosteroids.

Drug therapy for multisystem disorders (continued)

Drugs	Indications	Adverse reactions	Practice pointers
Antibiotics			
Ceftizoxime Ceftriaxone	• Serious infections of the lower respiratory and urinary tracts • Intra-abdominal, bone and joint, skin, and gynecological infections • Bacteremia • Septicemia	• Leukopenia • Hypersensitivity reactions • Serum sickness • Anaphylaxis • Phlebitis or thrombophlebitis • Diarrhea • Thrombocytopenia • Pseudomembranous colitis	• Obtain a specimen for culture and sensitivity tests before giving first dose. • Monitor prothrombin time and International Normalized Ratio in patients with impaired vitamin K synthesis or low vitamin K stores. Vitamin K therapy may be needed.
Other			
Drotrecogin alfa (activated) Activated protein C	• Severe sepsis associated with organ failure	• Bleeding • Stroke	• Don't administer to a patient with an epidural catheter in place. • Don't use concurrently with heparin.

infused. With the concern over acquired immunodeficiency syndrome and other blood-borne diseases, the use of autologous transfusion is currently on the rise.

Autologous transfusion may be indicated for:
• elective surgery (where the patient donates blood over an extended period of time before surgery)
• nonelective surgery (where the patient's blood is withdrawn immediately before surgery)
• perioperative and emergency blood salvage during and after thoracic or cardiovascular surgery and hip, knee, or liver resection
• perioperative and emergency blood salvage for traumatic injury of the lungs, liver, chest wall, heart, pulmonary vessels, spleen, kidneys, inferior vena cava, and iliac, portal, or subclavian veins.

Refuse to transfuse?

In some cases, a patient may refuse a blood transfusion. For example, a Jehovah's Witness may refuse a transfusion because of his religious beliefs. A competent adult has the right

> With the concern over blood-borne diseases, the use of autologous transfusion is on the rise.

(Text continues on page 610.)

Transfusing blood and blood components

This chart outlines indications, crossmatching concerns, and nursing considerations for transfusing blood and selected blood components.

Blood component	Indications	Compatibility	Nursing considerations
Whole blood Complete (pure) blood Volume: 450 to 500 ml	• To restore blood volume lost from hemorrhaging, trauma, or burns	• ABO identical: Type A receives A; type B receives B; type AB receives AB; type O receives O • Rh match necessary	• Keep in mind that whole blood is seldom administered. • Use a blood administration set to infuse blood within 4 hours. • Warm blood if giving a large quantity.
Packed red blood cells (RBCs) Same RBC mass as whole blood but with 80% of the plasma removed Volume: 250 ml	• To restore or maintain oxygen-carrying capacity • To correct anemia and blood loss that occurs during surgery • To increase RBC mass	• Type A receives A or O • Type B receives B or O • Type AB receives AB, A, B, or O • Type O receives O • Rh match necessary	• Use a blood administration set to infuse blood within 4 hours. • Bear in mind that packed RBCs provide the same oxygen-carrying capacity as whole blood with less risk of volume overload. • Give packed RBCs, as ordered, to prevent potassium and ammonia buildup, which may occur in stored plasma. • Avoid administering packed RBCs for anemic conditions correctable by nutritional or drug therapy.
Platelets Platelet sediment from RBCs or plasma Volume: 35 to 50 ml/unit	• To treat thrombocytopenia caused by decreased platelet production, increased platelet destruction, or massive transfusion of stored blood • To treat acute leukemia and marrow aplasia • To improve platelet count preoperatively in a patient whose count is 100,000/µl or less	• ABO identical when possible • Rh match preferred	• Use a filtered component drip administration set to infuse 100 ml over 15 minutes. • As prescribed, premedicate with antipyretics and antihistamines if the patient's history includes a platelet transfusion reaction. • Avoid administering platelets when the patient has a fever. • Prepare to draw blood for a platelet count, as ordered, 1 hour after the platelet transfusion to determine platelet transfusion increments. • Keep in mind that the doctor seldom orders a platelet transfusion for conditions in which platelet destruction is accelerated, such as idiopathic thrombocytopenic purpura and drug-induced thrombocytopenia.

Transfusing blood and selected components (continued)

Blood component	Indications	Compatibility	Nursing considerations
Fresh frozen plasma (FFP) Uncoagulated plasma separated from RBCs and rich in coagulation factors V, VIII, and IX Volume: 180 to 300 ml	• To treat postoperative hemorrhage or shock • To correct an undetermined coagulation factor deficiency • To replace a specific factor when that factor alone isn't available • To correct factor deficiencies resulting from hepatic disease	• ABO compatibility required • Rh match preferred	• Use a straight-line I.V. set and administer the infusion rapidly. • Keep in mind that large-volume transfusions of FFP may require correction for hypocalcemia because citric acid in FFP binds calcium.
Albumin 5% (buffered saline); albumin 25% (salt poor) A small plasma protein prepared by fractionating pooled plasma Volume: 5% = 12.5 g/250 ml; 25% = 12.5 g/50 ml	• To replace volume lost because of shock from burns, trauma, surgery, or infections • To replace volume and prevent marked hemoconcentration • To treat hypoproteinemia (with or without edema)	• Unnecessary	• Use the blood administration set supplied by the manufacturer with rate and volume dictated by the patient's condition and response. • Remember that reactions to albumin (fever, chills, nausea) are rare. • Avoid mixing albumin with protein hydrolysates and alcohol solutions. • Consider delivering albumin as a volume expander until the laboratory completes crossmatching for a whole blood transfusion. • Keep in mind that albumin is contraindicated in severe anemia and administered cautiously in cardiac and pulmonary disease because heart failure may result from circulatory overload.
Cryoprecipitate Insoluble portion of plasma recovered from FFP Volume: approximately 30 ml (freeze-dried)	• To control bleeding associated with hypofibrinogenemia or dysfibrinogenemia • To treat significant factor XIII deficiency	• ABO compatibility unnecessary but preferable • Rh match unnecessary	• Use a blood administration set to infuse. • Keep in mind that cryoprecipitate must be administered within 6 hours of thawing. • Be aware that patients with hemophilia A or von Willebrand's disease should only be treated with cryoprecipitate when appropriate factor VIII concentrates are not availble.

to refuse treatment. You may be able to use other treatment options if the patient refuses the blood transfusion, such as using blood-conservation strategies during surgery or providing erythropoietin iron and folic acid supplements preoperatively and postoperatively. Using available alternative treatments supports the patient's right of self-determination and honors the patient's wishes. A court order requiring the patient to undergo the standard treatment can also be obtained.

What to do

- Obtain doctor's orders and signed consent.
- Notify the doctor if the patient refuses the blood transfusion.
- Obtain baseline vital signs and start an I.V. line if one isn't already started. Use a 20G or larger-diameter catheter.

Double-check identity

- Identify the patient and check the blood bag identification number, ABO blood group, Rh compatibility, and expiration date of the blood product. This step should be confirmed by another licensed professional. Follow your facility's policy for blood administration.
- Obtain the patient's vital signs after the first 15 minutes and then every 30 minutes (or according to the facility's policy) for the remainder of transfusion therapy.
- If administering platelets or fresh frozen plasma, administer each unit immediately after obtaining it.
- Although some microaggregate filters can be used for up to 10 units of blood, always replace the filter and tubing if more than 1 hour elapses between transfusions. When administering multiple units of blood under pressure, use a blood warmer to avoid hypothermia.

Rapid replacement

- For rapid blood replacement, use a pressure bag or rapid transfusion device if necessary. Be aware that excessive pressure may develop, leading to broken blood vessels and extravasation with hematoma and hemolysis of the infusing RBCs.
- Obtain follow-up laboratory tests as ordered to determine the effectiveness of therapy.
- Record the date and time of the transfusion (time started and completed); the type and amount of transfusion product; the type and gauge of the catheter used for infusion; the patient's vital signs before, during, and after transfusion; a verification check of all identification data (including the individuals' names verifying the information); and the patient's response.
- Document the patient's transfusion reaction and the treatment (if any) required. (See *Guide to transfusion reactions.*)

A patient may refuse a transfusion because of religious beliefs. If necessary, a court order that requires the patient to undergo the transfusion may be obtained.

Remember to always replace the filter and tubing if more than 1 hour elapses between transfusions.

Guide to transfusion reactions

Any patient receiving a transfusion of processed blood products can experience a transfusion reaction. Transfusion reactions typically occur from antigen-antibody reactions; however, they may also occur as a result of bacterial contamination.

Reaction and causes	Signs and symptoms	Nursing interventions
Allergic • Allergen in donor blood • Donor blood hypersensitive to certain drugs	Anaphylaxis (chills, facial swelling, laryngeal edema, pruritus, urticaria, wheezing), fever, nausea, and vomiting	• Administer antihistamines as prescribed. • Monitor the patient for anaphylactic reaction, and administer epinephrine and corticosteroids if indicated.
Bacterial contamination • Organisms that can survive cold, such as Pseudomonas and Staphylococcus	Chills, fever, vomiting, abdominal cramping, diarrhea, shock, signs of renal failure	• Provide broad-spectrum antibiotics, corticosteroids, or epinephrine as prescribed. • Maintain strict blood storage control. • Change blood administration set and filter every 4 hours or after every 2 units. • Infuse each unit of blood over 2 to 4 hours; stop the infusion if the time span exceeds 4 hours. • Maintain sterile technique when administering blood products.
Febrile • Bacterial lipopolysaccharides • Antileukocytic recipient antibodies directed against donor white blood cells	Temperature up to 104° F (40° C), chills, headache, facial flushing, palpitations, cough, chest tightness, increased pulse rate, flank pain	• Relieve symptoms with an antipyretic, an antihistamine, or meperidine, as prescribed. • If the patient requires further transfusions, use frozen red blood cells, add a special leukocyte removal filter to the blood line, or premedicate him with acetaminophen, as prescribed, before starting another transfusion.
Hemolytic • ABO or Rh incompatibility • Intradonor incompatibility • Improper crossmatching • Improperly stored blood	Chest pain, dyspnea, facial flushing, fever, chills, shaking, hypotension, flank pain, hemoglobinuria, oliguria, bloody oozing at the infusion site or surgical incision site, burning sensation along vein receiving blood, shock, renal failure	• Monitor blood pressure. • Manage shock with I.V. fluids, oxygen, epinephrine, a diuretic, and a vasopressor, as prescribed. • Obtain posttransfusion-reaction blood samples and urine specimens for analysis. • Observe for signs of hemorrhage resulting from disseminated intravascular coagulation.
Plasma protein incompatibility • Immunoglobulin-A incompatibility	Abdominal pain, diarrhea, dyspnea, chills, fever, flushing, hypotension	• Administer oxygen, fluids, epinephrine, or a corticosteroid as prescribed.

• If administering multiple units of banked blood, be alert for signs of hypocalcemia caused by the citrate preservative.

Fluid replacement

Fluid replacement is a vital part of treating multisystem illnesses. To maintain the patient's health, the fluid and electrolyte balance in the intracellular and extracellular spaces needs to remain relatively constant. Whenever a person experiences an illness or a condition that prevents normal fluid intake or causes excessive fluid loss, I.V. fluid replacement may be necessary.

So predictable

I.V. therapy provides the patient with life-sustaining fluids, electrolytes, and medications and offers the advantage of immediate and predictable therapeutic effects. Solutions used for I.V. fluid replacement fall into the broad categories of crystalloids and colloids. (See *Understanding electrolytes.*)

Easy flowing

Crystalloids are solutions with small molecules that flow easily from the bloodstream into cells and tissues. There are three types of crystalloids:
• *Isotonic crystalloids* contain about the same concentration of osmotically active particles as extracellular fluid, so fluid doesn't shift between the extracellular and intracellular areas.
• *Hypotonic crystalloids* are less concentrated than extracellular fluid so they move from the bloodstream into the cell, causing the cell to swell.
• *Hypertonic crystalloids* are more highly concentrated than extracellular fluid, so fluid is pulled into the bloodstream from the cell, causing the cell to shrink. (See *A look at I.V. solutions*, pages 614 and 615.)

Water movers

Hypertonic solutions called *colloids* may be used to increase blood volume. Colloids draw water from the interstitial space into the vasculature. Examples of colloid solutions are plasma, albumin, hetastarch, and dextran.

The effects of colloids last several days if the lining of the capillaries is normal. The patient needs to be closely monitored during a colloid infusion for increased blood pressure, dyspnea, and bounding pulse, which are all signs of hypervolemia.

I provide immediate and predictable therapeutic effects!

During colloid infusion, be sure to monitor the patient for signs of hypervolemia.

Understanding electrolytes

Electrolytes help regulate water distribution, govern acid-base balance, and transmit nerve impulses. They also contribute to energy generation and blood clotting. The lists here summarize what the body's major electrolytes do. Check the illustration below to see how electrolytes are distributed in and around the cell.

Potassium (K)
- Main intracellular fluid (ICF) cation
- Regulates cell excitability
- Permeates cell membranes, thereby affecting the cell's electrical status
- Helps to control ICF osmolality and, consequently, ICF osmotic pressure

Magnesium (Mg)
- A leading ICF cation
- Contributes to many enzymatic and metabolic processes, particularly protein synthesis
- Modifies nerve impulse transmission and skeletal muscle response (unbalanced Mg concentrations dramatically affect neuromuscular processes)

Phosphorus (P)
- Main ICF anion
- Promotes energy storage and carbohydrate, protein, and fat metabolism
- Acts as a hydrogen buffer

Sodium (Na)
- Main extracellular fluid (ECF) cation
- Helps govern normal ECF osmolality (A shift in Na concentrations triggers a fluid volume change to restore normal solute and water ratios.)
- Helps maintain acid-base balance
- Activates nerve and muscle cells
- Influences water distribution (with chloride)

Chloride (Cl)
- Main ECF anion
- Helps maintain normal ECF osmolality
- Affects body pH
- Plays a vital role in maintaining acid-base balance; combines with hydrogen ions to produce hydrochloric acid

Calcium (Ca)
- A major cation in teeth and bones; found in fairly equal concentrations in ICF and ECF
- Also found in cell membranes, where it helps cells adhere to one another and maintain their shape
- Acts as an enzyme activator within cells (muscles must have Ca to contract)
- Aids coagulation
- Affects cell membranes permeability and firing level

Bicarbonate (HCO$_3$⁻)
- Present in ECF
- Primary function is regulating acid-base balance

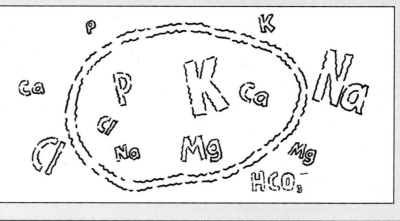

What to do

- Check the I.V. order for completeness and accuracy. Most I.V. orders expire after 24 hours. A complete order should specify the amount and type of solution, specific additives and their concentrations, and the rate and duration of the infusion.
- Keep in mind the size, age, and history of your patient when giving I.V. fluids to prevent fluid overload.

A look at I.V. solutions

This chart shows examples of commonly used I.V. fluids and includes some of the clinical uses and special consideration associated with their use.

Solution	Uses	Special considerations
Isotonic		
Dextrose 5% in water	• Fluid loss and dehydration • Hypernatremia	• Solution is isotonic initially; becomes hypotonic when dextrose is metabolized. • Don't use for resuscitation; can cause hyperglycemia. • Use cautiously in renal or cardiac disease; can cause fluid overload. • Doesn't provide enough daily calories for prolonged use; may cause eventual breakdown of protein.
0.9% sodium chloride (normal saline)	• Shock • Hyponatremia • Blood transfusions • Resuscitation • Fluid challenges • Metabolic alkalosis • Hypercalcemia • Fluid replacement in patients with diabetic ketoacidosis (DKA)	• Because this replaces extracellular fluid, use cautiously in patients with heart failure, edema, or hypernatremia; can lead to overload.
Lactated Ringer's	• Dehydration • Burns • Lower GI tract fluid loss • Acute blood loss • Hypovolemia due to third-space shifting	• Electrolyte content is similar to serum but doesn't contain magnesium. • Contains potassium; don't use with renal failure; can cause hyperkalemia. • Don't use in liver disease because the patient can't metabolize lactate; a functional liver converts it to bicarbonate; don't give if patient's pH is greater than 7.5.
Hypotonic		
0.45% sodium chloride (half-normal saline)	• Water replacement • DKA after initial normal saline solution and before dextrose infusion • Hypertonic dehydration • Sodium and chloride depletion • Gastric fluid loss from nasogastric suctioning or vomiting	• Use cautiously; may cause cardiovascular collapse or increased intracranial pressure. • Don't use in patients with liver disease, trauma, or burns.

A look at I.V. solutions *(continued)*

Solution	Uses	Special considerations
Hypertonic		
Dextrose 5% in half-normal saline	• DKA after initial treatment with normal saline solution and half-normal saline solution—prevents hypoglycemia and cerebral edema (occurs when serum osmolatity is reduced too rapidly)	• In DKA, use only when glucose falls below 250 mg/dl.
Dextrose 5% in normal saline	• Hypotonic dehydration • Temporary treatment of circulatory insufficiency and shock if plasma expanders aren't available • Syndrome of inappropriate antidiuretic hormone (or use 3% sodium chloride) • Addisonian crisis	• Don't use in cardiac or renal patients because of danger of heart failure and pulmonary edema.
Dextrose 10% in water	• Water replacement • Conditions in which some nutrition with glucose is required	• Monitor serum glucose levels.

• Change the site, dressing, and tubing as often as your institution's policy requires. Solutions should be changed at least every 24 hours.
• Monitor the I.V. site for signs of complications, such as infiltration, phlebitis or thrombophlebitis, infection, and extravasation.
• Monitor the patient for signs of complications of I.V. therapy, such as an allergic reaction, air embolism, and fluid overload.
• Monitor intake and output. Notify the doctor if your patient's urine output falls below 30 ml/hour.
• Monitor the patient for potential fluid and electrolyte disturbances and check serum electrolyte values. (See *Interpreting serum electrolyte test results*, page 616.)
• Documentation for a patient receiving an I.V. infusion should include the date, time, and type of catheter inserted, the site of insertion and its appearance, the type and amount of fluid infused, the patient's tolerance and response to therapy.

Don't forget to document the type of catheter used!

Disorders

Multisystem disorders include burns, GVHD, hyperthermia, hypothermia, hypovolemic shock, multiple organ dysfunction syndrome (MODS), septic shock, and trauma.

Interpreting serum electrolyte test results

Use the quick-reference chart below to interpret serum electrolyte test results for adult patients.

Electrolyte	Results	Implications	Common causes
Serum sodium	135 to 145 mEq/L	Normal	—
	< 135 mEq/L	Hyponatremia	Syndrome of inappropriate antidiuretic hormone secretion
	> 145 mEq/L	Hypernatremia	Diabetes insipidus
Serum potassium	3.5 to 5 mEq/L	Normal	—
	< 3.5 mEq/L	Hypokalemia	Diarrhea
	> 5 mEq/L	Hyperkalemia	Burns and renal failure
Total serum calcium	8.5 to 10.5 mg/dL	Normal	—
	< 8.5 mg/dL	Hypocalcemia	Acute pancreatitis
	> 10.5 mg/dL	Hypercalcemia	Hyperparathyroidism
Ionized calcium	4.5 to 5.1 mg/dL	Normal	—
	< 4.5 mg/dL	Hypocalcemia	Massive transfusion
	> 5.1 mg/dL	Hypercalcemia	Acidosis
Serum phosphates	2.5 to 4.5 mg/dL or 1.8 to 2.6 mEq/L	Normal	—
	< 2.5 mg/dL or 1.8 mEq/L	Hypophosphatemia	Diabetic ketoacidosis
	> 4.5 mg/dL or 2.6 mEq/L	Hyperphosphatemia	Renal insufficiency
Serum magnesium	1.5 to 2.5 mEq/L	Normal	—
	< 1.5 mEq/L	Hypomagnesemia	Malnutrition
	> 2.5 mEq/L	Hypermagnesemia	Renal failure
Serum chloride	98 to 108 mEq/L	Normal	—
	< 98 mEq/L	Hypochloremia	Prolonged vomiting
	> 108 mEq/L	Hyperchloremia	Hypernatremia

Burns

Burns are tissue injuries that result from contact with thermal, chemical, or electrical sources or from friction or exposure to the sun. They can cause cellular skin damage and a systemic response that leads to altered body function. A major burn affects every body system and organ, usually requiring painful treatment and a long period of rehabilitation.

Thermal burns are the most common type of burn. They may result from fires, scalding accidents, and sometimes abuse.

What causes it

Thermal burns, the most common burn type, commonly result from:
- residential fires
- automobile accidents
- playing with matches
- improper handling of firecrackers
- scalding accidents and kitchen accidents
- abuse (in children or elderly people)
- clothes that have caught on fire.

Scorching brews

Chemical burns result from contact, ingestion, inhalation, or injection of acids, alkalis, or vesicants (blistering agents).

It's electric

Electrical burns usually result from contact with faulty electrical wiring and cords or high-voltage power lines.

Rubbing or sunning the wrong way

Friction or abrasion burns occur when the skin rubs harshly against a coarse surface. Sunburn results from excessive exposure to sunlight.

Pathophysiology

Specific pathophysiologic events depend on the cause and classification of the burn. (See *Visualizing burn depth*, page 618.) The injuring agent denatures cellular proteins. Some cells die because of traumatic or ischemic necrosis. Loss of collagen cross-linking also occurs with denaturation, creating abnormal osmotic and hydrostatic pressure gradients that cause intravascular fluid to move into interstitial spaces. Cellular injury triggers the release of mediators of inflammation, contributing to local and, in the case of major burns, systemic increases in capillary permeability.

Visualizing burn depth

The most widely used system of classifying burn depth and severity categorizes them by degree. However, it's important to remember that most burns involve tissue damage of multiple degrees and thicknesses. This illustration may help you to visualize burn damage at the various degrees.

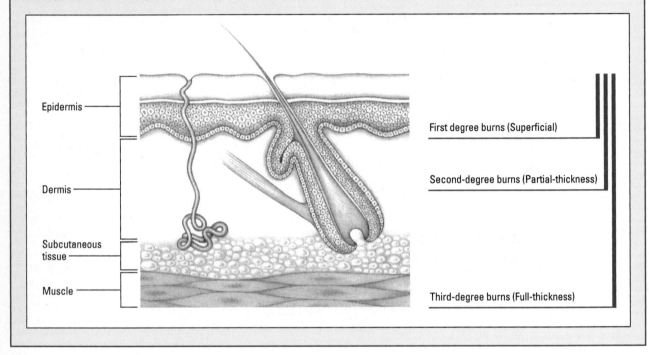

Epidermis

Dermis

Subcutaneous tissue

Muscle

First degree burns (Superficial)

Second-degree burns (Partial-thickness)

Third-degree burns (Full-thickness)

For your epidermis only

A *first-degree burn* causes localized injury or destruction to the skin's epidermis by direct contact (such as a chemical spill) or indirect contact (such as sunlight). The barrier function of the skin remains intact. This type of burn isn't life-threatening.

Barrier-breaking blisters

A *second-degree superficial partial-thickness burn* involves destruction to the epidermis and some dermis. Thin-walled, fluid-filled blisters develop within a few minutes of the injury. As these blisters break, the nerve endings become exposed to the air. Because pain and tactile responses remain intact, subsequent treatments are painful. The barrier function of the skin is lost.

Deep into the dermis

A *second-degree deep partial-thickness burn* involves the epidermis and dermis. The patient develops blisters and experiences mild-to-moderate edema and pain. The hair follicles remain intact, so the hair will regrow. Compared with a second-degree superficial partial-thickness burn, there's less pain sensation with this burn because the sensory neurons have undergone extensive destruction; however, because the barrier function of the skin is lost, sensitivity to pain remains in some areas around the burn.

Third layer, third degree

A *third-degree burn* extends through the epidermis and dermis and into the subcutaneous tissue layer. It may also involve muscle, bone, and interstitial tissues. Within hours, fluids and protein shift from capillary to interstitial spaces, causing edema. A person's body has an immediate immunologic response to a third-degree burn, making burn wound sepsis a potential threat. Finally, an increase in calorie demand after a third-degree burn increases the patient's metabolic rate.

Yowza! Those second-degree deep partial-thickness burns make it difficult for me to process sensations.

What to look for

Assessment provides a general idea of burn severity. First, determine the depth of tissue damage. A partial-thickness burn damages the epidermis and part of the dermis; a full-thickness burn also affects subcutaneous tissue. Traditionally, burns were gauged by degree. Today, however, most assessment findings use degrees and depth of tissue damage to describe a burn, as previously discussed.

Assessment of the burn will give you an idea of the degree and depth of the tissue damage.

Tracking burn traits

Signs and symptoms depend on the type of burn and may include:
• localized pain and erythema, usually without blisters in the first 24 hours (first-degree burn)
• chills, headache, localized edema, and nausea and vomiting (more severe first-degree burn)
• thin-walled, fluid-filled blisters appearing within minutes of the injury, with mild-to-moderate edema and pain (second-degree superficial partial-thickness burn)
• white, waxy appearance to damaged area (second-degree deep partial-thickness burn)
• white, brown, or black leathery tissue and visible thrombosed vessels due to destruction of skin elasticity (dorsum of hand, most common site of thrombosed veins), without blisters (third-degree burn)
• silver-colored, raised or charred area, usually at the site of electrical contact (electrical burn).

Configure this!

Inspection also reveals the location and extent of the burn. Note the burn's configuration. If the patient has a circumferential burn on an extremity, he runs the risk of edema occluding the circulation in that extremity. If he has burns on his neck, he may suffer airway obstruction; burns on the chest can lead to restricted respiratory excursion.

More to it than just skin

Inspect the patient for other injuries that may complicate recovery such as signs of pulmonary damage from smoke inhalation, including singed nasal hairs, mucosal burns, voice changes, coughing, wheezing, soot in the mouth or nose, and darkened sputum.

> Check a burn victim for pulmonary damage and smoke inhalation. These factors may complicate recovery.

Estimating the extent of a burn

You can estimate the extent of an adult patient's burn by using the Rule of Nines. This method quantifies BSA in multiples of nine, thus the name. To use this method, mentally transfer the burns on your patient to the body charts shown below. Add the corresponding percentages for each body section burned. You can use the total—a rough estimate of burn extent—to calculate fluid replacement needs.

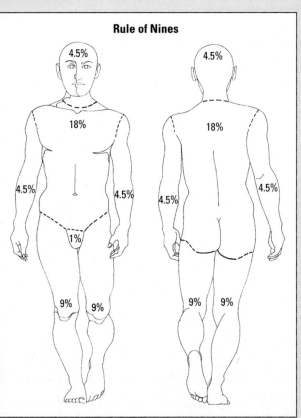

Rule of Nines

4.5% 4.5%
18% 18%
4.5% 4.5% 4.5% 4.5%
1%
9% 9% 9% 9%

What tests tell you

An assessment methods that can be used to determine the size of a burn is the Rule of Nines chart, which determines the percentage of body surface area (BSA) covered by the burn. (See *Estimating the extent of a burn*.)

A matter of class

Burns may be classified into three categories: major, moderate, and minor.

Major burns include:
- third-degree burns on more than 10% of BSA
- second-degree burns on more than 25% of BSA
- burns on hands, face, feet, or genitalia
- burns complicated by fractures or respiratory damage
- electrical burns
- burns in poor-risk patients.

Moderate burns include:
- third-degree burns on 2% to 10% of BSA
- second-degree burns on 15% to 25% of BSA.

Minor burns include:
- third-degree burns on less than 2% of BSA
- second-degree burns on less than 15% of BSA.

Back in the lab

Here are some additional diagnostic tests results regarding burns:
- Arterial blood gas (ABG) levels may be normal in the early stages but may reveal hypoxemia and metabolic acidosis later.
- Carboxyhemoglobin level may reveal the extent of smoke inhalation due to the presence of carbon monoxide.
- Complete blood count (CBC) may reveal a decreased Hb (due to hemolysis), increased HCT (secondary to hemoconcentration), and leukocytosis (resulting from a systemic inflammatory response or the possible development of sepsis).
- Electrolyte levels may show hyponatremia (from massive fluid shifting) and hyperkalemia (from fluid shifting and cell lysis). Other laboratory tests may reveal elevated blood urea nitrogen (BUN) levels (secondary to fluid loss or increased protein breakdown) and decreased total protein and albumin (resulting from plasma proteins leaking into the interstitial spaces).
- Creatine kinase (CK) and myoglobin levels may be elevated. Keep in mind that CK and myoglobin are helpful indicators of muscle damage. Therefore, the higher the CK or myoglobin level, the more extensive the muscle damage. The presence of myoglobin in urine may lead to acute tubular necrosis.

Creatine kinase and myoglobin are helpful indicators of muscle damage — the higher their levels, the more extensive the muscle damage.

A closer look at fluid replacement

Fluid replacement is essential for the patient with burns because of the massive fluid shifts that occur. However, extreme caution is needed because of the risk of overreplacement.

How much?
Numerous formulas may be used to determine the amount of fluid replacement to be administered during the first 24 hours after a burn injury. Typically, these formulas use body weight and the percentage of body surface area (BSA) burned. One of the most common formulas used is the Parkland formula shown here:

$$\frac{\text{2 to 4 ml of lactated Ringer's solution/kg}}{\text{percentage of BSA burned}}$$

Over how long?
Typically, one-half of the calculated amount is administered during the first 8 hours following the injury. (Note that the time of injury—not the time of the patient's arrival in the emer-gency department—is used as the initial start time of the 8-hour duration.) The remaining one-half of the amount is then administered over the next 16 hours.

What fluids?
During the first 24 hours, crystalloid solutions are commonly used because capillary perme-ability is greatly increased, allowing proteins to leak into the interstitial tissues. After the first 24 hours, colloid solutions can be included. Giving colloids before the initial 24 hour period would supply additional protein that could leak into the interstitial tissue.

Too much or too little?
During fluid replacement, always be alert for indications of overreplacement and underre-placement. Signs and symptoms of heart fail-ure and pulmonary edema suggest overre-placement. Assessment findings of hypo-volemic shock suggest underreplacement.

How it's treated

Initial burn treatments are based on the type of burn and may include:
- removing the source of the burn and any items that retain heat, such as clothing and jewelry
- maintaining an open airway; assessing airway, breathing, and circulation (ABCs)
- administering supplemental humidified oxygen
- controlling active bleeding
- covering partial-thickness burns that are over 30% of BSA or full-thickness burns that are over 5% of BSA with a clean, dry, sterile bed sheet (because of the drastic reduction in body temperature, don't cover large burns with saline-soaked dressings)
- fluid replacement (see *A closer look at fluid replacement*)
- antimicrobial therapy (for all patients with major burns)
- pain medication as needed
- anti-inflammatory medications

Partial-thickness burns that are over 30% of BSA or full-thickness burns that are over 5% of BSA should be covered with a clean, dry, sterile bed sheet.

Advice from the experts

Electrical burn care

Keep these tips in mind when caring for a patient with an electrical burn:
• Be alert for ventricular fibrillation as well as cardiac and respiratory arrest caused by the electrical shock; begin cardiopulmonary resuscitation immediately.
• Get an estimate of the voltage that caused the injury.
• Tissue damage from an electrical burn is difficult to assess because internal destruction along the conduction pathway usually is greater than the surface burn would indicate.
• An electrical burn that ignites the patient's clothes may also cause thermal burns.

• laboratory tests, such as CBC, electrolyte, glucose, BUN, and serum creatinine levels; ABG analysis; typing and crossmatching; urinalysis for myoglobinuria and hemoglobinuria
• close monitoring of intake and output and vital signs
• surgical intervention, including skin grafts and more thorough surgical debridement for major burns
• tetanus prophylaxis as ordered
• nutritional therapy.

What to do

• Immediately assess the patient's ABCs. Institute emergency resuscitative measures as necessary. Monitor arterial oxygen saturation and serial ABG values and anticipate the need for endotracheal (ET) intubation and mechanical ventilation should the patient's respiratory status deteriorate, especially with facial or neck burns.

Listen to the lungs

• Auscultate lung sounds for crackles, rhonchi, or stridor. Observe for signs of laryngeal edema or tracheal obstruction, including labored breathing, severe hoarseness, and dyspnea.
• Administer supplemental humidified oxygen as ordered.
• Perform oropharyngeal or tracheal suctioning as indicated by the patient's inability to clear his airway or evidence of abnormal breath sounds.
• Monitor the patient's cardiac and respiratory status closely, at least every 15 minutes, or more frequently, depending on his condition. Also monitor the patient for cardiac arrhythmias. Assess his level of consciousness (LOC) for changes, such as increasing confusion, restlessness, or decreased responsiveness. (See *Electrical burn care*.)

• If the patient has a chemical burn, irrigate the wound with copious amounts of water or normal saline solution. If the chemical entered the patient's eyes, remove contact lenses if necessary and flush the eyes with large amounts of water or normal saline solution for at least 30 minutes. Have the patient close his eyes and cover them with a dry, sterile dressing. Note the type of chemical that caused the burn and any noxious fumes. If necessary, refer the patient for an ophthalmologic examination.

• Place the patient in semi-Fowler's position to maximize chest expansion. Keep him as quiet and comfortable as possible to minimize oxygen demands.

• Prepare the patient for an emergency escharotomy of the chest and neck for deep burns or circumferential injuries, if necessary, to promote lung expansion and decrease pulmonary compromise.

• Administer rapid fluid replacement therapy as ordered, using a large-bore peripheral catheter or central venous catheter as indicated.

Shocking results

• Monitor the patient's vital signs and hemodynamic parameters for changes indicating hypovolemic shock or evidence of fluid overload and pulmonary edema.

• Assess the patient's intake and output every hour; insert an indwelling urinary catheter as indicated to ensure accurate urine measurement.

• Assess the patient's level of pain including nonverbal indicators, and administer analgesics such as morphine sulfate I.V. as ordered. Avoid I.M. injections because tissue damage associated with the burn injury may impair absorption of the drug when given I.M.

• Keep the patient calm, provide periods of uninterrupted rest in between procedures, and use nonpharmacologic pain relief measures as appropriate.

• Obtain daily weights and monitor intake, including daily calorie counts. Provide a high-calorie, high-protein diet. Assess the patient's abdomen for distention and presence of bowel sounds. If he's on nothing-by-mouth status, administer enteral feedings as ordered.

• Administer histamine-2 receptor antagonists, as ordered, to reduce the risk of ulcer formation.

• Assess the patient for signs and symptoms of infection, including fever, elevated WBC count, and changes in burn wound appearance or drainage. Obtain a wound culture, and administer antipyretic and antimicrobial agents as ordered.

• Administer tetanus prophylaxis, if indicated.

• Perform burn wound care as ordered. Prepare the patient for possible grafting as indicated.

> A burn patient needs a high-calorie, high-protein diet.

• Assess the neurovascular status of the injured area, including pulses, reflexes, paresthesia, color, and temperature of the injured area at least every 2 to 4 hours, or more frequently, if indicated.

• Assist with splinting, positioning, compression therapy, and exercise to the burned area as indicated. Maintain the burned area in a neutral position to prevent contractures and minimize deformity.

• Explain all procedures to the patient before performing them. Encourage him to actively participate in his care as much as possible, and provide opportunities for him to voice his concerns, especially about altered body image.

Graft-versus-host disease

GVHD, also known as *organ rejection*, can occur when an immunologically impaired recipient receives a graft from an immunocompetent donor.

100-day division

GVHD can be acute or chronic:

• Acute GVHD occurs within the first 100 days after a transplant. It's is a major contributing factor to mortality after bone marrow transplantation.

• Chronic GVHD occurs after day 100 of a transplant and involves an autoimmune response that affects multiple organs. Older patients and those who have suffered previous acute GVHD face the greatest risk of chronic GVHD. Patients who develop chronic GVHD immediately following acute GVHD have the highest mortality rates.

What causes it

Causes of GVHD include impaired immune function, transplantation from an incompatible donor, or transfusion of an incompatible blood product containing viable lymphocytes.

Less than 50% of organ recipients with histocompatibility identical to the donor develop GVHD. This incidence increases to more than 60% when there's one antigen mismatch. Death in patients with GVHD is commonly due to sepsis.

Pathophysiology

Three criteria are necessary for the development of GVHD:

immunologically competent cells in the graft

graft recognition of the host as foreign

inability of the host to react to the graft.

When graft cells attack

If graft and host cells aren't histocompatible, the graft cells become sensitive to the host's class II antigens and may launch an attack against the host cells. The exact mechanism by which this occurs remains unclear, although biopsy of active GVHD lesions usually reveals infiltration by eosinophils and mononuclear, phagocytic, and histiocytic cells.

Keep your guard up! Graft cells may attack host cells if the two aren't histocompatible.

What to look for

Signs and symptoms of acute GVHD include:
- skin rash (10 to 30 days after transplant)
- abdominal cramps and severe diarrhea
- GI bleeding
- jaundice.
    Signs of chronic GVHD include:
- skin changes resembling scleroderma that can ultimately lead to ulcerations
- joint contractures
- impaired esophageal motility.

What tests tell you

Although graft survival typically hinges on early detection of transplant rejection, no single test or combination of tests has proven to be definitive for doing this. Tests reveal only nonspecific evidence, which may easily be attributed to other causes, especially infection. Diagnosis commonly becomes a matter of exclusion and depends on the careful evaluation of signs and symptoms along with results from specific organ function tests, standard laboratory studies, and tissue biopsy.

Boffo biopsy

Tissue biopsy provides the most accurate, reliable diagnostic information, especially in heart, liver, and kidney transplants. Biopsy usually reveals immunocompetent T cells along with the extent of lymphocytic infiltration and tissue damage. Repeat biopsies help to identify early histologic changes characteristic of rejection, determine the degree of change from previous biopsies, and monitor the course and success of treatment.

A posttransplant biopsy may reveal immunocompetent T cells, which may indicate organ rejection.

Looking at the liver

Liver function studies reveal elevated levels of bilirubin, serum alkaline phosphatase, alanine aminotransferase, and aspartate aminotransferase.

How it's treated

Because GVHD may be fatal, initial interventions must focus on prevention.

Treatment may include:
• immunosuppressant therapy with methotrexate (with or without prednisone [Deltasone]), antithymocyte globulin (Atgam), cyclosporine (Sandimmune), cyclophosphamide (Cytoxan), or tacrolimus (Prograf) for the first 3 to 12 months after a transplant
• T-cell depletion in donor marrow (selective removal of T cells from the donor graft), which has been shown to reduce the severity and incidence of GVHD; however, patients have experienced an increase in graft failure and recurrent leukemia.

What to do

• Institute appropriate measures after bone marrow transplantation or organ transplant.
• Inspect the patient's skin closely for the development of skin erythema. Pay special attention to the soles of the feet and palms of the hands. Provide meticulous skin care if erythema occurs.
• Assess the patient's skin color for evidence of jaundice, especially the sclera of the eyes. Report any darkened urine or clay-colored stools.
• Monitor the patient's vital signs at least every 4 hours. Notify the doctor if the patient's temperature rises.
• Assess fluid balance status. Monitor intake and output frequently. Maintain hydration status with I.V. fluids as ordered. Anticipate the need for hemodynamic monitoring to assess the patient's status.
• Administer immunosuppressive agents as ordered.
• Monitor liver function results closely for changes in enzyme levels.
• Assess the patient's bowel elimination pattern and auscultate bowel sounds. Be alert for severe diarrhea. (See *Electrolyte and acid-base imbalances.*)
• Obtain blood and stool cultures as ordered to evaluate for possible sources of infection.
• Assess the patient for signs and symptoms of sepsis.

Take charge!

Electrolyte and acid-base imbalances

Follow these instructions when caring for a patient with graft-versus-host disease:
• Be alert for the development of electrolyte and acid-base imbalances secondary to losses from diarrhea.
• Expect to administer fluid electrolyte replacement therapy based on laboratory results.
• Keep in mind that potassium is a major electrolyte that's lost with diarrhea; anticipate the need for continuous cardiac monitoring to detect possible arrhythmias secondary to hypokalemia.

Hyperthermia

Hyperthermia, also known as *heat syndrome*, refers to an elevation in body temperature over 99° F (37.2° C). It may result from environmental or internal conditions that increase heat production or impair heat dissipation.

What causes it

Hyperthermia may result from conditions that increase heat production, such as excessive exercise, infection, and drugs (for example, amphetamines).

It may also result from impairment of heat dissipation ability. Factors that impair heat dissipation include:

- high temperatures or humidity
- lack of acclimatization
- excess clothing
- cardiovascular disease
- obesity
- dehydration
- sweat gland dysfunction
- drugs (such as phenothiazines and anticholinergics).

High temperatures or humidity can make it harder for your body to release heat.

Pathophysiology

Humans normally adjust to excessive temperatures by complex cardiovascular and neurologic changes that are coordinated by the hypothalamus. Heat loss offsets heat production to regulate the body temperature. It does this by evaporation or vasodilation, which cools the body's surface by radiation, conduction, and convection. However, when heat loss mechanisms fail to offset heat production, the body retains heat.

Goodbye fluid, hello hypovolemic shock

If body temperature remains elevated, fluid loss becomes excessive and may lead to hypovolemic shock. If untreated, the patient's thermoregulatory mechanisms can fail. (See *The skin's role in thermoregulation.*)

Feeling hot hot hot

Hyperthermia occurs in varying degrees:

- Mild hyperthermia (heat cramps) occurs with excessive perspiration and loss of salt from the body.
- Moderate hyperthermia (heat exhaustion) occurs when the body is subjected to high temperatures and blood accumulates in the skin in an attempt to decrease the body's temperature. This causes a decrease in the circulating blood volume, which decreases cerebral blood flow. Syncope then occurs.
- Critical hyperthermia (heat stroke) occurs when the body's temperature continues to rise and internal organs become damaged, eventually resulting in death. (See *Heat stroke in elderly patients*, page 630.)

The hypothalamus coordinates how the body adjusts to excessive temperatures.

The skin's role in thermoregulation

Abundant nerves, blood vessels, and eccrine glands within the skin's deeper layer aid thermoregulation (control of body temperature). The first flow chart shows how the body conserves body heat. The second flow chart shows how the body reduces body heat. Here's how the skin does its job.

It's time to warm up

The skin becomes exposed to cold or the internal body temperature falls.

Blood vessels constrict in response to autonomic nervous system.

Blood flow decreases through the skin and body heat is conserved.

Now let's cool things off

Increased blood flow reduces body heat. If this doesn't lower temperature, the eccrine glands act to increase sweat production, and evaporation cools the skin.

Small arteries in the second skin layer dilate (expand).

The skin becomes too hot or the internal body temperature rises.

Senior moment

Heat stroke in elderly patients

With aging, an individual's thirst mechanism and ability to sweat decreases. These factors put elderly patients at risk for heat stroke, especially during hot summer days. Heat stroke is a medical emergency and must be treated rapidly to prevent serious complications or death. To help prevent heat stroke, teach your older patient to follow these instructions:
• Reduce activity in hot weather, especially outdoor activity.
• Wear lightweight, loose-fitting clothing during hot weather; when outdoors, wear a hat and sun glasses and avoid wearing dark colors that absorb sunlight.

• Drink plenty of fluids, especially water, and avoid tea, coffee, and alcohol because they can cause dehydration.
• Use air conditioning or open windows (making sure that a secure screen is in place) and use a fan to help circulate air. (If the patient doesn't have air conditioning at home, suggest that during periods of excessive heat he go to community resources that have air conditioning, such as senior centers, libraries, and churches. Some community centers may even provide transportation for the patient.)

What to look for

Assessment findings vary with the degree of hyperthermia. (See *Hyperthermia signs and symptoms.*)

What tests tell you

No single diagnostic confirms hyperthermia, but these test results may help support the diagnosis:
• ABG results may reveal respiratory alkalosis and hypoxemia.
• CBC may reveal leukocytosis and increased HCT secondary to hemoconcentration.
• Electrolyte levels may show hypokalemia. Other blood studies may reveal elevated BUN levels, increased bleeding and clotting times, and fibrinolysis.
• Urinalysis may show concentrated urine, with elevated protein levels, tubular casts, and myoglobinuria.

How it's treated

Mild and moderate hyperthermia are treated by providing a cool environment and allowing the patient to rest. Oral or I.V. fluid and electrolyte replacement is administered as ordered.

Hyperthermia signs and symptoms

Hyperthermia, also know as *heat syndrome,* may be classified as mild (heat cramps), moderate (heat exhaustion), or critical (heat stroke). This table highlights the major assessment findings associated with each classification.

Classification	Assessment findings
Mild hyperthermia (heat cramps)	• Mild agitation (central nervous system findings otherwise normal) • Mild hypertension • Moist, cool skin and muscle tenderness; involved muscle groups possibly hard and lumpy • Muscle twitching and spasms • Nausea, abdominal cramps • Report of prolonged activity in a very warm or hot environment, without adequate salt intake • Tachycardia • Temperature ranging from 99° to 102° F (37.2° to 38.9° C)
Moderate hyperthermia (heat exhaustion)	• Dizziness • Headache • Hypotension • Muscle cramping • Nausea, vomiting • Oliguria • Pale, moist skin • Rapid thready pulse • Syncope or confusion • Thirst • Weakness • Temperature elevated up to 104° F (40° C)
Critical hyperthermia (heat stroke)	• Atrial or ventricular tachycardia • Confusion, combativeness, delirium • Fixed, dilated pupils • Hot, dry, reddened skin • Loss of consciousness • Seizures • Tachypnea • Temperature greater than 106° F (41.1° C)

To help treat patients with critical hyperthermia, fan them with cool air.

Critical measures

Measures for treating critical hyperthermia include:
• removing the patient's clothing and applying cool water to the skin, then fanning the patient with cool air

- controlling shivering by giving diazepam (Valium) or chlorpromazine (Thorazine).
- applying hypothermia blankets and ice packs to the groin and axillae, if necessary.

Treatment continues until the patient's body temperature drops to 102.2° F (39° C).

In addition to the cool down

Supportive measures for hyperthermia include:
- oxygen therapy
- central venous pressure (CVP) and pulmonary artery wedge pressure (PAWP) monitoring
- ET intubation, if necessary.

What to do

- Assess the patient's ABCs and initiate emergency resuscitative measures as indicated. Remove as much of the patient's clothing as possible.
- Assess oxygen saturation and administer supplemental oxygen as indicated and ordered. Monitor the patient's pulmonary status closely, including respiratory rate and depth and lung sounds; anticipate the need for ET intubation and mechanical ventilation if respiratory status deteriorates.
- Monitor vital signs continuously, especially core body temperature. Although the goal is to reduce the patient's temperature rapidly, too rapid a reduction can lead to vasoconstriction, which can cause shivering. Shivering increases metabolic demand and oxygen consumption and should be avoided.
- Employ external cooling measures, such as cool, wet sheets; tepid baths; and cooling blankets.
- Assess neurologic and cardiac status closely, including heart rate and rhythm. Institute continuous cardiac monitoring to evaluate for arrhythmias secondary to electrolyte imbalances. Monitor hemodynamic parameters, assess peripheral circulation, including skin color, peripheral pulses, and capillary refill.
- Monitor fluid and electrolyte balance and laboratory test results. Assess renal function studies to evaluate for rhabdomyolysis.

BRRRRR! Reducing a patient's temperature too quickly can cause shivering, which increases metabolic demand and oxygen consumption.

Hypothermia

Hypothermia is defined as a core body temperature below 95° F (35° C). It may be classified as mild (89.6° to 95° F [32° to 35° C]), moderate (86° to 89.6° F [30° to 32° C]), or severe (77° to 86° F [25° to 30° C]). Severe hypothermia can be fatal.

What causes it

Hypothermia commonly results from near drowning in cold water, prolonged exposure to cold temperatures, disease or debility that alters homeostasis, and the administration of large amounts of cold blood or blood products.

Likely candidates

The risk of serious cold injury, especially hypothermia, increases with youth, old age, lack of insulating body fat, wet or inadequate clothing, drug abuse, cardiac disease, smoking, fatigue, malnutrition and depletion of caloric reserves, and excessive alcohol intake.

Excessive alcohol intake can increase the risk of hypothermia.

Pathophysiology

In hypothermia, metabolic changes slow the functions of most major organ systems, resulting in decreased renal blood flow and decreased glomerular filtration. Vital organs are physiologically affected. Severe hypothermia results in depression of cerebral blood flow, diminished oxygen requirements, reduced cardiac output, and decreased arterial pressure.

What to look for

Obtaining the history of a patient with a cold injury may reveal:
• cause of hypothermia
• temperature to which the patient was exposed
• length of exposure.

Temperature dependent

Assessment findings in a patient with hypothermia vary with the patient's body temperature:
• Mild hypothermia includes severe shivering, slurred speech, and amnesia.
• Moderate hypothermia includes unresponsiveness, peripheral cyanosis, and muscle rigidity. If the patient was improperly rewarmed, he may show signs of shock.
• Severe hypothermia includes absence of palpable pulses, no audible heart sounds, dilated
pupils, and rigor-mortis-like state. In addition, ventricular fibrillation and a loss of deep tendon reflexes commonly occur.

What tests tell you

• Technetium 99m pertechnetate scanning shows perfusion defects and deep tissue damage and can be used to identify nonviable bone.
• Doppler and plethysmographic studies help determine pulses and the extent of frostbite after thawing.

How it's treated

Treatment for hypothermia consists of supportive measures and specific rewarming techniques, including:
• passive rewarming (the patient rewarms on his own)
• active external rewarming with heating blankets, warm water immersion, heated objects such as water bottles, and radiant heat
• active core rewarming with heated I.V. fluids, genitourinary tract irrigation, extracorporeal rewarming, hemodialysis, and peritoneal, gastric, and mediastinal lavage.

Cardiac concerns

Arrhythmias that develop usually convert to normal sinus rhythm with rewarming. If the patient has no pulse or respirations, CPR is needed until rewarming raises the core temperature to at least 89.6° F (32° C).

Measure dependent on monitoring

The administration of oxygen, ET intubation, controlled ventilation, I.V. fluids, and treatment for metabolic acidosis depend on test results and careful patient monitoring.

What to do

• Assess ABCs. Initiate CPR as appropriate. Keep in mind that hypothermia helps protect the brain from anoxia, which normally accompanies prolonged cardiopulmonary arrest. Therefore, even if the patient has been unresponsive for a long time, CPR may resuscitate him, especially after a cold-water near drowning.
• Assist with rewarming techniques as necessary. In moderate to severe hypothermia, only experienced personnel should attempt aggressive rewarming.
• During rewarming, provide supportive measures as ordered, including mechanical ventilation and heated, humidified therapy to maintain tissue oxygenation, and I.V. fluids that have been warmed with a warming coil to correct hypotension and maintain urine output.
• Continuously monitor the patient's core body temperature and other vital signs during and after initial rewarming. Continuously monitor his cardiac status, including continuous cardiac monitoring for evidence of arrhythmias.
• If using a hyperthermia blanket, discontinue the warming when the core body temperature is within 1° to 2° F (0.6° to 1.1° C) of the desired temperature. The patient's temperature will continue to rise even with the device turned off.
• If the patient has been hypothermic for longer than 45 to 60 minutes, administer additional fluids as ordered to compensate for the expansion of the vascular space that occurs during vasodi-

Here's a warm thought: hypothermia helps protect the brain from anoxia, so even if the patient has been unresponsive for a long time, CPR may resuscitate him.

lation in rewarming. Monitor the patient's heart rate and hemodynamic parameters closely to evaluate fluid needs and response to treatment.

• Monitor the patient's hourly output, fluid balance, and serum electrolyte levels, especially potassium. Be alert for signs and symptoms of hyperkalemia. If hyperkalemia occurs, administer calcium chloride, sodium bicarbonate, glucose, and insulin as ordered. Anticipate the need for sodium polystyrene sulfonate enemas. If his potassium levels are extremely elevated, prepare the patient for dialysis.

Hypovolemic shock

Hypovolemic shock most commonly results from acute blood loss — about 20% of total volume. Without sufficient blood or fluid replacement, hypovolemic shock may lead to irreversible damage to organs and systems.

> Hypovolemic shock most commonly results from acute blood loss.

What causes it

Massive volume loss may result from:
• GI bleeding, internal or external hemorrhage, or any condition that reduces circulating intravascular volume or other body fluids
• intestinal obstruction
• peritonitis
• acute pancreatitis
• ascites
• dehydration from excessive perspiration, severe diarrhea or protracted vomiting, diabetes insipidus, diuresis, or inadequate fluid intake.

Pathophysiology

Potentially life-threatening, hypovolemic shock stems from reduced intravascular blood volume, which leads to decreased cardiac output and inadequate tissue perfusion. The subsequent tissue anoxia prompts a shift in cellular metabolism from aerobic to anaerobic pathways. This results in an accumulation of lactic acid, which produces metabolic acidosis.

The road to shockville

When compensatory mechanisms fail, hypovolemic shock occurs in this sequence:

decreased intravascular fluid volume

diminished venous return, which reduces preload and decreases stroke volume

reduced cardiac output

decreased mean arterial pressure

impaired tissue perfusion

decreased oxygen and nutrient delivery to cells

multisystem organ failure.

What to look for

The specific signs and symptoms exhibited by the patient depend on the amount of fluid loss. (See *Estimating fluid loss.*)

Oh where oh where has the blood volume gone?

Typically, the patient's history includes conditions that reduce blood volume, such as GI hemorrhage, trauma, and severe diarrhea and vomiting.

Assessment findings may include:
* pale skin
* decreased sensorium

Estimating fluid loss

The following assessment parameters indicate the severity of fluid loss.

Minimal fluid loss
Intravascular volume loss of 10% to 15% is regarded as minimal. Signs and symptoms include:
* slight tachycardia
* normal supine blood pressure
* positive postural vital signs, including a decrease in systolic blood pressure > 10 mm Hg or an increase in pulse rate > 20 beats/minute
* increased capillary refill time > 3 seconds
* urine output > 30 ml/hour
* cool, pale skin on arms and legs
* anxiety.

Moderate fluid loss
Intravascular volume loss of about 25% is regarded as moderate. Signs and symptoms include:
* rapid, thready pulse
* supine hypotension
* cool truncal skin
* urine output 10 to 30 ml/hour
* severe thirst
* restlessness, confusion, or irritability.

Severe fluid loss
Intravascular volume loss of about 40% or more is regarded as severe. Signs and symptoms include:
* marked tachycardia
* marked hypotension
* weak or absent peripheral pulses
* cold, mottled, or cyanotic skin
* urine output < 10 ml/hour
* unconsciousness.

- rapid, shallow respirations
- urine output below 25 ml/hour
- rapid, thready peripheral pulses
- cold, clammy skin
- mean arterial pressure below 60 mm Hg and a narrowing pulse pressure
- decreased CVP, right atrial pressure, PAWP, and cardiac output.

What tests tell you

No single diagnostic test confirms hypovolemic shock, but these test results help to support the diagnosis:
- low HCT
- decreased Hb level
- decreased RBC and platelet counts
- elevated serum potassium, sodium, lactate dehydrogenase, creatinine, and BUN levels
- increased urine specific gravity (greater than 1.020) and urine osmolality; urine sodium levels less than 50 mEq/L
- decreased urine creatinine levels
- decreased pH and partial pressure of arterial oxygen and increased partial pressure of arterial carbon dioxide ($Paco_2$)
- gastroscopy, X-rays, aspiration of gastric contents through a nasogastric tube, and tests for occult blood
- coagulation studies for coagulopathy from disseminated intravascular coagulation (DIC).

Fluid and blood replacement is crucial to restoring intravascular volume and raising blood pressure in patients with hypovolemic shock.

How it's treated

Emergency treatment relies on prompt and adequate fluid and blood replacement to restore intravascular volume and to raise blood pressure and maintain it above 80 mm Hg. Rapid infusion of normal saline or lactated Ringer's solution and, possibly, albumin or other plasma expanders may expand volume adequately until whole blood can be matched.

Treatment may also include application of a pneumatic antishock garment (although controversial), oxygen administration, control of bleeding, dopamine or another inotropic drug and surgery, if appropriate.

What to do

- Assess the patient for the extent of fluid loss and begin fluid replacement as ordered. Obtain a type and crossmatch for blood component therapy.

ABCs and ABGs

* Assess ABCs. If the patient experiences cardiac or respiratory arrest, start CPR.
* Administer supplemental oxygen as ordered. Monitor oxygen saturation and ABG studies for evidence of hypoxemia and anticipate the need for ET intubation and mechanical ventilation should the patient's respiratory status deteriorate. Place the patient in semi-Fowler's position to maximize chest expansion. Keep the patient as quiet and comfortable as possible to minimize oxygen demands.
* Monitor vital signs, neurologic status, and cardiac rhythm continuously for changes such as cardiac arrhythmias or myocardial ischemia. Observe skin color and check capillary refill. Notify the doctor if capillary refill is greater than 2 seconds. (See *When blood pressure drops.*)
* Monitor hemodynamic parameters, including CVP, PAWP, and cardiac output and input, frequently — as often as every 15 minutes — to evaluate the patient's status and response to treatment.
* Monitor intake and output closely. Insert an indwelling urinary catheter and assess urine output hourly. If bleeding from the GI tract is suspected as the cause, check all stools, emesis, and gastric drainage for occult blood. If output falls below 30 ml/hour in an adult, expect to increase the I.V. fluid infusion rate, but watch for signs of fluid overload such as elevated PAWP. Notify the doctor if urine output doesn't increase.
* Administer blood component therapy as ordered; monitor serial Hb values and HCT to evaluate effects of treatment.
* Administer dopamine or norepinephrine I.V., as ordered, to increase cardiac contractility and renal perfusion.
* Watch for signs of impending coagulopathy (such as petechiae, bruising, and bleeding or oozing from gums or venipuncture sites) and report them immediately.
* Provide emotional support and reassurance appropriately in the wake of massive fluid losses.
* Prepare the patient for surgery as appropriate.

When blood pressure drops

A drop below 80 mm Hg in systolic blood pressure usually signals inadequate cardiac output from reduced intravascular volume. Such a drop usually results in inadequate coronary artery blood flow, cardiac ischemia, arrhythmias, and other complications of low cardiac output. If the patient's systolic blood pressure drops below 80 mm Hg and his pulse is thready, increase the oxygen flow rate and notify the doctor immediately.

Multiple organ dysfunction syndrome

MODS is a condition that occurs when two or more organs or organ systems are unable to function in their role of maintaining homeostasis. Intervention is necessary to support and maintain organ function. MODS isn't an illness itself; rather, it's a manifestation of another progressive underlying condition.

MODS isn't an illness itself. It's a manifestation of another underlying condition.

What causes it

MODS develops when widespread systemic inflammation, a condition known as systemic inflammatory response syndrome (SIRS), overtaxes a patient's compensatory mechanisms. SIRS can be triggered by infection, ischemia, trauma, reperfusion injury, or multisystem injury. If allowed to progress, SIRS can lead to organ inflammation and ultimately, MODS.

Pathophysiology

MODS is classified as primary or secondary:
• Primary MODS involves organ or organ system failure that's caused by a direct injury (such as trauma, aspiration, or near drowning) or a primary disorder (such as pneumonia or pulmonary embolism). Primary MODS commonly involves the lungs. Patients typically develop acute respiratory distress syndrome (ARDS), which progresses to encephalopathy and coagulopathy. As the syndrome continues, other organ systems are affected.
• Secondary MODS involves organ or organ system failure that's due to sepsis. Typically the infection source isn't associated with the lungs. The most common infection sources include intra-abdominal sepsis, extensive blood loss, pancreatitis, or major vascular injuries. ARDS develops sooner and progressive involvement of other organs and organ systems occurs more rapidly than in primary MODS.

What to look for

The assessment findings associated with MODS typically reveal an acutely ill patient with signs and symptoms associated with SIRS. Early findings may include:
• fever, usually greater than 101° F (38.3° C)
• tachycardia
• narrowed pulse pressure
• tachypnea
• decreased pulmonary artery pressure (PAP), PAWP, and CVP, and increased cardiac output.

As time goes by

As SIRS progresses, findings reflect impaired perfusion of the tissues and organs, such as:
• decreased LOC
• respiratory depression
• diminished bowel sounds
• jaundice
• oliguria or anuria
• increased PAP and PAWP and decreased cardiac output.

What tests tell you

No single test confirms MODS, and test results depend on the cause, such as trauma, aspiration, pulmonary embolism, or sepsis:
• ABG analysis may reveal hypoxemia with respiratory acidosis or metabolic acidosis.
• CBC may reveal decreased Hb level and HCT as well as leukocytosis.
• X-rays may reveal fractures, a cervical spine injury, pulmonary infiltrates, or abnormal air or fluid in the chest or abdominal organs.
    Additional tests that may be performed include MRI, a CT scan, and angiography.

How it's treated

Treatment focuses on supporting respiratory and circulatory function and includes:
• mechanical ventilation and supplemental oxygen
• hemodynamic monitoring
• fluid infusion (crystalloids and colloids)
• vasopressors
• measuring intake and output
• serial laboratory values
• dialysis
• antimicrobial agents.

Treatment for MODS focuses on supporting respiratory and circulatory function.

What to do

• Keep in mind that nursing care for the patient with MODS is primarily supportive.
• Maintain the patient's airway and breathing with the use of mechanical ventilation and supplemental oxygen.
• Monitor his vital signs, oxygen saturation, hemodynamic parameters, and cardiac rhythm for arrhythmias.
• Administer I.V. fluids as ordered.
• Monitor laboratory values.
• Monitor intake and output.
• Administer appropriate medications as ordered.
• Provide emotional support to the patient and family; explain diagnostic tests and treatments.

Septic shock

Low systemic vascular resistance and an elevated cardiac output characterize septic shock. The disorder is thought to occur in response to infections that release microbes or immune mediators such as tumor necrosis factor or interleukin-1.

What causes it

Any pathogenic organism can cause septic shock. Gram-negative bacteria, such as *Escherichia coli*, *Klebsiella pneumoniae*, *Serratia*, *Enterobacter*, and *Pseudomonas* rank as the most common causes and account for up to 70% of all cases. Opportunistic fungi cause about 3% of cases. Rare causative organisms include mycobacteria and some viruses and protozoa.

Septic shock can occur in any person with impaired immunity, but elderly people are at greatest risk.

Pathophysiology

Septic shock is a type of distributive shock.

Endotoxins started it!

An immune response is triggered when bacteria release endotoxins. In response, macrophages secrete tumor necrosis factor (TNF) and interleukins. These mediators, in turn, are responsible for increased release of platelet-activating factor (PAF), prostaglandins, leukotrienes, thromboxane A_2, kinins, and complement.

Compromised capillaries and more

The consequences of this immune activity are vasodilation and vasoconstriction, increased capillary permeability, reduced systemic vascular resistance, microemboli, and an elevated cardiac output. Endotoxins also stimulate the release of histamine, further increasing capillary permeability.

Deepening depression

Moreover, myocardial depressant factor, TNF, PAF, and other factors depress myocardial function. Cardiac output falls, resulting in multisystem organ failure.

What to look for

The patient's history may include a disorder or treatment that causes immunosuppression, or it may include a history of invasive tests or treatments, surgery, or trauma. At onset, the patient may have fever and chills, although 20% of patients may be hypothermic.

Phase facts

The patient's signs and symptoms will reflect either the hyperdynamic (warm) phase of septic shock or the hypodynamic (cold) phase.

Pathogens like me can cause septic shock. Shocking, huh?

A patient with septic shock may have a history of immunosuppression, invasive tests or treatments, surgery, or trauma.

Warm form

The hyperdynamic phase is characterized by:
- increased cardiac output
- peripheral vasodilation
- decreased systemic vascular resistance
- altered LOC
- rapid, shallow respirations
- decreased urine output
- rapid, full, bounding pulse.

Coolin' (no foolin')

The hypodynamic phase is characterized by:
- decreased cardiac output
- peripheral vasoconstriction
- increased systemic vascular resistance
- inadequate tissue perfusion
- pale and possibly cyanotic skin color
- mottling of extremities
- decreased LOC
- rapid, shallow respirations
- decreased or absent urine output
- absence of peripheral pulses or a rapid, weak, thready pulse
- cold and clammy skin
- hypotension, usually with a systolic pressure below 90 mm Hg or 50 to 80 mm Hg below the patient's previous level.
- crackles or rhonchi if pulmonary congestion is present
- reduced or normal PAWP.

What tests tell you

These findings aid in the diagnosis of septic shock:
- Blood cultures are positive for the offending organism.
- CBC shows the presence or absence of anemia and leukopenia, severe or absent neutropenia, and usually the presence of thrombocytopenia.
- ABG studies may reveal metabolic acidosis, hypoxemia, and low $Paco_2$ that progresses to increased $Paco_2$ (thereby indicating respiratory acidosis).
- BUN and creatinine levels are increased and creatinine clearance is decreased.
- Prothrombin time, partial thromboplastin time, and bleeding time are increased; platelets are decreased and fibrin split products are increased.
- Chest X-rays reveal evidence of pneumonia (as the underlying infection) or ARDS (indicating progression of septic shock).
- ECG shows ST depression and inverted T waves.

Chest X-rays that reveal the presence of ARDS indicate progression of septic shock.

- Amylase and lipase levels may show pancreatic insufficiency.
- Hepatic enzyme levels are elevated due to liver ischemia.
- Blood glucose levels are initially elevated and then decrease.
- CT scan reveals abscesses or sources of possible infection.

How it's treated

Location and treatment of the underlying sepsis is essential to treating septic shock. This includes:
- removing the source of infection, such as I.V., intra-arterial, or urinary drainage catheters
- aggressive antimicrobial therapy appropriate for the causative organism
- culture and sensitivity tests of urine and wound drainage
- surgery, if appropriate
- reducing or discontinuing immunosuppressive drug therapy
- possible granulocyte transfusions in patients with severe neutropenia
- oxygen therapy and mechanical ventilation if necessary
- colloid or crystalloid infusions
- administering a vasopressor such as dopamine.

What to do

- Assess ABCs. Monitor cardiopulmonary status closely.
- Administer supplemental oxygen as ordered.
- Monitor oxygen saturation and ABG values for evidence of hypoxemia and anticipate the need for ET intubation and mechanical ventilation should the patient's respiratory status deteriorate. Place the patient in semi-Fowler's position to maximize chest expansion. Keep the patient as quiet and comfortable as possible to minimize oxygen demands.

Vital moves

- Monitor the patient's vital signs continuously for changes. Observe his skin color and check capillary refill. Notify the doctor if capillary refill is greater than 2 seconds.
- Keep in mind that the patient's temperature is usually elevated in the early stages of septic shock and that he commonly experiences shaking chills. As the shock progresses, the temperature typically drops and the patient experiences diaphoresis.
- If the patient's systolic blood pressure drops below 80 mm Hg, increase the oxygen flow rate, and notify the doctor immediately. Alert the doctor and increase the infusion rate if the patient experiences a progressive drop in blood pressure accompanied by a thready pulse.

Temperature is usually elevated in the early stages of septic shock; however, as shock progresses, temperature drops.

• Remove I.V., intra-arterial, or urinary drainage catheters and send them to the laboratory to culture for the presence of the causative organism (prepare to reinsert or assist with reinsertion of new devices). Obtain blood cultures as ordered and begin antimicrobial therapy as ordered. Monitor the patient for possible adverse effects of therapy.

• Institute continuous cardiac monitoring to evaluate for possible arrhythmias, myocardial ischemia, or adverse effects of treatment.

• Monitor the patient's intake and output closely. Notify the doctor if his urine output is less than 30 ml/hour.

• Administer I.V. fluid therapy as ordered, usually normal saline or lactated Ringer's solution. Monitor hemodynamic parameters to determine response to therapy.

• Be alert for signs and symptoms of possible fluid overload, such as dyspnea, tachypnea, crackles, peripheral edema, jugular vein distention, and increased PAP.

• Administer positive inotropic agents as ordered.

• Allow for frequent rest periods to minimize the patient's oxygen demands.

• Institute infection control precautions; use strict aseptic technique for all invasive procedures.

• Provide nutritional support therapy.

• Monitor laboratory test results, especially coagulation studies and hepatic enzyme levels, for changes indicative of DIC and hepatic failure, respectively.

• Provide emotional support to the patient and his family.

• Prepare the patient for surgery as appropriate.

To put it bluntly, trauma may be considered blunt, penetrating, or perforating, depending on the extent of the injury.

Trauma

Trauma is a physical injury or wound that's inflicted by an external or violent act. Trauma may be intentional or unintentional. Multiple traumas involve injuries to more than one body area or organ and are the leading cause of death in persons younger than age 45.

What's your type?

The type of trauma determines the extent of injury:

• blunt trauma — leaves the body intact

• penetrating trauma — disrupts the body surface

• perforating trauma — leaves entrance and exit wounds as an object passes through the body.

What causes it

Trauma may be caused by weapons, automobile crashes, physical confrontation, falls, or any other unnatural occurrence to the body.

Pathophysiology

Traumatic wounds include:
• abrasion—the skin is scraped, with partial loss of the skin surface
• laceration—the skin is torn, causing jagged, irregular edges; the severity of a laceration depends on its size, depth, and location
• puncture wound—when a pointed object, such as a knife or glass fragment, penetrates the skin
• traumatic amputation—part of the body (a limb or part of a limb) is removed.

> Physical confrontation is one cause of trauma.

What to look for

Assessment findings will vary according to the type and extent of trauma. A conscious patient with multiple injuries may be able to help focus the assessment on areas that need immediate attention, such as difficulty breathing or neurologic symptoms.

Primary assessment

During the primary assessment the patient is assessed for life-threatening problems involving his airway, breathing, circulation, disability, and exposure (ABCDEs). (See *Primary assessment of the trauma patient*, page 646.)

Sport some life support

Monitor cardiac rhythm, initiate CPR, and administer drugs and electrical shock therapy (defibrillation and synchronized cardioversion) as appropriate for cardiac arrhythmias.

Secondary assessment

After completing the primary assessment and treating life-threatening conditions, perform a secondary assessment. This includes taking a history and performing a physical examination.

Skip to the important stuff...

During an emergency, you won't have time to obtain all of the patient's regular history. Focus on the most important information, including:
• signs and symptoms related to the present condition
• allergies to drugs, foods, latex, or environmental factors

Primary assessment of the trauma patient

This chart shows what to look for (ABCDEs) and what to do during the trauma patient's primary assessment.

Parameter	Assessment	Interventions
A = Airway	• Airway patency	• Position the patient. • To open the airway, make sure that the neck is midline and stabilized and then perform the jaw-thrust maneuver.
B = Breathing	• Respirations (rate, depth, effort) • Breath sounds • Chest wall movement and chest injury • Position of trachea (midline or deviation)	• Administer 100% oxygen with bag-valve-mask. • Use airway adjuncts (such as oral or nasal airway, endotracheal tube, esophageal-tracheal combitube, cricothyrotomy). • Suction as needed. • Remove foreign bodies that may obstruct breathing. • Treat life-threatening conditions (pneumothorax, tension pneumothorax).
C = Circulation	• Pulse and blood pressure • Bleeding or hemorrhage • Capillary refill, color of skin and mucous membranes • Cardiac rhythm	• Administer cardiopulmonary resuscitation, medications, and defibrillation or synchronized cardioversion. • Control hemorrhaging with direct pressure or pneumatic devices. • Establish I.V. access and fluid therapy (isotonic fluids and blood). • Treat life-threatening conditions such as cardiac tamponade.
D = Disability	• Neurological assessment, including level of consciousness, pupils, and motor and sensory function	• Institute cervical spine immobilization until X-rays confirm the absence of cervical spine injury.
E = Exposure and environment	• Injuries and environmental exposure (extreme cold or heat)	• Institute appropriate therapy (warming therapy for hypothermia or cooling therapy for hyperthermia).

• medication history, including prescription and over-the-counter medications, herbs, and supplements
• past medical history
• last meal
• events leading to the injury or condition.

...then fill in the blanks

When the patient's condition is stabilized, fill in the other components of the normal health history. Remember to include a history of blood transfusions and tetanus immunization if the patient has an open wound.

Illicit or otherwise

Question the patient about alcohol and drug use. Patients in substance withdrawal may exhibit behavioral changes and be more difficult to manage. Determine the frequency of substance use to assess whether the patient may experience withdrawal postoperatively.

In the know from head to toe

During the secondary assessment you may choose to perform a rapid head-to-toe examination that concentrates on areas relating to the patient's cheif complaint rather than a body-systems examination because it's quicker. The head-to-toe examination includes assessing the patient's general appearance and vital signs, head and neck, chest and back, abdomen, perineal area, and extremities.

All systems go

When the patient is stable, perform a body-system examination according to your facility's policy and procedure. A thorough assessment helps systematically identify and correct problems and establishes a baseline for future comparison.

What tests tell you

The diagnostic tests performed are based on the body system affected by the trauma. For example, a patient with a blunt chest injury would require a chest X-ray to detect rib and sternal fractures, pneumothorax, flail chest, pulmonary contusion, and a lacerated or ruptured aorta. Angiography studies would also be performed with suspected aortic laceration or rupture. Diagnostic tests for a patient with head trauma may include a CT scan, cervical spine X-rays, skull X-rays, or an angiogram.

Here are some other diagnostic tests that may performed on the patient with multiple trauma:
• ABG analysis is used to evaluate respiratory status and determines acidotic and alkalotic states.
• CBC indicates the amount of blood loss.
• Coagulation studies are used to evaluate clotting ability.
• Serum electrolyte levels may indicate the presence of electrolyte imbalances.

How it's treated

Trauma care basics include:
• triage
• assessing and maintaining ABCs
• protecting the cervical spine

> **Memory jogger**
>
> To help remember what information to obtain during assessment of the trauma patient, use the acronym **SAMPLE:**
>
> **S** Signs and symptoms
>
> **A** Allergies
>
> **M** Medications
>
> **P** Past medical history
>
> **L** Last meal
>
> **E** Events leading to injury

> You may choose to perform a head-to-toe examination when assessing a patient with multiple traumas because it's quicker than a body-systems examination.

- assessing the LOC
- preparing the patient for transport and possible surgery.

Taking type into consideration

Management of traumatic wounds usually depends on the specific type of wound and degree of contamination. Treatment may include:
- controlling bleeding, usually by applying firm, direct pressure and elevating the extremity
- cleaning the wound
- administering pain medication
- administering antibiotic therapy
- surgery.

Additional treatment is based on the body system that's affected by the trauma and the extent of injury. For example, treatment of a blunt chest injury may include maintaining a patent airway, providing adequate ventilation, maintaining fluid and electrolyte balance, and inserting a chest tube for pneumothorax, hemothorax, or tension pneumothorax.

What to do

- Assess ABCs and initiate emergency measures if necessary; administer supplemental oxygen as ordered.
- Immobilize the head and neck with an immobilization device, sandbags, backboard, and tape. Assist with cervical spine X-rays.
- Monitor vital signs and note significant changes.
- Monitor oxygen saturation and cardiac rhythm for arrhythmias.
- Assess neurologic status including LOC and pupillary and motor response.
- Obtain blood studies, including type and crossmatch.
- Insert two I.V. large bore catheters and infuse normal saline or lactated Ringer's solution.
- Quickly and carefully assess for multiple injuries.
- Assess wounds and provide wound care as appropriate. Cover open wounds and control bleeding by applying pressure and elevating extremities.
- Assess for increased abdominal distention and increased diameter of extremities.
- Administer blood products as appropriate.
- Monitor for signs of hypovolemic shock.
- Provide pain medication, as appropriate.
- Provide reassurance to the patient and his family.
- Explain diagnostic test and treatments.

Quick quiz

1. To expand plasma volume or to replace clotting factors, you would expect to give:

    A.   albumin.
    B.   FFP.
    C.   whole blood.
    D.   packed RBCs.

Answer: B. FFP is the product of choice for replacing clotting factors.

2. Hypertonic solutions cause fluids to move from the:

    A.   interstitial space to the intracellular space.
    B.   intracellular space to the extracellular space.
    C.   extracellular space to the intracellular space.
    D.   intracellular space to the interstitial space.

Answer: B. Because of their increased osmolality, hypertonic solutions draw fluids out of the cells and into the extracellular space.

3. Your patient has second- and third-degree burn injuries to his anterior chest, anterior abdomen, and entire right arm. Using the Rule of Nines, the percent of total body surface area involved can be estimated at:

    A.   18%.
    B.   27%.
    C.   45%.
    D.   50%.

Answer: B. The anterior chest and abdomen constitute 18% of the BSA, and the entire right arm is 9%, for a total of 27%.

4. What is the first step you should take for a patient with hypovolemic shock?

    A.   Assess for dehydration.
    B.   Administer I.V. fluids.
    C.   Insert a urinary catheter.
    D.   Obtain blood for a CBC.

Answer: B. Hypovolemic shock is an emergency that requires rapid infusion of I.V. fluids.

5.   Signs of septic shock include:
    A.   clear, watery sputum.
    B.   severe hypertension.
    C.   hypotension.
    D.   increased urine output.

Answer: C. Hypotension is a sign of hypodynamic septic shock, along with pale and possibly cyanotic skin color; mottling of extremities; decreased LOC; rapid, shallow respirations; decreased or absent urine output; absence of peripheral pulses; or a rapid, weak, pulse.

Scoring

☆☆☆   If you answered all five questions correctly, way to go! You are multitalented when it comes to multisystem issues.

☆☆   If you answered four questions correctly, good work! This last quick quiz must not have been too traumatic for you.

☆   If you answered fewer than four questions correctly, don't go into shock. You can always review the chapter again.

Woo-hoo! You finished the last quick quiz of the book!

Appendices and index

Web resources for critical care nursing

Agency for Healthcare Research and Quality
www.ahcpr.gov

American Association of Critical Care Nurses
www.aacn.org

American Burn Association
www.ameriburn.org

American Cancer Society
www.cancer.org

American Diabetes Association
www.diabetes.org

American Heart Association
www.americanheart.org

American Holistic Nurses' Association
ahna.org

American Lung Association
www.lungusa.org

American Nurses Association
www.nursingworld.org

American Pain Society
www.ampainsoc.org

Centers for Disease Control and Prevention
www.cdc.gov

Intravenous Nurses Society
www.ins1.org

National Institute of Neurological Disorders and Stroke
www.ninds.nih.gov

National Kidney Foundation
www.kidney.org

National League for Nursing
www.nln.org

PubMed
www.ncbi.nlm.nih.gov/PubMed

Sigma Theta Tau, International
www.nursingsociety.org

Wound Ostomy and Continence Nurses Society
www.wocn.org

Glossary

acid-base balance: mechanism by which the body's acids and bases are kept in balance

acidosis: condition resulting from the accumulation of acid or the loss of base

advance directive: document used as a guideline for life-sustaining medical care of a patient with an advanced disease or disability, who is no longer able to indicate his own wishes; includes living wills and durable powers of attorney for health care

afterload: resistance that the left ventricle must work against to pump blood through the aorta

agranulocyte: leukocyte (white blood cell) not made up of granules or grains; includes lymphocytes, monocytes, and plasma cells

aldosterone: adrenocortical hormone that regulates sodium, potassium, and fluid balance

alkalosis: condition resulting from the accumulation of base or the loss of acid

allergen: substance that induces an allergy or a hypersensitivity reaction

anaphylaxis: severe allergic reaction to a foreign substance

aneurysm: sac formed by the dilatation of the wall of an artery, a vein, or the heart

anoxia: absence of oxygen in the tissues

antibody: immunoglobulin molecule that reacts only with the specific antigen that induced its formation in the lymph system

antidiuretic hormone: hormone made by the hypothalamus and released by the pituitary gland that decreases the production of urine by increasing the reabsorption of water by the renal tubules

antigen: foreign substance, such as bacteria or toxins, that induces antibody formation

aphasia: language disorder characterized by difficulty expressing or comprehending speech

arrhythmia: disturbance of the normal cardiac rhythm from the abnormal origin, discharge, or conduction of electrical impulses

ataxia: uncoordinated actions when voluntary muscle movements are attempted

atrial kick: amount of blood pumped into the ventricles as a result of atrial contraction; contributes approximately 30% of total cardiac output

autologous transfusion (autotransfusion): reinfusion of the patient's own blood or blood components

automaticity: ability of a cardiac cell to initiate an impulse on its own

borborygmus: loud, gurgling, splashing sounds caused by gas passing through the intestine; normally heard over the large intestine

bruit: abnormal sound heard over peripheral vessels that indicates turbulent blood flow

capture: successful pacing of the heart, represented on the electrocardiogram tracing by a pacemaker spike followed by a P wave or QRS complex

cardiac cycle: the period from the beginning of one heartbeat to the beginning of the next; includes two phases, systole and diastole

cardiac output: amount of blood ejected from the left ventricle per minute; normal value is 4 to 8 L/minute

cardioversion: restoration of normal rhythm by electric shock or drug therapy

cerebral edema: increase in the brain's fluid content; may result from correcting hypernatremia too rapidly

Chvostek's sign: abnormal spasm of facial muscles that may indicate hypocalcemia or tetany; tested by lightly tapping the facial nerve (upper cheek, below the zygomatic bone)

colloid: large molecule, such as albumin, that normally doesn't cross the capillary membrane

complement system: major mediator of inflammatory response; a functionally related system made up of 20 proteins circulating as functionally inactive molecules

conduction: transmission of electrical impulses through the myocardium

conductivity: ability of one cardiac cell to transmit an electrical impulse to another cell

contractility: ability of a cardiac cell to contract after receiving an impulse

critical pathway: documentation tool used in managed care and case management in which a time line is defined for the patient's condition and for the achievement of expected outcomes; used by caregivers to determine where the patient should be in his progress toward optimal health

crystalloid: solute, such as sodium or glucose, that crosses the capillary membrane in solution

cytotoxic: destructive to cells

deep tendon reflex: involuntary muscle contraction in response to a sudden stretch that can be elicited by a hammer or finger tap on a tendon at its insertion

defibrillation: termination of ventricular fibrillation by electrical shock

dehydration: condition in which the loss of water from cells causes them to shrink

demyelination: destruction of a nerve's myelin sheath, which interferes with normal nerve conduction

depolarization: response of a myocardial cell to an electrical impulse that causes movement of ions across the cell membrane, which triggers myocardial contraction

diastole: phase of the cardiac cycle when both atria (atrial diastole) or both ventricles (ventricular diastole) are at rest and filling with blood

diplopia: double vision

distal: farthest away

durable power of attorney for health care: legal document whereby a patient authorizes another person to make medical decisions for him should he become incompetent to do so

dysarthria: speech defect commonly related to a motor deficit of the tongue or speech muscles

dysphagia: difficulty swallowing

enhanced automaticity: condition in which pacemaker cells increase the firing rate above their inherent rate

excitability: ability of a cardiac cell to respond to an electrical stimulus

extravasation: leakage of intravascular fluid into surrounding tissue; can be caused by such medications as chemotherapeutic drugs, dopamine, and calcium solutions that produce blistering and, eventually, tissue necrosis

granulocyte: any cell containing granules, especially a granular leukocyte (white blood cell)

hematopoiesis: production of red blood cells in the bone marrow

homeostasis: dynamic, steady state of internal balance in the body

hormone: chemical substance produced in the body that has a specific regulatory effect on the activity of specific cells or organs

host defense system: elaborate network of safeguards that protects the body from infectious organisms and other harmful invaders

hypervolemia: excess of fluid and solutes in extracellular fluid, can be caused by increased fluid intake, fluid shifts in the body, or renal failure

hypotonic: solution that has fewer solutes than another solution

hypovolemia: condition marked by the loss of fluid and solutes from extracellular fluid that, if left untreated, can progress to hypovolemic shock

hypoxemia: oxygen deficit in arterial blood (lower than 80 mm Hg)

hypoxia: oxygen deficit in the tissues

immunocompetence: ability of cells to distinguish antigens from substances that belong to the body and to launch an immune response

immunodeficiency disorder: disorder caused by a deficiency of the immune response due to hypoactivity or decreased numbers of lymphoid cells

immunoglobulin: serum protein synthesized by lymphocytes and plasma cells that has known antibody activity; main component of humoral immune response

intrinsic: naturally occurring electrical stimulus from within the heart's conduction system

ischemia: decreased blood supply to a body organ or tissue

isotonic solution: solution that has the same concentration of solutes as another solution

leukocyte: white blood cell that protects the body against microorganisms that cause disease

living will: witnessed document indicating a patient's desire to be allowed to die a natural death, rather than be kept alive by life-sustaining measures; applies to decisions that will be made after a terminally ill patient is incompetent and has no reasonable possibility of recovery

lymph node: structure that filters the lymphatic fluid that drains from body tissues and is later returned to the blood as plasma; removes noxious agents from the blood

lymphocyte: leukocyte produced by lymphoid tissue that participates in immunity

macrophage: highly phagocytic cells that are stimulated by inflammation

metabolic acidosis: condition in which excess acid or reduced bicarbonate in the blood drops the arterial blood pH below 7.35

metabolic alkalosis: condition in which excess bicarbonate or reduced acid in the blood increases the arterial blood pH above 7.45

nephron: structural and functional unit of the kidney that forms urine

neuron: highly specialized conductor cell that receives and transmits electrochemical nerve impulses

nursing diagnosis: clinical judgment made by a nurse about a patient's responses to actual or potential health problems or life processes; describes a patient problem that the nurse can legally solve; may apply to families and communities as well as individual patients

nursing process: systematic approach to identifying a patient's problems and then taking nursing actions to address them; steps include assessing the patient's problems, forming a diagnostic statement, identifying expected outcomes, creating a plan to achieve expected outcomes and solve the patient's problems, implementing the plan or assigning others to implement it, and evaluating the plan's effectiveness

nystagmus: involuntary, rhythmic movement of the eye

oliguria: low urine output, less than 400 ml/24 hours

orthostatic hypotension: drop in blood pressure and increase in heart rate

that occur when the body changes position; can be caused by a loss of circulating blood volume

paroxysmal: episode of an arrhythmia that starts and stops suddenly

peristalsis: sequence of muscle contractions that propels food through the GI tract

petechiae: minute hemorrhagic spots in the skin

pH: measurement of the percentage of hydrogen ions in a solution; normal pH is 7.35 to 7.45 of arterial blood

phagocytosis: engulfing of microorganisms, other cells, and foreign particles by a phagocyte

point of maximal impulse: point at which the upward thrust of the heart against the chest wall is greatest, usually over the apex of the heart

practice guidelines: sequential instructions for treating patients with specific health problems

preload: stretching force exerted on the ventricular muscle by the blood it contains at the end of diastole

refractory period: brief period during which excitability in a myocardial cell is depressed

renin: enzyme produced by the kidneys in response to an actual or perceived decline in extracellular fluid volume; an important part of blood pressure regulation

repolarization: recovery of the myocardial cells after depolarization during which the cell membrane returns to its resting potential

respiratory acidosis: acid-base disturbance caused by failure of the lungs to eliminate sufficient carbon dioxide;

partial pressure of arterial carbon dioxide above 45 mm Hg and pH below 7.35

respiratory alkalosis: acid-base imbalance that occurs when the lungs eliminate more carbon dioxide than normal; partial pressure of arterial carbon dioxide below 35 mm Hg and pH above 7.45

rhabdomyolysis: disorder in which skeletal muscle is destroyed; causes intracellular contents to spill into extracellular fluid

systole: phase of the cardiac cycle when both of the atria (atrial systole) or the ventricles (ventricular systole) are contracting

telangiectasis: permanently dilated small blood vessels that form a weblike pattern; may be the result of scleroderma, lupus erythematosus, or cirrhosis or may be normal in healthy, older adults

thrill: palpable vibration felt over the heart or vessel that results from turbulent blood flow

thrombolytic: clot dissolving

Trousseau's sign: carpal (wrist) spasm elicited by applying a blood pressure cuff to the upper arm and inflating it to a pressure 20 mm Hg above the patient's systolic blood pressure; indicates the presence of hypocalcemia

vasopressor: drug that stimulates contraction of the muscular tissue of the capillaries and arteries

V̇/Q̇ ratio: ratio of ventilation (amount of air in the alveoli) to perfusion (amount of blood in the pulmonary capillaries); expresses the effectiveness of gas exchange

water intoxication: condition in which excess water in the cells results in cellular swelling

Selected references

American Heart Association. "Guidelines 2000 for Cardiopulmonary Resuscitation and Emergency Cardiovascular Care," *Supplement to Circulation* 102(8):I1-21, August 2000.

Andrews, M., and Boyle, J. *Transcultural Concepts in Nursing Care*, 4th ed. Philadelphia: Lippincott Williams & Wilkins, 2003.

Berry, B.E., and Pinard, A.E. "Assessing Tissue Oxygenation," *Critical Care Nurse* 22(3): 22-40, June 2002.

Better ElderCare: A Nurse's Guide to Caring for Older Adults. Springhouse, Pa.: Springhouse Corp., 2002.

Bickley, L.S., and Szilagyi, P.G. *Bates' Guide to Physical Examination and History Taking*, 8th ed. Philadelphia: Lippincott Williams & Wilkins, 2003.

Braunwald, E., et al. (eds.). *Harrison's Principles of Internal Medicine*, 15th ed. New York: McGraw-Hill Book Co., 2001.

Bullock, B.L., and Henze, R.L. *Focus on Pathophysiology.* Philadelphia: Lippincott Williams & Wilkins, 2000.

Catalano, J. *Guide to ECG Analysis*, 2nd ed. Philadelphia: Lippincott Williams & Wilkins, 2002.

Craven, R., and Hirnle, C. *Fundamentals of Nursing Human Health and Function*, 4th ed. Philadelphia: Lippincott Williams & Wilkins, 2003.

Critical Care Challenges: Disorders, Treatments, and Procedures. Philadelphia: Lippincott Williams & Wilkins, 2003.

Eliopoulos, C. *Gerontological Nursing*, 5th ed. Philadelphia: Lippincott Williams & Wilkins, 2001.

Fischbach, F.A. *Manual of Laboratory Diagnostic Tests*, 6th ed. Philadelphia: Lippincott, Williams & Wilkins, 2000.

Grap, M.J. "Pulse Oximetry," *Critical Care Nurse* 22(3):69-76, June 2002.

Handbook of Diagnostic Tests, 3rd ed. Philadelphia: Lippincott Williams & Wilkins, 2003.

Hickey, J.V. *The Clinical Practice of Neurological and Neurosurgical Nursing*, 5th ed. Philadelphia: Lippincott Williams & Wilkins, 2003.

Hickey, J.V., et al. *Advanced Practice Nursing, Changing Roles and Clinical Applications*, 2nd ed. Philadelphia: Lippincott Williams & Wilkins, 2000.

Huff, J. *ECG Workout Exercises in Arrhythmia Interpretation*, 4th ed. Philadelphia: Lippincott Williams & Wilkins, 2002.

Karch, A.M. *2003 Lippincott's Nursing Drug Guide.* Philadelphia: Lippincott Williams & Wilkins, 2003.

Lynn-McHale, D.J., and Carlson, K.K. (eds.). *AACN Procedure Manual for Critical Care*, 4th ed. Philadelphia: W.B. Saunders Co., 2001.

Mastering ACLS. Springhouse, Pa.: Springhouse Corp., 2002.

Morton, P., and Gonce Morton, P. *Critical Care Nursing: A Holistic Approach*, 8th ed. Philadelphia: Lippincott Williams & Wilkins, 2003.

Nursing2004 Drug Handbook, 24th ed. Philadelphia: Lippincott Williams & Wilkins, 2004.

Nursing Procedures & Protocols. Philadelphia: Lippincott Williams & Wilkins, 2003.

Pagana, K.D., and Pagana, T.J. *Mosby's Diagnostic and Laboratory Test Reference*, 6th ed. St. Louis: Mosby Year–Book, Inc, 2003.

Professional Guide to Pathophysiology. Philadelphia: Lippincott Williams & Wilkins, 2003.

Schell, H., and Puntillo, K. *Critical Care Nursing Secrets.* Philadelphia: Hanley & Belfus, 2001.

SkillMasters: Expert ECG Interpretation. Philadelphia: Lippincott Williams & Wilkins, 2003.

Springhouse Review for Critical Care Nursing Certification, 3rd ed. Philadelphia: Lippincott Williams & Wilkins, 2002.

St. Marie, B. (ed). *Core Curriculum for Pain Management Nursing.* Philadelphia: W.B. Saunders Co., 2002.

Index

i refers to an illustration; t refers to a table; boldface refers to full-color pages.

i refers to an illustration; t refers to a table; boldface refers to full-color pages.

i refers to an illustration; t refers to a table; boldface refers to full-color pages.

i refers to an illustration; t refers to a table; boldface refers to full-color pages.

i refers to an illustration; t refers to a table; boldface refers to full-color pages.

i refers to an illustration; t refers to a table; boldface refers to full-color pages.

XYZ

Notes